ATLAS OF ULTRASOUND IN OBSTETRICS AND GYNECOLOGY

A MULTIMEDIA REFERENCE

ATLAS OF ULTRASOUND IN OBSTETRICS AND GYNECOLOGY

A MULTIMEDIA REFERENCE

PETER M. DOUBILET, MD, PHD

Professor of Radiology
Harvard Medical School;
Vice-Chair of Radiology
Department of Radiology
Brigham and Women's Hospital
Boston, Massachusetts

CAROL B. BENSON, MD

Professor of Radiology
Harvard Medical School;
Director of Ultrasound
Co-Director of High-Risk Obstetrical Ultrasound
Department of Radiology
Brigham and Women's Hospital
Boston, Massachusetts

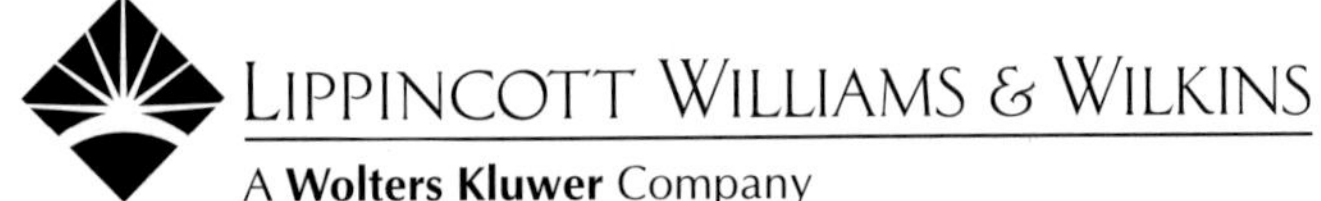

Philadelphia • Baltimore • New York • London
Buenos Aires • Hong Kong • Sydney • Tokyo

Acquisitions Editor: Joyce-Rachel John
Developmental Editor: Julia Seto
Production Editor: Rakesh Rampertab
Manufacturing Manager: Benjamin Rivera
Cover Designer: Armen Kojoyian
Compositor: Lippincott Williams & Wilkins Desktop Division
Printer: Asia Pacific

530 Walnut Street
Philadelphia, PA 19106 USA
LWW.com

Printed in China

Library of Congress Cataloging-in-Publication Data

Doubilet, Peter M.
Atlas of ultrasound in obstetrics and gynecology / Peter M. Doubilet, Carol B. Benson.
p. ; cm.
Includes bibliographical references and index.
ISBN 0-7817-3633-1 (alk. paper)
1. Generative organs, Female—Ultrasonic imaging—Atlases. 2. ultrasonics in obstetrics—Atlases. 3. Fetus—Diseases—Diagnosis—Atlases. I. Benson, Carol B. II. Title.
DNLM: 1. Ultrasonography, Prenatal—Atlases. 2. Fetal Diseases—ultrasonography—atlases. 3. Genital Diseases, Female—ultrasonography—atlases. 4. Pregnancy Complications—ultrasonography—Atlases. WQ 17 D726a 2003]
RG107.5.U4 D68 2003
618.2'07543—dc21

2002035290

---

10 9 8 7 6 5 4 3 2

Each of us dedicates this atlas to our spouse, for patiently tolerating the long hours spent in writing it.

COMPACT DISKETTE ICON

Figure legends with compact diskette (CD) icon have real-time ultrasound video clips in the corresponding figure on the CD version of the atlas.

CONTENTS

Nonfetal Abnormalities

Pathology

Procedures

PREFACE

Ultrasound emerged as a major tool in medical imaging in the 1970s, and it has been on a sustained trajectory of technological improvement ever since. As sonography has moved from static to real-time, from black-and-white to shades of gray, and from unidimensional (A-mode) to two to three to four dimensional, its utility and range of applications have grown impressively.

Nowhere has the impact of ultrasound been more dramatic than in obstetrics and gynecology. The ability of sonography to detect fetal abnormalities prior to delivery, to diagnose gynecological diseases without surgery, and to direct minimally invasive therapy, has revolutionized these fields of medicine. The marked improvement in ultrasound image quality in recent years and the ability to store high quality digital images and video clips have enhanced ultrasound's role in obstetrics and gynecology. These advances have prompted us to produce this atlas. In particular, we feel that video clips are now an integral part of sonography. Our atlas, with a compact diskette (CD) that contains video clips, depicts key elements of sonography, including its dynamic real-time aspect.

Ultrasound interpretation depends heavily on pattern recognition: identifying normal structures and establishing specific diagnoses from patterns of abnormal anatomy. As such, we anticipate that this atlas will be useful in both clinical and educational settings. In the clinical arena, the atlas can serve as a reference, to be pulled off the shelf when there is an abnormal sonographic finding for which the diagnosis is unclear. On the educational front, the atlas can serve as a learning and study tool, as it offers up-to-date images and clips covering a wide range of obstetrical and gynecological entities. We hope that the atlas, in both its book and CD formats, is a useful addition to the growing body of ultrasound literature.

ACKNOWLEDGMENTS

We are grateful to our colleagues and co-workers in the Brigham and Women's Hospital Radiology Department Ultrasound Section, as well as the joint Radiology-Obstetrics High-Risk Obstetrical Ultrasound Unit. Their expertise and hard work have made our institution a center of excellence in ultrasound.

We wish to express our gratitude to Gareth Ballester, whose creativity, technical expertise, and tireless efforts were critical to putting together the CD version of this atlas. His knowledge and skills made the CD possible, and his cheerful demeanor made its creation a pleasant task.

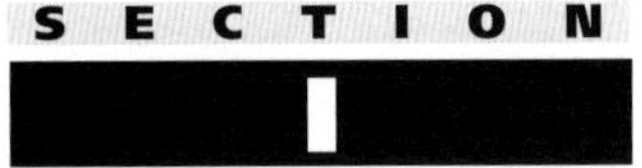

OBSTETRICAL ULTRASOUND

1

FIRST TRIMESTER

1.1. NORMAL PREGNANCY AT 5–6 WEEKS GESTATION

Description and Clinical Features

Within a week after fertilization (~3 weeks gestational age, because gestational age corresponds to time elapsed since last menstrual period), the gestational sac and embryo implant within the uterus. In response to hormonal stimulation from the corpus luteum (the remnant of the ovarian follicle that released the ovum before fertilization), the endometrium thickens (decidualizes) to support the developing gestational sac. When a pregnancy is present, beta-human chorionic gonadotropin (β-HCG) can be detected in the maternal blood and urine. The β-HCG is first detectable in the blood at approximately 4 weeks gestational age, close to the expected time of menses.

The gestational sac is approximately 2 mm in mean diameter at 5.0 weeks gestation, growing to 10 mm at 6.0 weeks. It is surrounded by the chorion with its chorionic villi. The amnion, a second, thinner membrane, initially forms a small cavity containing the developing embryo, immediately adjacent to the yolk sac. The yolk sac is located in the fluid space between the chorion and the amnion. Before 6.0 weeks gestation, the embryo is microscopic in size (<1 mm).

Sonography

The gestational sac can first be visualized at approximately 5.0 weeks gestation when scanning transvaginally. It should be identifiable in a normal pregnancy by the time the maternal serum β-HCG concentration reaches a level of 1,000 mIU/mL (first or third International Preparation). At this stage, the gestational sac appears as a fluid collection in the uterus adjacent to the uterine cavity (Figure 1.1-1). It is typically surrounded in part by two echogenic rings, representing two layers of decidua. The yolk sac, a circular structure that is normally less than 6 mm in diameter, is first identifiable within the gestational sac by transvaginal sonography at approximately 5.5 weeks (Figure 1.1-2). When scanning transabdominally, the gestational sac and yolk sac are visualized approximately one-half week later than they are transvaginally.

The corpus luteum can usually be seen on ultrasound in one of the ovaries. It can have a number of sonographic appearances, including a simple cyst, a thick-walled or complex cyst, or a hypoechoic structure (Figure 1.1-3). It typically measures 2–3 cm in diameter.

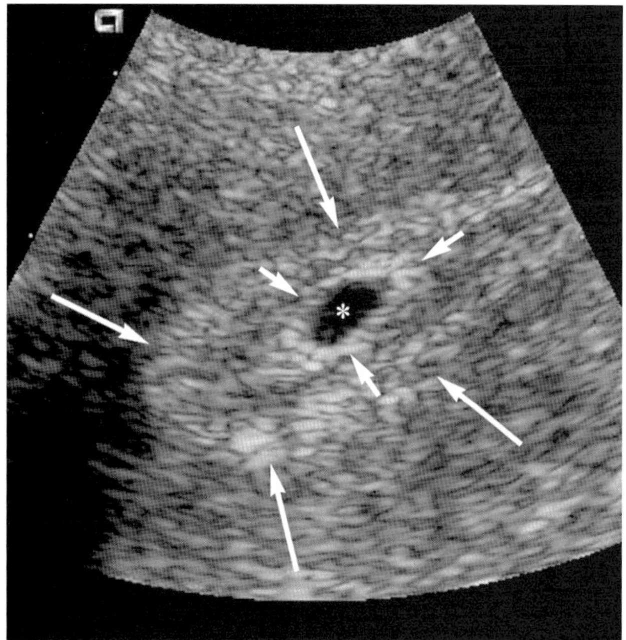

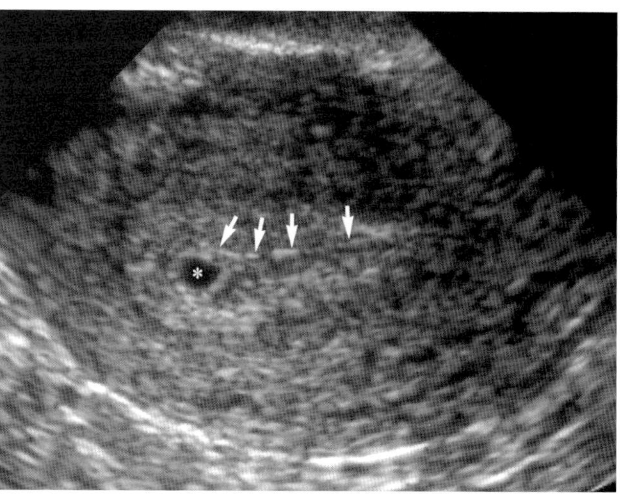

FIGURE 1.1-1. Gestational sacs at 5.0 weeks gestation. The gestational sacs *(*)* in these two cases are visible as rounded fluid collections within the endometrium, with no structures within them. In both cases, there are features that identify these fluid collections as gestational sacs, as opposed to blood or secretions in the uterine cavity. **A:** The gestational sac is surrounded by two echogenic rings, an inner ring *(short arrows)*, and an outer ring *(long arrows)*, corresponding to two layers of decidua. **B:** The gestational sac is adjacent to, and not within, the echogenic stripe representing the uterine cavity *(arrows)*.

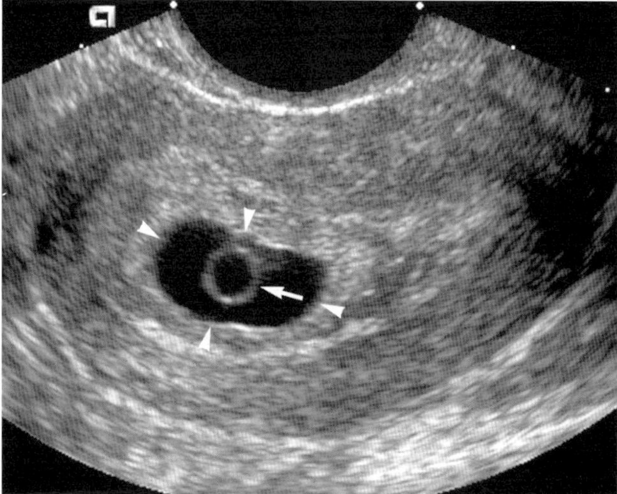

FIGURE 1.1-2. Gestational sac at 5.5 weeks gestation. The gestational sac *(arrowheads)* contains a yolk sac *(arrow)*, but no embryo is yet visible.

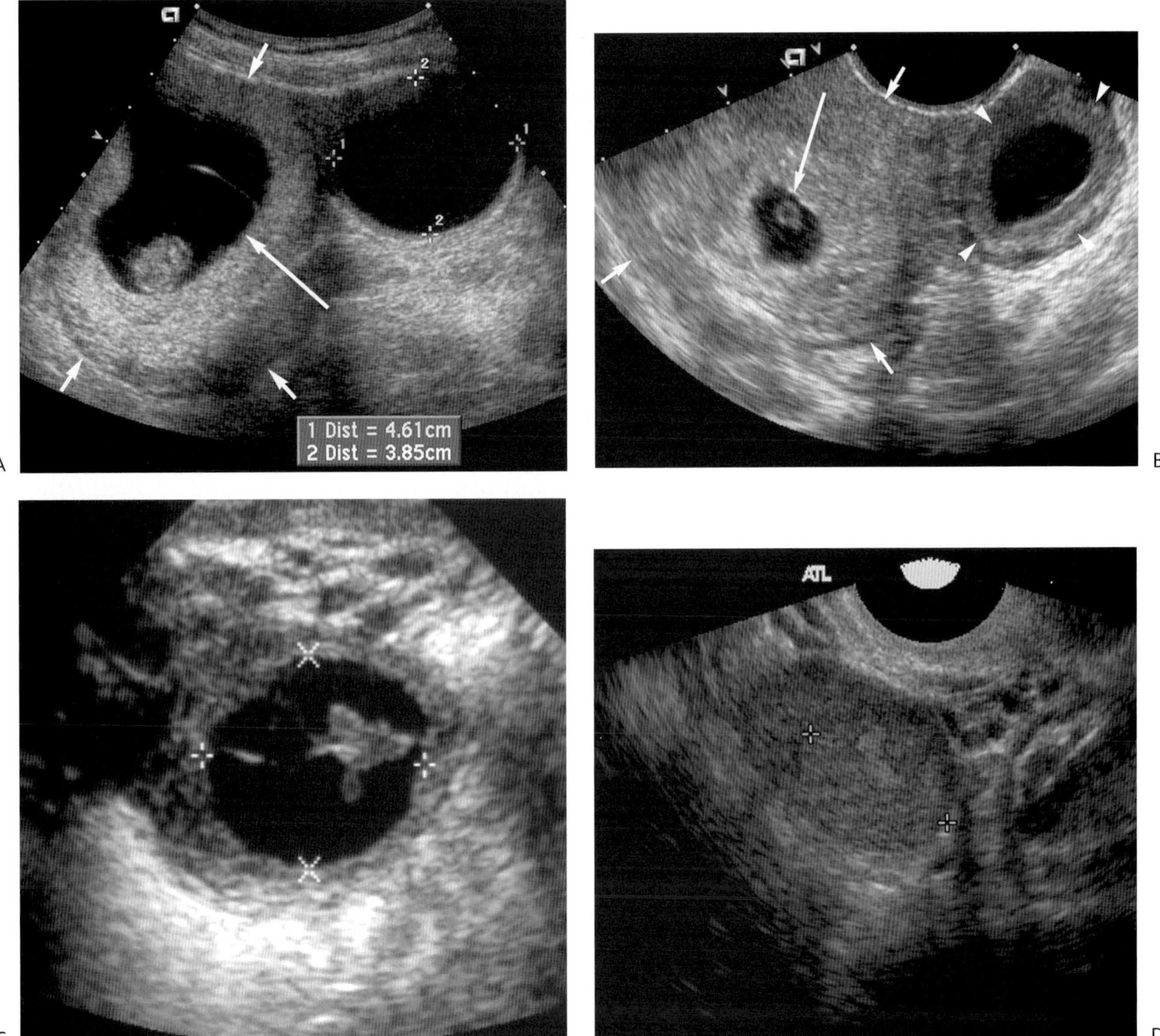

FIGURE 1.1-3. Corpus luteum. The range of sonographic appearances of the corpus luteum includes a thin-walled cyst *(calipers)* **(A)**, a thick-walled cyst *(arrowheads)* **(B)**, a cyst with internal debris *(calipers)* **(C)**, a structure with diffuse internal echoes *(calipers)* **(D)**. On images **(A)** and **(B)**, the corpus luteum is seen adjacent to the uterus *(short arrows)* containing a gestational sac *(long arrow)*.

1.2. NORMAL PREGNANCY AT 6–10 WEEKS GESTATION

Description and Clinical Features

Between 6 and 10 weeks gestational age, the embryo undergoes rapid growth and development. It increases approximately 15-fold in length, from 2 mm at 6.0 weeks gestation to 30 mm at 10.0 weeks. The internal organs differentiate, with organogenesis largely complete by 10 weeks. In particular, by 10 weeks, the cardiac chambers and valves are well formed, and the rectum is separate from the urogenital sinus, so that the gastrointestinal and genitourinary systems are distinct. The kidneys have begun their ascent from the pelvis, and the midgut herniates into the base of the umbilical cord.

The external appearance of the embryo also undergoes major changes during this stage. By 10 weeks, facial features are recognizable, and limbs, including fingers and toes, are formed.

During the 6–10-week time period, the chorionic villi at the implantation site proliferate, whereas those opposite the implantation site regress. This results in two portions of the chorion: the thick chorion frondosum, where the villi have proliferated, and the smooth membranous chorion laeve, where the villi have degenerated. The chorion frondosum interdigitates with the maternal decidua to form the placenta.

Sonography

The embryonic heartbeat can first be seen on transvaginal sonography at approximately 6.0 weeks gestational age. Initially, it is seen as a flickering movement adjacent to the yolk sac (Figure 1.2-1). Within 2–3 days, the heartbeat can be seen to lie within a clearly visible embryo (Figure 1.2-2). The heart rate is normally at least 100 beats per minute before 6.3 weeks [corresponding to a crown-rump length (CRL) of <5 mm] and at least 120 beats per minute from 6.3 to 7.0 weeks (corresponding to a CRL of 5–9 mm).

The embryo initially appears on ultrasound as an undifferentiated structure, without identifiable parts (other than the beating heart). By 7–8 weeks, the head and trunk can

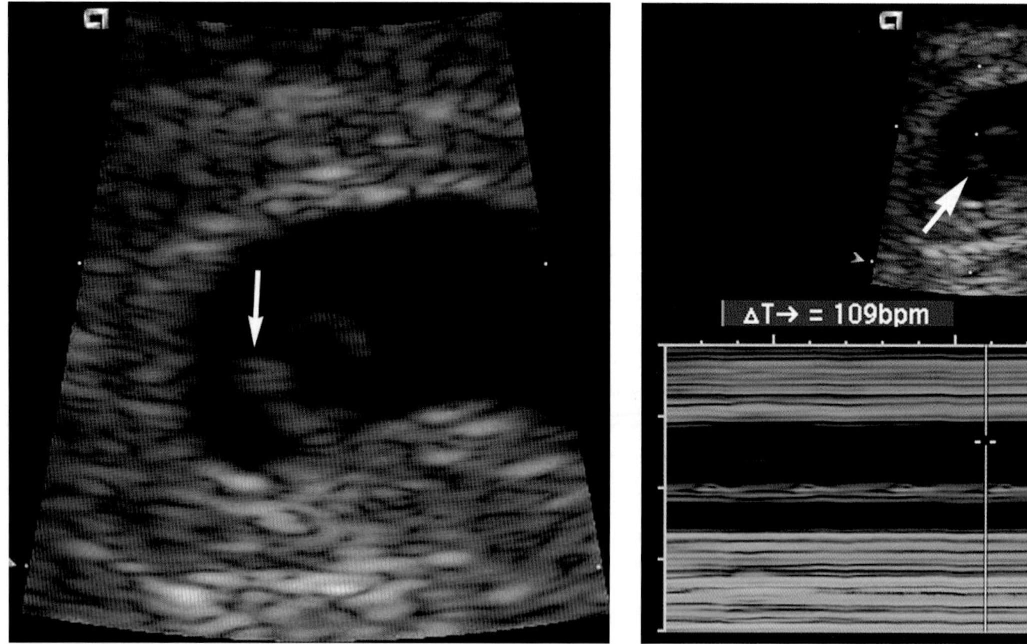

FIGURE 1.2-1. Embryonic cardiac activity at 6.0 weeks gestation. A: The embryo *(arrow)* is visible as a small focal echogenic structure adjacent to the yolk sac. **B:** Cardiac activity in the embryo *(arrow)* is documented by M-mode to be at a rate of 109 beats per minute *(calipers)*.

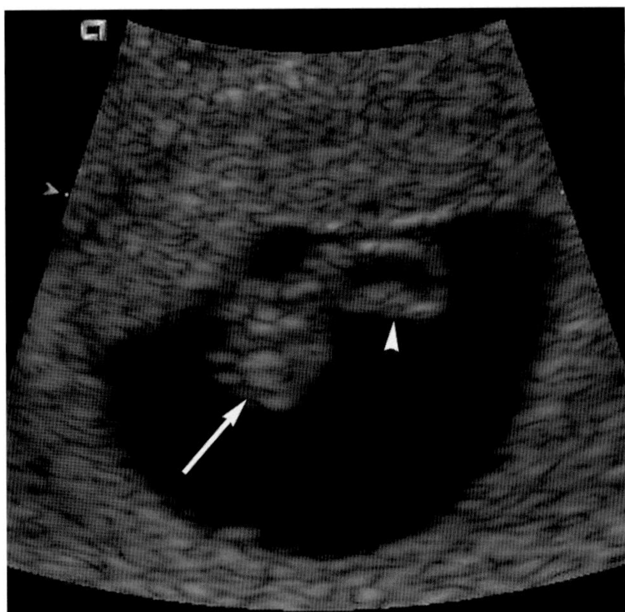

FIGURE 1.2-2. **6.5-Week embryo.** The embryo *(arrow)*, approximately 5 mm in length, is clearly identifiable adjacent to the yolk sac *(arrowhead)*. Cardiac activity was seen within the embryo on real-time sonography.

be separately identified, and an intracranial cystic structure is identifiable, corresponding to the developing rhombencephalon (Figure 1.2-3). By 10 weeks, at which time the CRL is approximately 30 mm, limb buds can be identified sonographically.

The yolk sac continues to be visible during this period (Figure 1.2-4). The amnion is seen within the gestational sac as a thin, smooth, curvilinear structure surrounding the embryo/fetus. Anechoic fluid is seen within the amniotic sac and between the amnion and chorion. By 9–10 weeks, the placenta is identifiable as a homogeneously echogenic structure surrounding a portion of the gestational sac (Figure 1.2-5).

A

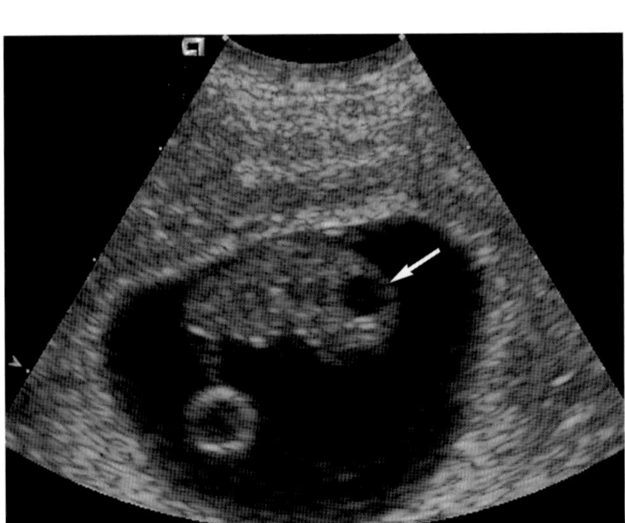

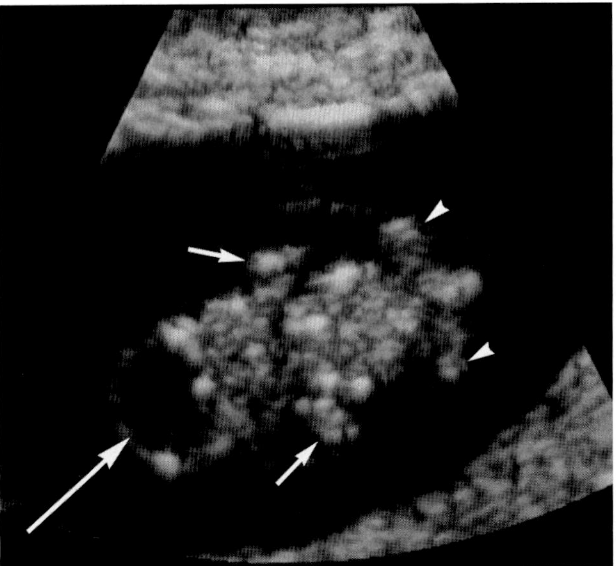

B

FIGURE 1.2-3. Fetus in the mid first trimester. A: The rhombencephalon *(arrow)* is visible in this 8-week fetus. **B:** Anatomic structures visible by 10 weeks gestational age include rhombencephalon *(long arrow)* and limb buds *(short arrows, upper extremities; arrowheads, lower extremities)*. The fetal head and body are clearly distinct.

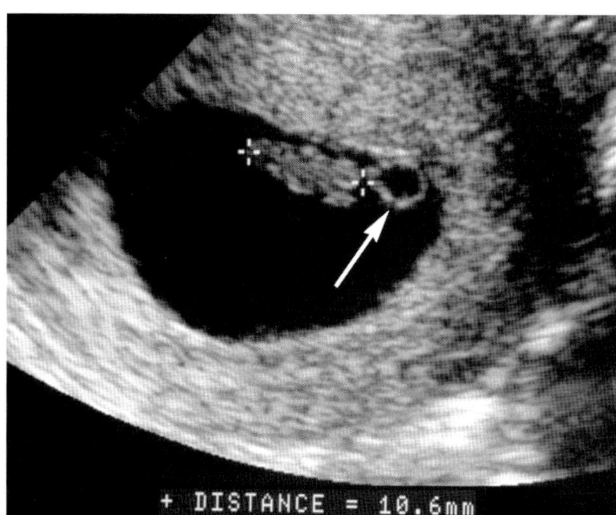

FIGURE 1.2-4. Yolk sac. The yolk sac *(arrow)* is seen in close proximity to the 7-week embryo. The yolk sac must not be included in the measurement of the crown-rump length *(calipers)*.

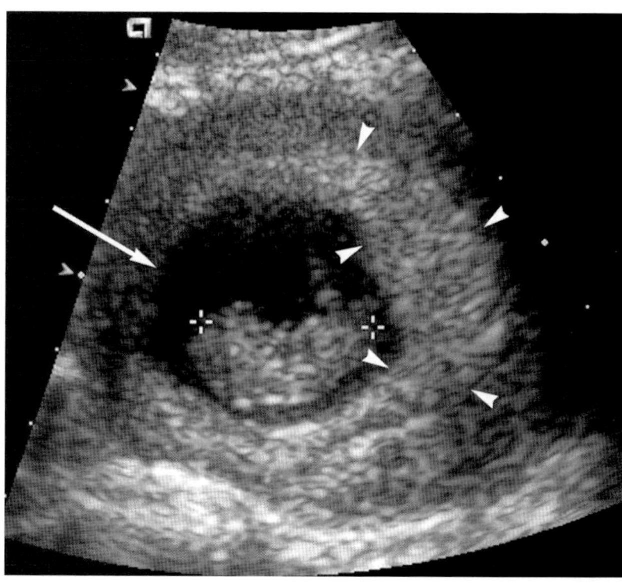

FIGURE 1.2-5. Placenta at 9 weeks gestation. The placenta *(arrowheads)* is seen as a thick echogenic structure surrounding part of the gestational sac. No thickening is seen on the opposite side of the gestational sac *(arrow)*, where the chorionic villi have regressed. The fetus *(calipers)* is seen within the gestational sac.

1.3. NORMAL PREGNANCY AT 10–13 WEEKS GESTATION

Description and Clinical Features

By 10 weeks gestation, the term *embryo* is replaced by *fetus*. During the 10–13 week time period, no major new structures develop because organogenesis is complete, but there is considerable growth of the fetus and its internal organs. The fetus more than doubles in length, from a CRL of 30 mm at 10.0 weeks to 65 mm at 13.0 weeks.

The external configuration of the fetus changes somewhat during this stage. The facial features take on a more human-like appearance, with the eyes beginning in a relatively lateral location and moving medially. The body proportions change, as the head, which accounts for a fairly large proportion of the total fetal size at 10 weeks, decreases in proportion to the rest of the body thereafter. The bulge at the base of the umbilical cord in the 10-week fetus, representing the herniated midgut, resolves by approximately 12 weeks, as the intestines return to their normal intra-abdominal location.

Sonography

On sonography at 10–13 weeks, the fetus has clearly distinct head, trunk, and limbs. By the end of this period, considerable detail of a number of fetal structures can often be identified (Figure 1.3-1). These include the four cardiac chambers, stomach, bladder, extremities (including hands and feet), skeleton, and face.

There is a lucent zone in the posterior aspect of the fetal neck, termed the nuchal translucency, that measures up to approximately 2.5 mm in thickness (Figure 1.3-2). A soft-tissue mass, generally less than 7 mm in maximum diameter, is seen projecting from the anterior abdominal wall into the base of the umbilical cord (Figure 1.3-3), corresponding to the presence of bowel in this location during normal embryologic development.

The amnion may still be visible within the gestational sac, close to the chorion. The placenta is visible as an echogenic structure surrounding part of the gestational sac (Figure 1.3-4).

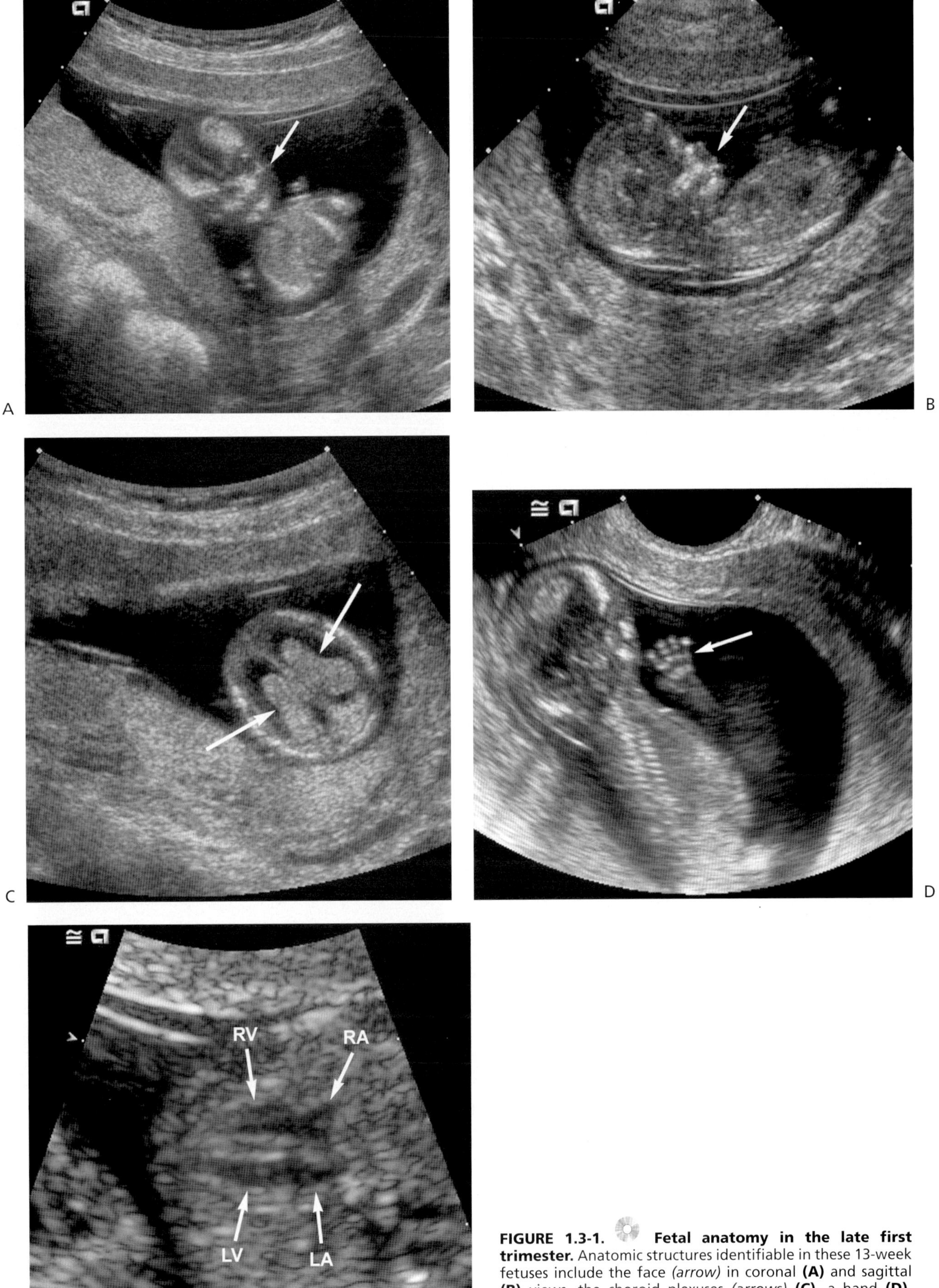

FIGURE 1.3-1. **Fetal anatomy in the late first trimester.** Anatomic structures identifiable in these 13-week fetuses include the face *(arrow)* in coronal **(A)** and sagittal **(B)** views, the choroid plexuses *(arrows)* **(C)**, a hand **(D)**, four-chamber view of the heart *(RV arrow, right ventricle; LV arrow, left ventricle; RA arrow, right atrium; LA arrow, left atrium)* **(E)**.

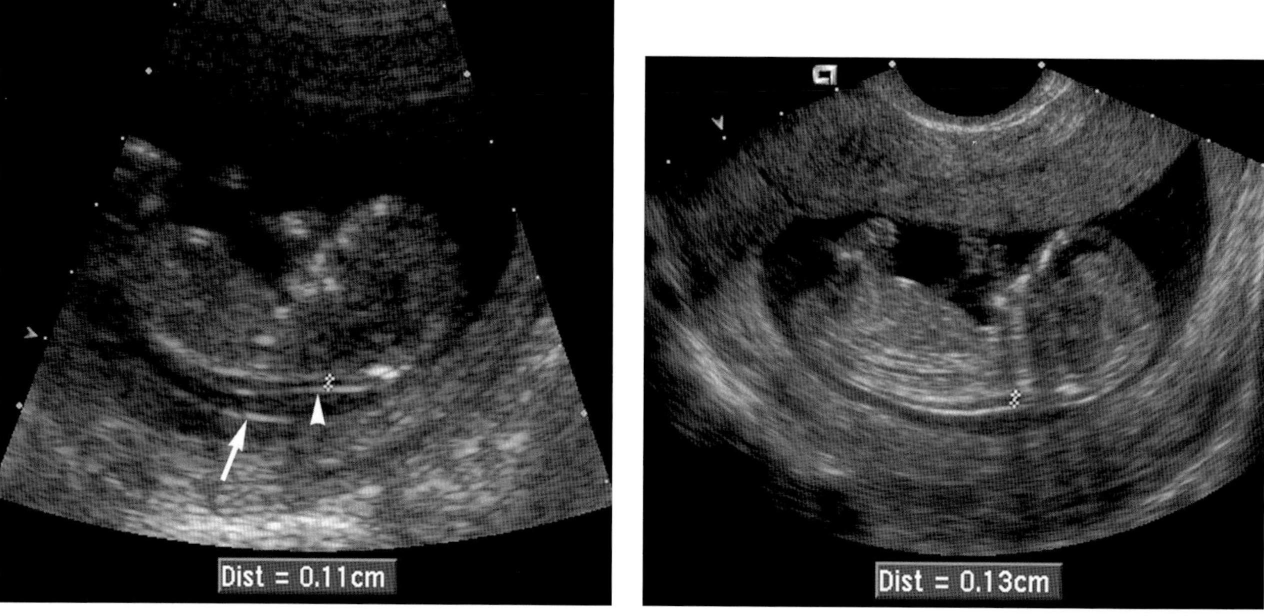

FIGURE 1.3-2. Nuchal translucency. A: Transabdominal nuchal lucency measurement. Measurement *(calipers)* is taken of the lucent area in the posterior neck, with the posterior caliper placed just inside the echogenic skin *(arrowhead)*. The amnion *(arrow)* should not be mistaken for the skin. **B:** Transvaginal nuchal lucency measurement *(calipers)*.

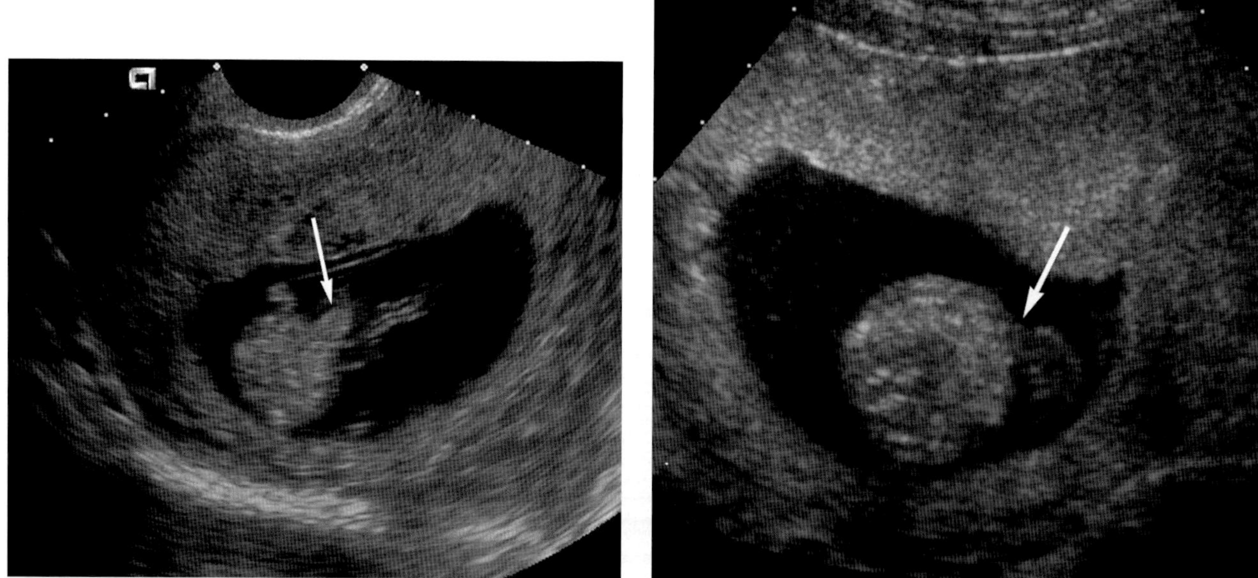

FIGURE 1.3-3. Physiologic bowel herniation. A: Transverse view of the fetal abdomen at 11.5 weeks gestation demonstrates echogenic material extending into the base of the umbilical cord *(arrow)*. **B:** At 14 weeks, the herniation into the base of the umbilical cord has resolved, leading to a normal umbilical insertion site *(arrow)* into the ventral abdominal wall.

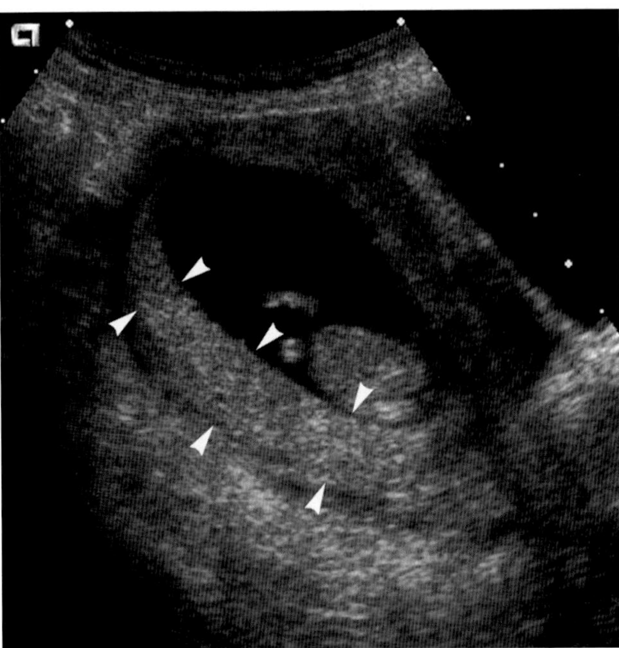

FIGURE 1.3-4. Placenta at 11 weeks. The placenta *(arrowheads)* appears as a homogeneous echogenic structure surrounding a part of the gestational sac.

SUGGESTED READINGS

1. Benson CB, Doubilet PM. Fetal measurements, normal and abnormal fetal growth. In: Rumack C, Charbonneau W, Wilson S, eds. *Diagnostic ultrasound*, 2nd ed. St. Louis: Yearbook Medical Publishers, 1998:1013–1031.
2. Bowerman RA. Sonography of fetal midgut herniation: normal size criteria and correlation with crown-rump length. *J Ultrasound Med* 1993;12:251–254.
3. Bradley WG, Fiske CE, Filly RA. The double sac sign of early intrauterine pregnancy: use in exclusion of ectopic pregnancy. *Radiology* 1982;143:223–226.
4. Bree RL, Edwards M, Bohm-Velez M, et al. Transvaginal sonography in the evaluation of normal early pregnancy: correlation with HCG level. *AJR Am J Roentgenol* 1989;153:75–79.
5. Doubilet PM, Benson CB. Embryonic heart rate in the early first trimester: what rate is normal? *J Ultrasound Med* 1995;14:431–434.
6. Doubilet PM, Benson CB. Emergency obstetrical ultrasound. *Semin Roentgenol* 1998;33:339–450.
7. Fleischer AC, Kepple DM. Transvaginal sonography of early intrauterine pregnancy. In: Fleischer AC, Manning FA, Jeanty P, et al., eds. *Sonography in obstetrics & gynecology: principles and practice*, 6th ed. New York: McGraw-Hill, 2001:61–88.
8. Goldstein I, Zimmer EA, Tamir A, et al. Evaluation of normal gestational sac growth: appearance of embryonic heartbeat and embryo body movements using the transvaginal technique. *Obstet Gynecol* 1991;77:885–888.
9. Hertzberg BS, Mahony BS, Bowie JD. First trimester fetal cardiac activity: sonographic documentation of a progressive early rise in heart rate. *J Ultrasound Med* 1988;7:573–575.
10. Laing FC, Frates MC. Ultrasound evaluation during the first trimester of pregnancy. In: Callen PW, ed. *Ultrasonography in obstetrics and gynecology*, 4th ed. Philadelphia: WB Saunders, 2000:105–145.
11. Lyons EA, Levi CS, Dashefsky SM. The first trimester. In: Rumack CM, Wilson SR, Charboneau JW, eds. *Diagnostic ultrasound*, 2nd ed. St. Louis: Mosby, 1998:975–1011.
12. Moore KL, Persaud TVN. *The developing human*, 5th ed. Philadelphia: WB Saunders, 1993.
13. Nyberg DA, Laing FC, Filly RA, et al. Ultrasonic differentiation of the gestational sac of early pregnancy from the pseudogestational sac of ectopic pregnancy. *Radiology* 1983;146:755–759.
14. Schats R, Jansen CAM, Wladimiroff JW. Embryonic heart activity: appearance and development in early human pregnancy. *Br J Obstet Gynaecol* 1990;97:989–994.

2

SECOND AND THIRD TRIMESTER FETAL ANATOMY

2.1. CENTRAL NERVOUS SYSTEM, SPINE, AND FACE

Description and Clinical Features

By the beginning of the second trimester, the fetal brain, cranium, spinal cord, vertebral column, and facial structures are well formed, although these organs and structures will continue to develop morphologically and will undergo extensive growth during the second and third trimesters. In particular, during the third trimester, the brain undergoes rapid growth and, toward term, develops sulci and gyri. Each spinal vertebra is formed with three ossification centers: a central ossification center that will become the vertebral body and two posterior ossification centers that will become the laminae and pedicles. Measurements of the fetal head are used to assess gestational age and fetal growth.

Sonography

On second and third trimester sonography, the fetal cranium and its contents are evaluated using three key images: the biparietal diameter measurement view, an image demonstrating the lateral ventricles, and one showing the posterior fossa. The biparietal diame-

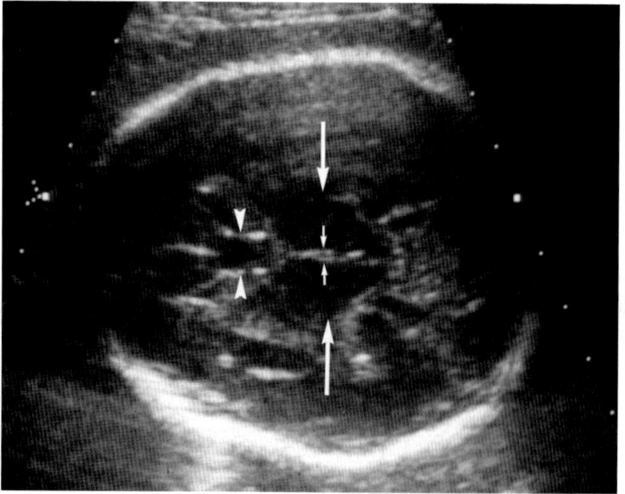

FIGURE 2.1-1. Level of biparietal diameter. Axial view of the fetal head, at the level used for measurement of the biparietal diameter, demonstrates the paired thalami *(large arrows)* with the slit-like third ventricle between them *(small arrows)*, and the cavum septum pellucidum *(arrowheads)*.

ter measurement is taken on an axial view at the level of the paired thalami and the cavum septum pellucidum (Figure 2.1-1) by placing the calipers on the leading edges of the cranium (Figure 2.1-2). The occipitofrontal diameter is measured on the same view, from the middle of the cranium frontally to the middle occipitally (Figure 2.1-2). On this view, the head circumference can also be measured using the electronic ellipse function to trace the outer contour of the cranium (Figure 2.1-3). Important intracranial structures identified on this view include the thalami, third ventricle, and cavum septum pellucidum (Figure 2.1-1). The third ventricle is normally a narrow slit of fluid between the heart-shaped, paired thalami. The cavum septum pellucidum is a square-shaped fluid space between the frontal horns of the lateral ventricles.

The lateral ventricles and choroid plexuses are assessed on an axial view at the level of the occipital horns and atria of the lateral ventricles. The measurement of the lateral ventricle is taken by placing calipers across the ventricle at the atrium, near the posterior tip of the choroid plexus, perpendicular to the axis of the lateral ventricle (Figure 2.1-4).

Axial views of the posterior fossa allow assessment of the cerebellum, fourth ventricle, and cisterna magna. The normal cerebellum has a posterior contour like the side of a peanut, with the hypoechoic, rounded, cerebellar hemispheres on either side of the narrower, more echogenic, cerebellar vermis (Figure 2.1-5). The cisterna magna, the fluid space between the vermis and the occipital bone (Figure 2.1-6), normally measures less than 10 mm in anteroposterior dimension. When evaluating the cisterna magna, care must be taken to image it in a near-axial plane that has a slightly coronal angulation. If the image plane is angled coronally more than 15 degrees, the cisterna magna may appear artificially enlarged to greater than 10 mm (Figure 2.1-7). The fourth ventricle is a small fluid space located anterior to the cerebellar vermis and posterior to the midbrain (Figure 2.1-6).

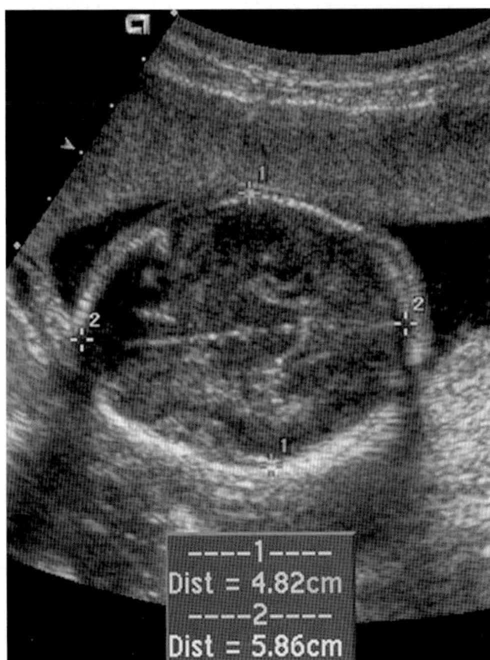

FIGURE 2.1-2. Biparietal and occipitofrontal diameter measurements. The + calipers labeled 1 are placed on the leading edge of the cranial bone at the near and far sides of the skull to measure the biparietal diameter. The + calipers labeled 2 are placed in the middle of the visible cranial bone anteriorly and posteriorly to measure the occipitofrontal diameter.

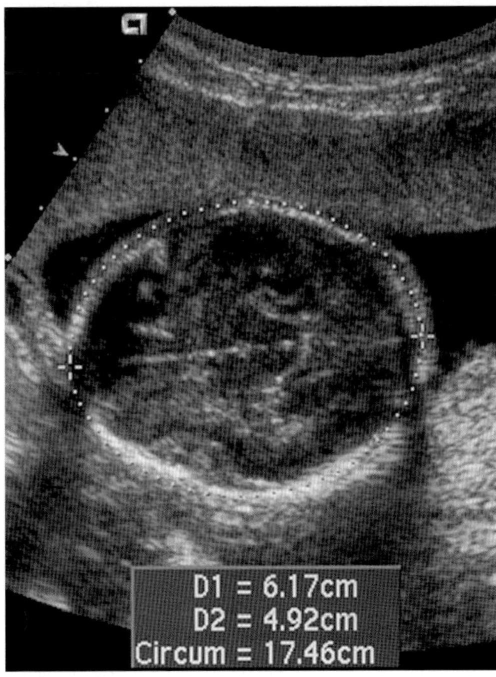

FIGURE 2.1-3. Head circumference measurement. On an image at the same level as the biparietal diameter, the head circumference is measured with electronic ellipse calipers (+ . . . . . +) around the outer rim of the ossified cranium.

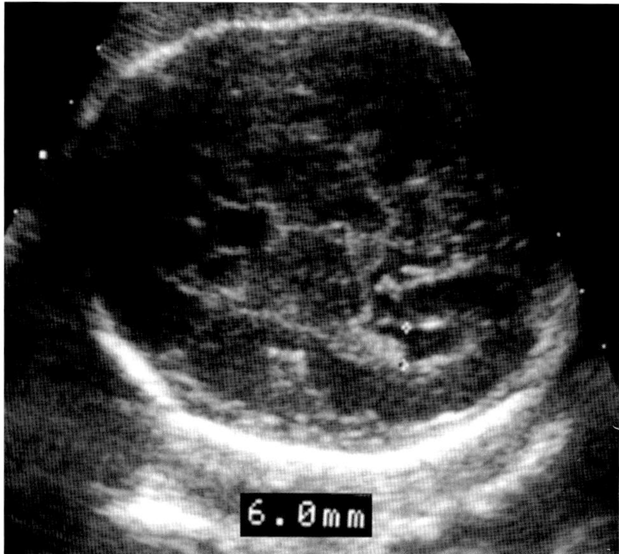

FIGURE 2.1-4. Lateral ventricular measurement. Axial view of the head demonstrates measurement of the width of the lateral ventricle at the level of the atrium, with + calipers placed on the ventricular wall.

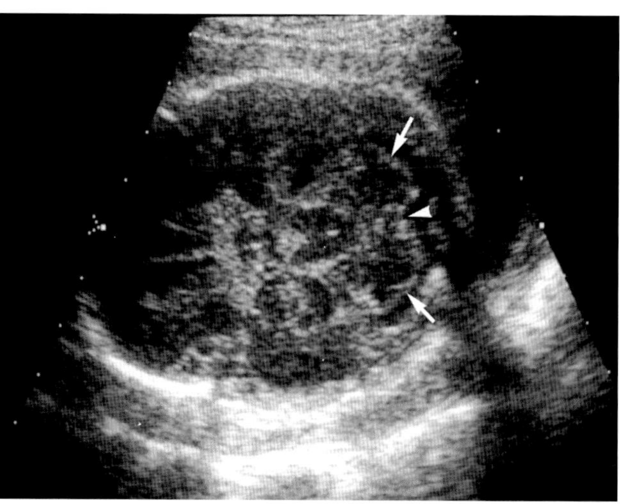

FIGURE 2.1-5. Cerebellum. Axial view of the posterior fossa demonstrates the contour of the normal cerebellum, with rounded cerebellar hemispheres *(arrows)* on either side of the more echogenic vermis *(arrowhead)*.

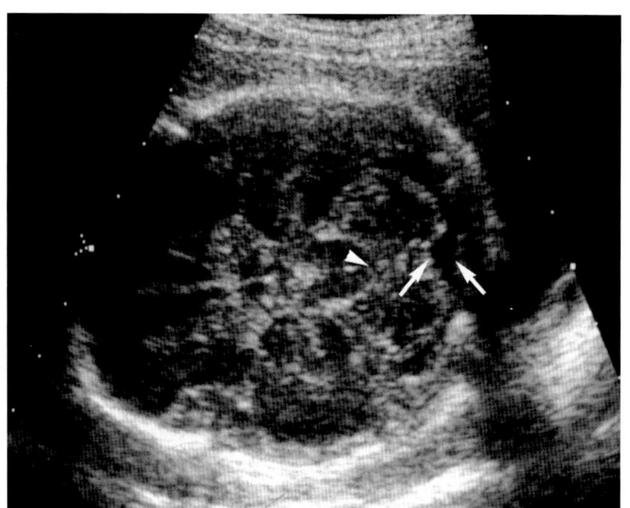

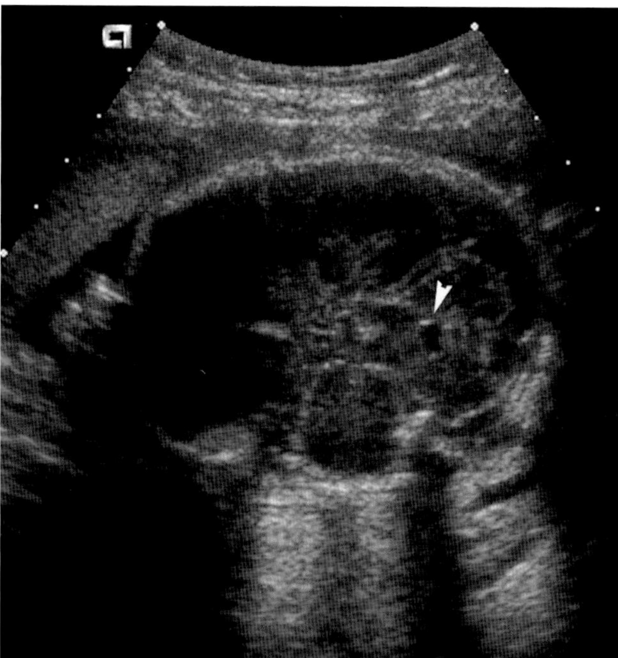

FIGURE 2.1-6. Cisterna magna and fourth ventricle. A: Axial view of the posterior fossa similar to that in Figure 2.1-5 demonstrates the fluid-filled cisterna magna *(arrows)* and the location of the fourth ventricle *(arrowhead)*. **B:** Axial image of posterior fossa demonstrates a small amount of fluid in the fourth ventricle *(arrowhead)*.

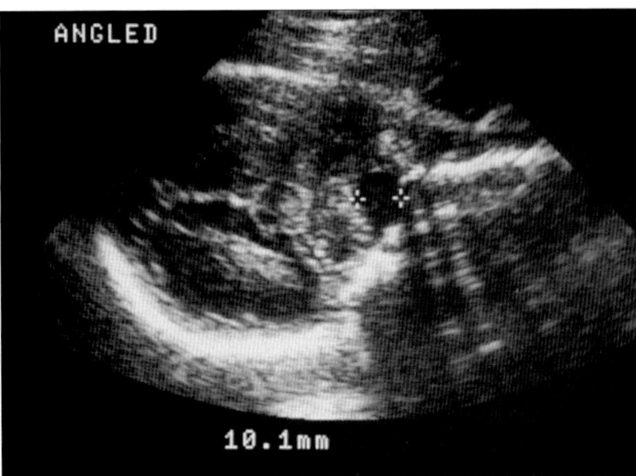

FIGURE 2.1-7. Pseudo megacisterna magna. Steeply angled axial view of the posterior fossa falsely enlarges the width of the cisterna magna (+ calipers) to greater than 10 mm.

The fetal spine should be assessed from the cervical spine through the sacrum in both longitudinal and transverse planes. The three ossification centers of each vertebra are brightly echogenic. The central ossification center, which forms the vertebral body, is located midline and anterior to the two posterior ossification centers, which form the posterior elements. On transverse view, the three ossification centers form a C or U shape at each level (Figure 2.1-8), with skin covering posteriorly. On longitudinal views, the ossification centers are aligned in parallel until they converge at the lower sacrum (Figure 2.1-9). Only two of the three ossification centers can be seen on a longitudinal image. On a sagittal image, the central ossification center and one posterior ossification center are visualized for each vertebra. On a coronal image, both posterior ossification centers are seen at each level. There should be a one-to-one correspondence between ossification centers on either view. The spine should be straight from side to side and have a normal thoracic kyphosis and lumbar lordosis.

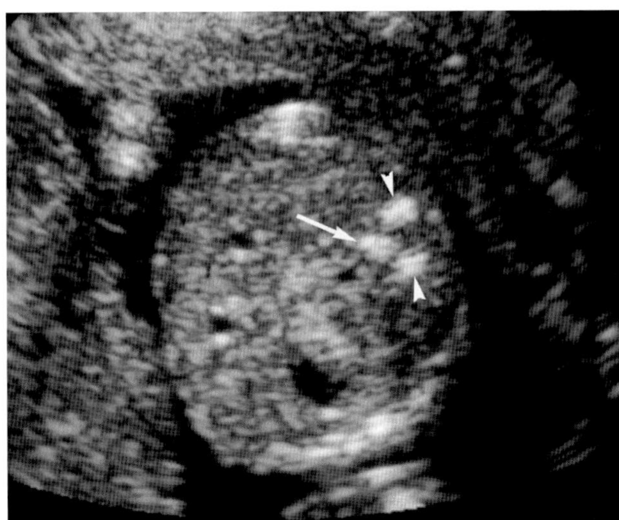

FIGURE 2.1-8. **Spine.** Transverse view of a lumbar vertebra demonstrates its three ossification centers: two posterior *(arrowheads)* and one anterior *(arrow)*. Skin covers the spine posteriorly.

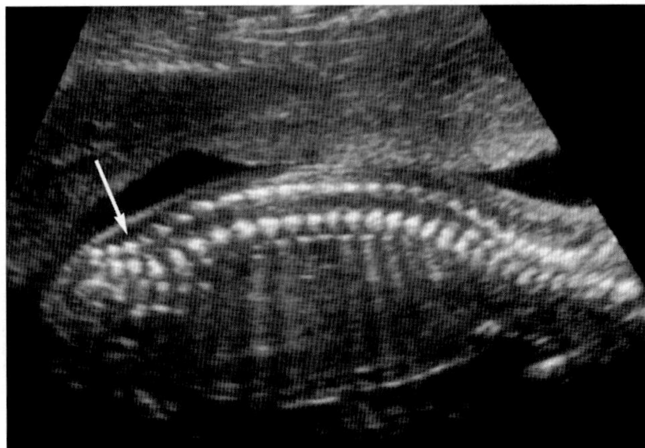

FIGURE 2.1-9. Spine. Longitudinal image of the entire spine demonstrates parallel alignment of posterior ossification centers until they converge at the sacrum *(arrow)*.

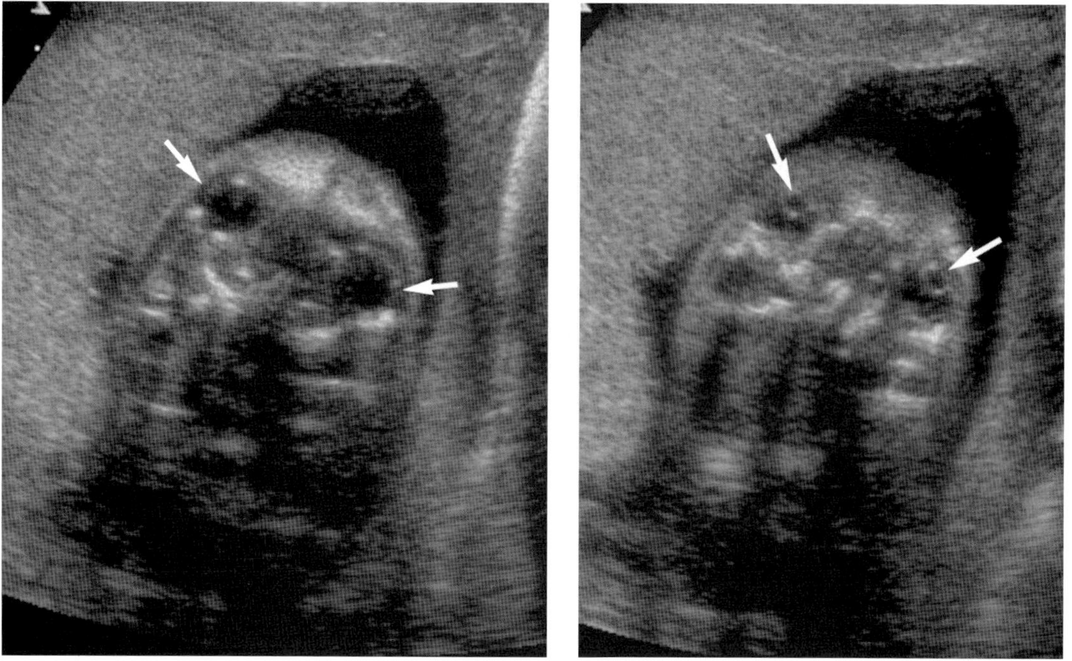

FIGURE 2.1-10. Orbits. A: Coronal images through the face demonstrate both orbits *(arrows)*. **B:** The lens of each eye is seen as a small bright circle in each globe *(arrows)*.

The fetal face is assessed in sagittal, coronal, and transverse views. The presence and position of the orbits and globes are best evaluated on transverse or coronal images (Figure 2.1-10). On a coronal view, the nose and lips are well seen (Figure 2.1-11). Sagittal views of the face demonstrate formation of the mandible, maxilla, and nasal bones as well as the soft tissues overlying these bones (Figure 2.1-12).

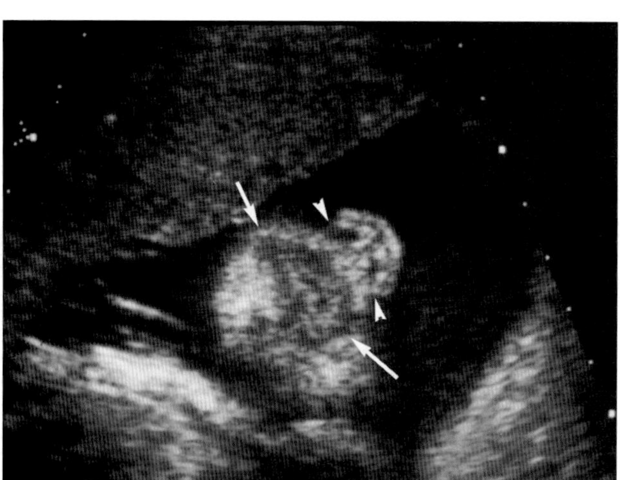

FIGURE 2.1-11. Nose and lips. Coronal view of the lower face demonstrates the upper and lower lips *(arrows)* and the lower contour of the nose with both nostrils *(arrowheads)*.

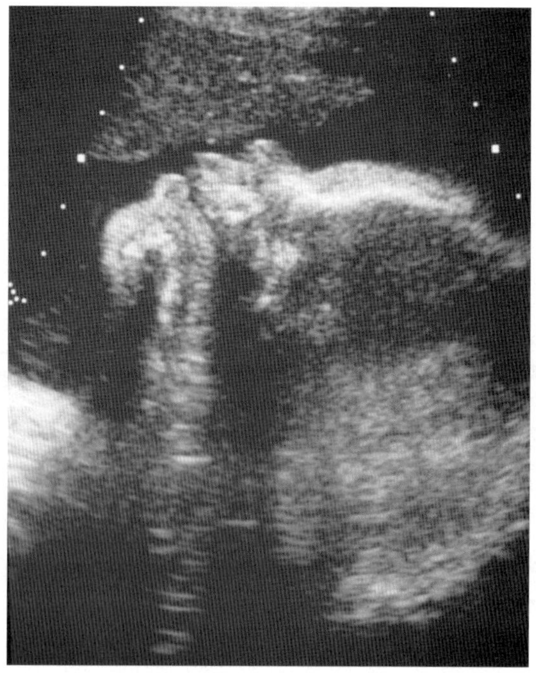

FIGURE 2.1-12. Facial profile. Sagittal view shows the soft tissues of the face overlying the echogenic bones that support it.

2.2. THORAX AND HEART

Description and Clinical Features

The thorax is supported by the spine and ribs and contains the heart, lungs, and mediastinal structures. Thoracic contents are separated from the abdominal cavity by the diaphragm.

The fetal heart comprises four chambers: the right and left ventricles and right and left atria. The right and left ventricles are similar in size and wall thickness, as are the right and left atria. The atrial and ventricular septa separate the right and left sides of the heart. The foramen ovale is an opening in the atrial septum through which blood flows from the right to the left atrium *in utero*. After birth, normal hemodynamic changes in cardiopulmonary function cause closure of this physiologic opening.

The aorta arises from the left ventricle, coursing superiorly and toward the right. The anterior wall of the ascending aorta is continuous with the interventricular septum. The main pulmonary artery arises from the right ventricle anterior and slightly to the left of the aorta and trifurcates into the right and left pulmonary arteries and the ductus arteriosus. *In utero*, the ductus arteriosus carries blood from the pulmonary artery to the descending aorta. Like the foramen ovale, the ductus arteriosus closes after birth.

Sonography

On the transverse view of the thorax at the level of the heart, the thorax is round. The heart is located slightly to the left of midline, and the lungs have homogeneous echotexture (Figure 2.2-1). The diaphragm, best seen on longitudinal view, is convex upward on each side. Episodes of fetal breathing, as demonstrated by regular diaphragmatic motion, are commonly seen, particularly toward term (Figure 2.2-2).

The four chambers of the heart are best imaged on an axial view of the thorax (Figures 2.2-1 and 2.2-3). The apex of the heart points to the left, such that the right ventricle lies directly posterior to the sternum and the left atrium sits anterior to the descending aorta and spine. The atria are similar in size and wall thickness, as are the ventricles. The left ventricle has a more conical shape and smoother inner surface than the right ven-

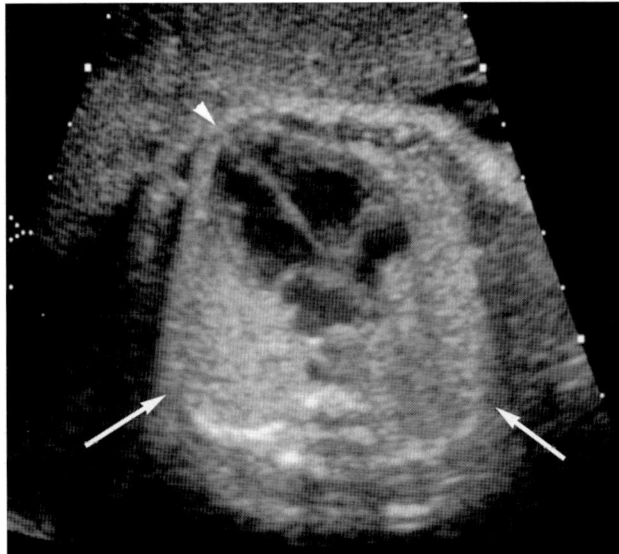

FIGURE 2.2-1. Thorax. Transverse view at the level of the four-chamber view of the heart demonstrates homogeneous lung tissue *(arrows)* filling the thorax around the heart *(arrowhead)*.

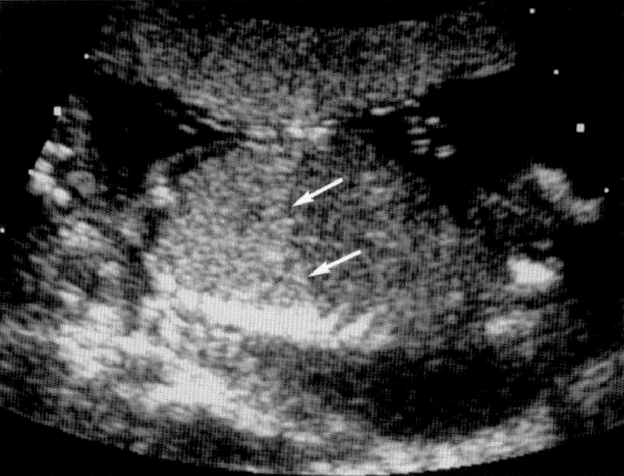

FIGURE 2.2-2. Diaphragm. Sagittal view of the fetal trunk demonstrates the dome-shaped diaphragm *(arrows)* separating the liver from more echogenic lung tissue. With fetal breathing motion, the diaphragm can be seen to move up and down rhythmically.

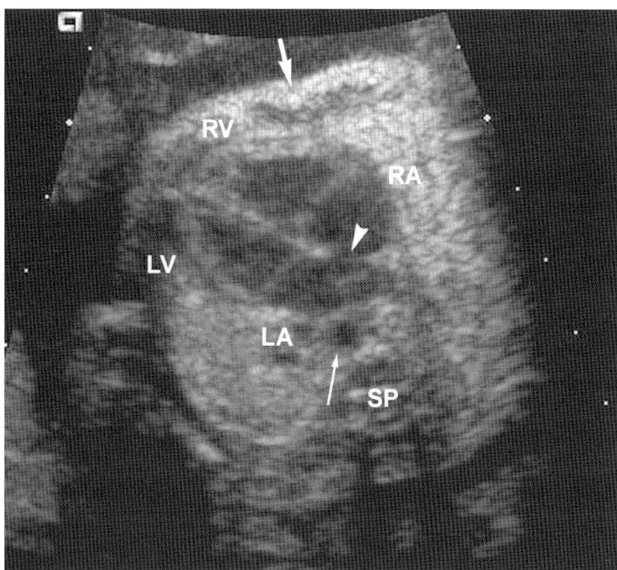

FIGURE 2.2-3. **Four-chamber view of the heart.** Transverse view of the fetal thorax demonstrates the four chambers of the heart (LV, left ventricle; RV, right ventricle; LA, left atrium, RA, right atrium), with the foramen ovale *(arrowhead)* seen as an opening between the right and left atria. The right ventricle is positioned just posterior to the sternum *(large arrow)*. The left atrium is located anterior to the descending aorta *(small arrow)*, which is just anterior to the spine (SP).

tricle. The foramen ovale, located between the atria, appears as a valve-like opening in the atrial septum (Figure 2.2-3).

The left ventricular outflow tract is best imaged on an oblique view of the left ventricle demonstrating the long axis of the ventricle and the aortic root. The entire length of the ventricular septum is visible, and the septum should be intact and continuous with the anterior wall of the aorta (Figure 2.2-4). Transverse views of the right ventricular outflow tract demonstrate the division of the main pulmonary artery into the right pulmonary artery, which courses behind the aorta, and the ductus arteriosus (Figure 2.2-5).

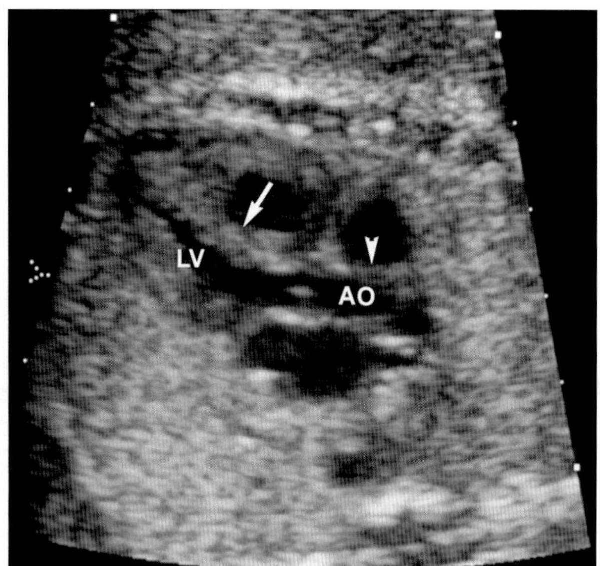

FIGURE 2.2-4. Left ventricular outflow tract. Oblique axial view of the heart demonstrates the aorta (AO) arising from the left ventricle (LV). The ventricular septum *(arrow)* is continuous with the anterior aortic wall *(arrowhead)*. The aortic valve appears as a bright dot in the lumen at the junction of the aorta with the left ventricle.

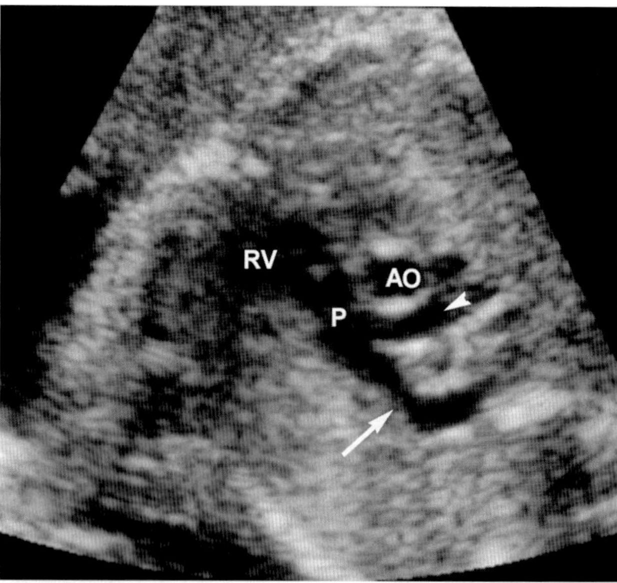

FIGURE 2.2-5. Right ventricular outflow tract. Transverse view of the heart superior to the four-chamber view demonstrates the pulmonary artery (P) arising from the right ventricle (RV), branching into the ductus arteriosus *(arrow)* and the right pulmonary artery *(arrowhead)*, which courses behind the ascending aorta (AO).

2.3. ABDOMEN

Description and Clinical Features

The fetal abdomen contains the gastrointestinal and genitourinary tracts as well as a number of major blood vessels. It is bounded by the abdominal wall and the diaphragm. Measurements of the fetal abdomen provide important information about fetal size and growth.

Fluid is normally present within the fetal stomach in the right upper quadrant, and bowel fills the mid to lower abdomen. The umbilical cord enters the abdomen at the umbilicus. The umbilical vein courses through the liver to the left portal vein and ductus venosum. The paired umbilical arteries course on either side of the urinary bladder to their origins at the iliac arteries.

The fetal kidneys are normally located in the renal fossas on either side of the spine, whereas the urinary bladder is located in the lower abdomen and pelvis.

Sonography

The fetal abdomen is evaluated during the second and third trimester sonographic examination on four key images: the abdominal measurement view and images of the umbilical cord insertion site, the kidneys, and the urinary bladder. The abdominal diameter or circumference is measured on an axial view of the abdomen at the level of the stomach and intrahepatic portion of the umbilical vein (Figure 2.3-1). The abdomen should be round and smooth in contour. On this view, the stomach should be seen as a fluid-filled structure in the left upper quadrant. The liver is seen in the right upper quadrant, and the gallbladder is usually seen just inferior to the liver (Figure 2.3-2). Abdominal diameter measurements are obtained by placing perpendicular pairs of calipers on the outer edge of the fetal abdomen across the abdomen anteroposteriorly and transversely (Figure 2.3-3). The abdominal circumference measurement is obtained on the same view of the abdomen, using electronic ellipse calipers to trace the outer edge of the abdomen (Figure 2.3-4).

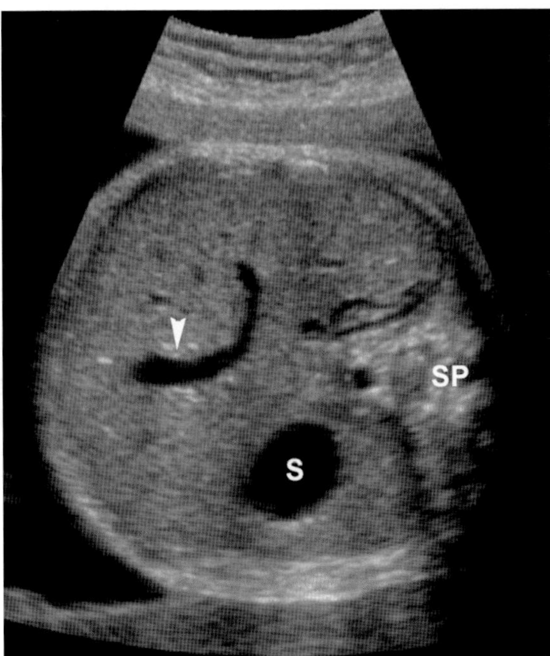

FIGURE 2.3-1. Abdomen. Transverse view of the abdomen at the level of the stomach (S) and intrahepatic portion of the umbilical vein *(arrowhead)* as it joins the left portal vein. The spine (SP) is seen in transverse posteriorly.

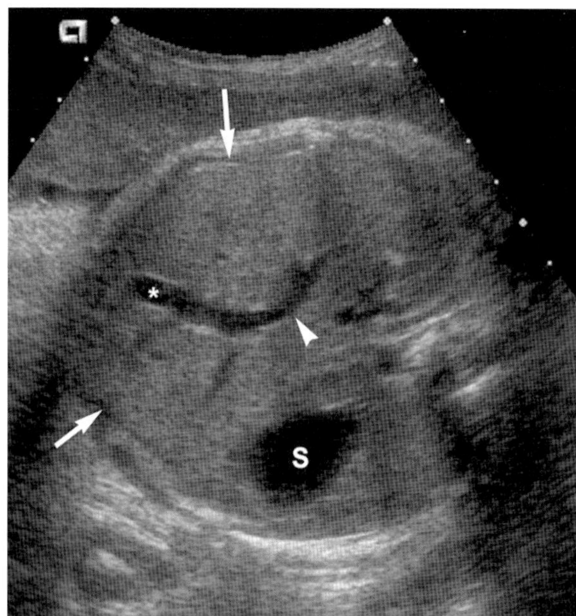

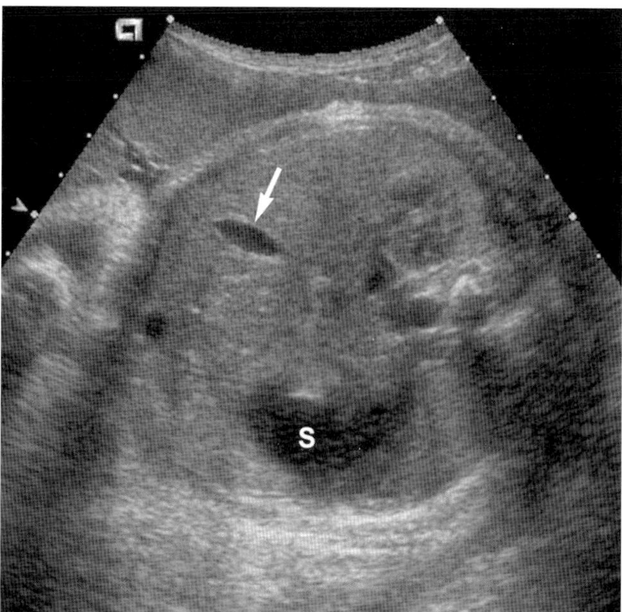

FIGURE 2.3-2. Liver and gallbladder. A: Transverse view of abdomen demonstrates the liver *(arrows)* filling the right upper quadrant and the stomach (S) in the left upper quadrant. Within the liver, the umbilical vein *(*)* is seen joining the left portal vein *(arrowhead)*. **B:** Transverse image inferior to **(A)** demonstrates the gallbladder *(arrow)* in the right upper quadrant. The stomach (S) is in the left upper quadrant.

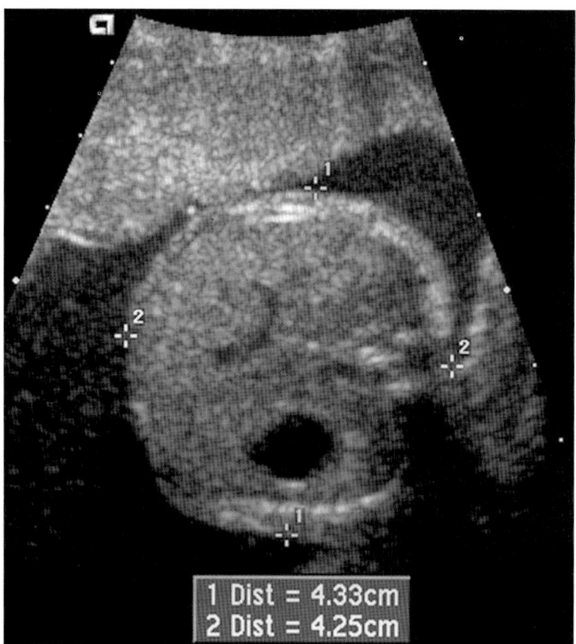

FIGURE 2.3-3. Abdominal diameter measurements. The + calipers labeled 1 measure the transverse dimension of the fetal abdomen. The + calipers labeled 2, perpendicular to those labeled 1, measure the anteroposterior diameter. These two measurements are used to estimate the size of the fetal abdomen and calculate the fetal weight.

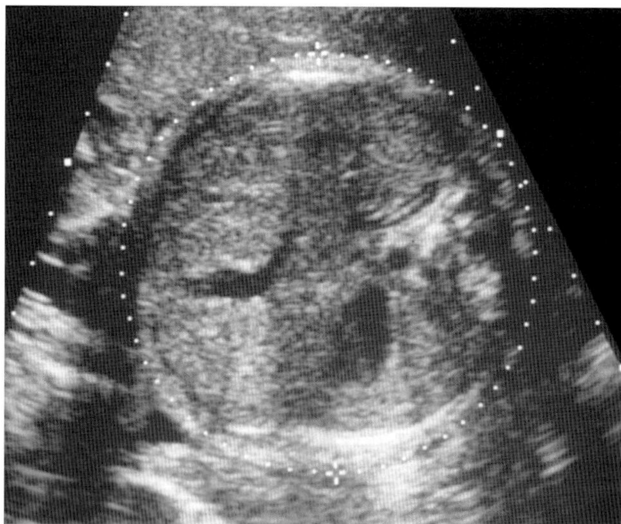

FIGURE 2.3-4. Abdominal circumference measurement. The + calipers and connecting dots trace the outer perimeter of the abdomen on a transverse view to measure the abdominal circumference.

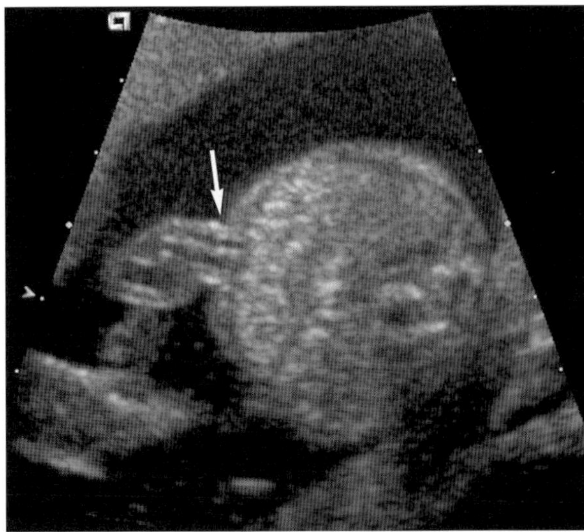

FIGURE 2.3-5. Umbilical cord insertion. Transverse view of fetal abdomen at the level of the umbilical cord insertion *(arrow)* demonstrates an intact anterior abdominal wall.

The umbilical cord enters the fetal abdomen at the umbilicus (Figure 2.3-5). The abdominal wall should be otherwise intact.

The kidneys can be seen on a transverse view of the abdomen on both sides of the lumbar spine (Figure 2.3-6). On longitudinal views, each kidney appears as a reniform structure with an echogenic capsule and central echoes of the renal sinus (Figure 2.3-7). A small amount of fluid is sometimes seen within the renal pelvis (Figure 2.3-6). In the third trimester, the medullary pyramids may be visible as hypoechoic areas within the renal parenchyma (Figure 2.3-7).

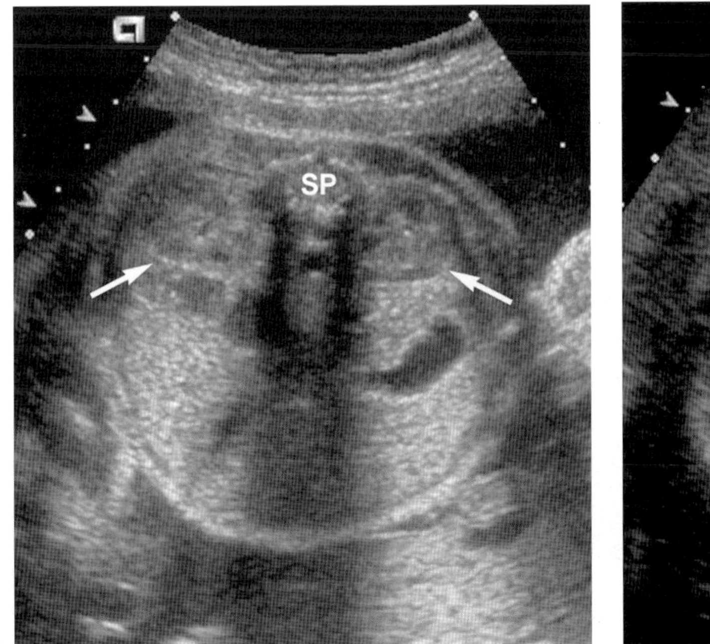

A

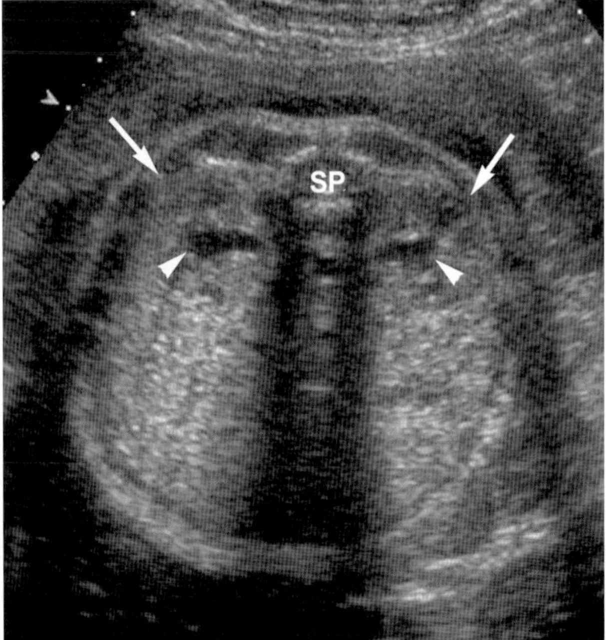

B

FIGURE 2.3-6. Kidneys. A: Transverse view of the fetal abdomen demonstrates a kidney *(arrows)* on either side of the spine (SP). The kidney has a thin, bright capsule and is less echogenic than the bowel and liver anterior to it. **B:** The normal kidneys *(arrows)* on either side of the spine (SP) on this transverse view have a small amount of fluid in each renal pelvis *(arrowheads).*

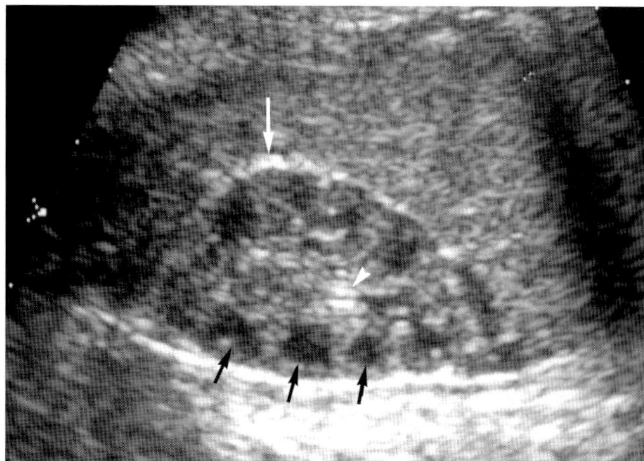

FIGURE 2.3-7. Kidney. Longitudinal image of one kidney demonstrates its reniform shape, with its echogenic capsule *(white arrow)* and bright echoes of the renal sinus *(arrowhead)* noted centrally. In the renal parenchyma are evenly spaced hypoechoic regions representing medullary pyramids *(black arrows)*.

The urinary bladder is an anechoic structure in the fetal pelvis and lower abdomen (Figure 2.3-8).

The bowel and mesentery fill much of the lower abdomen and are usually slightly more echogenic than the liver and less echogenic than bone. Individual loops are rarely identified in normal fetuses, except near term, when the colon may become visible, either hypoechoic or hyperechoic, forming the periphery of the bowel (Figure 2.3-9).

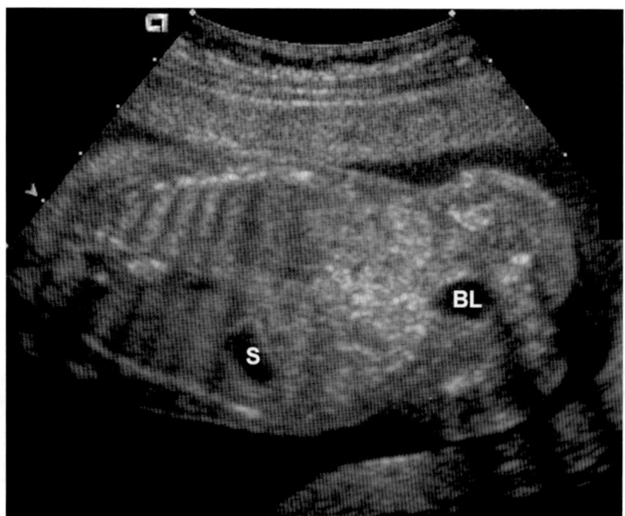

FIGURE 2.3-8. Urinary bladder. Longitudinal image of fetal abdomen demonstrating urinary bladder (BL) in pelvis and lower abdomen. The stomach (S) is seen in the left upper quadrant.

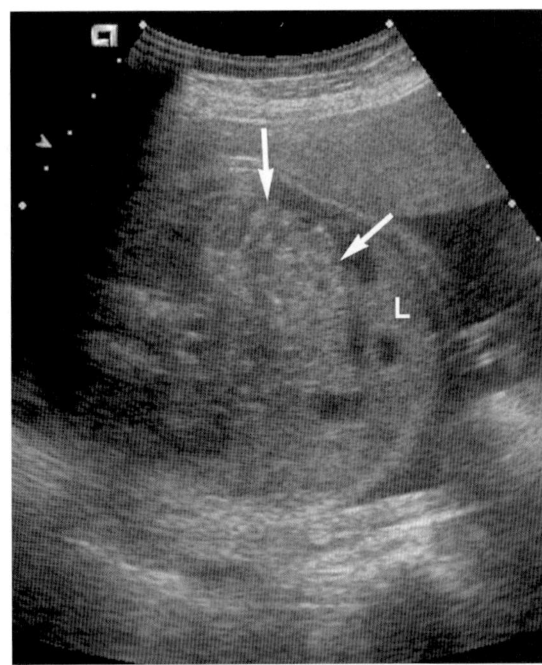

A

FIGURE 2.3-9. **Bowel. A:** Transverse image of the lower abdomen demonstrates heterogeneous bowel *(arrows)*, more echogenic than the liver (L). **B:** An isolated hypoechoic loop of colon *(arrow)* is seen at the periphery of the abdomen in this third-trimester fetus. **C:** Echogenic colon *(arrows)* is seen at the periphery of the abdomen in this term fetus.

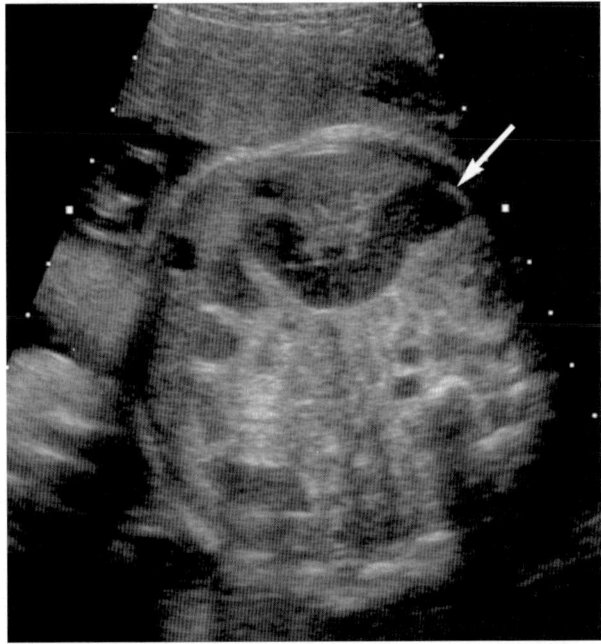

B

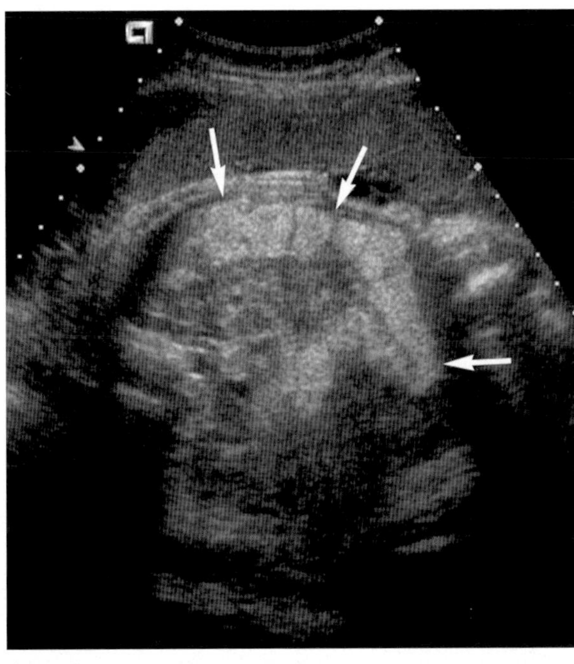

C

2.4. SKELETON

Description and Clinical Features

During the second and third trimesters, the skeletal system undergoes rapid growth and progressive ossification. The diaphyses of the long bones in the upper and lower extremities are ossified by the end of the first trimester. Secondary, or epiphyseal, ossification centers form after birth, except for the distal femur, proximal tibia, and proximal humerus, which can begin to ossify near term. The bones of the skull begin to ossify in the first trimester and become increasingly ossified during the second and third trimesters, but the sutures and fontanelles do not close until several months after birth. Each vertebra forms from three ossification centers: a central ossification center that becomes the vertebral body and right and left posterior ossification centers that become the pedicles and laminae. The length of the long bones, especially the femur, is used to estimate gestational age and to assess fetal growth.

Sonography

During routine second and third trimester sonograms, the cranium is imaged on several views of the brain, the spine is imaged in its entirety in longitudinal and transverse planes, and the femur is measured to assess gestational age. The cranium should be oval in shape and intact. Normal spaces are seen between the cranial bones at the cranial sutures (Figure 2.4-1). The spine should contain parallel ossification centers on coronal and sagittal views (Figure 2.4-2).

The diaphyses of all the long bones of the upper and lower extremities are well ossified by the second trimester, making it easy to confirm the presence of the radius and ulna in the forearm, the tibia and fibula in the lower leg (Figure 2.4-3), the humerus in each upper arm, and the femur in each thigh. The femur measurement is taken on a longitudinal view of the femur with the calipers placed at either end of the ossified portion of the diaphysis (Figure 2.4-4). The hands are often closed, but with fetal activity, it is common to see the fetus open the hands (Figure 2.4-5). The feet (Figure 2.4-6) are normally aligned perpendicular to the plane of the tibia and fibula.

A
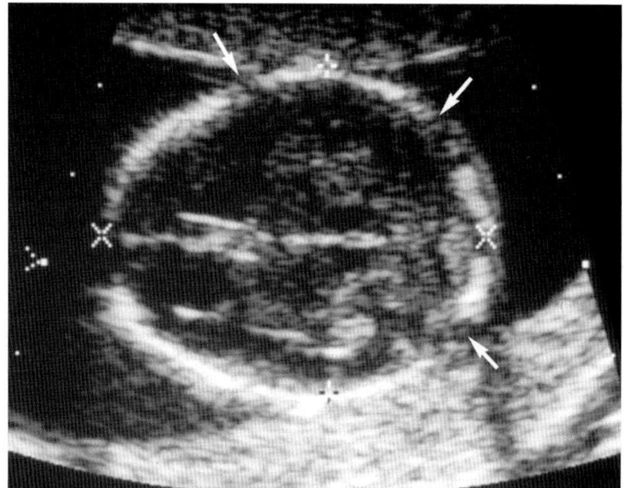

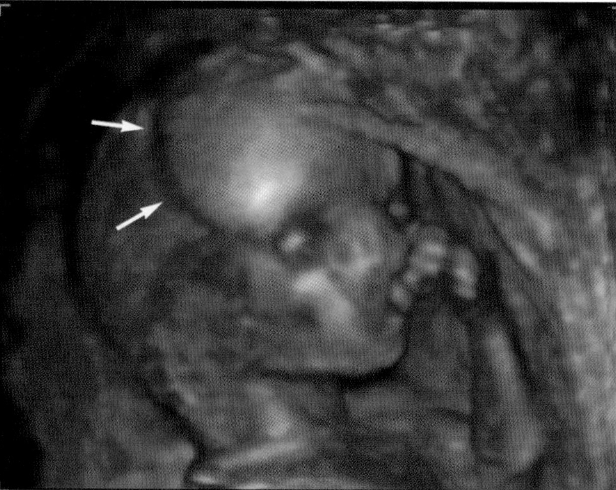
B

FIGURE 2.4-1. Cranial sutures. A: Normal discontinuity of the ossified cranium represents the cranial sutures *(arrows)*. **B:** Three-dimensional sonogram of a 16-week fetal head demonstrates a cranial suture *(arrows)*.

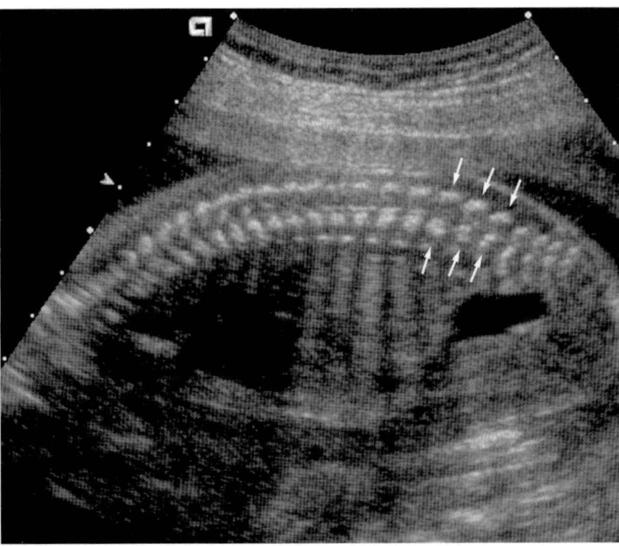

FIGURE 2.4-2. Lumbosacral spine. Longitudinal image of spine demonstrates parallel ossification centers *(small arrows)* at each level.

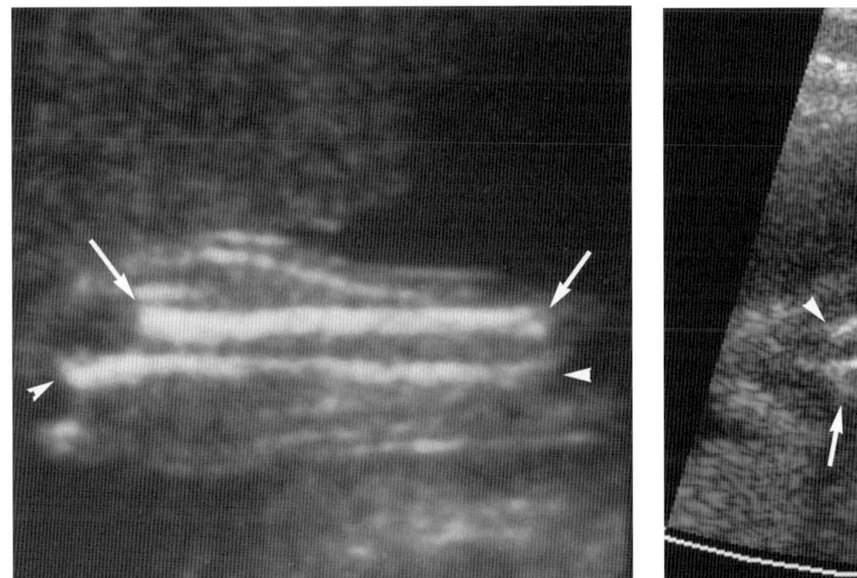

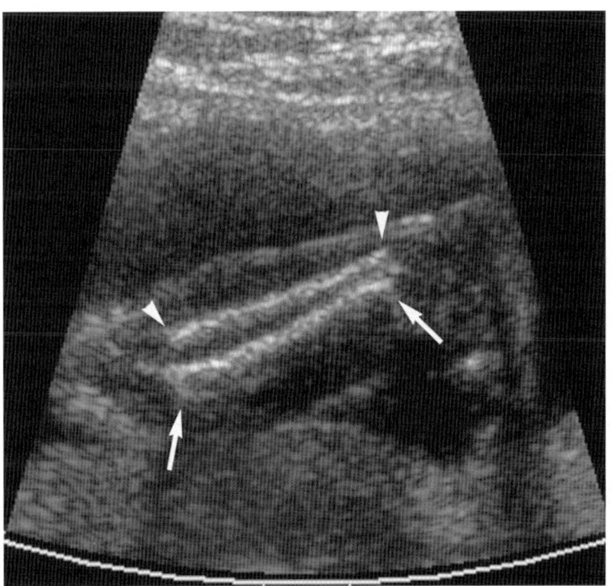

FIGURE 2.4-3. Long bones of the forearm and lower leg. A: Image of forearm demonstrates the radius *(arrows)* and ulna *(arrowheads)* lying in parallel. **B:** Image of the lower leg demonstrates the tibia *(arrows)* and fibula *(arrowheads)*.

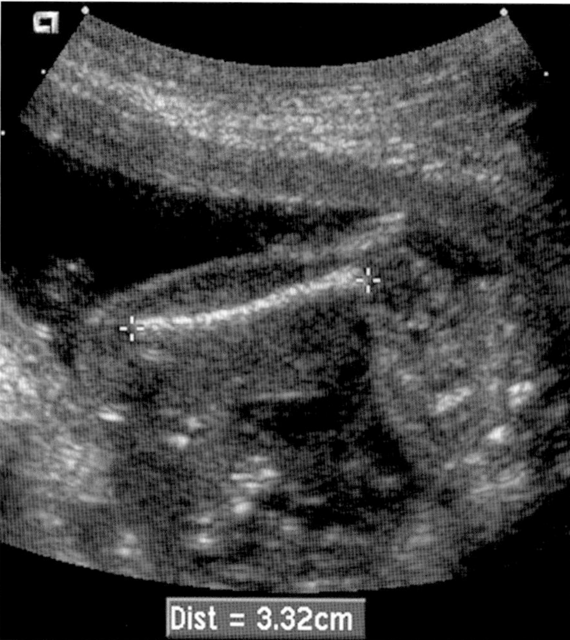

FIGURE 2.4-4. Femur with measurement. + calipers mark the ends of the ossified femoral diaphysis to measure the femur length in this 20-week fetus.

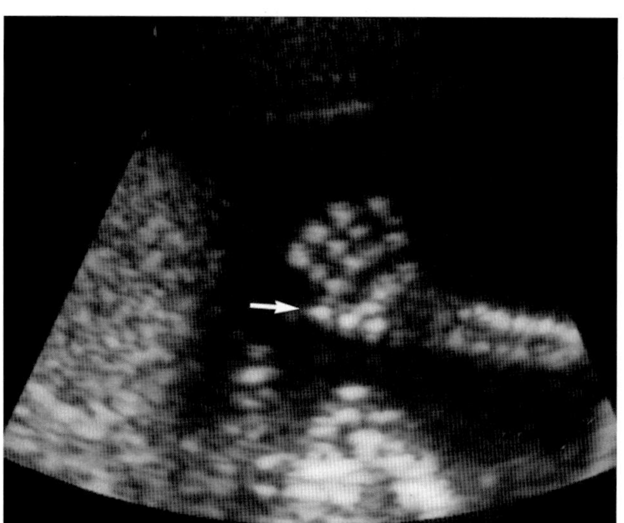

FIGURE 2.4-5. Hand. Open hand demonstrates three phalanges in each finger and two in the thumb *(arrow)*.

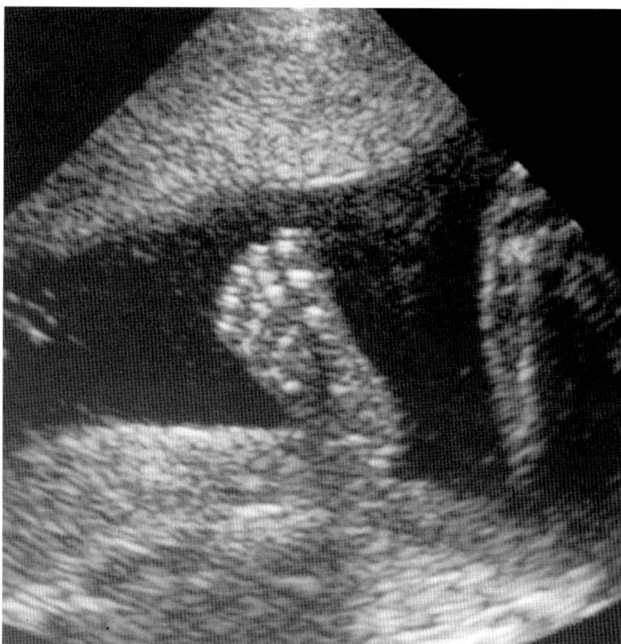

FIGURE 2.4-6. Foot. Image of foot demonstrates normal shape and five toes.

SUGGESTED READINGS

1. Benson CB. Ruling out fetal anomalies. In: Benson CB, Arger P, Bluth EI, eds. *Ultrasound in obstetrics and gynecology, a practical approach*. New York: Thieme Medical and Scientific Publishers, 2000: 145–154.
2. Brown DL, Di Salvo DN, Frates MC, et al. Normal variants and pitfalls in the sonographic evaluation of fetal heart. *AJR Am J Roentgenol* 1993;160:1251–1255.
3. Filly RA, Feldstein VA. Ultrasound evaluation of normal fetal anatomy. In: Callen PW, ed. *Ultrasonography in obstetrics and gynecology*, 4th ed. Philadelphia: WB Saunders, 2000:221–276.
4. Hadlock FP, Deter RL, Harrist RB, et al. Fetal biparietal diameter: rational choice of plane of section for sonographic measurement. *AJR Am J Roentgenol* 1982;138:871–874.
5. Haimovici JA, Doubilet PM, Benson CB, et al. Clinical significance of isolated enlargement of the cisterna magna (>10 mm) on prenatal sonography. *J Ultrasound Med* 1997;16:731–734.
6. Hilpert PL, Hall BE, Kurtz AB. The atria of the fetal lateral ventricles: a sonographic study of normal atrial size and choroid plexus volume. *AJR Am J Roentgenol* 1995;164:731–734.
7. Jeanty P, Rodesch F, Delbeke D, et al. Estimation of gestational age from measurements of fetal long bones. *J Ultrasound Med* 1984;3:75–79.
8. Laing FC, Frates MC, Brown DL, et al. Sonography of the fetal posterior fossa: false appearance of mega cisterna magna and Dandy Walker variant. *Radiology* 1994;192:247–251.
9. Mahony BS, Callen PW, Filly RA. The distal femoral epiphyseal ossification center in the assessment of third-trimester menstrual age: sonographic identification and measurement. *Radiology* 1985;155: 201–204.

3

SECOND AND THIRD TRIMESTER NONFETAL COMPONENTS

3.1. UMBILICAL CORD

Description and Clinical Features

The umbilical cord contains the blood vessels that carry blood between the fetus and the placenta. Its outermost component is a membrane that is continuous with the amnion. Within this membrane lie the umbilical blood vessels bathed in Wharton's jelly. The normal cord contains one vein and two arteries.

The umbilical arteries connect to the internal iliac arteries in the fetal pelvis. With each fetal systolic contraction, blood flows in the umbilical arteries away from the fetus toward the placenta. Blood returns to the fetus through the umbilical vein, which drains via the left portal vein into the inferior vena cava through the ductus venosum.

Sonography

Except in cases of severe oligohydramnios, the umbilical cord is visible as a serpiginous structure surrounded by amniotic fluid, extending from the placenta to the fetus (Figure

A

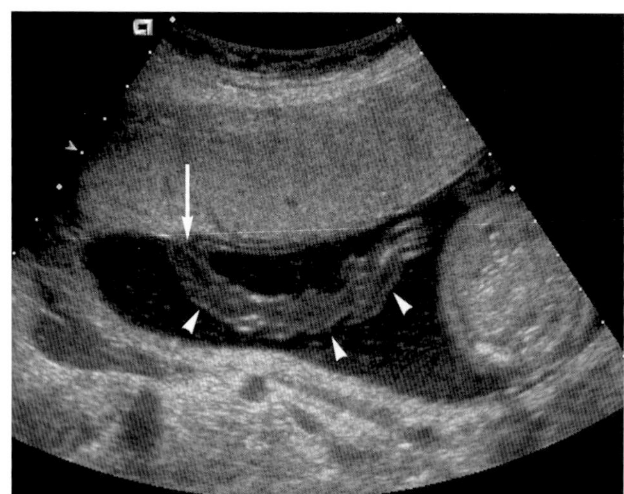

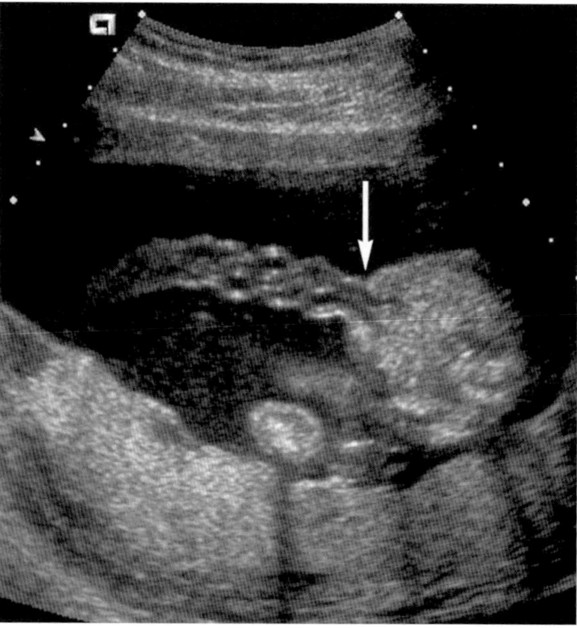

B

FIGURE 3.1-1. Umbilical cord. A: The umbilical cord is seen as a thin-walled curvilinear structure *(arrowheads)* extending from its placental insertion site *(arrow)* toward the fetus. **B:** Umbilical cord insertion *(arrow)* into the fetus is shown.

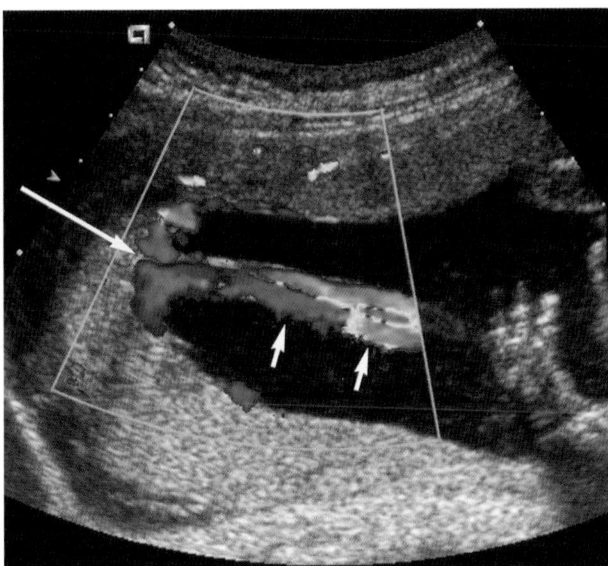

FIGURE 3.1-2. Color Doppler of the umbilical cord. A portion of the umbilical cord *(short arrows)* and its insertion into the placenta *(long arrow)* are demonstrated.

3.1-1). In most cases, both the placental and fetal cord insertion sites can be identified. Visualization of the cord may be enhanced using color Doppler (Figure 3.1-2). If a transverse section through a single loop of cord can be imaged, one large and two small circles are seen, the former representing the umbilical vein and the latter the umbilical arteries (Figure 3.1-3).

The intrafetal extensions of these vessels can be imaged via color Doppler. In particular, the existence of two umbilical arteries can be confirmed by demonstration of two umbilical arteries adjacent to the fetal bladder (Figure 3.1-4).

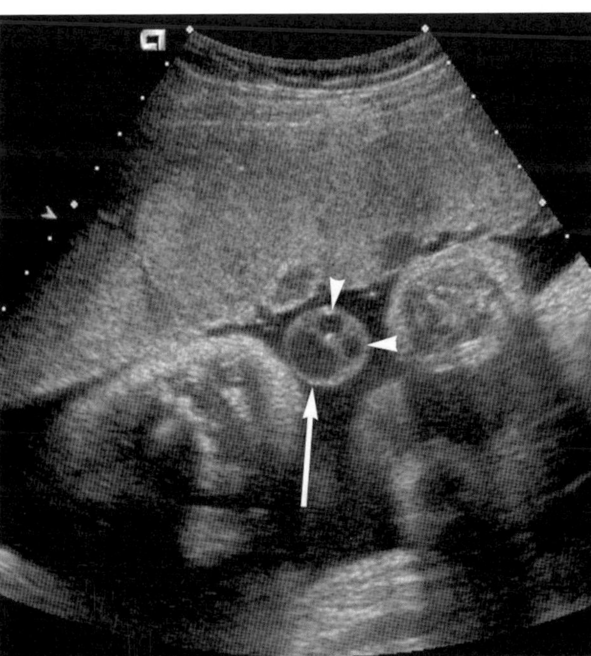

A

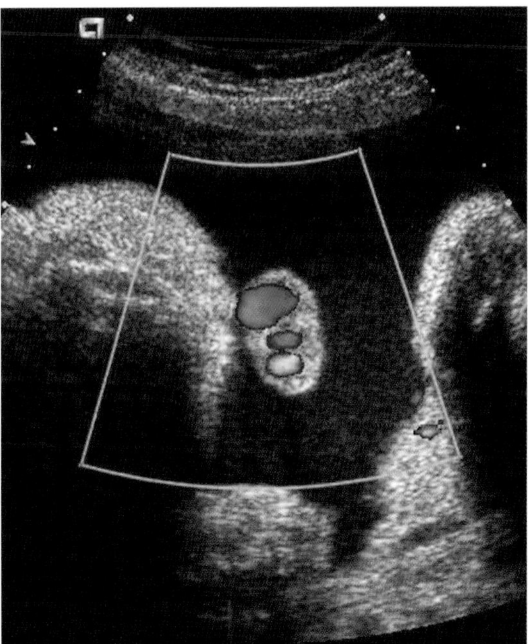

B

FIGURE 3.1-3. Vascular composition of the cord. A: Cross-section of the umbilical cord reveals two arteries *(arrowheads)* and one vein *(arrow)*. **B:** Color Doppler of a cross-section of the umbilical cord reveals two arteries *(small red dots)* and one vein *(larger blue structure)*.

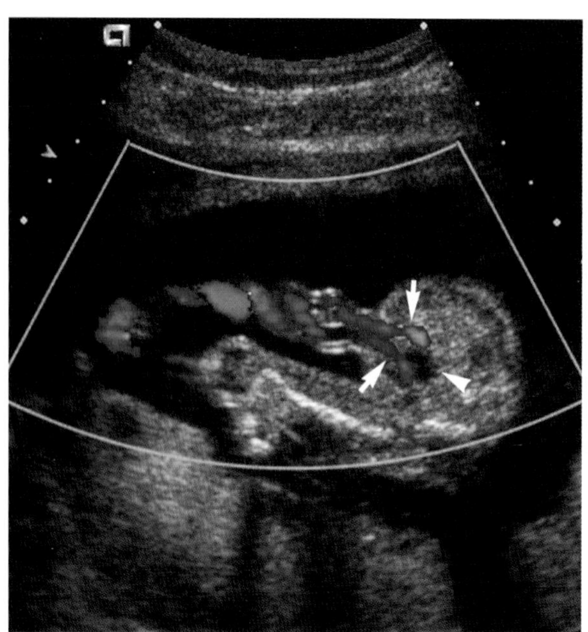

FIGURE 3.1-4. Doppler demonstration of two umbilical arteries in the fetal pelvis. Color Doppler in the fetal pelvis reveals two umbilical arteries *(arrows)* coursing laterally to the fetal bladder *(arrowhead)*.

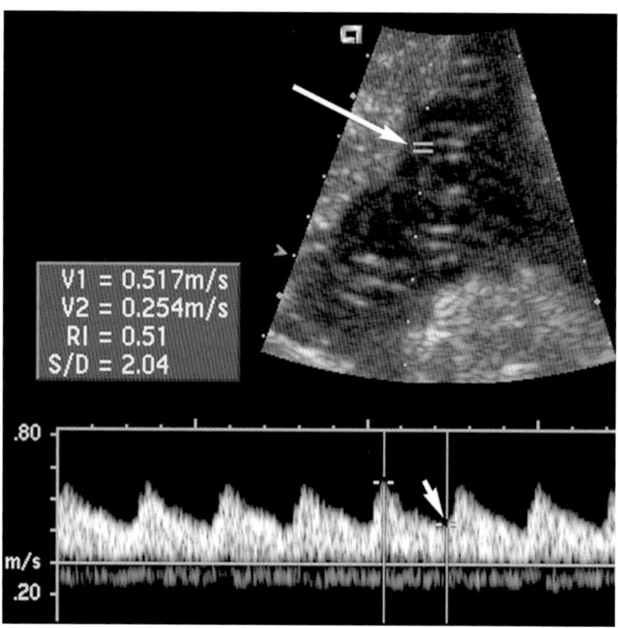

FIGURE 3.1-5. Umbilical arterial spectral Doppler. Spectral Doppler gate *(long arrow)* is placed within the umbilical artery. On the resulting spectral waveform, there is a normal pulsatile pattern with forward blood flow throughout the cardiac cycle, including diastole *(short arrow)*. The systolic/diastolic ratio is 2.04, which is within normal limits.

Spectral Doppler of the umbilical arteries demonstrates pulsatile flow (Figure 3.1-5). Flow normally continues in a forward direction throughout the fetal cardiac cycle. The systolic/diastolic ratio tends to decrease as pregnancy proceeds and is normally <4 at 26–30 weeks gestation, <3.5 at 30–34 weeks, and <3 from 34 weeks onward.

3.2. CERVIX IN PREGNANCY

Description and Clinical Features

The cervix is the most caudal portion of the uterus. It normally remains long and closed until term. When labor ensues, the cervix becomes effaced, leading to shortening and dilation of the cervical canal.

Sonography

The cervix can be evaluated sonographically using a transabdominal, translabial, or transvaginal approach. The transvaginal approach provides the highest resolution view and the most consistent visualization of the cervix, but the transabdominal approach is generally adequate in the low-risk patient. If the cervix cannot be adequately visualized transabdominally, as may happen when the fetal presenting part shadows out the cervix, translabial or transvaginal sonography may be necessary to assess the cervix.

With any of these approaches, the normal cervix appears as a fairly homogeneous echogenic structure at least 3 cm in length (Figure 3.2-1). The endocervical canal is generally visible as a thin line running the length of the cervix that may be hypo- or hyperechoic with respect to the rest of the cervix. Its appearance derives from the apposition of the anterior and posterior walls of the canal, and cervical mucous within the canal. One or more Nabothian cysts may be seen within the cervix.

A number of pitfalls must be avoided to obtain an accurate measurement of the cervical length. Measurement when there is a lower uterine segment contraction will falsely increase the measurement (Figure 3.2-2). Rectal gas shadowing may lead to a falsely short measurement on a translabial scan (Figure 3.2-3).

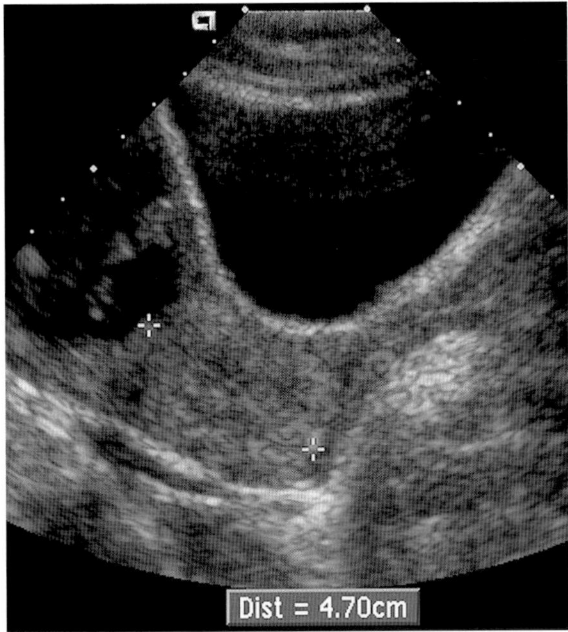

A

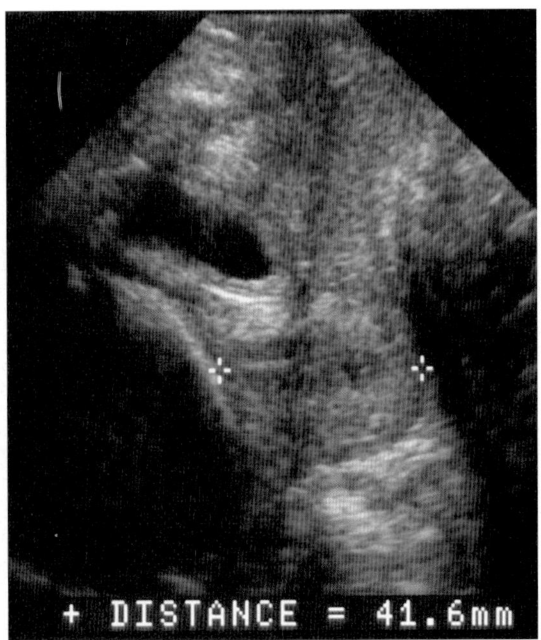

B

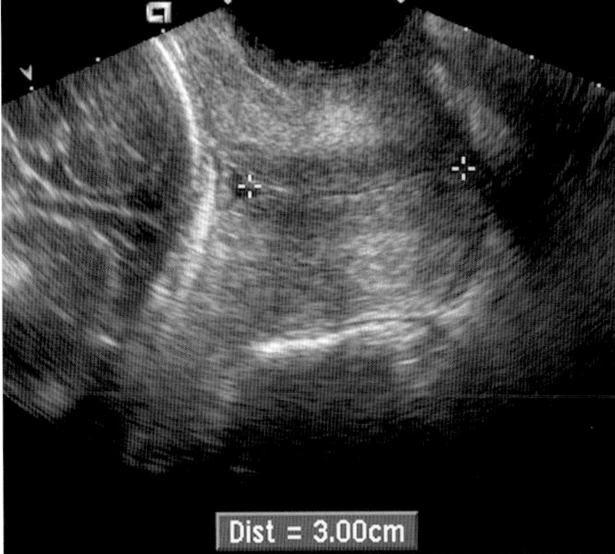

C

FIGURE 3.2-1. Normal cervix. The cervix is normal in configuration and length *(calipers)* on transabdominal **(A)**, translabial **(B)**, and transvaginal sonograms **(C)**, measuring at least 3 cm on each of these sagittal images.

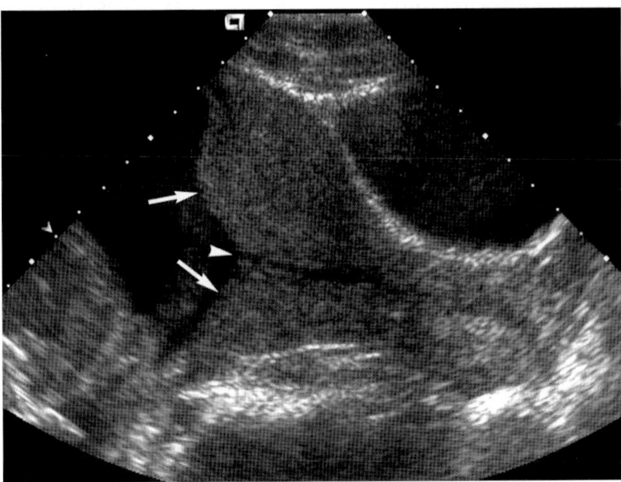

FIGURE 3.2-2. Pitfall in cervical length measurement: lower uterine segment contraction. Sagittal view of the lower uterus demonstrates circumferential thickening of the uterine wall in the lower segment *(arrows)*, representing a uterine contraction. The contraction apposes the anterior and posterior walls of the lower segment. If the innermost point of apposition *(arrowhead)* is mistaken for the internal os, an erroneously large measurement of cervical length will be obtained.

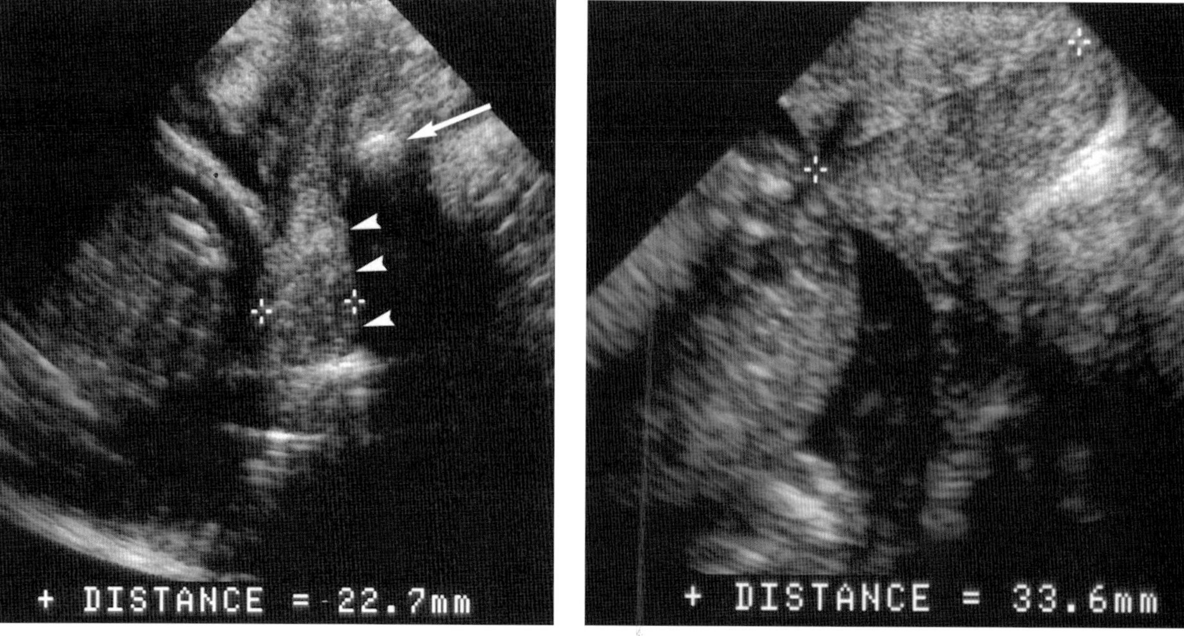

FIGURE 3.2-3. Pitfall in cervical length measurement: rectal gas shadowing on a translabial view. A: On this translabial view, rectal gas *(arrow)* casts a shadow that obscures the external portion of the cervix. A cervical measurement of 22.7 mm is erroneous because the outer caliper is positioned on the edge of the gas shadow *(arrowheads)*. **B:** Transvaginal scan performed immediately thereafter demonstrates the true length of the cervix to be 33.6 mm *(calipers)*.

3.3. PLACENTA

Description and Clinical Features

The placenta is the organ in which the fetal and maternal circulations comingle, permitting oxygen and nutrients to be passed from the mother to the fetus and fetal wastes to travel in the opposite direction. The placenta is composed of multiple cotyledons. The umbilical cord normally inserts near the mid portion of the placenta. From the insertion site, the umbilical arteries and vein divide into multiple branches that run along the surface of the placenta and then penetrate the cotyledons.

The placenta is contiguous with the maternal endometrium and is continuous with the chorionic membrane surrounding the gestational sac. The endometrium, if intact and unscarred, prevents the placenta from growing into the myometrium. The location of the placenta evolves over the course of gestation as areas of the placenta proliferate and other areas atrophy, leading to apparent migration or shifting of the placental position.

Sonography

In the second and most of the third trimesters, the placenta (Figure 3.3-1) appears on ultrasound as a homogeneously echogenic structure surrounding part of the gestational sac. The umbilical cord insertion site into the placenta can be identified, unless it is obscured from view by the fetus. Visualization of the insertion site is important if percutaneous umbilical blood sampling is planned. Gray-scale sonography is usually sufficient to identify the insertion site, but color Doppler is helpful (or necessary) in some cases.

In the third trimester, it is common to visualize calcifications within the placenta (Figure 3.3-2). By the latter part of this trimester, the calcifications may encircle the cotyledons.

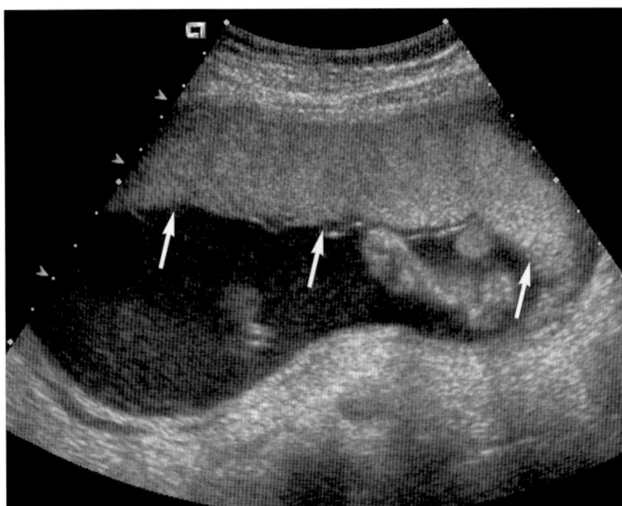

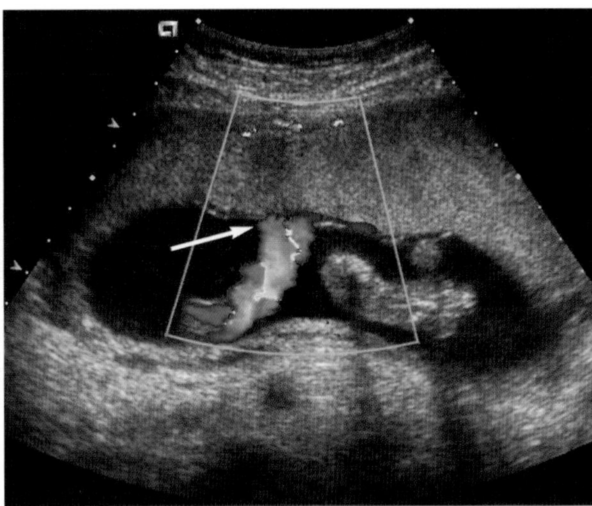

FIGURE 3.3-1. Normal placenta. A: The placenta in this 22-week gestation is a homogeneously echogenic structure *(arrows)* covering the anterior aspect of the gestational sac. **B:** The umbilical cord insertion site into the placenta *(arrow)* is clearly identified using color Doppler.

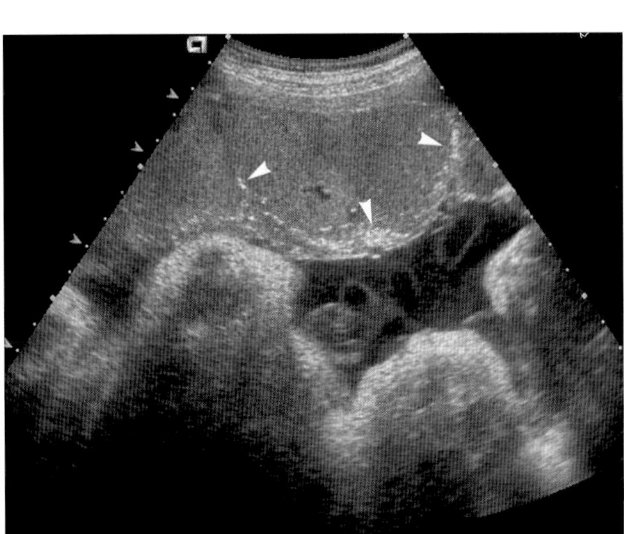

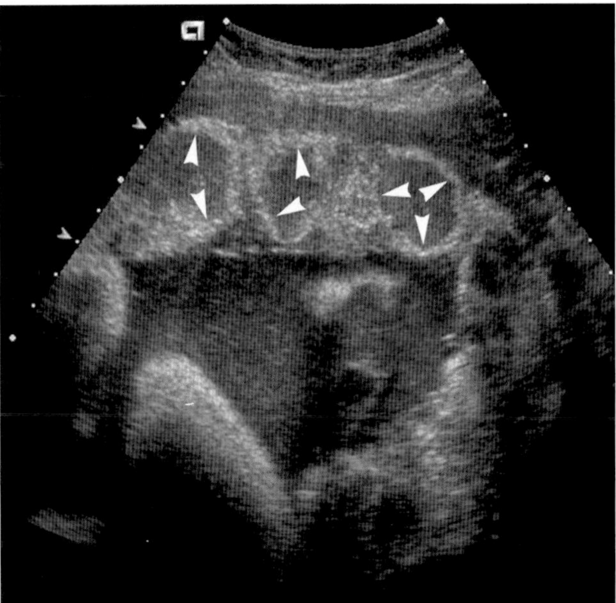

FIGURE 3.3-2. Calcified placentas. A: In this 32-week gestation, speckled calcifications *(arrowheads)* are seen along the borders of placental cotyledons. **B:** The cotyledons are surrounded by dense calcifications *(arrowheads)* in this 40-week gestation.

3.4. AMNIOTIC FLUID

Description and Clinical Features

Amniotic fluid fills the amniotic cavity and surrounds the developing fetus, providing room for the fetus to grow and cushioning it from external trauma. In the first and early second trimesters, amniotic fluid derives from flow of fluid across the amniotic membrane. From approximately 16 weeks of gestation onward, amniotic fluid is produced mainly by fetal urine. At this stage, amniotic fluid volume is determined by a dynamic balance of production and consumption: production via fetal urination, consumption via fetal swallowing and gastrointestinal tract absorption.

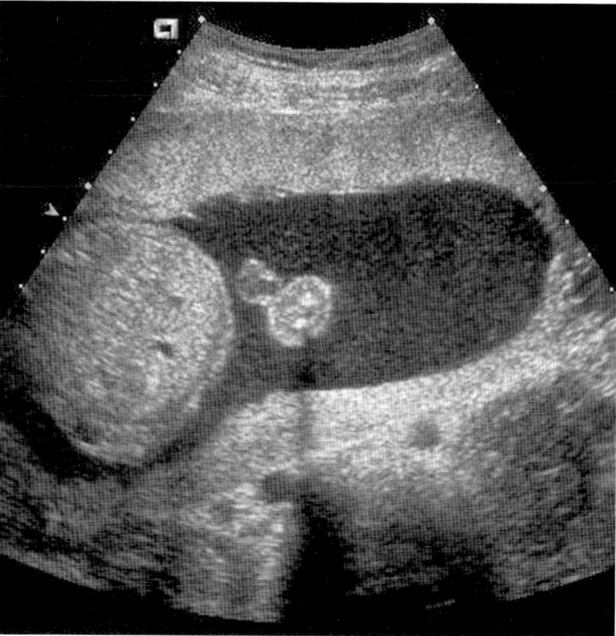

FIGURE 3.4-1. **Vernix in amniotic fluid.** The amniotic fluid is filled with small echogenic particles, which were seen to be swirling on real-time sonography.

Sonography

Amniotic fluid is normally anechoic until the mid third trimester, after which it is common to see swirling echogenic particles of vernix within the fluid (Figure 3.4-1). Sonographic assessment of amniotic fluid volume is most commonly performed using one of the following approaches:

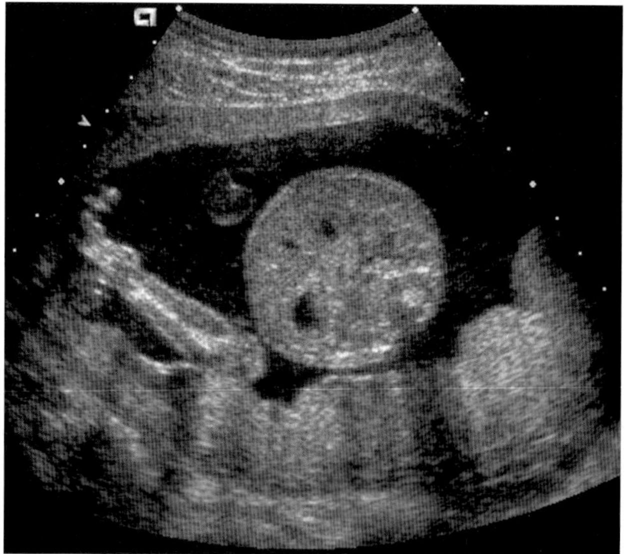

FIGURE 3.4-2. **Subjective assessment of amniotic fluid volume.** On this single image, the volume of amniotic fluid is subjectively within the normal range for the gestational age of 20 weeks. The full assessment, however, is based on a real-time sweep through the gravid uterus and not on any single image.

Subjective assessment: The gestational sac is scanned in its entirety, and the operator makes a judgment as to whether the total amount of amniotic fluid is within the normal range for gestational age (Figure 3.4-2).

Single-deepest pocket measurement: The deepest pocket of fluid, measured vertically (anteroposteriorly) is normally between 2 and 8 cm (Figure 3.4-3).

Four-quadrant amniotic fluid index: The amniotic fluid index is determined by dividing the uterus into four quadrants via transverse and sagittal lines through the maternal umbilicus, measuring the deepest vertical pocket of fluid in each quadrant, and summing the four numbers. The amniotic fluid index is normally 5–18 cm (Figure 3.4-3).

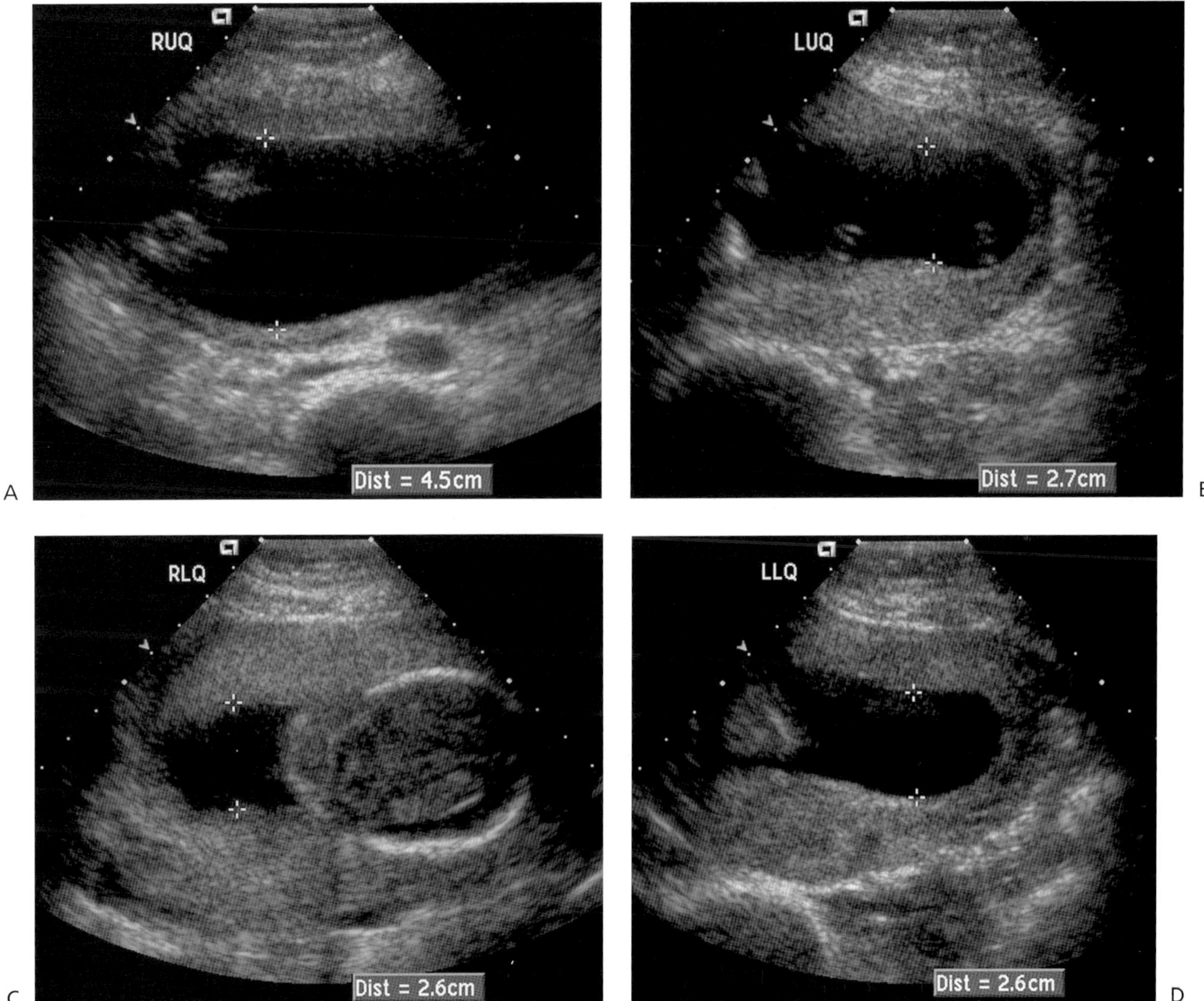

FIGURE 3.4-3. Deepest pocket measurement and amniotic fluid index for assessment of amniotic fluid volume. The four images **(A–D)** demonstrate the deepest vertical pocket *(calipers)* in each of the four quadrants of the uterus (RUQ, right upper quadrant; LUQ, left upper quadrant; RLQ, right lower quadrant; LLQ, left lower quadrant), with the quadrants defined by transverse and sagittal lines through the umbilicus. The single deepest pocket measurement is 4.5 cm, in the right upper quadrant **(A)**. The amniotic fluid index, obtained by summing the four measurements, is 12.4 cm.

SELECTED READINGS

1. Brace RA, Wolf EJ. Normal amniotic fluid volume changes throughout pregnancy. *Am J Obstet Gynecol* 1989;161:382–388.
2. Callen PW. Amniotic fluid: its role in fetal health and disease. In: Callen PW, ed. *Ultrasonography in obstetrics and gynecology*, 4th ed. Philadelphia: WB Saunders, 2000:638–659.
3. Di Salvo DN, Benson CB, Laing FC, et al. Sonographic evaluation of the placental cord insertion site. *AJR Am J Roentgenol* 1998;170:1295–1298.
4. Fleischer AC. Sonography of the umbilical cord and intrauterine membranes. In: Fleischer AC, Manning FA, Jeanty P, et al., eds. *Sonography in obstetrics & gynecology: principles and practice*, 6th ed. New York: McGraw-Hill, 2001:225–245.
5. Gervasi MT, Romero R, Maymon E, et al. Ultrasound examination of the uterine cervix during pregnancy. In: Fleischer AC, Manning FA, Jeanty P, et al., eds. *Sonography in obstetrics & gynecology: principles and practice*, 6th ed. New York: McGraw-Hill, 2001:821–841.
6. Goldstein RB, Filly RA. Sonographic estimation of amniotic fluid volume: subjective assessment versus pocket measurements. *J Ultrasound Med* 1988;7:363–369.
7. Harris RD, Alexander RD. Ultrasound of the placenta and umbilical cord. In: Callen PW, ed. *Ultrasonography in obstetrics and gynecology*, 4th ed. Philadelphia: WB Saunders, 2000:597–625.
8. Hertzberg BS, Livingston E, DeLong DM, et al. Ultrasonographic evaluation of the cervix: transperineal versus endovaginal imaging. *J Ultrasound Med* 2001;20:1071–1078.
9. Iams JD, Goldenberg RL, Meis PJ, et al. The length of the cervix and the risk of spontaneous premature delivery. *N Engl J Med* 1996;334:567–572.
10. Iams JD. Cervical ultrasonography. *Ultrasound Obstet Gynecol* 1997;10:156–160.
11. Jackson GM, Ludmir J, Bader TJ. The accuracy of digital examination and ultrasound in the evaluation of cervical length. *Obstet Gynecol* 1992;79:214–218.
12. Jauniaux E. The placenta. In: Dewbury K, Meire H, Cosgrove D, et al., eds. *Ultrasound in obstetrics and gynaecology*, 2nd ed. London: Churchill-Livingstone, 2001:527–555.
13. Leerentveld RA, Gilberts EC, Arnold MJ, et al. Accuracy and safety of transvaginal sonographic placental localization. *Obstet Gynecol* 1990;76:759–762.
14. Magann EF, Chauhan SP, Whitworth NS, et al. Subjective versus objective evaluation of amniotic fluid volume of pregnancies of less than 24 weeks' gestation. *J Ultrasound Med* 2001;20:191–195.
15. Moore TR, Cayle JE. The amniotic fluid index in normal human pregnancy. *Am J Obstet Gynecol* 1990;162:1168–1173.
16. Moore TR. Superiority of the four-quadrant sum over the single-deepest-pocket technique in ultrasonographic identification of abnormal amniotic fluid volumes. *Am J Obstet Gynecol* 1990;163:762–767.
17. Rutherford SE, Phelan JP, Smith CV, et al. The four-quadrant assessment of amniotic fluid volume: an adjunct to antepartum fetal heart rate testing. *Obstet Gynecol* 1987;70:353–356.
18. Scheerer LJ, Bartolucci L. Ultrasound evaluation of the cervix. In: Callen PW, ed. *Ultrasonography in obstetrics and gynecology*, 4th ed. Philadelphia: WB Saunders, 2000:577–596.
19. Sherer DM, Langer O. Oligohydramnios: use and misuse in clinical management. *Ultrasound Obstet Gynecol* 2001;18:411–419.
20. Sonek J, Shellhaas C. Cervical sonography: a review. *Ultrasound Obstet Gynecol* 1998;11:71–78.
21. Spirt BA, Gordon LP. Sonography of the placenta. In: Fleischer AC, Manning FA, Jeanty P, et al., eds. *Sonography in obstetrics & gynecology: principles and practice*, 6th ed. New York: McGraw-Hill, 2001:195–224.
22. To MS, Skentou C, Cicero S, et al. Cervical assessment at the routine 23-weeks' scan: problems with transabdominal sonography. *Ultrasound Obstet Gynecol* 2000;15:292–296.
23. Westergaard HB, Langhoff-Roos J, Lingman G, et al. A critical appraisal of the use of umbilical artery Doppler ultrasound in high-risk pregnancies: use of meta-analyses in evidence-based obstetrics. *Ultrasound Obstet Gynecol* 2001;17:466–476.

4

CENTRAL NERVOUS SYSTEM

4.1. HYDROCEPHALUS

Description and Clinical Features

Hydrocephalus is defined as increased volume of cerebrospinal fluid within the cerebral ventricles. This is manifested by dilation of some or all of the cerebral ventricles, most often the lateral ventricles. Hydrocephalus may result from a variety of causes, including genetic syndromes, congenital anomalies of the brain and spinal cord, and *in utero* infection or exposure to teratogens. Hydrocephalus is commonly associated with other fetal abnormalities, often involving intracranial structures or the spine.

The prognosis for a fetus with hydrocephalus is related to the degree and severity of associated abnormalities and to the cerebral cortical thickness.

Sonography

Hydrocephalus is diagnosed sonographically when there is abnormal dilation of the cerebral ventricles. From 18 weeks gestation onward, criteria for hydrocephalus include width of the lateral ventricle at the atrium measuring more than 10 mm (Figure 4.1-1) and choroid plexus dangling from its medial attachment (Figures 4.1-1 and 4.1-2) toward the lateral wall of the lateral ventricle.

A

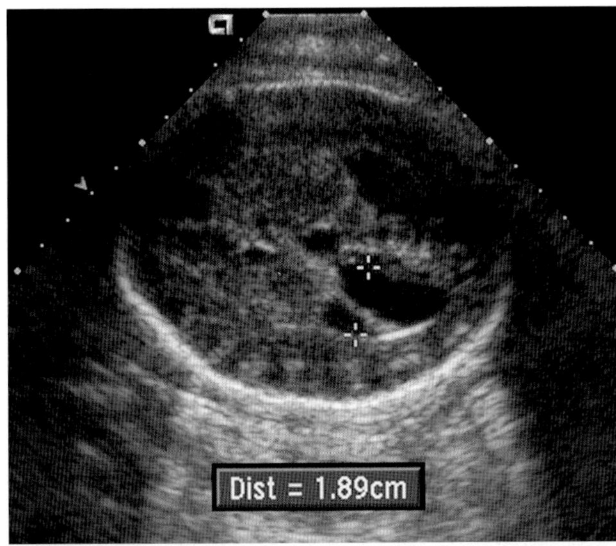

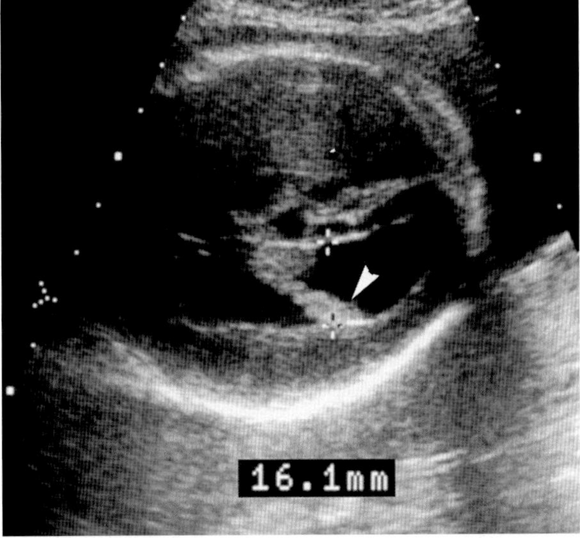

B

FIGURE 4.1-1. Hydrocephalus. A: Axial view of a fetal head at 35 weeks gestation demonstrates a dilated lateral ventricle with + calipers measuring width of atrium of lateral ventricle as 18.9 mm. The calipers are aligned perpendicular to the axis of the ventricle. **B:** A 30-week fetus with dilated ventricles *(+ calipers)*. Choroid plexus *(arrowhead)* is seen outlined by fluid, extending from its medial wall attachment to the lateral wall of the ventricle.

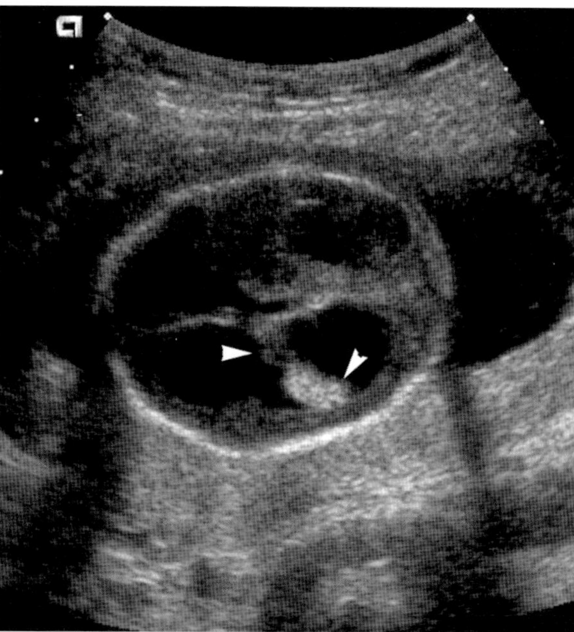

FIGURE 4.1-2. Hydrocephalus with a dangling choroid plexus. Axial view of an 18-week fetus with hydrocephalus demonstrates the choroid plexus *(arrowheads)* dangling from its medial attachment toward the lateral wall of the ventricle.

Before 18 weeks, the diagnosis of hydrocephalus is based on the appearance of the lateral ventricle and dangling choroid plexus because ventricular dilation may be present with a ventricular width less than 10 mm (Figure 4.1-3).

When hydrocephalus is diagnosed based on dilation of the lateral ventricles, it is important to assess the third and fourth ventricles for dilation. A dilated third ventricle is diagnosed when there is abnormal separation of the walls of the third ventricle by cerebrospinal fluid (Figure 4.1-4). Increased fluid in the fourth ventricle is best seen on axial or sagittal views of the posterior fossa.

Because hydrocephalus is commonly associated with other anomalies of the central nervous system, the fetal cranium and posterior fossa should be evaluated. The cranium should be assessed, looking for a lemon shape that would suggest a meningomyelocele or an opening with herniated tissue that would indicate an encephalocele. The posterior fossa should be assessed for evidence of a Dandy-Walker malformation or the Chiari II

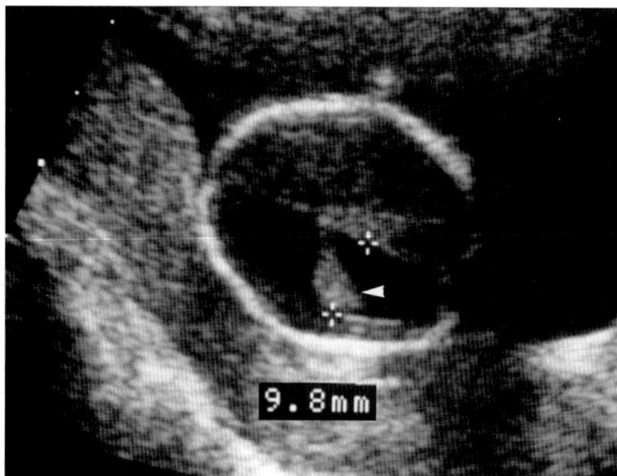

FIGURE 4.1-3. Hydrocephalus in a 16-week fetus. Severely dilated ventricle *(+ calipers)* with dangling choroid plexus *(arrowhead)*. Measurement is less than 10 mm (9.8 mm) despite the presence of hydrocephalus, because of the early gestational age.

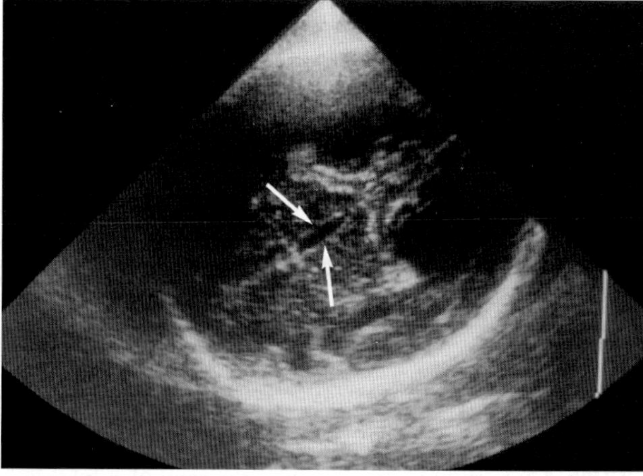

FIGURE 4.1-4. Dilated third ventricle with hydrocephalus. Axial view of the head at the level of the thalami and third ventricle *(arrows)* the demonstrates dilation in this fetus with hydrocephalus from congenital toxoplasmosis.

malformation associated with meningomyelocele. If the posterior fossa is normal, the diagnosis of aqueductal stenosis should be considered.

4.2. AQUEDUCTAL STENOSIS

Description and Clinical Features

Aqueductal stenosis is obstruction of the cerebral ventricular system at the aqueduct of Sylvius, which lies between the third and fourth ventricles. Aqueductal stenosis leads to hydrocephalus, with dilation of the lateral and third ventricles. The fourth ventricle and posterior fossa are normally formed. Aqueductal stenosis is sometimes the result of an X-linked recessive genetic trait and, therefore, is more commonly found in males than females. Other causes of aqueductal stenosis include *in utero* infections (e.g., toxoplasmosis, cytomegalovirus, and syphilis), teratogen exposure, or an intracranial tumor obstructing the aqueduct.

Sonography

With aqueductal stenosis, both lateral ventricles and the third ventricle are dilated, whereas the posterior fossa and fourth ventricle are normal (Figure 4.2-1).

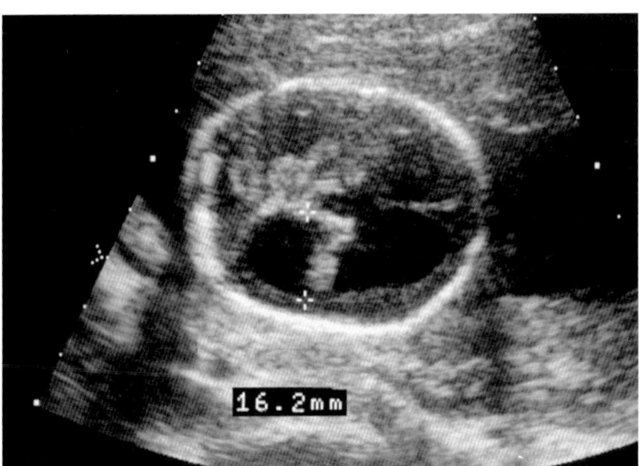

A

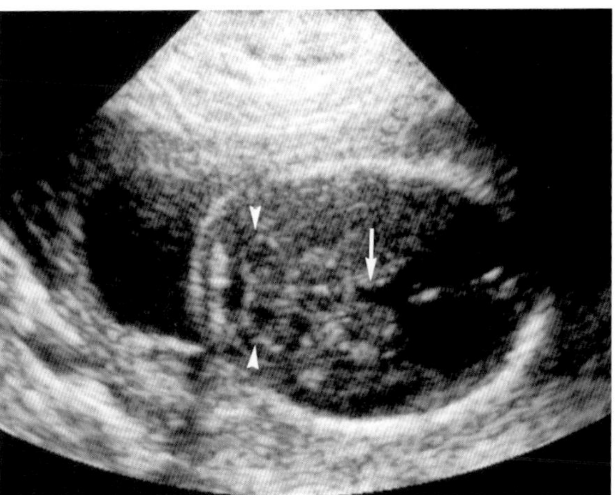
B

FIGURE 4.2-1. Aqueductal stenosis. Axial views of a fetal head demonstrating marked dilation of the lateral ventricle to 16 mm *(calipers)* **(A)** and a dilated third ventricle *(arrow)* with a normal posterior fossa and cerebellum *(arrowheads)* **(B)**.

4.3. DANDY-WALKER MALFORMATION

Description and Clinical Features

The Dandy-Walker malformation is characterized by a posterior fossa cyst that communicates with the fourth ventricle, agenesis or hypoplasia of the cerebellar vermis, and hydrocephalus. The posterior fossa cyst, or Dandy-Walker cyst, is a fluid collection that extends from the fourth ventricle between the cerebellar hemispheres to the cisterna magna. The cerebellar hemispheres are separated by the fluid of the Dandy-Walker cyst, and they often are abnormally formed. The degree of hydrocephalus is variable.

Dandy-Walker malformations are associated with a variety of genetic syndromes and chromosomal abnormalities. They can also result from *in utero* infection.

Sonography

When a Dandy-Walker malformation is present, fluid is seen between the cerebellar hemispheres and the cerebellar vermis is absent or hypoplastic (Figure 4.3-1). The

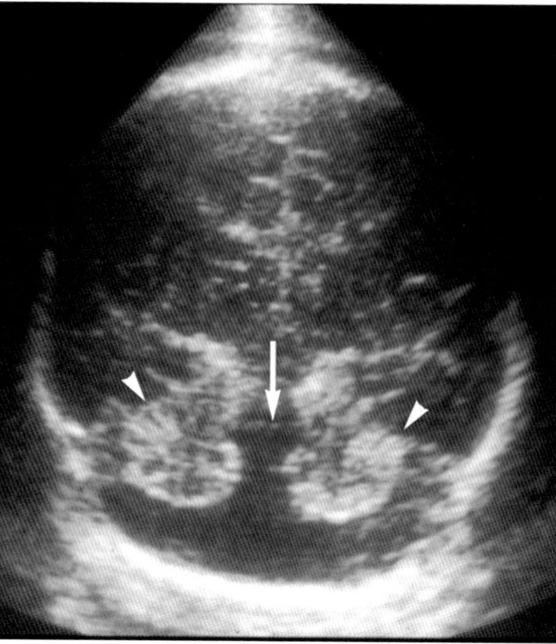

FIGURE 4.3-1. Dandy-Walker malformation. Angled coronal view through the head demonstrates a keyhole-shaped defect *(arrow)* between the cerebellar hemispheres *(arrowheads)* owing to the absence of the cerebellar vermis, permitting communication between the fourth ventricle and the cisterna magna.

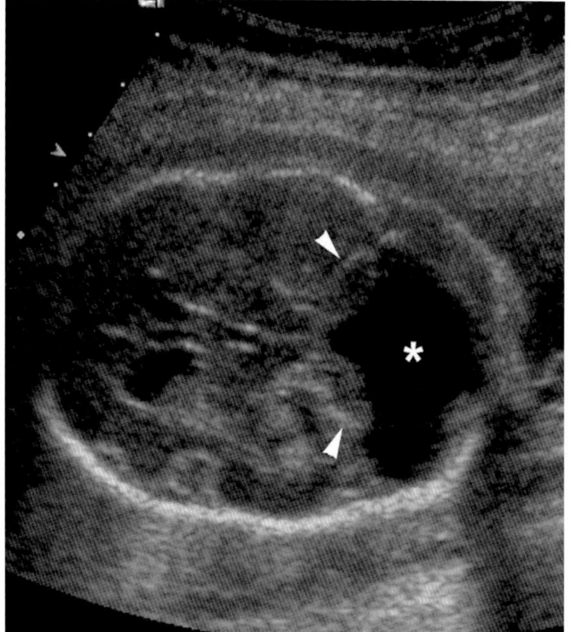

A

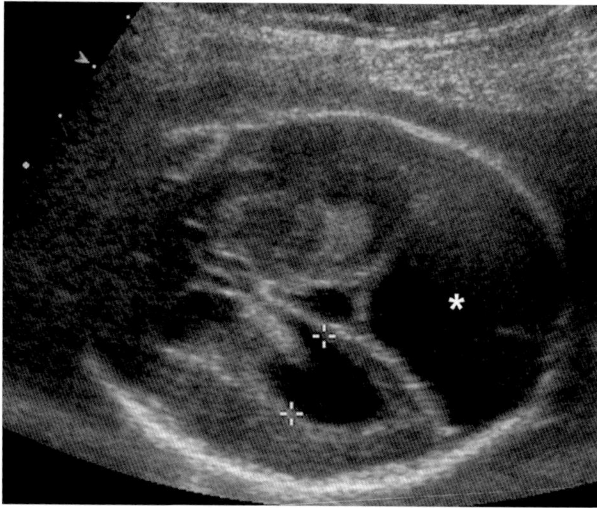

B

FIGURE 4.3-2. Dandy-Walker malformation with large posterior fossa cyst and hydrocephalus. A: Axial image of the posterior fossa demonstrates absence of the cerebellar vermis as well as splaying and flattening of the cerebellar hemispheres *(arrowheads)* by a large fluid-filled space *(*)* connecting the fourth ventricle to the cisterna magna. **B:** Axial image superior to **(A)** demonstrates a dilated lateral ventricle *(calipers)*, representing hydrocephalus, and the large posterior fossa cyst *(*)*.

Dandy-Walker cyst often has a characteristic keyhole shape between the cerebellar hemispheres. The posterior aspect of the cyst may be quite large (Figure 4.3-2). The cerebellar hemispheres are sometimes flattened (Figure 4.3-2) rather than having their normally rounded shape. Hydrocephalus (Figure 4.3-2) often accompanies the posterior fossa abnormalities.

4.4. ARACHNOID CYSTS

Description and Clinical Features

Arachnoid cysts are cysts that form in the layers of the arachnoid membrane. The cysts are often midline but can arise anywhere within the cranial vault. The cysts may obstruct the normal flow of cerebrospinal fluid, causing hydrocephalus, particularly when located in the posterior fossa. Interhemispheric cysts may be associated with agenesis of the corpus callosum. Cysts on the surface of the brain may cause compression of the brain beneath the cyst.

Sonography

An arachnoid cyst appears as a rounded fluid collection within the cranial vault (Figure 4.4-1). Surrounding structures may be displaced or compressed (Figure 4.4-2), and there may be associated hydrocephalus if the cyst obstructs the flow of cerebrospinal fluid (Figure 4.4-3). The distinction between an arachnoid cyst and a Dandy-Walker malformation may sometimes be difficult to determine with sonography. Careful assessment of the cerebellum for the presence of the cerebellar vermis assists in the diagnosis. Associated agenesis of the corpus callosum may be difficult to diagnose until the third trimester.

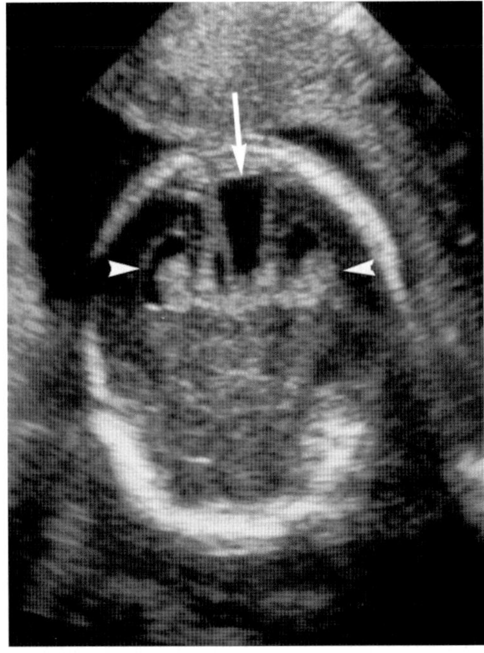

FIGURE 4.4-1. Interhemispheric arachnoid cyst. Angled axial view through the head demonstrates an anechoic cyst *(arrow)* between the cerebral hemispheres posteriorly. The occipital horns *(arrowheads)* are visible at this level.

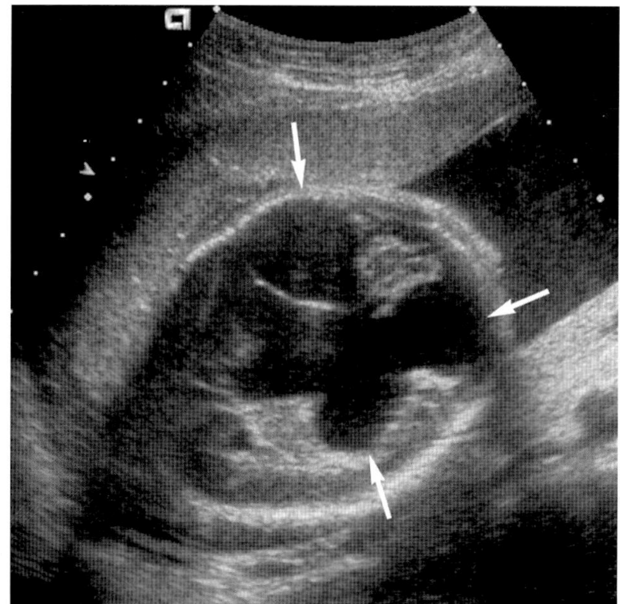

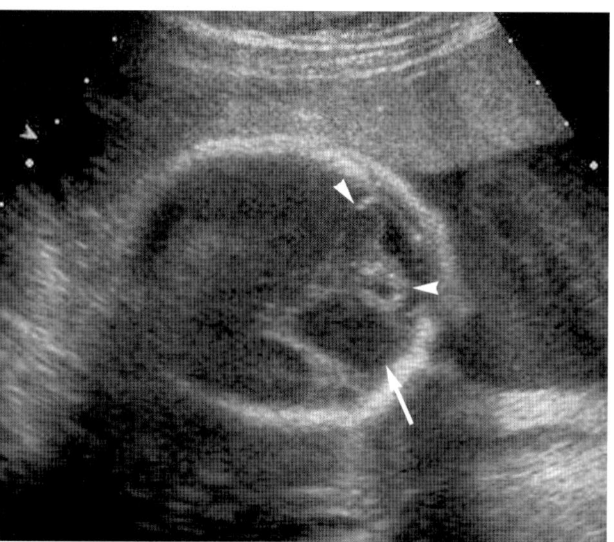

FIGURE 4.4-2. Arachnoid cyst compressing surrounding structures. A: Axial view of the head demonstrates a large irregular cyst *(arrows)* within the cranium posteriorly. **B:** Image of the posterior fossa demonstrates displacement and compression of the cerebellum *(arrowheads)* by the cyst *(arrow)*.

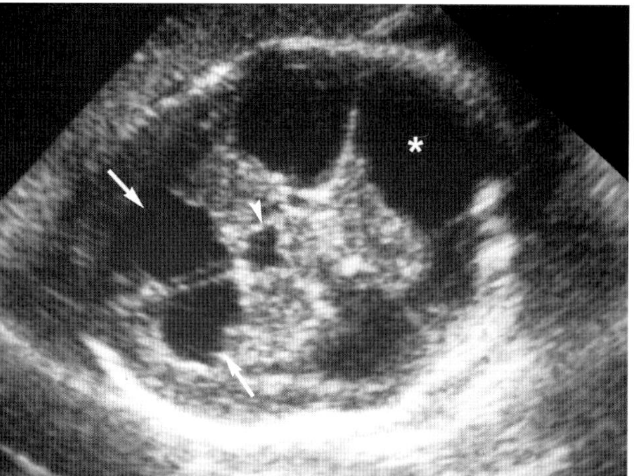

FIGURE 4.4-3. Posterior fossa arachnoid cyst with hydrocephalus. Axial image of the head demonstrates a posterior fossa cyst *(*)* causing hydrocephalus, with dilation of the frontal horns of the lateral ventricles *(arrows)* and the third ventricle *(arrowhead)*.

4.5. ANENCEPHALY

Description and Clinical Features

Anencephaly is a neural tube defect involving the fetal head, characterized by absence of the cranium. Dystrophic brain tissue may form in the empty shell behind the face, but this tissue tends to atrophy as pregnancy progresses. The face, from the orbits down, is usually normally formed. Anencephaly makes up approximately 45% of all neural tube defects.

This large open defect causes very high maternal serum α-fetoprotein levels. As a result, many cases of anencephaly are detected prenatally owing to widespread screening with maternal serum α-fetoprotein.

Fetuses with anencephaly are often very active because they lack cortical suppression. Polyhydramnios is commonly present because fetal swallowing is impaired.

The prognosis is dismal, with virtually all fetuses dying at birth.

Sonography

Absence of the fetal cranium is the hallmark of anencephaly. The lower face will be seen, with no skull above the orbits anteriorly (Figure 4.5-1) or above the cervical spine posteriorly (Figure 4.5-2). Occasionally, dystrophic brain tissue is seen floating above the face

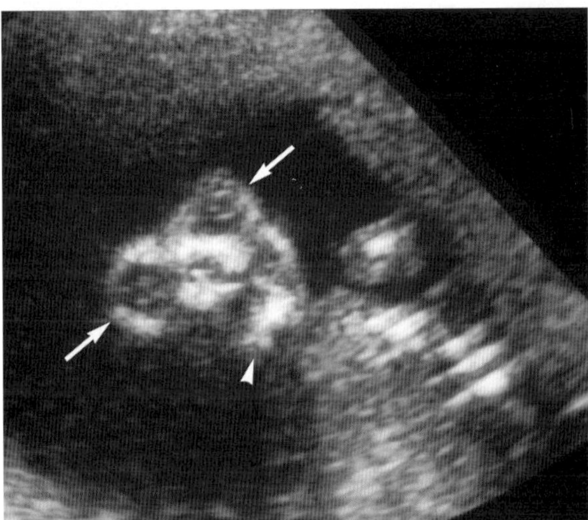

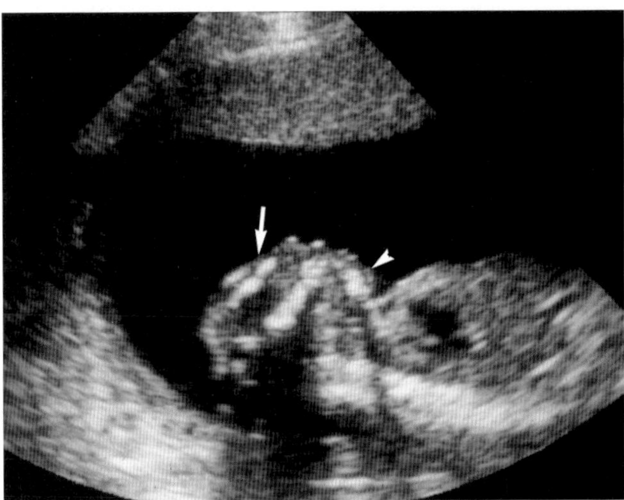

FIGURE 4.5-1. Anencephaly. A: Coronal image of the fetal face demonstrates absence of the forehead and cranium above the orbits *(arrows)*. The lower face and mandible *(arrowhead)* are normally formed. **B:** Sagittal image of the fetus demonstrates absence of the forehead and cranium *(arrow)*. The mandible *(arrowhead)* and lower face are normal.

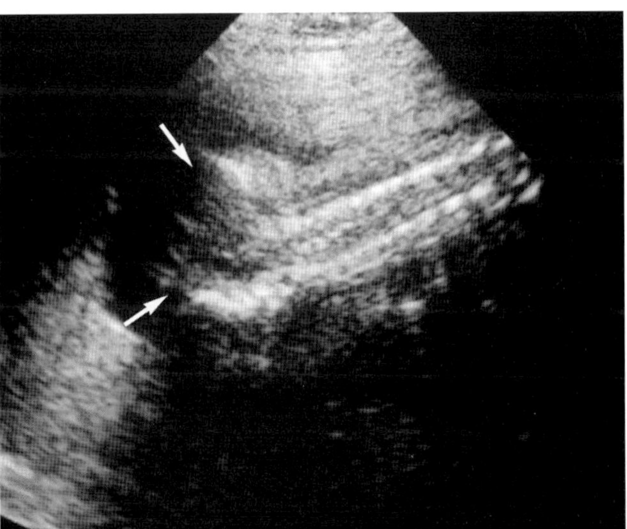

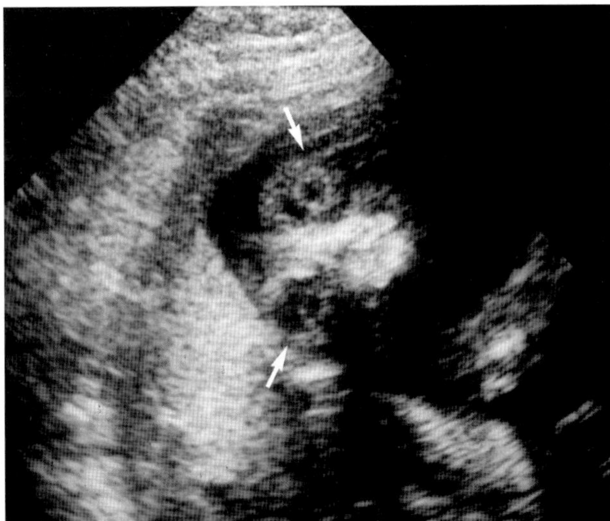

FIGURE 4.5-2. Anencephaly with no cranium above the cervical spine. A: Longitudinal view of the upper cervical spine shows absence of the cranium and a large open defect above the spine *(arrows)*. **B:** Coronal image of the face of the same fetus demonstrates absence of the forehead above the orbits *(arrows)*.

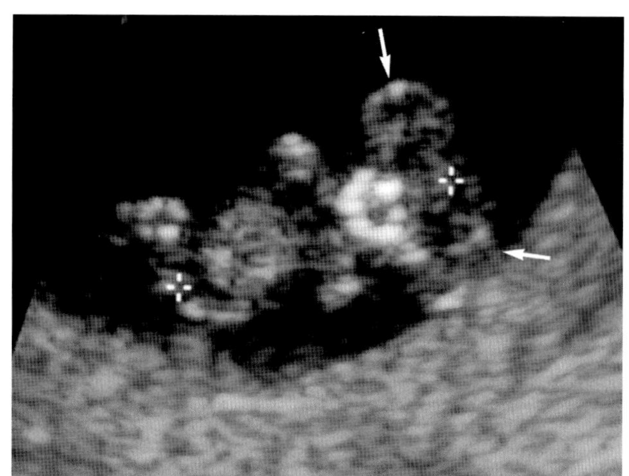

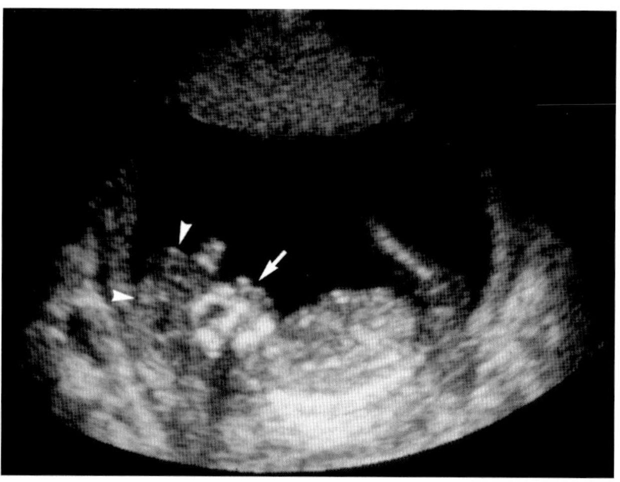

FIGURE 4.5-3. Anencephaly with dystrophic brain tissue in the region of the absent cranium. A: Twelve-week fetus *(calipers)* with anencephaly demonstrates amorphous mass of brain tissue *(arrows)* where the cranium should be. **B:** Sagittal image of a 15-week fetus shows amorphous soft-tissue mass *(arrowheads)* in the region of the absent cranium above the face *(arrow)*.

(Figure 4.5-3), particularly when anencephaly is diagnosed in the late first trimester or early second trimester. After the early second trimester, it is uncommon to see any tissue in the expected region of the cranial vault. Polyhydramnios may be present, and the fetus is often very active.

4.6. ENCEPHALOCELE

Description and Clinical Features

Encephalocele is characterized by a defect in the cranium through which the intracranial contents herniate outside the skull. Occipital encephaloceles are a form of neural tube defect, comprising approximately 5% of neural tube defects. Encephaloceles can also result from amniotic band syndrome and may be found with Meckel-Gruber syndrome, an autosomal recessive genetic syndrome. The findings with Meckel-Gruber syndrome include encephalocele, polycystic kidneys, polydactyly, cleft palate, cardiac anomalies, and liver cysts. Severe oligohydramnios is usually present, owing to the polycystic kidneys.

Like other neural tube defects, maternal serum α-fetoprotein levels are usually elevated with encephaloceles. Occasionally, the defect is closed, covered by the scalp, in which case the maternal serum α-fetoprotein may be normal.

Most encephaloceles are located in the midline, most commonly posterior involving the occiput, less commonly parietal or frontal. Encephaloceles that result from amniotic band syndrome may involve any part of the skull and are often not in the midline.

The herniated sac may contain dystrophic brain tissue or may only contain meninges and fluid. Within the head, there may be associated hydrocephalus, and, in some cases, the "lemon" sign may be seen during the second trimester.

The prognosis is variable, depending on the location of the encephalocele and the amount of brain tissue herniated into the encephalocele sac.

Sonography

The cranial defect of an encephalocele appears as an interruption in the bony skull (Figure 4.6-1). The intracranial contents are seen herniating through the defect (Figure 4.6-1). The herniated sac is usually rounded and contains tissue as well as fluid. With an ante-

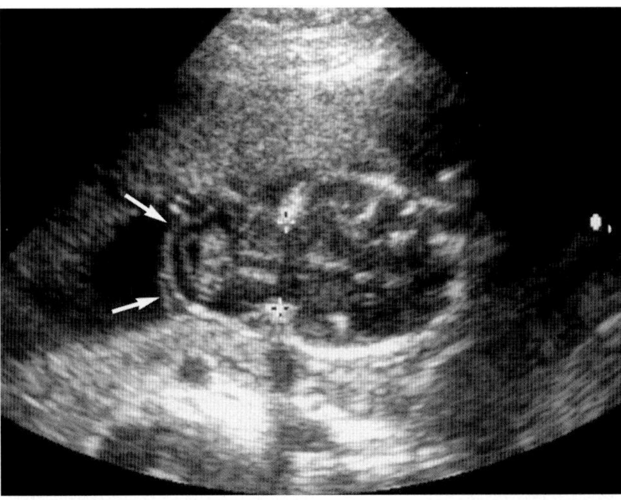

FIGURE 4.6-1. Occipital encephalocele. Calipers mark a bony defect in the occiput through which intracranial contents herniate outside the skull into the encephalocele sac *(arrows)*.

rior encephalocele, a soft-tissue mass will be seen protruding anteriorly through a defect in the frontal bones between the orbits (Figure 4.6-2). Hypertelorism, or widening of the normal distance between the orbits, may be present. On a sagittal midline view of the fetal face, the encephalocele may be seen as a protrusion of soft tissue between the forehead and the tip of the nose (Figure 4.6-2).

Encephaloceles seen with Meckel-Gruber syndrome are often difficult to visualize because of severe oligohydramnios (Figure 4.6-3). In such cases, the fetal kidneys will also be abnormal, appearing enlarged and echogenic.

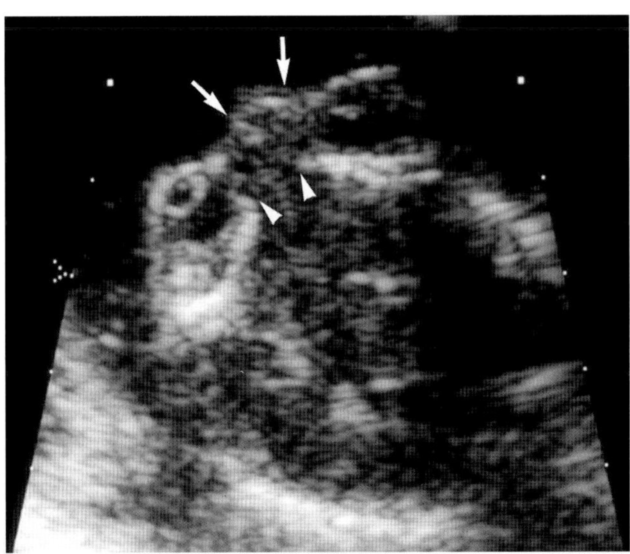

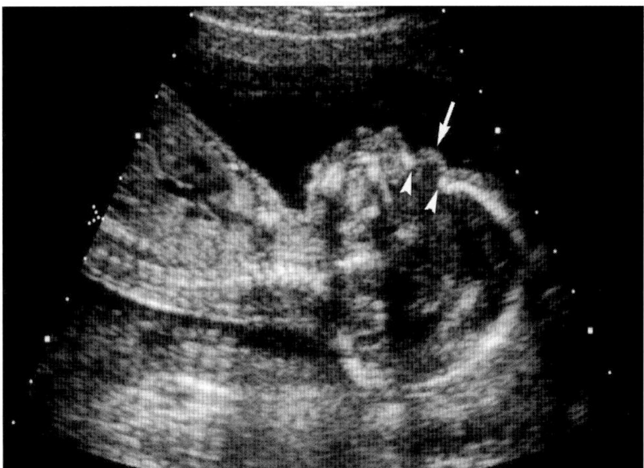

FIGURE 4.6-2. Anterior encephalocele. A: Axial image through the orbits demonstrates a defect in nasofrontal bone *(arrowheads)*, with a small encephalocele sac *(arrows)* protruding between the orbits anteriorly. **B:** Sagittal image of the facial profile shows a nasofrontal bony defect *(arrowheads)* and protruding anterior encephalocele sac *(arrow)*.

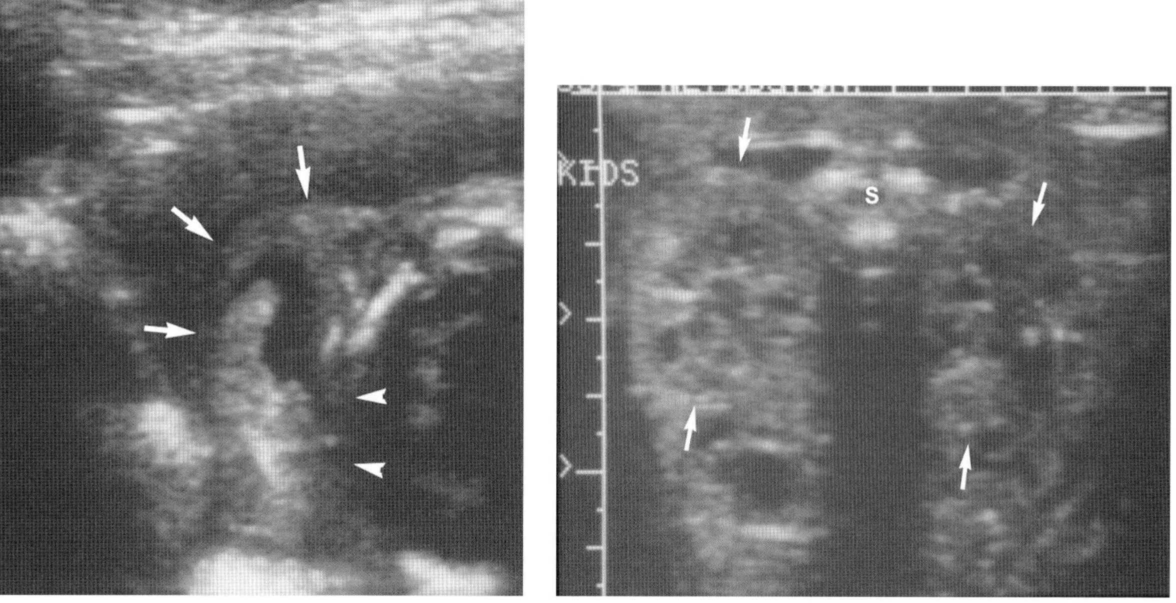

FIGURE 4.6-3. Meckel-Gruber syndrome. A: Image of the posterior head demonstrates a large occipital defect *(arrowheads)*, with herniated brain, fluid, and meninges in the encephalocele sac *(arrows)* outside the cranium. **B:** Transverse image of bilateral enlarged echogenic kidneys *(arrows)* on either side of the spine (S) demonstrates polycystic kidneys associated with this autosomal recessive syndrome. There is also severe oligohydramnios.

4.7. HOLOPROSENCEPHALY

Description and Clinical Features

Holoprosencephaly is a developmental anomaly of the brain in which the prosencephalon (forebrain) fails to cleave normally into two cerebral hemispheres. This results in complete or partial fusion of the cerebral hemispheres and communication of the lateral ventricles across the midline. The falx is underdeveloped or absent. The corpus callosum is usually absent. The thalami may be partially or completely fused.

Holoprosencephaly can have varying degrees of severity, depending on the extent of failure of cleavage of the prosencephalon. Alobar holoprosencephaly is the most severe form, characterized by complete failure of cleavage, fusion of the cerebral hemispheres, complete absence of the falx, and a large central cerebral ventricle. The thalami are usually fused. Semilobar holoprosencephaly has partial cleavage of the prosencephalon, with a rudimentary falx indenting the midline of the fused cerebral hemispheres. The ventricles have a wide connection across the midline, and the thalami may be partially fused. With lobar holoprosencephaly, the least severe form, the falx is present although incomplete; the cerebral hemispheres are partially separated and partially fused. The ventricles have a narrow communication across the midline.

Holoprosencephaly is commonly associated with an abnormal karyotype, often trisomy 13, and with fetal anomalies, particularly midline facial clefts, hypotelorism, and a proboscis.

Sonography

With holoprosencephaly, the configuration of the cerebral ventricles is abnormal. In particular, the ventricles communicate across the midline (Figure 4.7-1) and are dilated. The third ventricle is often absent. The falx is absent or rudimentary, and the cerebral hemi-

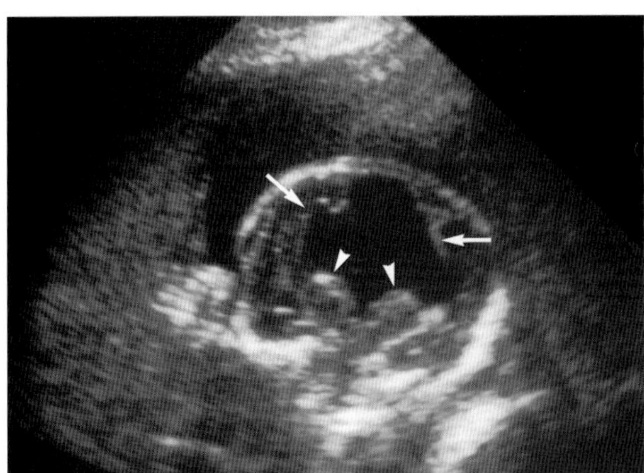

FIGURE 4.7-1. Holoprosencephaly. Coronal image of a head demonstrates fusion of lateral ventricles into a central monoventricle *(arrows)*. The thalami are partially splayed *(arrowheads)*, and the falx is absent.

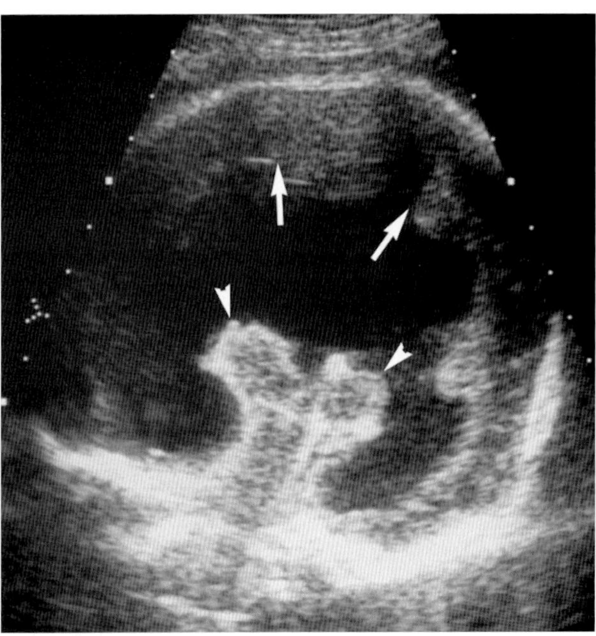

FIGURE 4.7-2. Holoprosencephaly. The cerebral cortex *(arrows)* is fused across the midline and the falx is absent. The thalami are partially fused *(arrowheads)*.

spheres are fused across the midline (Figure 4.7-2). The thalami are partially or completely fused (Figure 4.7-2). With alobar holoprosencephaly the fused ventricle is large and centrally located and the thalami are usually completely fused (Figure 4.7-3), whereas with semilobar holoprosencephaly, the ventricles are smaller and have a narrower communication across the midline (Figure 4.7-4). When holoprosencephaly is diagnosed, the face should be assessed for midline anomalies.

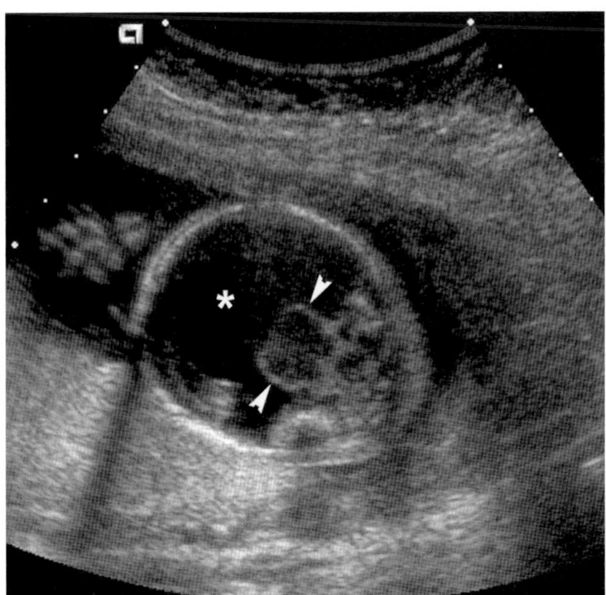

FIGURE 4.7-3. Alobar holoprosencephaly. Coronal image of a head demonstrates complete fusion of the thalami *(arrowheads)* and a large central fluid collection *(*)* representing the fused ventricles.

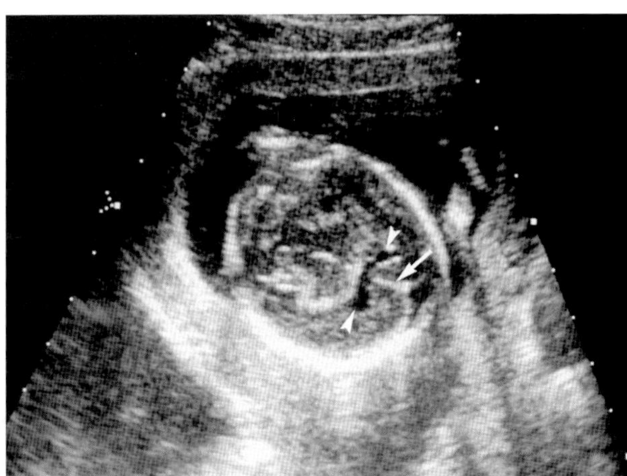

FIGURE 4.7-4. Semilobar holoprosencephaly. Angled axial image of ventricles demonstrates narrow communication between lateral ventricles across the midline *(arrowheads)*. The cerebral cortex is partially cleaved *(arrow)*.

4.8. SCHIZENCEPHALY

Description and Clinical Features

Schizencephaly is abnormal formation of the brain in which there are clefts or defects in the cerebral hemisphere that are filled with cerebrospinal fluid and communicate with the subarachnoid space or cerebral ventricles. Microcephaly is often present. Affected children are usually neurologically impaired, with developmental delays, mental retardation, or motor paralysis.

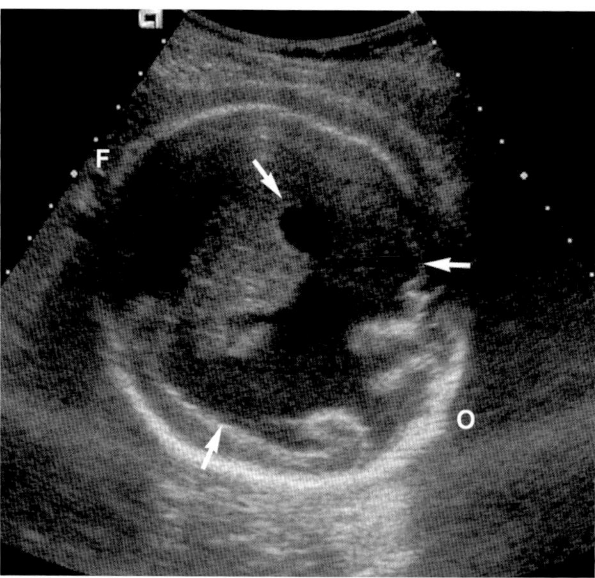

FIGURE 4.8-1. Schizencephaly. Axial image of the head, frontal bone (F) to occiput (O), demonstrates a large irregular asymmetric fluid space *(arrows)* replacing portions of the parietal lobes and occipital lobes on each side, representing a large cleft in the brain.

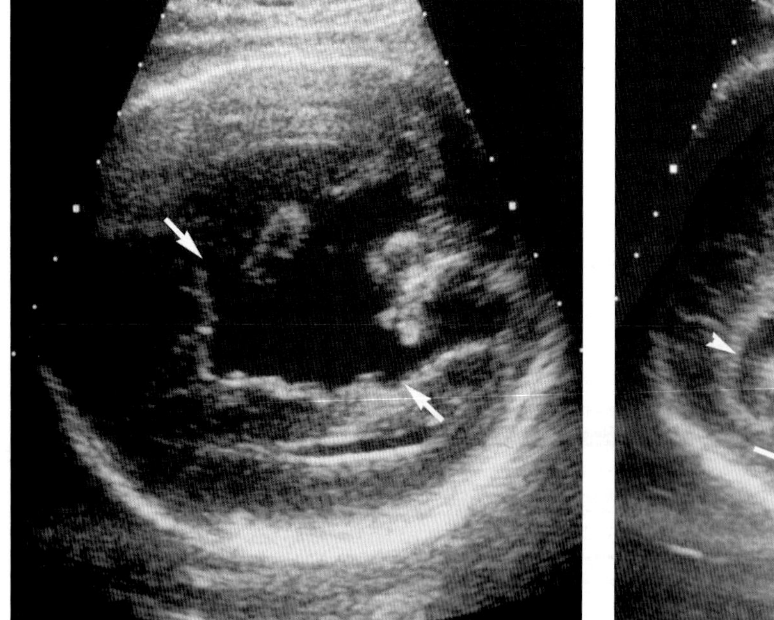

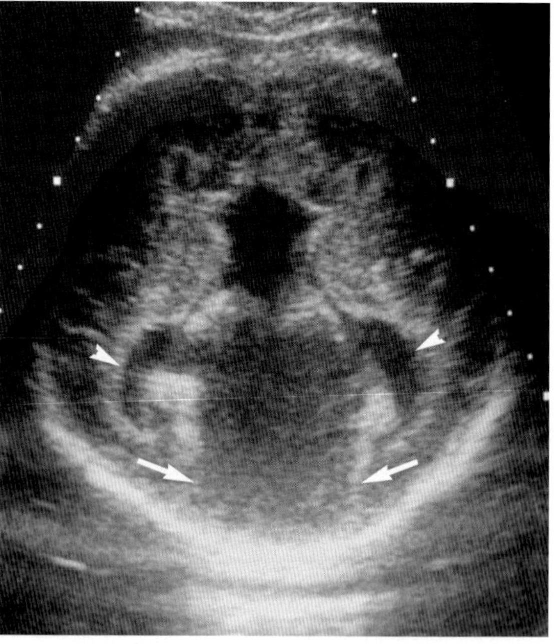

FIGURE 4.8-2. Schizencephaly. A: Axial image of the upper cranium demonstrates irregular fluid space *(arrows)* replacing cerebral cortical tissue. **B:** Coronal view through the cerebral cortex shows that the cleft in the brain communicates with the occipital horns of the lateral ventricles *(arrowheads)* and extends out to the cranium *(arrows)*.

Sonography

The clefts or defects in the cerebral hemispheres of schizencephaly are fluid-filled spaces that extend to the arachnoid space or communicate with the lateral ventricles (Figures 4.8-1 and 4.8-2). The defects are not usually symmetric. Microcephaly, diagnosed when measurements of the fetal head lag behind the expected range for gestational age, may be present.

4.9. AGENESIS OF THE CORPUS CALLOSUM

Description and Clinical Features

The corpus callosum is a band of neural tissue that connects the right and left cerebral hemispheres. Agenesis of the corpus callosum results from failure of formation of part of or all the corpus callosum. Because the anterior portion of the corpus callosum develops before the posterior portion, partial agenesis of the corpus callosum typically affects the posterior aspect.

Agenesis of the corpus callosum is often associated with intracranial and extracranial anomalies. A common associated anomaly is an interhemispheric cyst.

Sonography

The most common sonographic finding with agenesis of the corpus callosum is an abnormal configuration and location of the lateral ventricles. They are aligned parallel to the falx, instead of the normal convergence anteriorly, and are laterally displaced. The occipital horns are typically disproportionately dilated, a finding termed colpocephaly (Figure 4.9-1). The third ventricle is elevated and often mildly dilated. Cerebral sulci can be seen radiating from the roof of the third ventricle outward (Figure 4.9-2).

A
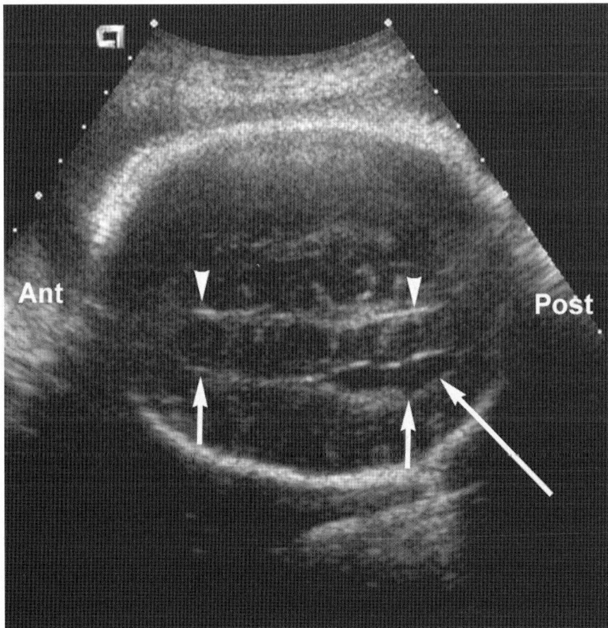

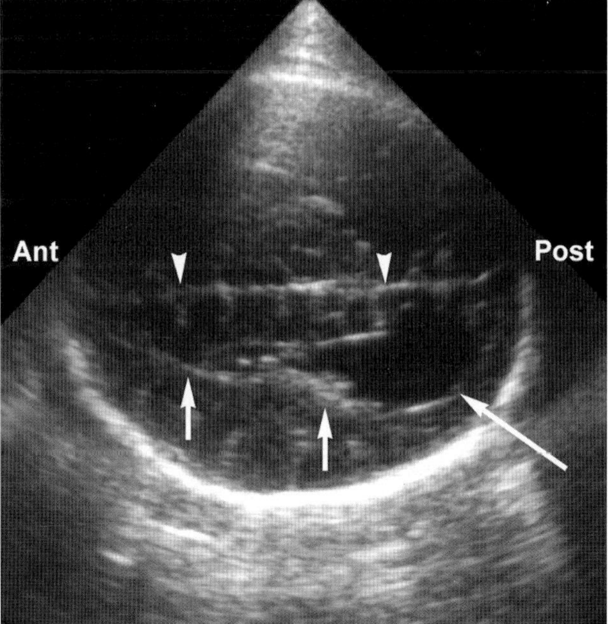

B

FIGURE 4.9-1. Agenesis of the corpus callosum with parallel alignment of the lateral ventricles and colpocephaly. A and B: Axial images of two different fetal heads demonstrate the lateral ventricle *(short arrows)* oriented parallel to the falx *(arrowheads)*. The occipital horn *(long arrow)* is dilated. Ant, anterior; Post, posterior.

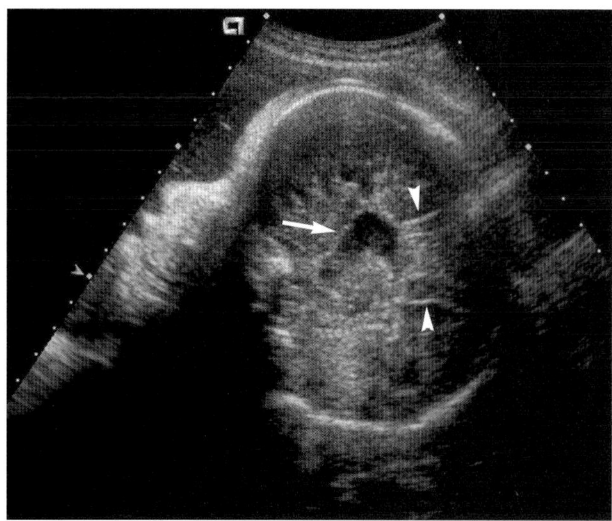

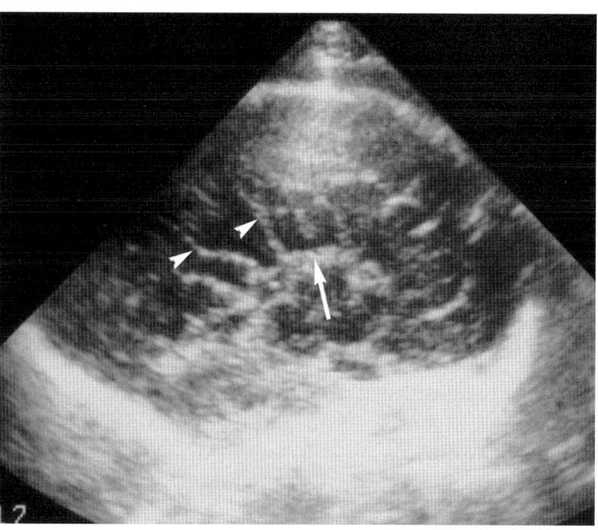

FIGURE 4.9-2. Agenesis of the corpus callosum with elevation of the third ventricle and sulci radiating from the roof of the third ventricle. A: Sagittal midline image of the head demonstrates the third ventricle *(arrow)* elevated and mildly dilated. Sulci *(arrowheads)* are seen radiating from the roof of the third ventricle. **B:** Sagittal midline image in another fetus demonstrates sulci *(arrowheads)* radiating from the roof of the third ventricle *(arrow)*.

The cavum septum pellucidum is absent with agenesis of the corpus callosum; thus, sonographic visualization of a cavum septum pellucidum excludes the diagnosis of complete agenesis. Prenatal diagnosis of partial agenesis of the corpus callosum is rarely made.

Because of the association with other anomalies, careful sonographic assessment for fetal anomalies is warranted when the diagnosis of agenesis of the corpus callosum is made.

4.10. INTRACRANIAL TUMORS

Description and Clinical Features

Fetal intracranial tumors are rare and usually benign. Teratomas are the most common intracranial tumor. Other masses include craniopharyngiomas, oligodendrogliomas, gangliocytomas, and lipomas of the corpus callosum. Tumors arising from the bony cranium may also occasionally be encountered. The prognosis for most intracranial tumors is poor because of rapid growth and replacement of normal brain tissue. Lipomas of the corpus callosum are often associated with agenesis of the corpus callosum.

Sonography

An intracranial tumor is diagnosed sonographically when a mass is seen within the cranium (Figure 4.10-1). The mass may be cystic, solid, or complex. It may arise within the brain or from the meninges or cranium (Figure 4.10-2). Occasionally, calcification will be noted. Depending on the size and location of the mass, the intracranial contents will be displaced or malformed. Hydrocephalus may develop if the mass obstructs the normal flow of cerebrospinal fluid. Occasionally, an intracranial tumor will erode the bony calvarium and protrude outside the skull, mimicking an encephalocele. Intracranial hemorrhage may mimic a tumor, causing a mass effect on the surrounding brain. In such cases, magnetic resonance imaging may be helpful in differentiating hemorrhage from a tumor.

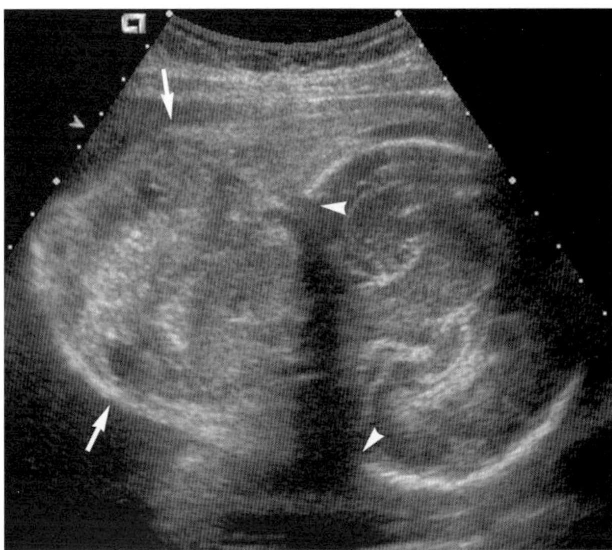

FIGURE 4.10-1. Intracranial and neck teratoma. Large teratoma *(arrows)* is growing through the cranium *(arrowheads)*, extending outside the head and along the neck.

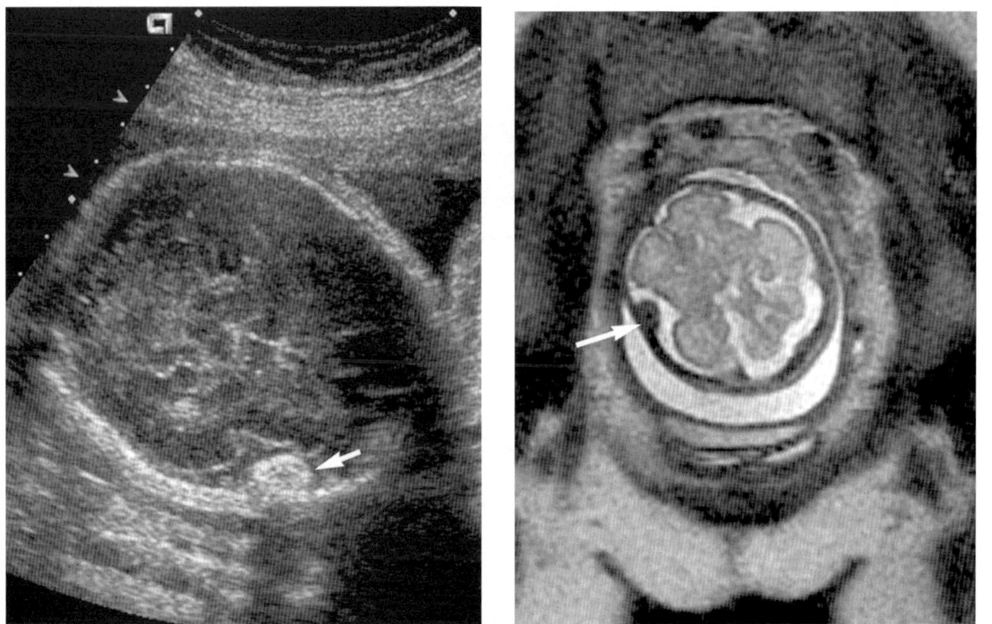

FIGURE 4.10-2. Cranial mass. A: Axial image of the head demonstrates an echogenic mass *(arrow)* with shadowing that appears to arise from the bony skull. **B:** Magnetic resonance image of the fetus demonstrates a mass *(arrow)* arising from the bony calvarium, indenting the subarachnoid space and separate from the brain.

4.11. VEIN OF GALEN ANEURYSM

Description and Clinical Features

A vein of Galen aneurysm is a vascular malformation in the head that leads to increased flow in the vein of Galen. The malformation is typically fed by several cerebral arteries. Because of marked arteriovenous shunting in the malformation, blood drains posteriorly into a dilated vein of Galen. The lesion is not a true aneurysm but rather a high-flow vascular malformation that results in enlargement of the vein of Galen. The high-flow nature of the lesion sometimes causes high-output congestive heart failure and hydrops in the fetus, which is associated with a poor outcome.

Sonography

A vein of Galen aneurysm appears as an anechoic cystic structure in the midline of the head, often without a mass effect on the surrounding structures (Figure 4.11-1). The cystic mass usually has an irregular contour. Spectral Doppler interrogation of the lesion demonstrates turbulent flow (Figure 4.11-2). Color Doppler can demonstrate the feeding arteries as well as increased flow in the vein draining the malformation (Figure 4.11-3). When a diagnosis of vein of Galen aneurysm is made, the fetus should be assessed for evidence of congestive heart failure, including cardiac dilation or signs of hydrops.

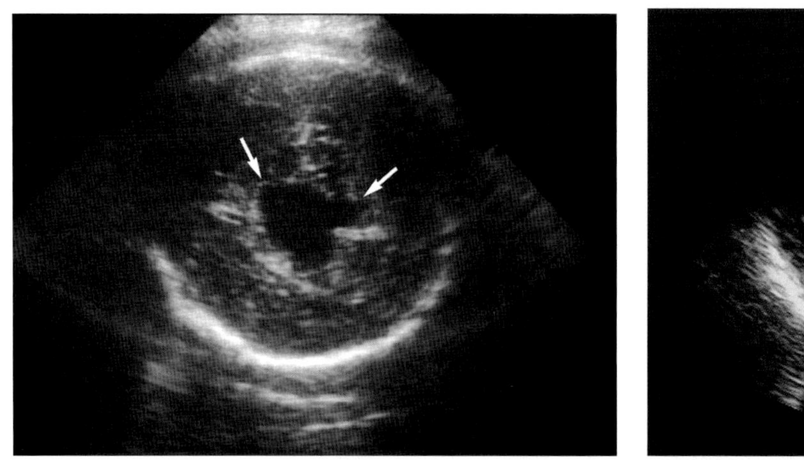

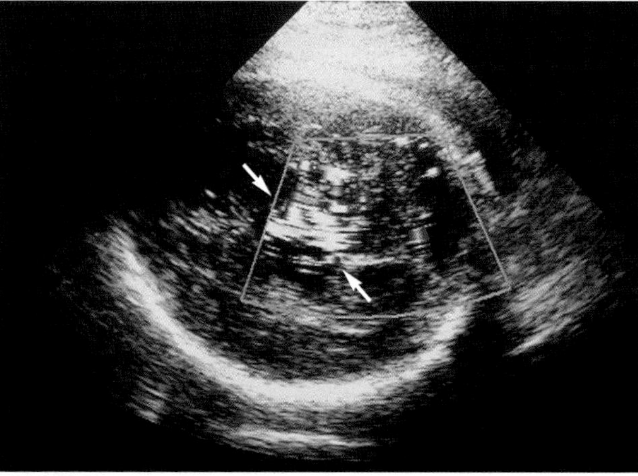

FIGURE 4.11-1. Vein of Galen aneurysm. A: Axial image of the head demonstrates an irregularly shaped cystic lesion *(arrows)* in midline. **B:** Color Doppler confirms the vascular nature of the lesion *(arrows)*.

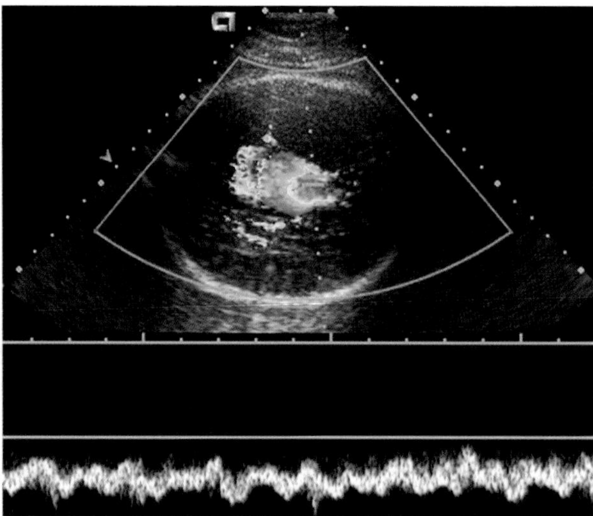

FIGURE 4.11-2. Doppler of a vein of Galen aneurysm. Color and spectral Doppler image of a vein of Galen aneurysm demonstrates a large amount of turbulent flow in the vascular lesion.

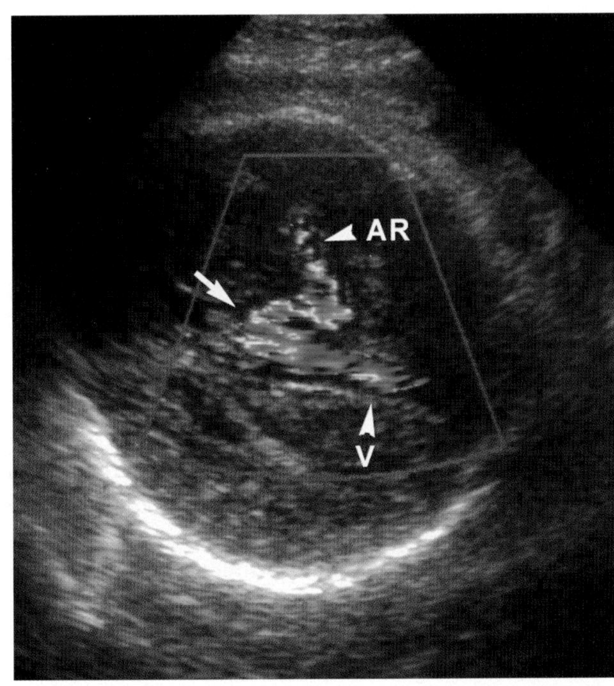

A

FIGURE 4.11-3. Feeding and draining vessels from vein of Galen aneurysm. A: Axial color Doppler image of the head shows turbulent flow in a large artery *(arrowhead AR)* feeding the vein of Galen aneurysm *(arrow)* and flow in the large draining vein *(arrowhead V)*. **B:** Color Doppler image of the circle of Willis in another case with a vein of Galen aneurysm demonstrates marked dilation of the arteries *(arrows)* in the circle and extending from it. **C:** Color Doppler image just superior to **(B)** demonstrates dilated draining veins *(arrow)*.

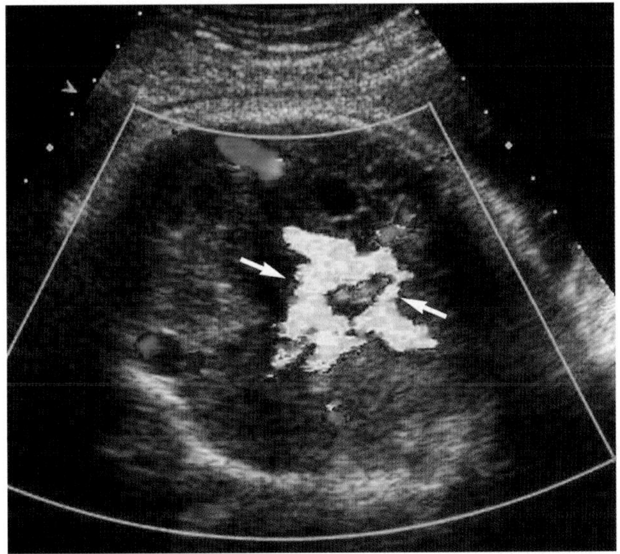

B

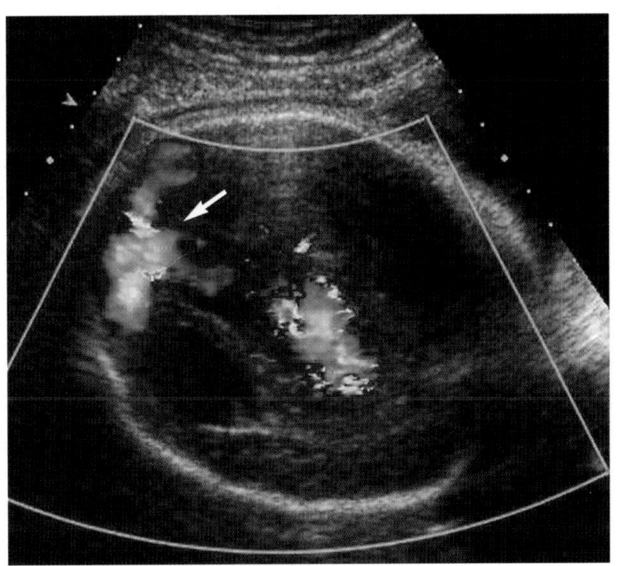

C

4.12. INTRACRANIAL HEMORRHAGE AND PORENCEPHALY

Description and Clinical Features

Intracranial hemorrhage is usually a complication of prematurity that occurs after birth. Rarely, however, intracranial hemorrhage occurs *in utero*, usually in the third trimester. Predisposing factors in the mother include alloimmune and idiopathic thrombocytopenia, anticoagulation therapy, cocaine or other drug abuse, and direct trauma to the fetus. Fetal abnormalities, such as twin-twin transfusion syndrome, death of a co-twin, and fetomaternal hemorrhage, can also be predisposing factors for intracranial hemorrhage.

As in the neonate, intracranial hemorrhage in the fetus usually occurs in the germinal matrix, into the lateral ventricles, or within the parenchyma surrounding the ventricles. As a result of the hemorrhage, the fetus may develop posthemorrhagic hydrocephalus. Parenchymal hemorrhages usually lead to loss of the affected brain tissue.

Porencephaly is an abnormality of the cerebral cortex in which there are cavities or cysts replacing normal brain tissue. These are thought to occur from *in utero* damage to the tissue, such as from a parenchymal hemorrhage. The cysts or cavities communicate with the lateral ventricles.

Fetuses with porencephaly typically have neurologic abnormalities. After intracranial hemorrhage, the prognosis for the fetus is related to the size of the hemorrhage and the amount of parenchymal loss.

Sonography

An intracranial hemorrhage appears as a hyperechoic region in the fetal brain or an echogenic structure in a ventricle. In the germinal matrix, the hemorrhage (Figure 4.12-1) is located in the caudothalamic notch adjacent to the frontal horns of the lateral ventricles. With an intraventricular hemorrhage, echoes are seen in the cerebrospinal fluid of the involved ventricle, and an echogenic mass, representing a clot, may be seen within the ventricle (Figure 4.12-2). Sometimes the clot will fill the lateral ventricle with a shape conforming to that of the ventricle (Figure 4.12-2). Subsequent to an intraventricular hemorrhage, the fetus may develop posthemorrhagic hydrocephalus (Figure 4.12-3), characterized by dilation of the lateral ventricles and the third ventri-

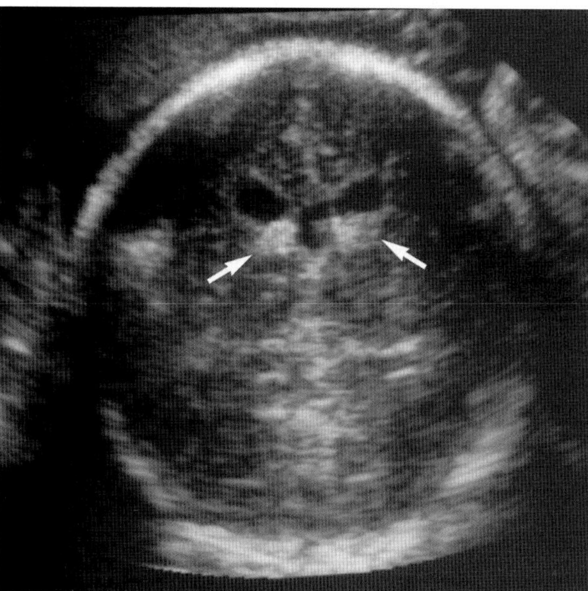

FIGURE 4.12-1. Germinal matrix hemorrhage. Coronal image through the head demonstrates bilateral echogenic areas in the region of the germinal matrices *(arrows)* adjacent to the frontal horns of the lateral ventricles, representing hemorrhage.

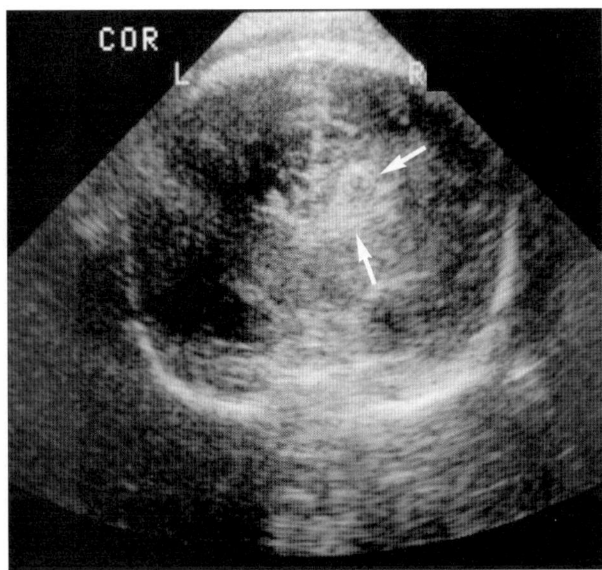

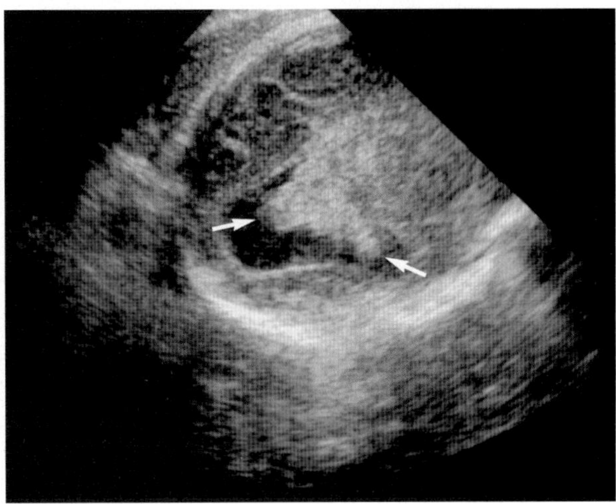

A B

FIGURE 4.12-2. Intraventricular hemorrhage. A: Coronal image of a fetal head obtained transvaginally demonstrates the right (R) frontal horn filled with echogenic blood and clot *(arrows)*. **B:** Sagittal image of the right lateral ventricle demonstrates a clot in the occipital horn *(arrows)*.

cle in some cases. A parenchymal hemorrhage is characterized by an area in the brain of increased echogenicity with poorly defined margins. Magnetic resonance imaging may be helpful in differentiating parenchymal hemorrhage from an intracranial tumor (Figure 4.12-4).

A porencephalic cyst appears as a cystic lesion within the brain that communicates with the lateral ventricle (Figure 4.12-3 and 4.12-5). A parenchymal hemorrhage may evolve into a porencephalic cyst over time.

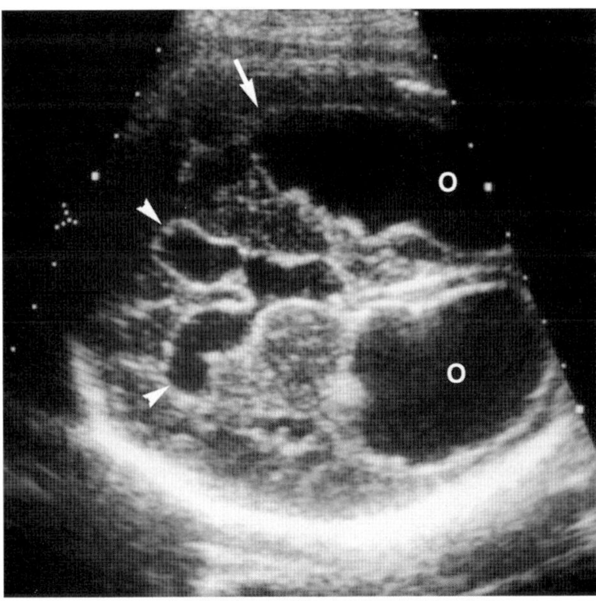

FIGURE 4.12-3. Posthemorrhagic hydrocephalus and porencephalic cyst. Axial image of the head demonstrates a dilated frontal *(arrowheads)* and occipital horns (O) of the lateral ventricles with extension of fluid from one ventricle into the cerebral parenchyma *(arrow)* owing to a porencephalic cyst. These changes resulted from intracranial hemorrhage earlier in gestation.

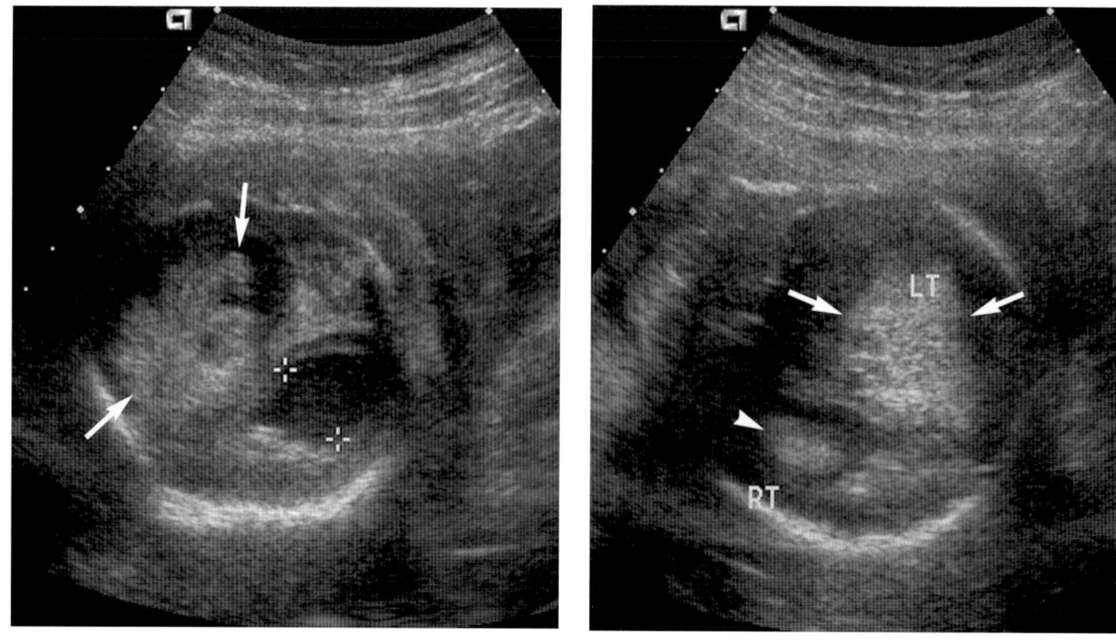

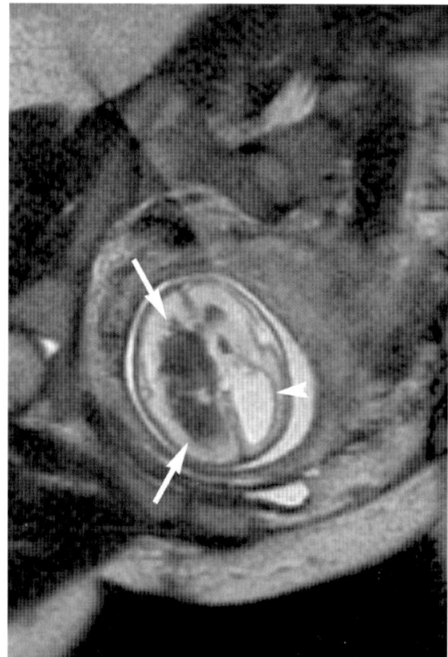

FIGURE 4.12-4. Intracranial hemorrhage with magnetic resonance imaging correlation. A: Axial image of the head demonstrates a poorly defined echogenic mass *(arrows)* with dilation of the contralateral ventricle *(calipers)*. **B:** Coronal image demonstrates an irregular echogenic mass *(arrows)* in the region of the left cerebral cortex. The choroid plexus *(arrowhead)* in the right ventricle has similar echogenicity. **C:** Fetal magnetic resonance imaging demonstrates the low signal of blood *(arrows)* in the ventricle and cerebral parenchyma on one side and the higher signal of fluid in the dilated lateral ventricle *(arrowhead)* on the other side.

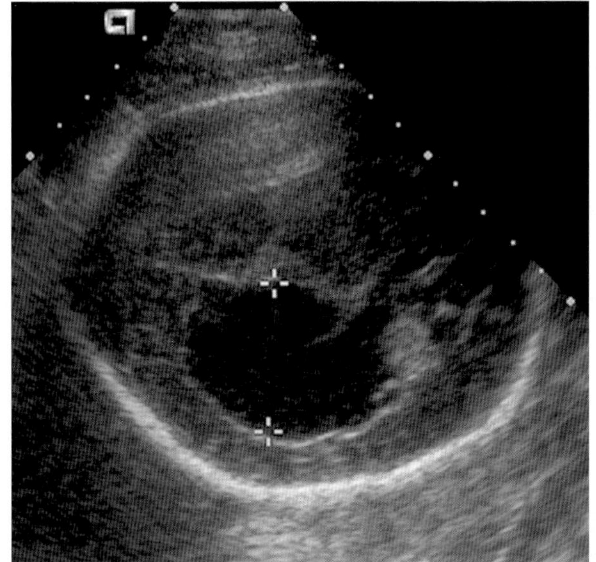
A

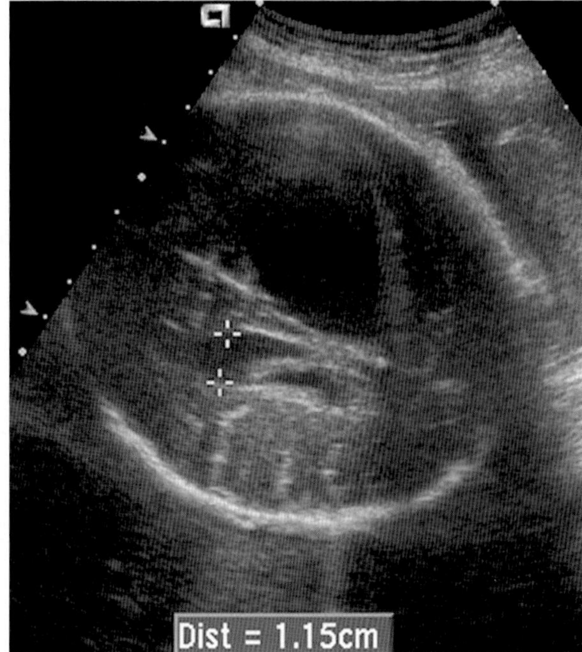

B

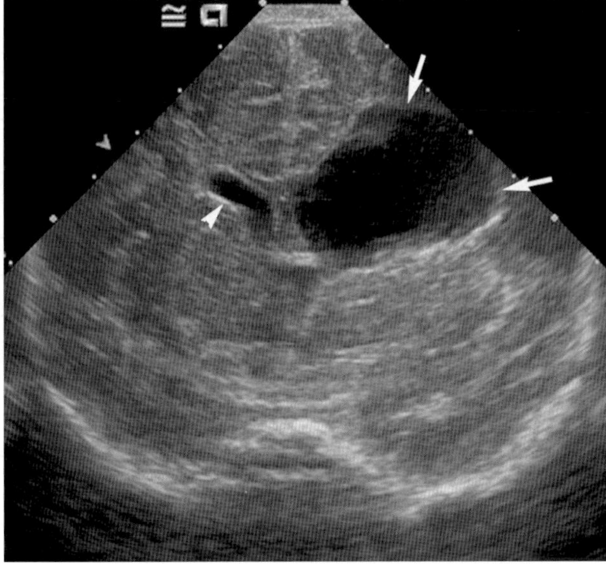
C

FIGURE 4.12-5. Porencephaly. A: Axial image of the head demonstrates enlargement of a lateral ventricle *(calipers)* owing to the loss of adjacent cerebral cortex, corresponding to porencephaly. **B:** Contralateral ventricle *(calipers)* is mildly dilated. **C:** Coronal image of the neonatal head demonstrates outpouching of the frontal horn *(arrows)* of the left lateral ventricle owing to porencephaly. The right frontal horn *(arrowhead)* has a normal configuration.

4.13. HYDRANENCEPHALY

Description and Clinical Features

Hydranencephaly, absence of the cerebral hemispheres, is a rare and devastating abnormality. It is thought to occur as a result of a massive vascular accident to the brain, such as carotid occlusion, that causes infarction of both cerebral hemispheres. The abnormality occurs after the brain has developed, in the late first trimester or further along in pregnancy. The necrotic brain tissue is resorbed and replaced by fluid that fills the fetal head. The falx is present.

The prognosis for fetuses with hydranencephaly is dismal. Because the midbrain is often preserved, neonates display many autonomic functions, such as breathing, sucking, and spontaneous reflexes but no higher cognitive functions.

Sometimes the fluid-filled cranium of a fetus with hydranencephaly grows rapidly, leading to macrocephaly. In such cases, vaginal delivery may be difficult or impossible.

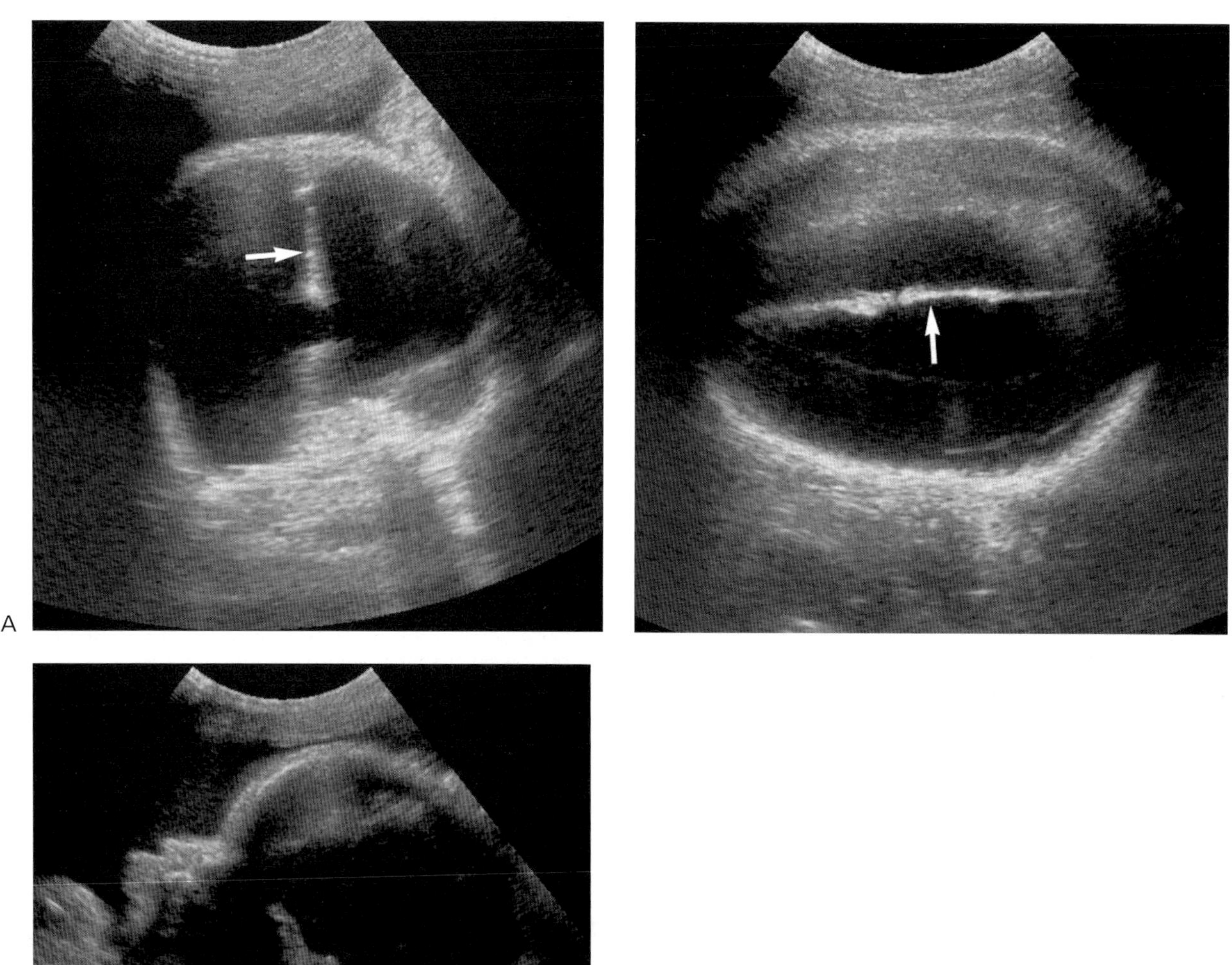

FIGURE 4.13-1. Hydranencephaly. Coronal **(A)**, axial **(B)**, and sagittal **(C)** images of head with fluid filling the cranium. No cerebral cortical tissue is visible, but the falx *(arrows)* is present.

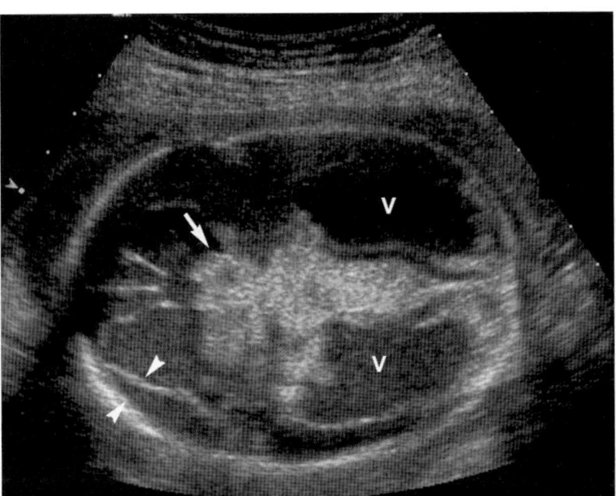

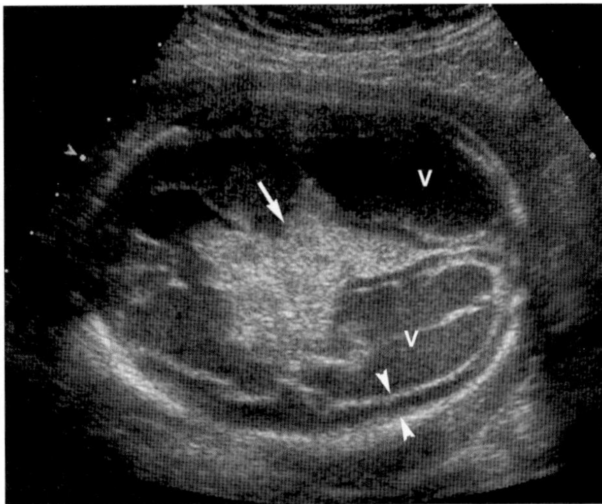

A B

FIGURE 4.13-2. Massive brain infarction. A, B: Axial images of head demonstrate dilated, irregularly shaped lateral ventricles (V) filled with echoes owing to blood. Bright echoes in the thalami and brainstem *(arrows)* represent hemorrhagic infarction. The residual cerebral cortex is thin *(arrowheads)*.

Sonography

The sonographic appearance of hydranencephaly is a fluid-filled fetal head with no identifiable cerebral cortical tissue (Figure 4.13-1). The presence of the falx differentiates this abnormality from alobar holoprosencephaly. The midbrain is seen in some cases.

If serial sonograms are performed on a fetus with evolving hydranencephaly, the evolution of the abnormality can be observed. The early sonographic finding of massive brain infarction is markedly altered echogenicity of the cerebral hemispheres, with areas of increased echogenicity owing to hemorrhage and complex cystic areas owing to necrosis (Figure 4.13-2). As the infarcted brain shrinks and liquefies, the size of the cerebral hemispheres decreases, with cortical thinning and dilation of the lateral ventricles (Figure 4.13-2). With time, the cerebral cortical tissue is broken down completely, until only debris and fluid are seen within the head (Figure 4.13-3).

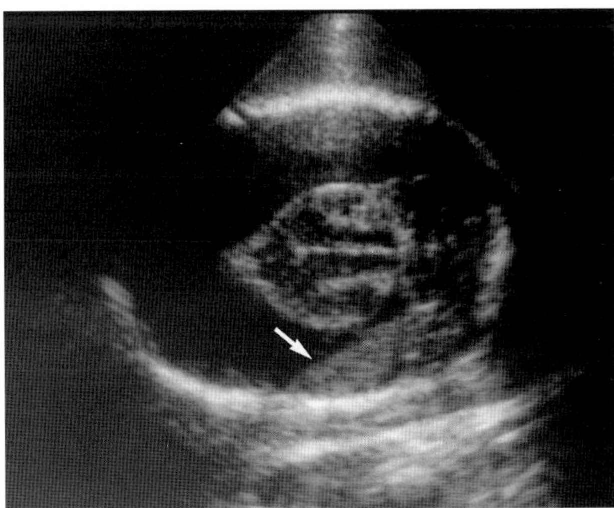

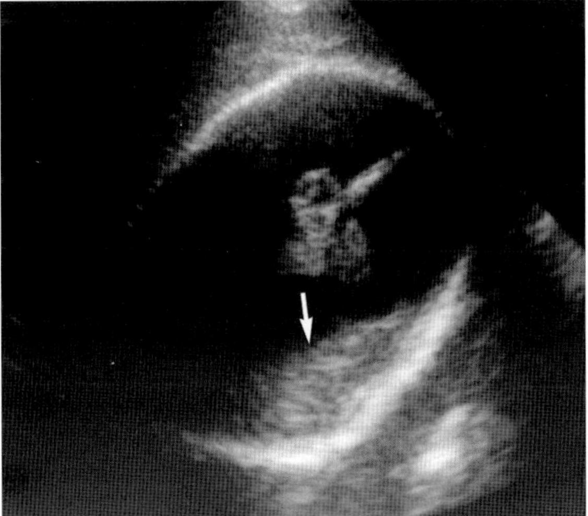

A B

FIGURE 4.13-3. Hydranencephaly with debris in the cranial vault. A: Axial image demonstrates the fluid-filled cranium with a small amount of debris layering posteriorly *(arrow)*. **B:** After changing maternal position, the debris layers more anteriorly *(arrow)*.

SUGGESTED READINGS

1. Babcook CJ, Goldstein RB, Barth RA, et al. Prevalence of ventriculomegaly in association with myelomeningocele: correlation with gestational age and severity of posterior fossa deformity. *Radiology* 1994;3:703–707.
2. Benacerraf BR, Stryker J, Frigoletto FD. Abnormal US appearance of the cerebellum (banana sign): indirect sign of spina bifida. *Radiology* 1989;171: 151–153.
3. Bennett GL, Bromley B, Benacerraf BR. Agenesis of the corpus callosum: prenatal detection usually is not possible before 22 weeks of gestation. *Radiology* 1996;199:447–450.
4. Cardoza JD, Filly RA, Podrasky AE. The dangling choroid plexus: a sonographic observation of value in excluding ventriculomegaly. *AJR Am J Roentgenol* 1988;151:767–770
5. Cardoza JD, Goldstein RB, Filly RA. Exclusion of fetal ventriculomegaly with a single measurement: the width of lateral ventricular atrium. *Radiology* 1988;169:711–714.
6. Chang MC, Russell SA, Callen PW, et al. Sonographic detection of inferior vermian agenesis in Dandy-Walker malformations: prognostic implications. *Radiology* 1994;193:765–770.
7. Durfee SM, Kim FM, Benson CB. Postnatal outcome of fetuses with the prenatal diagnosis of asymmetric hydrocephalus. *J Ultrasound Med* 2001;20:263–268.
8. Estroff JA, Scott MR, Benacerraf BR. Dandy-Walker variant: prenatal sonographic features and clinical outcome. *Radiology* 1992;185:755–758.
9. Filly RA, Cardoza JD, Goldstein RB, et al. Detection of fetal central nervous system anomalies: a practical level of effort for a routine sonogram. *Radiology* 1989;172:403–408.
10. Filly RA, Chinn DH, Callen PW. Alobar holoprosencephaly: ultrasonographic prenatal diagnosis. *Radiology* 1984;151:455–459.
11. McGahan JP, Nyberg DA, Mack LA. Sonography of facial features of alobar and semilobar holoprosencephaly. *AJR Am J Roentgenol* 1990;154:143–148
12. Nyberg DA, Mack LA, Hirsch J, et al. Abnormalities of fetal cranial contour in sonographic detection of spina bifida: evaluation of the "lemon" sign. *Radiology* 1988;167:387–392.
13. Pilu G, Falco P, Perolo A, et al. Ultrasound evaluation of the fetal neural axis. In: Callen PW, ed. *Ultrasonography in obstetrics and gynecology*, 4th ed. Philadelphia: WB Saunders, 2000:277–306.
14. Pilu G, Romero R, Gabrielli S, et al. Prenatal diagnosis of cerebrospinal anomalies. In: Fleischer AC, Manning FA, Jeanty P, et al., eds. *Sonography in obstetrics & gynecology: principles and practice*, 6th ed. New York: McGraw-Hill, 2001:375–388.
15. Toi A, Sauerbrei EE. The fetal brain. In: Rumack CM, Wilson SR, Charboneau JW, eds. *Diagnostic ultrasound*, 2nd ed. St. Louis: Mosby, 1998:1251–1282.

5

SPINE

5.1. SPINA BIFIDA AND MENINGOMYELOCELE

Description and Clinical Features

Spina bifida results from abnormal development of the neural tube, with failure of the posterior vertebral arches to close and form the bony sheath that surrounds the spinal cord. When the meninges, nerve roots, or spinal cord are exposed or protrude through the spina bifida defect, the abnormality is termed a *meningomyelocele*. A dorsal sac is present when these protruding tissues extend posteriorly behind the spinal defect. The bony defect can occur at any level of the spine but most commonly affects the lower lumbar and/or sacral spine. Hydrocephalus is commonly present and may require shunt placement after birth. The Chiari II malformation of the posterior fossa, characterized by a small posterior fossa, an enlarged foramen magnum, and downward herniation of the cerebellar tonsils and vermis, is virtually always present.

The incidence of spina bifida with meningomyelocele is approximately one to four per 1,000 births, but the incidence varies with geographic locations and race. Folic acid deficiency in early pregnancy has been identified as a risk factor. Most cases of spina bifida with meningomyelocele can be detected by screening pregnant women for elevated levels of maternal serum α-fetoprotein.

The prognosis depends on the level of the spinal defect. The higher the level is, the greater the neurologic deficit. In addition, many affected children have intellectual impairment.

Sonography

When spina bifida with meningomyelocele is present, sonographic abnormalities are usually visible in both the fetal head and spine. On a longitudinal view of the spine at the affected level, the ossification centers typically are widely spaced or disrupted (Figure 5.1-1). On a transverse view, the posterior ossification centers are splayed apart and diverge, disrupting the normal C or U shape (Figure 5.1-2). The dorsal sac protrudes posteriorly at the site of the defective posterior arch (Figures 5.1-1 and 5.1-2). The sac usually contains fluid and may also have solid material.

The fetal head is abnormal in most fetuses with meningomyeloceles. The posterior fossa is small, and the cerebellum is compressed against the occiput, obliterating the cisterna magna. During the second trimester, the small cerebellum is hypoechoic and curved around the cerebellar peduncles, with an appearance called the "banana" sign (Figure 5.1-3). Later in pregnancy, the cerebellum is larger and more echogenic, although it is still compressed against the occiput, and no fluid will be seen in the region of the cisterna magna (Figure 5.1-4).

Hydrocephalus is present in the majority of cases, with dilation of the lateral ventricles.

During the second trimester, the cranium of most fetuses with meningomyeloceles has an abnormal contour termed the "lemon" sign. This is characterized by flattening or concavity of the frontal bones (Figure 5.1-5). By the third trimester, the cranium is more ossified and usually has a normal oval configuration.

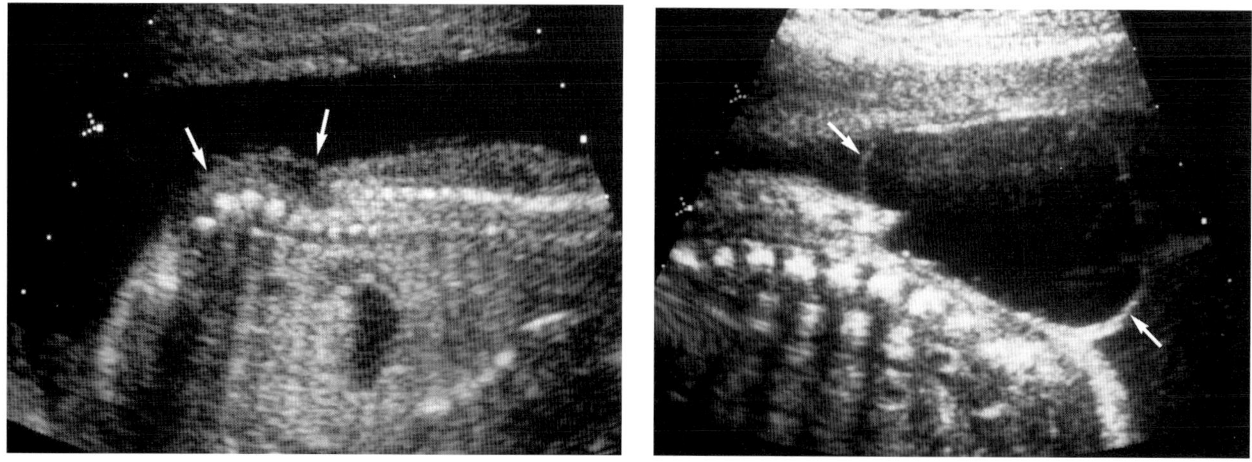

FIGURE 5.1-1. Meningomyelocele. A: Sagittal image of the spine with a meningomyelocele demonstrates disruption of the lower spine *(arrows)*. **B:** Sagittal image of a third-trimester fetus with a large spinal defect shows opening of the distal spine with a large cystic mass protruding posteriorly *(arrows)*.

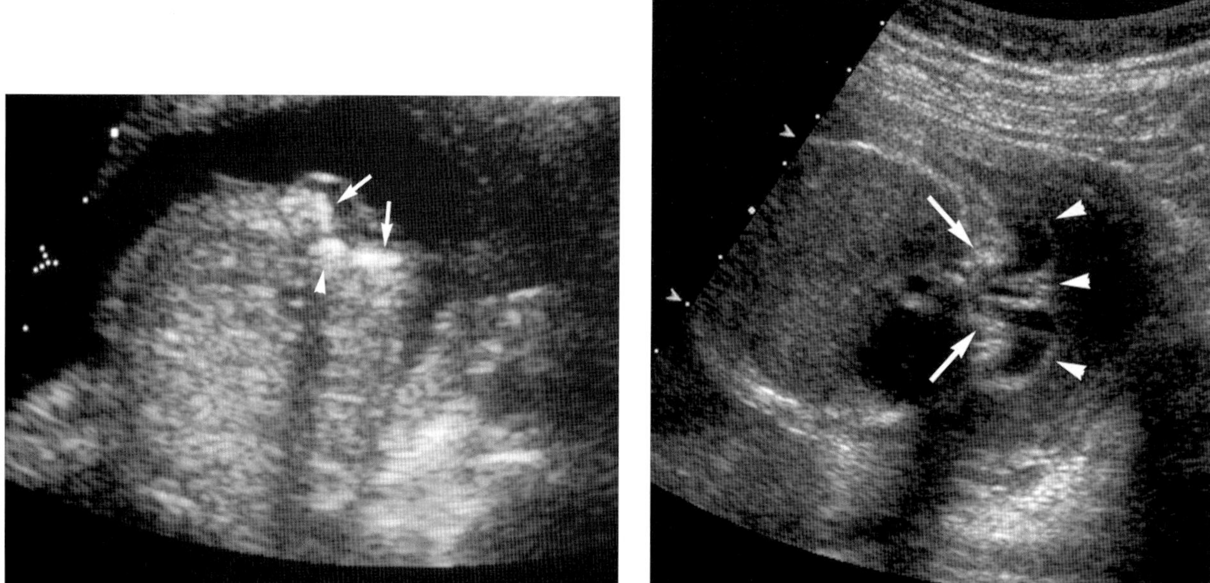

FIGURE 5.1-2. Meningomyelocele with splaying of the posterior ossification centers. A: Transverse image of the spine at the level of a meningomyelocele demonstrates marked splaying of the two posterior ossification centers *(arrows)*. The third ossification center *(arrowhead)* represents the vertebral body. **B:** Transverse image of a meningomyelocele demonstrates splayed posterior ossification centers *(arrows)* and a complex cystic mass protruding posteriorly *(arrowheads)*, representing the dorsal sac.

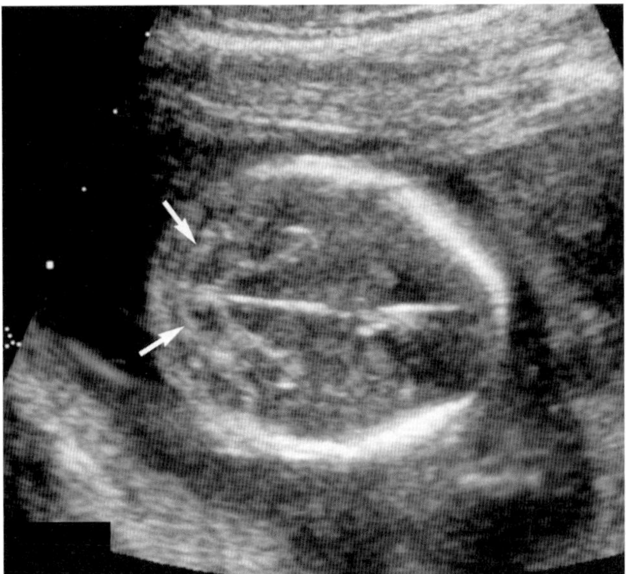

FIGURE 5.1-3. Banana sign associated with a meningomyelocele. Axial image of the posterior fossa demonstrates a banana-shaped cerebellum *(arrows)* in a small posterior fossa with effacement of the cisterna magna, owing to the Chiari II malformation. This fetus had a lumbosacral meningomyelocele.

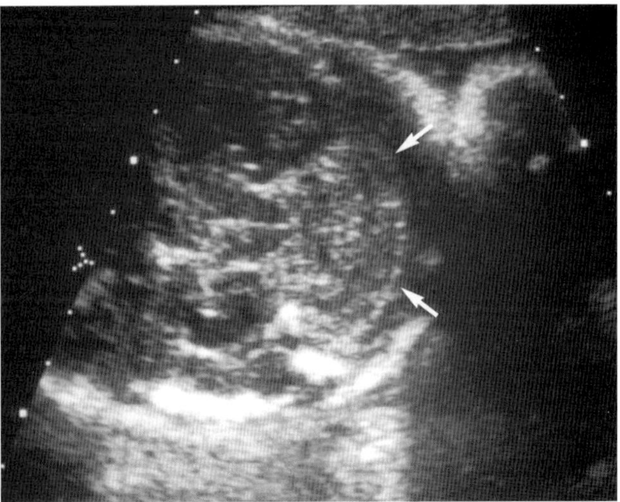

FIGURE 5.1-4. Chiari II malformation at 35 weeks gestation. Axial image of the posterior fossa in a fetus with a meningomyelocele demonstrates an echogenic cerebellum *(arrows)* compressed posteriorly against the occiput with complete effacement of the cisterna magna.

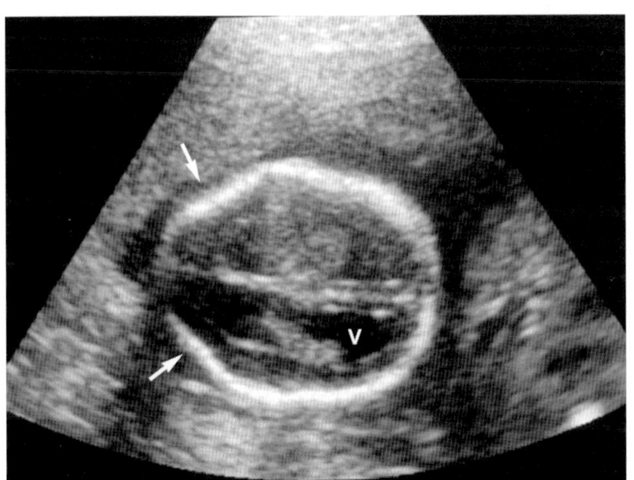

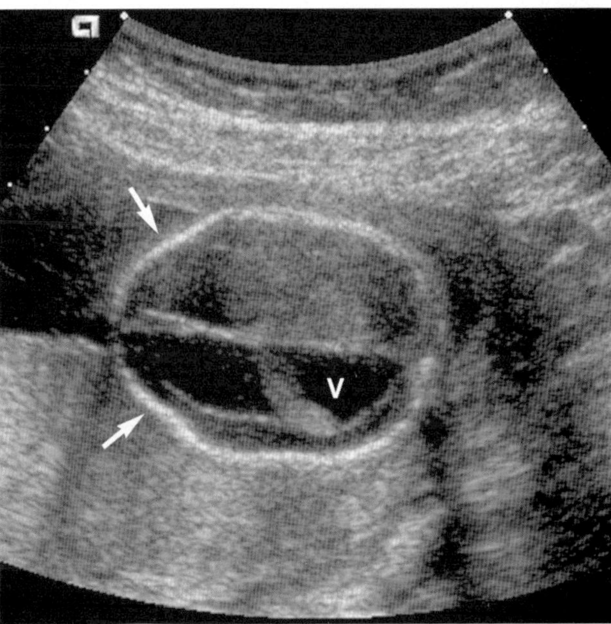

FIGURE 5.1-5. Lemon sign. A and B: Axial images of the heads of two different fetuses with meningomyeloceles demonstrate concavity of the frontal bones *(arrows)*, giving the head a lemon shape. The lateral ventricles (V) are dilated.

5.2. HEMIVERTEBRAE

Description and Clinical Features

Hemivertebrae are anomalous vertebrae in which part or all of one side of the vertebral body and posterior elements is absent. The result is a kink or bend in the spine at the affected level, causing scoliosis. The anomaly can affect a single or multiple vertebrae. Affected vertebral bodies have a wedge shape. Associated anomalies of the skeletal system are common, most often involving the ribs and extremities. In addition, hemivertebrae is a component of a variety of syndromes with anomalies affecting many organ systems, including the cardiovascular, gastrointestinal, central nervous, and genitourinary systems. The prognosis depends on the degree of severity of the associated anomalies.

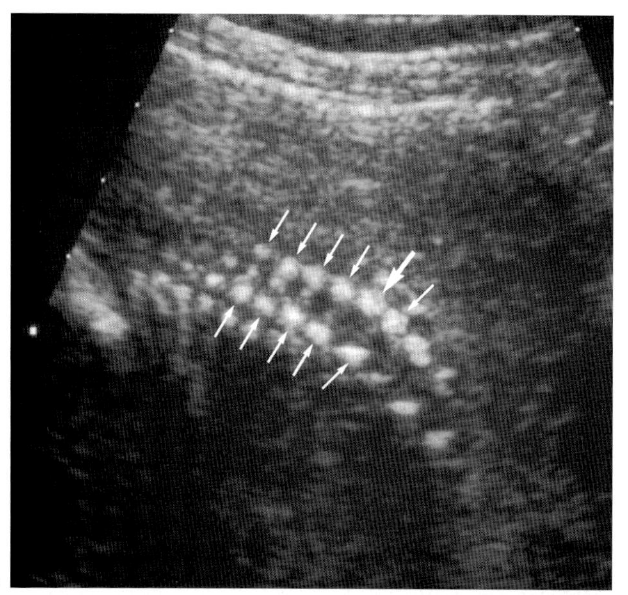
A

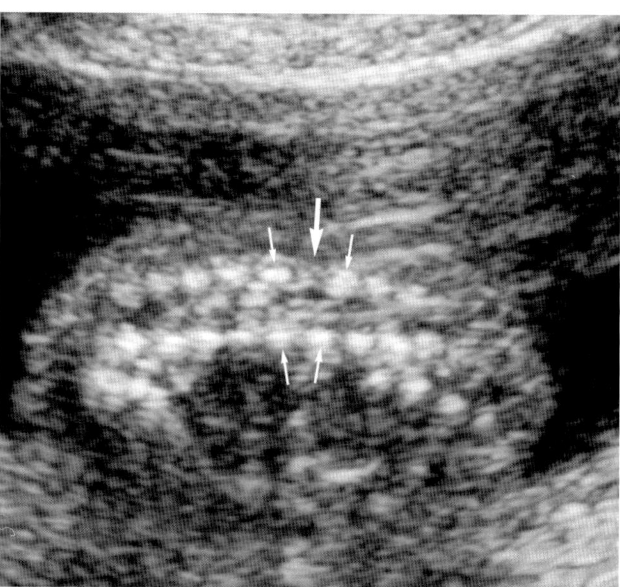
B

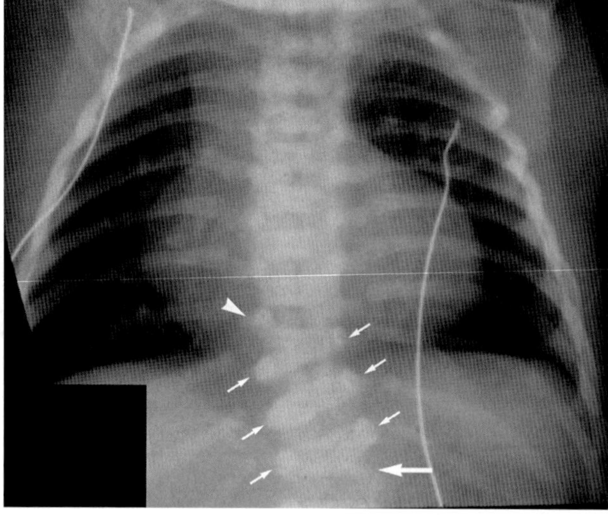
C

FIGURE 5.2-1. Hemivertebrae. A: Longitudinal image of the lower thoracic and upper lumbar spine demonstrates an extra ossification center on one side *(large arrow)* representing a hemivertebra. The posterior ossification centers *(small arrows)* for the other vertebral bodies correspond one to one. **B:** Longitudinal image of the lower thoracic spine demonstrates separation of the posterior ossification centers *(small arrows)* on one side by a hemivertebra *(large arrow)*. **C:** X-ray of the same patient as in **(B)** demonstrates the hemivertebra *(large arrow)* seen on ultrasound with matched posterior ossification centers *(small arrows)* superiorly. A second contralateral hemivertebra *(arrowhead)* is noted three levels above.

Sonography

On ultrasound, a hemivertebra is seen on a coronal view of the spine as a disruption of the normally paired posterior ossification centers. An extra ossification center will be seen on one side, without a matching center on the other (Figure 5.2-1). In addition, a kink or bend in the spine will be identified at that level.

5.3. SCOLIOSIS

Description and Clinical Features

Scoliosis is an abnormal lateral curvature of the spine. It can affect any level but most commonly involves the thoracic and upper lumbar spine. The abnormal spine often forms a lateral S shape. In many cases, no cause for the scoliosis can be found, although there is sometimes a family history of the disorder. Occasionally, congenital abnormalities of the vertebra, such as hemivertebrae, account for the spinal curvature. Some cases result from neuromuscular disorders, such as arthrogryposis, others from genetic syndromes, such as neurofibromatosis, and still others from a skeletal dysplasia.

Many cases of scoliosis are not detected *in utero* or even at birth but present later in childhood. The greater the severity of the scoliosis, the more likely it is that it will be detected prenatally.

Sonography

On ultrasound, scoliosis appears as an abnormal lateral curvature of the spine (Figure 5.3-1). When this is seen *in utero*, careful sonographic assessment of the fetus is warranted to look for bony abnormalities of the vertebrae, such as hemivertebrae, and to search for other anomalies in the fetus. Fetuses with arthrogryposis (Figure 5.3-2) usually have

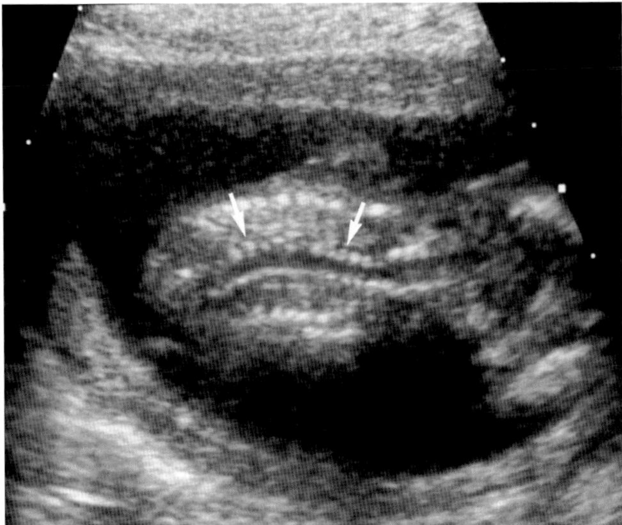

FIGURE 5.3-1. Scoliosis. Longitudinal image of the spine *(arrows)* demonstrates curvature from scoliosis. This fetus has trisomy 18.

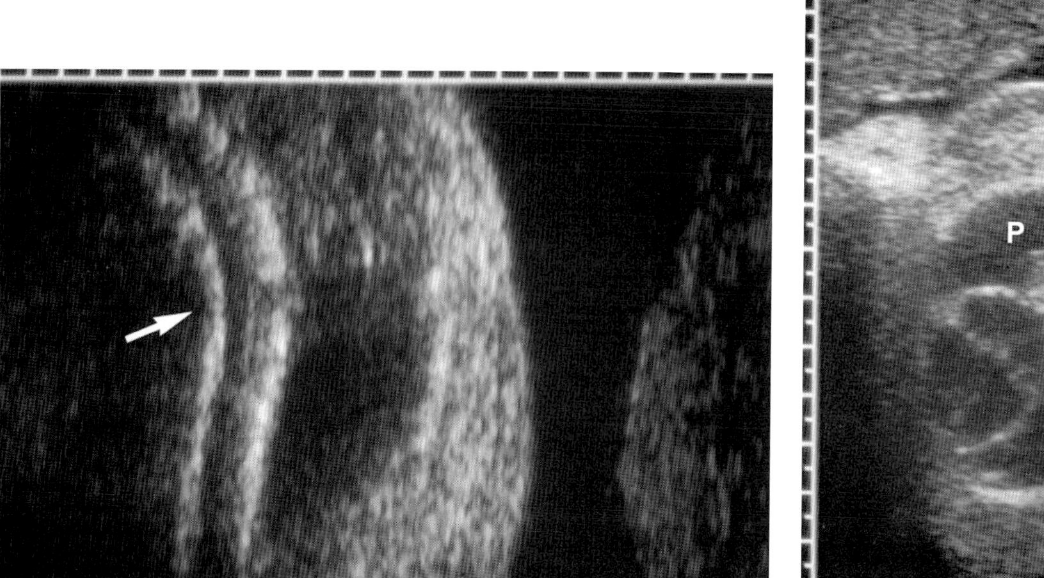

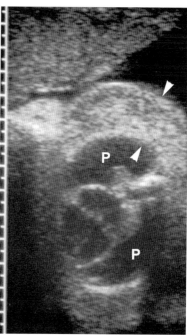

FIGURE 5.3-2. Arthrogryposis with scoliosis. A: Longitudinal image of the spine in a fetus with arthrogryposis demonstrates a marked curvature *(arrow)*. **B:** Transverse image of the thorax at the level of the four-chamber view of the heart in the same fetus shows bilateral pleural effusions (P) and extensive skin thickening *(arrowheads)*.

scoliosis, multiple limb contractures, and hydrops with skin thickening, pleural effusion, and ascites. Fetal movements are minimal.

5.4. CAUDAL REGRESSION AND SACRAL AGENESIS

Description and Clinical Features

Caudal regression refers to a spectrum of abnormalities involving the lower spine and, in some cases, the pelvis and lower extremities. Sacral agenesis, characterized by hypoplasia or absence of two or more sacral vertebrae, is a component of caudal regression. Caudal regression and sacral agenesis are found with increased frequency in fetuses of diabetic mothers, particularly those diabetic mothers with poor glucose control. The prognosis is related to the extent of absence and deformity of the lower spine and sacral nerves and to the degree of severity of other anomalies.

Sonography

The sonographic diagnosis of sacral agenesis is made when there is absence of some or all of the sacrum (Figure 5.4-1). More extensive forms of caudal regression are diagnosed when there is absence of a part of the lower spine in conjunction with a deformity of the pelvis or lower extremities.

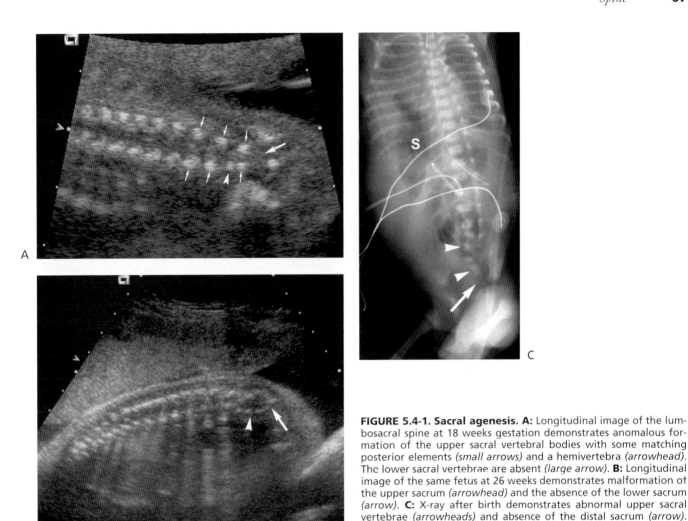

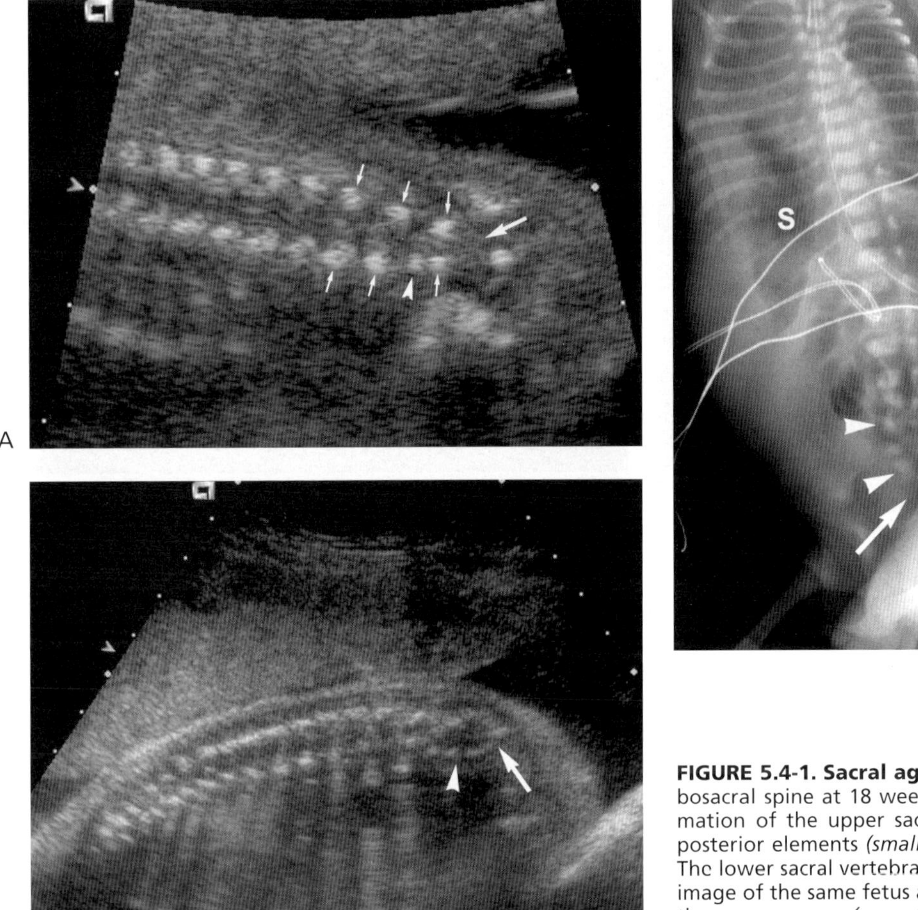

FIGURE 5.4-1. Sacral agenesis. A: Longitudinal image of the lumbosacral spine at 18 weeks gestation demonstrates anomalous formation of the upper sacral vertebral bodies with some matching posterior elements *(small arrows)* and a hemivertebra *(arrowhead)*. The lower sacral vertebrae are absent *(large arrow)*. **B:** Longitudinal image of the same fetus at 26 weeks demonstrates malformation of the upper sacrum *(arrowhead)* and the absence of the lower sacrum *(arrow)*. **C:** X-ray after birth demonstrates abnormal upper sacral vertebrae *(arrowheads)* and absence of the distal sacrum *(arrow)*. This baby also had a Morgagni diaphragmatic hernia with the stomach (S) seen in the right thorax.

5.5. SACROCOCCYGEAL TERATOMA

Description and Clinical Features

Sacrococcygeal teratomas are germ-cell tumors arising in the sacral region. These tumors may grow exophytically from the region of the lower sacrum, extending inferiorly and posteriorly from the fetal buttocks. Alternatively, these tumors may grow anteriorly into the pelvis. Those that grow within the pelvis may invade surrounding structures or cause mass effect, and can cause ureteral obstruction and hydronephrosis. Those that grow posteriorly may cause bony destruction of the sacrum and pelvic bones. In either case, sacral nerves may be destroyed, leading to neurogenic bladder and lower extremity paralysis.

Sacrococcygeal teratomas may grow very rapidly and be highly vascular. As a result, the fetus is at risk of developing high-output congestive heart failure, manifested by cardiomegaly and hydrops. The presence of hydrops with sacrococcygeal teratoma carries a poor prognosis.

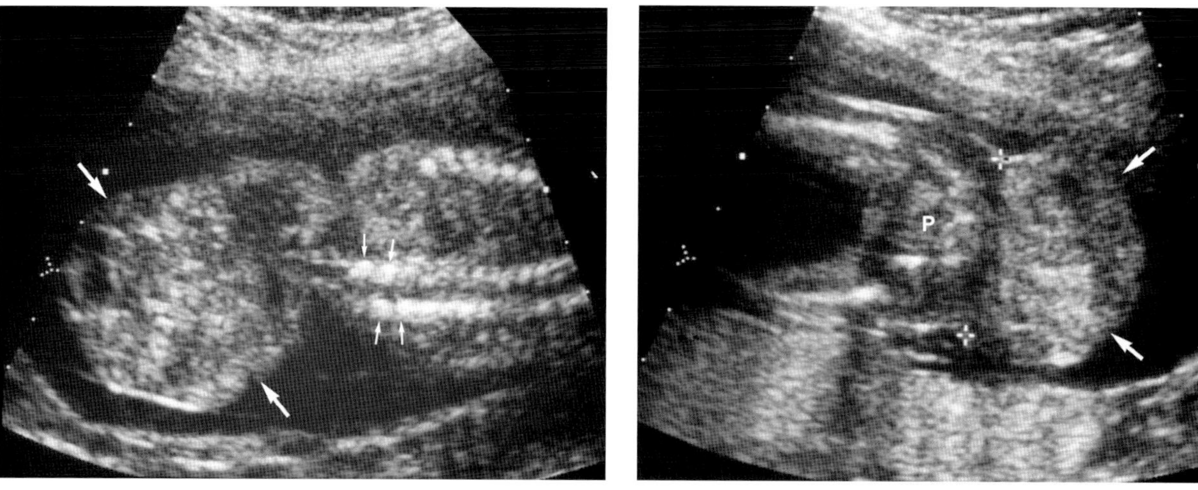

FIGURE 5.5-1. Exophytic sacrococcygeal teratoma. A: Longitudinal image of the lower spine demonstrates a large mass *(large arrows)* growing posteriorly and inferiorly from the lower sacrum. Posterior ossifications *(small arrows)* of several sacral vertebrae are visible. **B:** Transverse image of the pelvis (P) demonstrates a mass *(arrows)* growing posteriorly. Calipers mark the junction between the mass and the pelvis.

Sonography

An exophytic sacrococcygeal teratoma appears as a complex mass arising from the distal spine, extending posteriorly and inferiorly (Figure 5.5-1). The mass is usually hypervascular. When a sacrococcygeal teratoma extends anteriorly into the pelvis, the tumor margins may be difficult to delineate by ultrasound because of invasion of surrounding structures by the mass (Figure 5.5-2). Hydronephrosis (Figure 5.5-3) may be present owing to ureteral obstruction by growth of the mass into the pelvis or to a neurogenic bladder from sacral nerve damage.

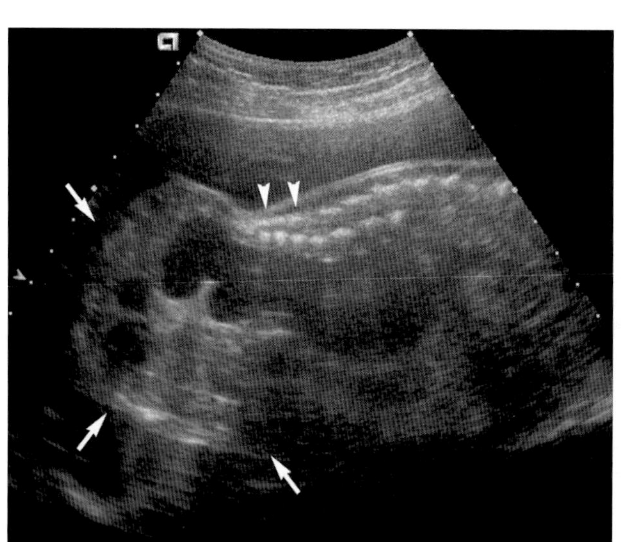

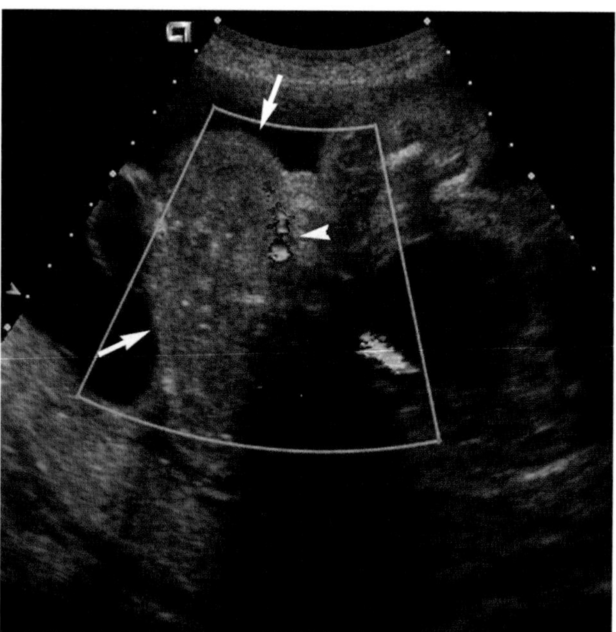

FIGURE 5.5-2. Sacrococcygeal teratoma invading the pelvis. A: Longitudinal image of the sacral spine *(arrowheads)* demonstrates a large complex mass *(arrows)* extending into the pelvis anteriorly and inferiorly. **B:** Transverse image of the pelvis with color Doppler demonstrates a large vessel *(arrowhead)* feeding the sacrococcygeal teratoma.

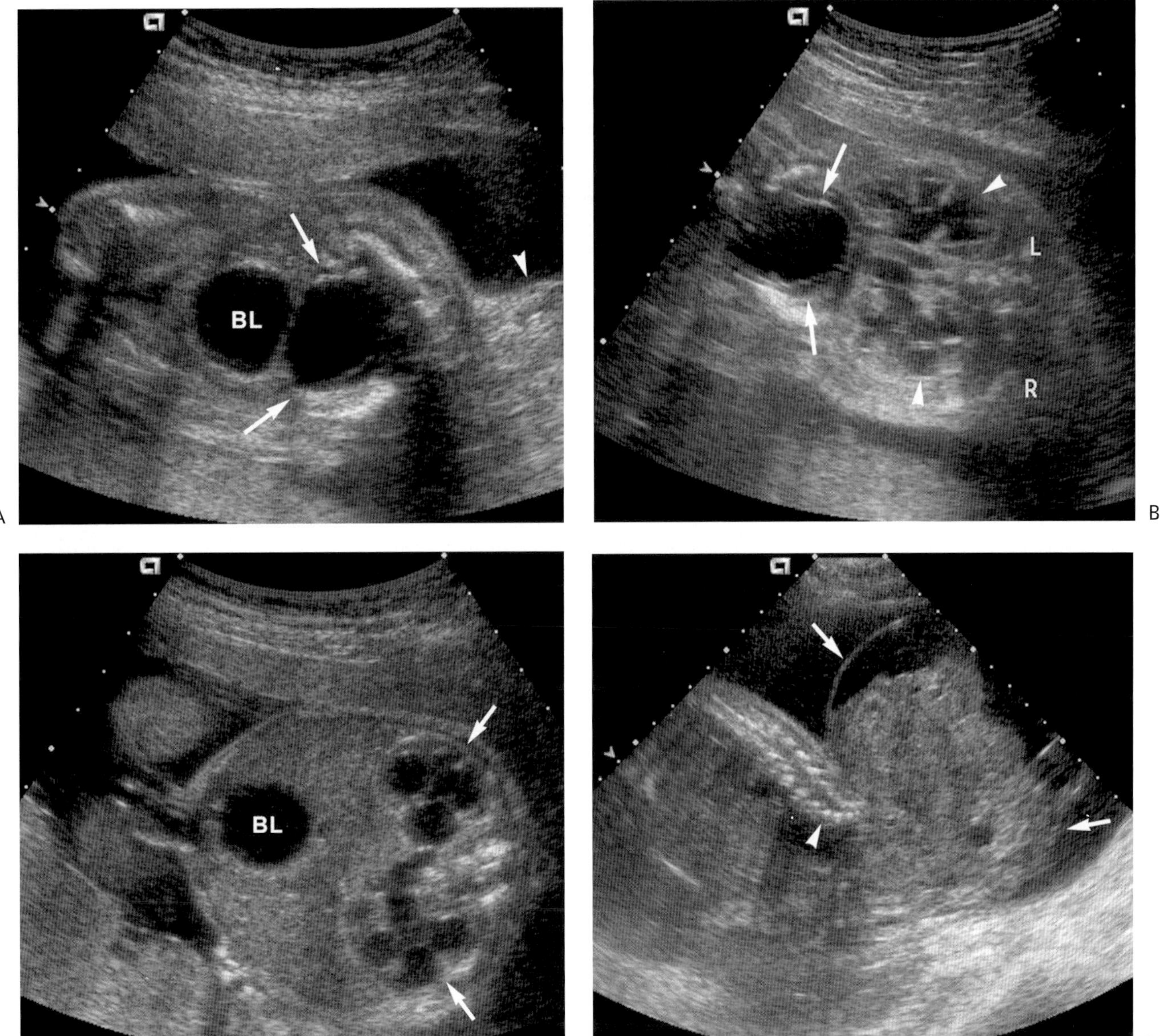

FIGURE 5.5-3. Bilateral hydronephrosis caused by sacrococcygeal teratoma invading pelvis. A: Transverse image of the pelvis demonstrates a cystic mass *(arrows)* posterior to the bladder (BL), representing extension of a large sacrococcygeal teratoma *(arrowhead)* into the pelvis. **B:** The posterior cystic mass *(arrows)* obstructs both kidneys (*arrowheads*; L, left kidney; R, right kidney). **C:** Transverse image through both kidneys *(arrows)* demonstrates marked hydronephrosis owing to obstruction from the pelvic tumor. The bladder (BL) is seen anteriorly. **D:** The large sacrococcygeal teratoma *(arrows)* also extends posteriorly and inferiorly below the sacrum *(arrowhead)*.

SUGGESTED READINGS

1. Babcook CJ, Goldstein RB, Barth RA, et al. Prevalence of ventriculomegaly in association with myelomeningocele: correlation with gestational age and severity of posterior fossa deformity. *Radiology* 1994;3:703–707.
2. Benacerraf BR, Stryker J, Frigoletto FD. Abnormal US appearance of the cerebellum (banana sign): indirect sign of spina bifida. *Radiology* 1989;171:151–153.
3. Filly RA. The "lemon" sign: a clinical perspective. *Radiology* 1988;167:573–575.
4. Gabbe SG, Mintz MC, Mennuti MT, et al. Detection of open spina bifida by the lemon sign: pathologic correlation. *J Clin Ultrasound* 1988;16:399–402.

5. Goldstein RB, Podrasky AE, Filly RA, et al. Effacement of the fetal cisterna magna in association with myelomeningocele. *Radiology* 1989;172:409–413.
6. Kollias SS, Goldstein RB, Cogen PH, et al. Prenatally detected myelomeningoceles: sonographic accuracy in estimation of the spinal level. *Radiology* 1992;185:109–112.
7. Nyberg DA, Mack LA. The spine and neural tube defects. In: Nyberg DA, Mahony BS, Pretorius DH, eds. *Diagnostic ultrasound of fetal anomalies: text and atlas*. Chicago: Year Book Medical Publishers, 1990:146–202.
8. Nyberg DA, Mack LA, Hirsch J, et al. Abnormalities of fetal cranial contour in sonographic detection of spina bifida: evaluation of the "lemon" sign. *Radiology* 1988;167:387–392.
9. Sauerbrei EE, Toi A. The fetal spine. In: Rumack CM, Wilson SR, Charboneau JW, eds. *Diagnostic ultrasound*, 2nd ed. St. Louis: Mosby, 1998:1283–1302.
10. Van den Hof MC, Nicolaides KH, Campbell J, et al. Evaluation of the lemon and banana signs in one hundred thirty fetuses with open spina bifida. *Am J Obstet Gynecol* 1990;162:322–327.

6

FACE

6.1. CLEFT LIP AND PALATE

Description and Clinical Features

Cleft lip is a congenital defect in the upper lip, often involving the anterior maxilla as well, that extends into the ipsilateral nostril. Cleft lip with cleft palate is a larger defect involving both the upper lip and anterior maxilla and part of the soft and hard palate. Isolated cleft palate is a defect of the posterior soft and hard palate, in which the maxilla and upper lip are normally formed. Cleft lip and/or cleft palate may be unilateral or bilateral, or may be a larger defect in the midline. Midline defects are associated with intracranial anomalies, particularly holoprosencephaly. Unilateral or bilateral cleft lips and/or cleft palates are associated with a variety of syndromes including genetic, nongenetic, and those related to abnormal karyotypes. Anomalies are found in association with isolated cleft lip in 20% of cases. Among fetuses with combined cleft lip and palate, 47% have an associated anomaly, almost half of which are chromosomal defects.

Cleft lip is found in approximately one per 1,000 livebirths. Males are affected more frequently than females, accounting for 60%–80% of cases. In the absence of other anomalies, the prognosis is excellent. When other anomalies are present, the prognosis is related to the severity of these anomalies.

The presence of cleft lip and/or cleft palate *in utero* causes impaired fetal swallowing. Thus, these pregnancies are often complicated by polyhydramnios.

Sonography

Unilateral cleft lip appears as a defect in one side of the upper lip extending to the ipsilateral nostril (Figure 6.1-1). Amniotic fluid outlines the defect. When a cleft palate is also present, the groove extends deeper than with cleft lip alone. With bilateral cleft lip, defects are seen on both sides of the upper lip, each extending into the ipsilateral nostril (Figure 6.1-2). The intervening midline portion of the upper lip and maxilla will sometimes protrude or become everted, an appearance called maxillary prominence (Figure 6.1-3). Midline cleft lips appear as central defects in the upper lip extending into the base of the nose and both nostrils (Figure 6.1-4). As with a unilateral cleft lip, when cleft palate accompanies midline cleft lip, the defect appears deeper. Diagnosis of cleft lip, whether unilateral, bilateral, or midline, is often facilitated by the presence of polyhydramnios, allowing amniotic fluid to surround the fetal face for better sonographic visualization.

The prenatal diagnosis of cleft palate in the absence of cleft lip is usually not possible because the bones of the face and skull obstruct the sonographic beam.

Because of the association with other anomalies, a careful fetal survey should be performed when a facial cleft is identified.

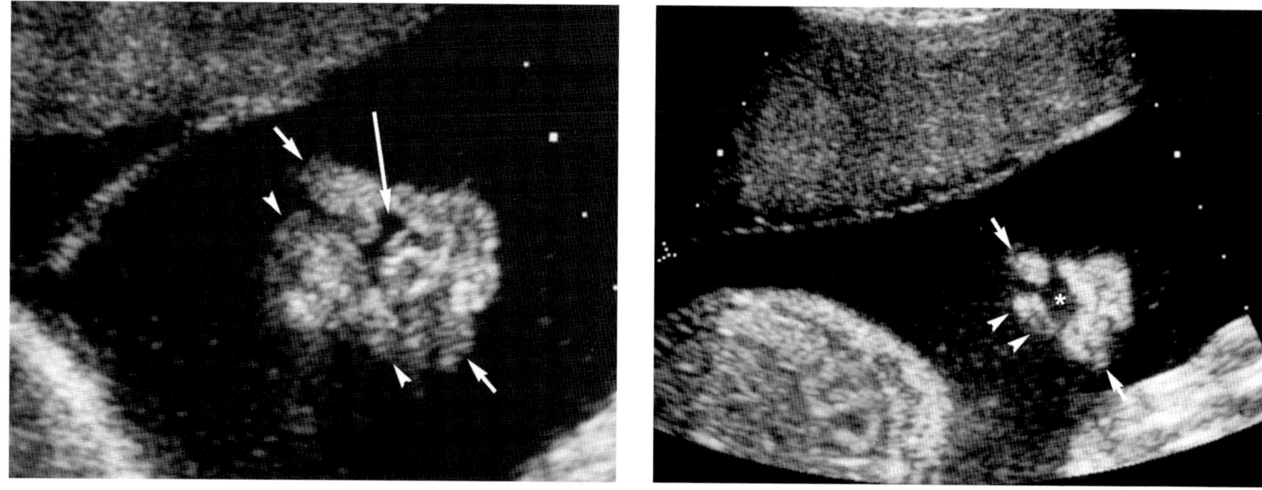

FIGURE 6.1-1. Unilateral cleft lip. A: Coronal image of the lower face demonstrates a large unilateral defect *(long arrow)* in the upper lip *(short arrows)* extending into the ipsilateral nostril. The lower lip *(arrowheads)* is seen inferior to the cleft. **B:** Coronal image of the mouth shows a large cleft (*) in the upper lip *(arrows)*. A portion of the lower lip *(arrowheads)* is visible beneath the cleft.

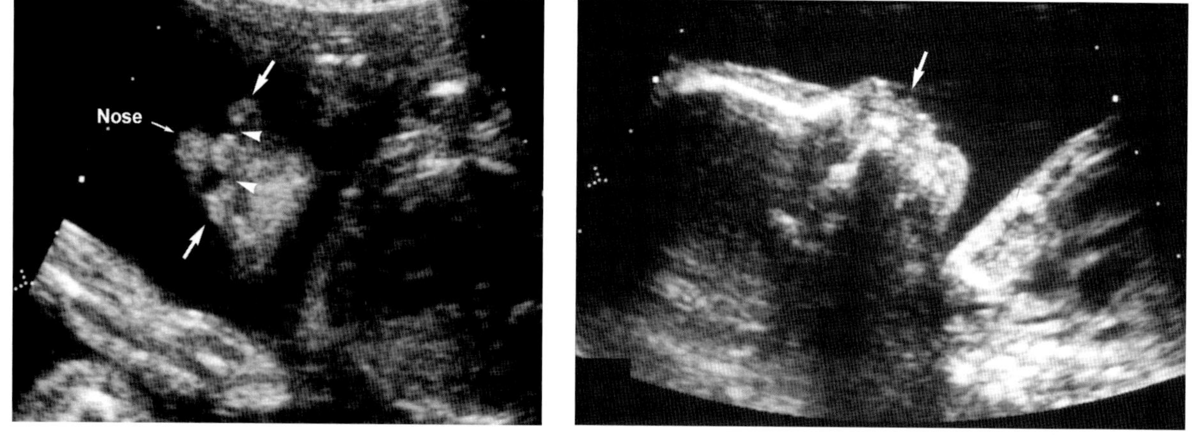

FIGURE 6.1-2. Bilateral cleft lip. A: Coronal image of the lower face demonstrates bilateral clefts *(arrowheads)* in the upper lip *(arrows)* with each cleft extending into the ipsilateral nostril of the nose (nose, *small arrow*). **B:** The facial profile is normal, without maxillary prominence *(arrow)*.

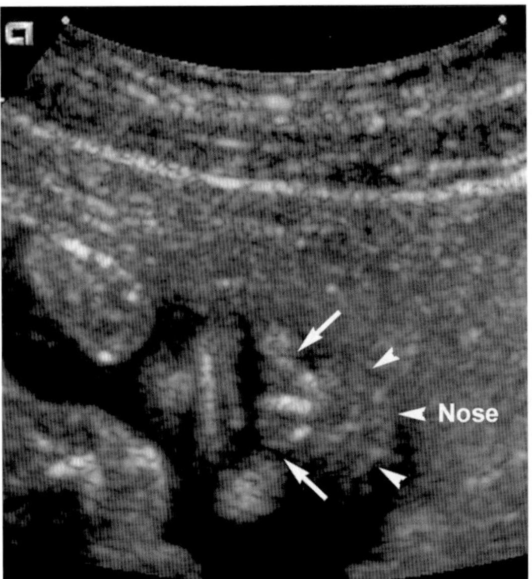

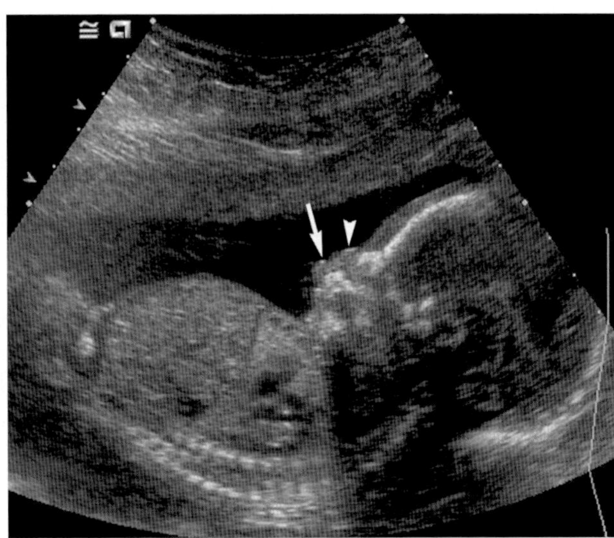

A B

FIGURE 6.1-3. Bilateral cleft lip and palate with maxillary prominence. A: Coronal image of the lower face demonstrates bilateral clefts in the upper lip *(arrows)* on either side of the bony protuberance, representing the maxillary prominence, inferior to the nose (nose, *arrowheads*). **B:** Sagittal image of the face demonstrates the maxillary protuberance *(arrow)* extending farther from the face than the nose *(arrowhead)*.

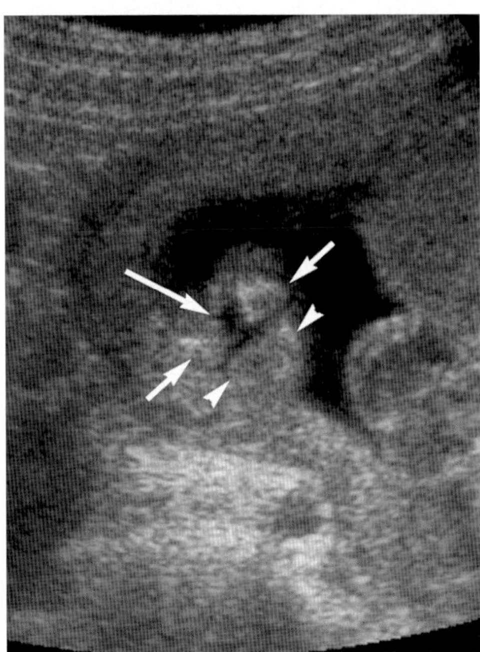

FIGURE 6.1-4. Midline facial cleft. Coronal image of the mouth demonstrates a central defect *(long arrow)* in the upper lip *(arrows)*. The lower lip *(arrowheads)* is inferior to the cleft.

6.2. MACROGLOSSIA

Description and Clinical Features

Macroglossia is an abnormally large tongue. It can occur in fetuses of diabetic mothers, fetuses with Beckwith-Wiedemann syndrome (a syndrome characterized by organomegaly and omphalocele), and fetuses with hypothyroidism. The enlarged tongue protrudes from the mouth and may interfere with swallowing, thus causing polyhydramnios.

Sonography

When macroglossia is present, the tongue persistently protrudes from the fetal mouth (Figure 6.2-1). When the tongue is seen protruding from the mouth, careful examination of the fetal mouth is warranted to determine whether the tongue itself is enlarged or the tongue is being displaced by an oral mass (Figures 6.2-2 and 6.2-3). Once the diagnosis of macroglossia is made, the fetus should be assessed for Beckwith-Wiedemann syndrome, with careful assessment of the ventral abdominal wall.

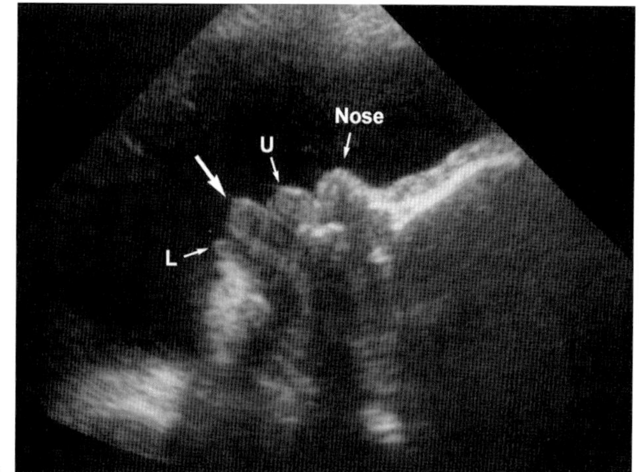

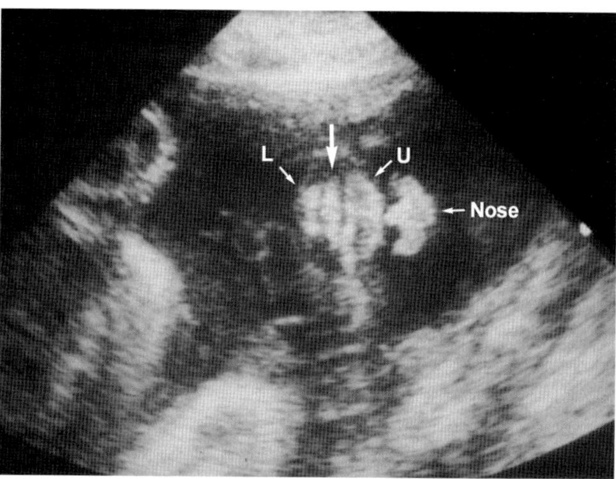

FIGURE 6.2-1. Macroglossia. Sagittal **(A)** and coronal **(B)** images of the face in a fetus with Beckwith-Wiedemann syndrome demonstrate a large tongue *(arrow)* protruding anteriorly between the upper (U) and lower (L) lips.

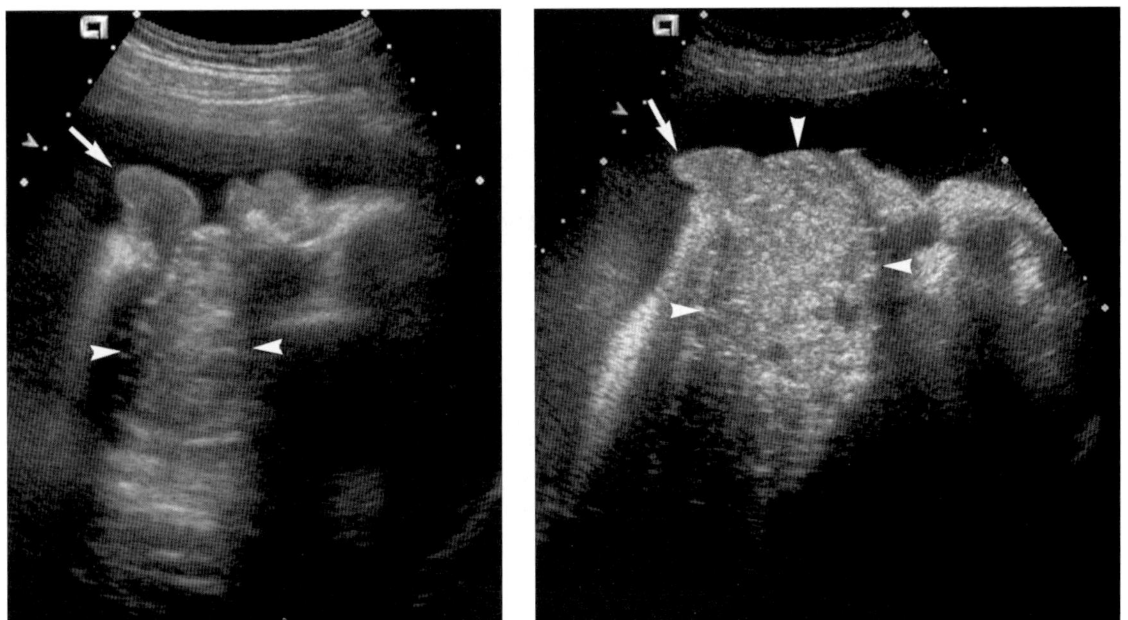

FIGURE 6.2-2. Tongue protruding from the mouth due to an oral tumor. Sagittal images of the face at 30 **(A)** and 32 **(B)** weeks demonstrate an enlarging oral mass *(arrowheads)* that is forcing the tongue *(arrow)* to protrude from the mouth.

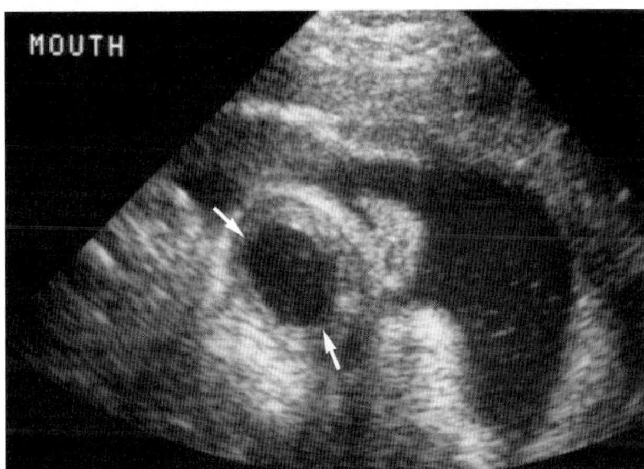

FIGURE 6.2-3. Salivary cyst. Coronal image of the nose and lips demonstrates a large cyst *(arrows)* that is forcing the mouth open and the tongue to protrude.

6.3. MICROGNATHIA

Description and Clinical Features

Micrognathia is defined as a small or hypoplastic mandible. This anomaly is associated with a variety of syndromes and chromosomal abnormalities. In particular, it is a common finding in fetuses with trisomy 18 and trisomy 13. Micrognathia is a component of a variety of skeletal dysplasias and dysostoses, such as Treacher Collins syndrome and Nager acrofacial dysostosis.

The presence of a small mandible may interfere with fetal swallowing. As a result, micrognathia may lead to polyhydramnios.

Sonography

The small mandible, characteristic of micrognathia, is best identified sonographically on a sagittal midline view of the fetal face demonstrating a small chin (Figure 6.3-1). Because of the association of micrognathia with aneuploidy, careful evaluation of the fetus is warranted once a small mandible is identified to look for sonographic findings associated with abnormal chromosomes.

A

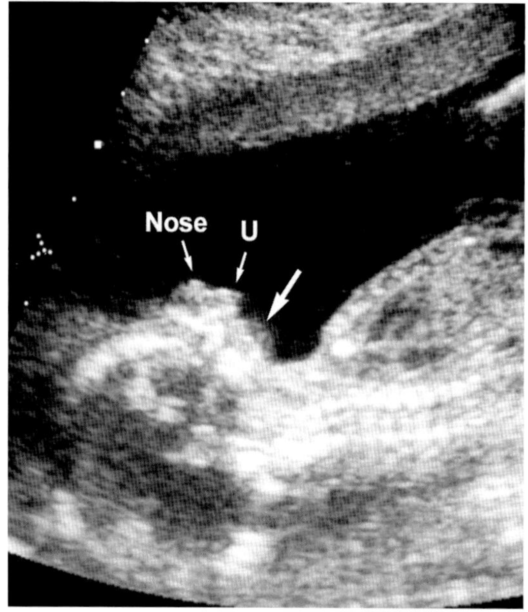

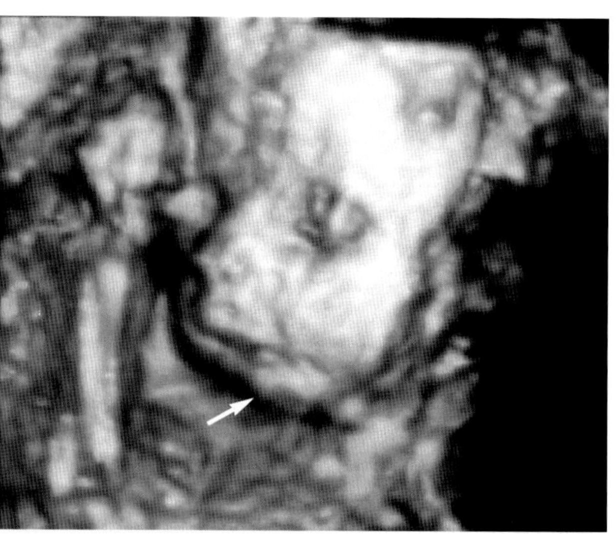

B

FIGURE 6.3-1. Micrognathia. A: Sagittal image of the face demonstrates a very small mandible and chin *(arrow)* beneath the upper lip (U) and nose. **B:** Three-dimensional ultrasound of another fetus demonstrates a small jaw *(arrow)*. (Courtesy of Dr. Beryl Benacerraf.)

6.4. HYPOTELORISM

Description and Clinical Features

Hypotelorism is characterized by the eyes being positioned closer together than normal. This anomaly is associated with anomalies of the brain, especially holoprosencephaly.

Sonography

The diagnosis of hypotelorism is made by identifying the eyes abnormally close together (Figure 6.4-1). This is accomplished by measuring the binocular distance and comparing it with norms for gestational age. Because of the strong association of hypotelorism and holoprosencephaly, careful evaluation of the fetal brain is warranted when hypotelorism is diagnosed.

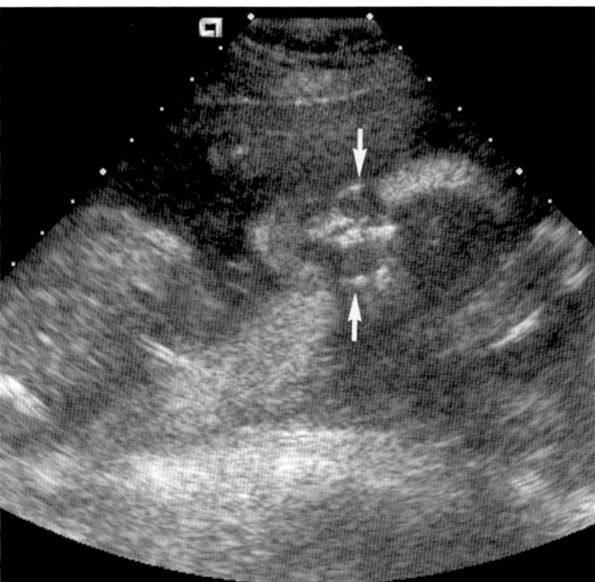

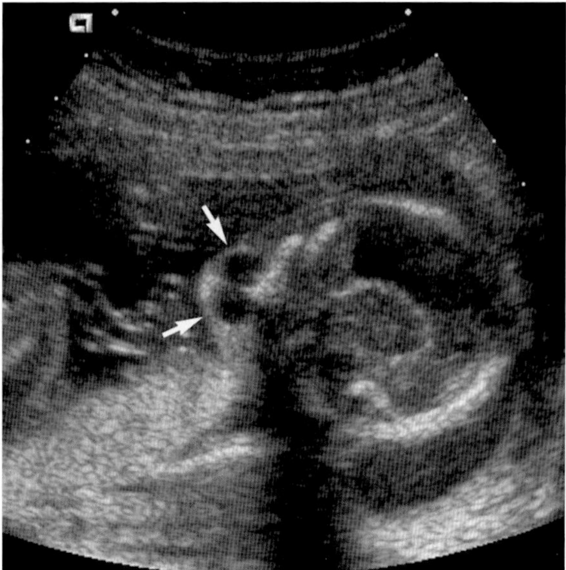

FIGURE 6.4-1. Hypotelorism. A: Coronal image of the face of a fetus with holoprosencephaly demonstrates the orbits *(arrows)* abnormally close together. **B:** The globes *(arrows)* of the eye, protruding from the orbits, are so close together that they touch each other.

6.5. CYCLOPIA AND PROBOSCIS

Description and Clinical Features

Cyclopia refers to fusion of the eyes into a single midline orbit. A proboscis is an abnormally formed nose that is long and thin, sometimes with a single nostril. It is located higher on the face than normal, sometimes at or above the level of the eyes. The presence of cyclopia and/or a proboscis indicates a high likelihood of holoprosencephaly.

Sonography

The face appears grossly abnormal sonographically in the presence of cyclopia and/or a proboscis. The single or fused eye is located in the middle of the face and the proboscis protrudes from the upper portion of the face (Figure 6.5-1 and 6.5-2). In some cases, a sin-

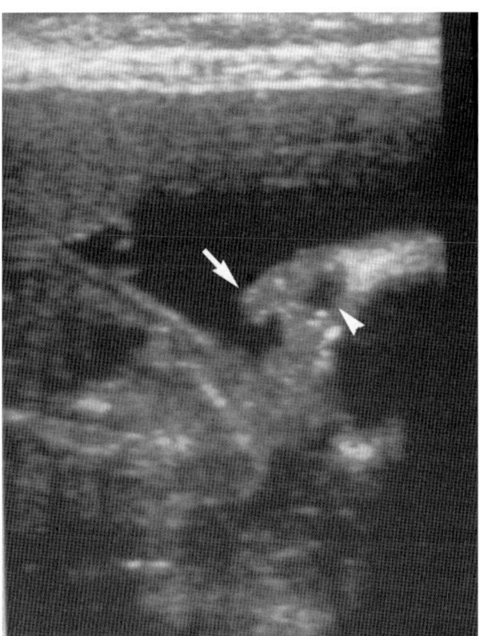

FIGURE 6.5-1. Cyclopia with a proboscis in a fetus with alobar holoprosencephaly. Sagittal image of the facial profile demonstrates a centrally located single orbit *(arrowhead)* and the nose *(arrow)* abnormally formed and located at the level of the eye. (From Benson CB, Jones TB, Lavery MJ, Platt L. *Atlas of obstetrical ultrasound.* Philadelphia: J.B. Lippincott, 1988, with permission.)

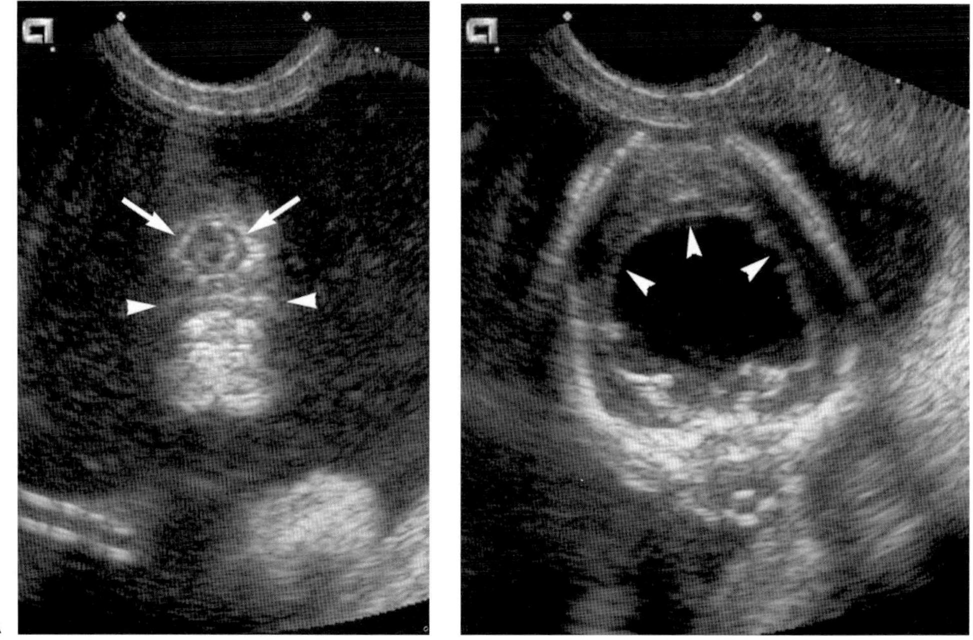

FIGURE 6.5-2. Cyclopia with alobar holoprosencephaly. A: Coronal image of the face demonstrates a single eye *(arrows)* in the midline, above the mouth *(arrowheads)*. **B:** Coronal image through the cranium demonstrates a monoventricle with fused cerebral tissue *(arrowheads)*.

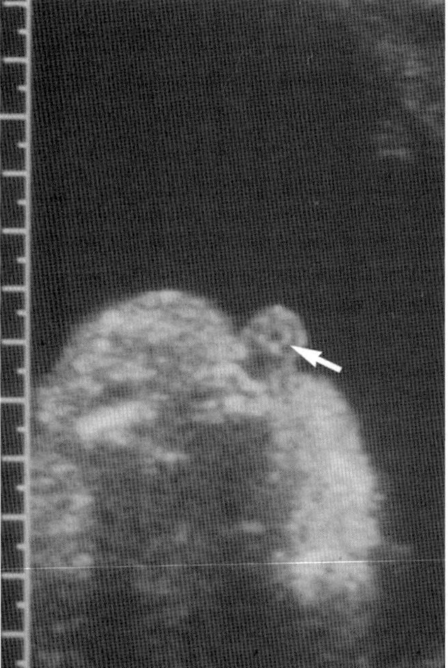

FIGURE 6.5-3. Single nostril in a fetus with holoprosencephaly. Axial image of the lower nose demonstrates a single nostril *(arrow)*.

gle nostril can be diagnosed on an axial view of the lower part of the nose (Figure 6.5-3). Because of the strong association between these facial anomalies and holoprosencephaly, careful sonographic examination of the fetal brain should be performed.

6.6. MICROPHTHALMIA AND ANOPHTHALMIA

Description and Clinical Features

The orbit can be congenitally small, termed microphthalmia, or completely absent, termed anophthalmia. This is a rare condition that results from the failure of the globe of the eye to develop, which, in turn, causes failure of the normal formation of the bony eye socket and eyelids. The ocular muscles and lacrimal glands also fail to develop. In addition to unilateral blindness, infants have a facial deformity that can be quite disfiguring.

This anomaly may be a sporadic abnormality or may result from *in utero* exposure to toxoplasmosis or rubella. It is sometimes seen with trisomy 18.

Sonography

The sonographic diagnosis of microphthalmia or anophthalmia is made when the orbit is abnormally small, and, at most, a small eyeball or lens is seen within it (Figure 6.6-1). Facial asymmetry is also a common finding.

A

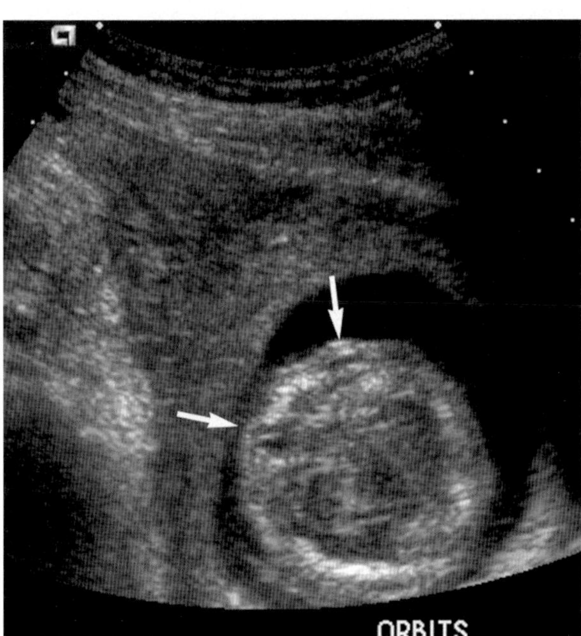

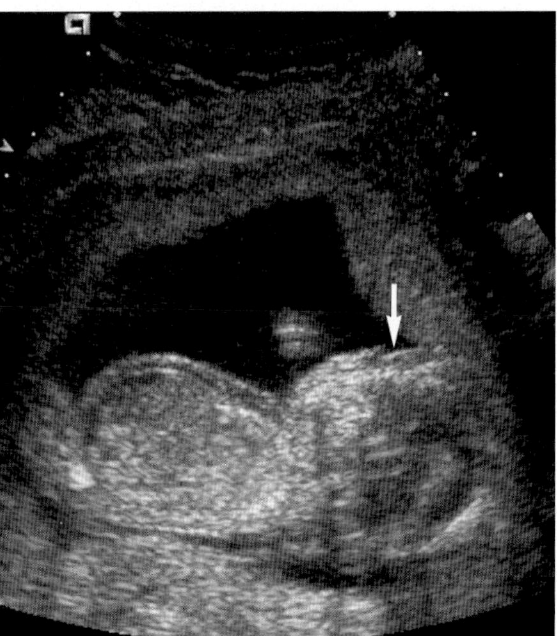

B

FIGURE 6.6-1. Microphthalmia in a fetus with trisomy 18. A: Axial image of the head at the level of the eyes demonstrates very small orbits *(arrows)*. **B:** Parasagittal image of the face demonstrates no visible orbit *(arrow)*.

6.7. CRANIAL SYNOSTOSIS

Description and Clinical Features

Cranial synostosis results from premature closure of one or more cranial sutures. This leads to deformity of the head that progresses as the fetus grows. Approximately 10%–20% of cases are associated with a recognized syndrome, such as Crouzon, Apert, Carpenter, and Chotzen syndromes. In the absence of a recognized syndrome, the prognosis is excellent if only a single suture closes prematurely. With two or more sutures involved, neurologic deficits and hydrocephalus are more likely to develop.

Surgical repair is often performed for cosmetic purposes and to prevent obstructive hydrocephalus.

Sonography

The diagnosis of cranial synostosis can be suggested when the shape of the fetal head is abnormal (Figure 6.7-1). The cranial deformity will vary, depending on which suture or sutures close prematurely. The face is often abnormal as well, with hypotelorism found in some cases.

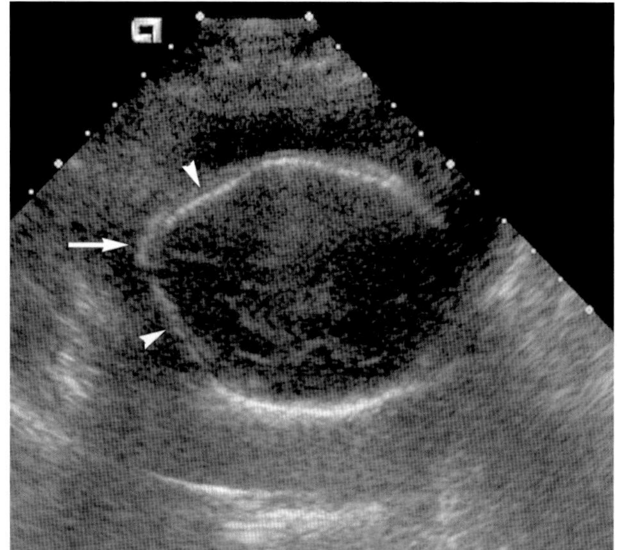

A

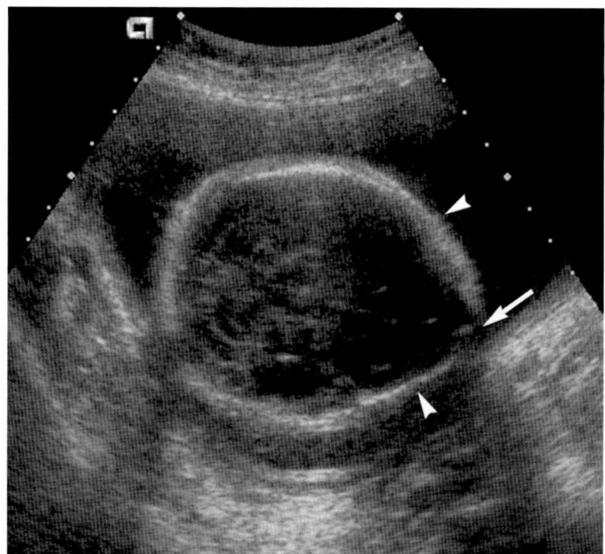

B

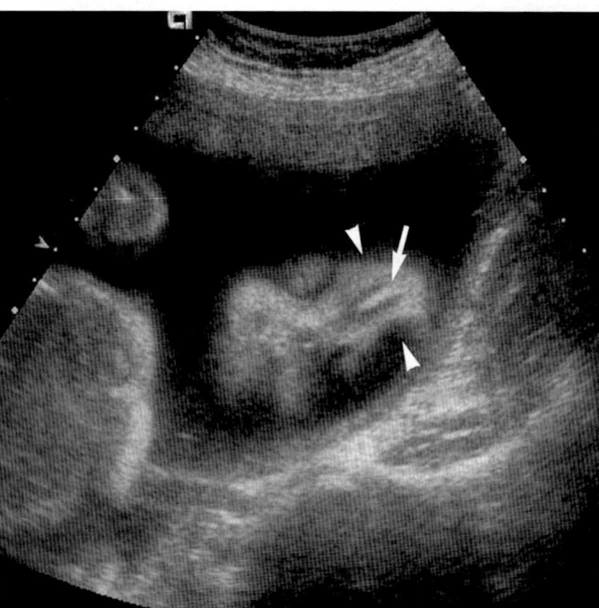

C

FIGURE 6.7-1. Cranial synostosis. A and B: Axial images of the head of a 28-week fetus demonstrate the abnormal shape of the cranium with flattening of the frontal bones *(arrowheads)* so that they converge at a point anteriorly *(arrow)*. **C:** Coronal image of the face demonstrates the abnormal forehead, pointed anteriorly *(arrow)* and flattened on the sides *(arrowheads)*.

SUGGESTED READINGS

1. Babcook CJ. The fetal face and neck. In: Callen PW, ed. *Ultrasonography in obstetrics and gynecology*, 4th ed. Philadelphia: WB Saunders, 2000:307–330.
2. Babcook CJ, McGahan JP. Axial ultrasonographic imaging of the fetal maxilla for accurate characterization of facial clefts. *J Ultrasound Med* 1997;16:619–625.
3. Babcook CJ, McGahan JP, Chong BW, et al. Evaluation of fetal midface anatomy related to facial clefts: use of US. *Radiology* 1996;201:113–118.
4. Clementi M, Tenconi R, Bianchi F, et al. and Euroscan Study Group. Evaluation of prenatal cleft lip with or without cleft palate and cleft palate by ultrasound: experience from 20 European registries. *Prenat Diagn* 2000;20:870–875.
5. McGahan JP, Nyberg DA, Mack LA. Sonography of facial features of alobar and semilobar holoprosencephaly. *AJR Am J Roentgenol* 1990;154:143–148.
6. Milerad J, Larson O, Hagberg C, et al. Associated malformations in infants with cleft lips and palate: a prospective, population-based study. *Pediatrics* 1997;100:180–186.
7. Nyberg DA, Hegge FN, Kramer D, et al. Premaxillary protrusion: a sonographic clue to bilateral cleft lip and palate. *J Ultrasound Med* 1993;12:331–335.
8. Nyberg DA, Sickler GK, Hegge FN, et al. Fetal cleft lip with and without cleft palate: US classification and correlation with outcome. *Radiology* 1995;195:677–684.
9. Robinson JN, Benson CB, McElrath TF, et al. Prenatal ultrasound and the diagnosis of fetal cleft lip. *J Ultrasound Med* 2001;20:1165–1170.
10. Savoldelli G, Schmid W, Schinzel A. Prenatal diagnosis of cleft lip and palate by ultrasound. *Prenat Diagnosis* 1982;2:313–317.
11. Toi A. The fetal face and neck. In: Rumack CM, Wilson SR, Charboneau JW, eds. *Diagnostic ultrasound*, 2nd ed. St. Louis: Mosby, 1998:1233–1250.

7

THORAX, NECK, AND LYMPHATICS

7.1. CYSTIC ADENOMATOID MALFORMATION

Description and Clinical Features

Congenital cystic adenomatoid malformation of the lung is a pulmonary mass that includes both cystic and solid components. There are usually multiple cysts within the lesion. The cysts vary in size, and cyst size is the basis for the categorization of cystic adenomatoid malformations into subtypes.

Type 1: some or all of the cysts are more than 2 cm in diameter
Type 2: cysts are approximately 1 cm in diameter
Type 3: cysts are microscopic in size

Cystic adenomatoid malformations are generally unilateral, often restricted to a single lobe. They receive their blood supply from the pulmonary circulation.

In the preultrasound era, cystic adenomatoid malformations (especially types 2 and 3) were thought to carry a poor prognosis. Since the advent and widespread use of ultrasound, much more is known about the natural history and prognosis of these lesions. In particular, cystic adenomatoid malformations diagnosed in the second or early third trimester sometimes remain stable in size or become smaller as pregnancy proceeds. These lesions have an excellent prognosis, and they may be so small in relation to the normal lung at the time of birth that they cause no symptoms. Large cystic adenomatoid malformations, however, may cause fetal hydrops and carry a poor prognosis.

Sonography

A cystic adenomatoid malformation appears sonographically as a unilateral pulmonary mass with one of the following characteristics:

Type 1: a mass with one or more large cysts (Figure 7.1-1)
Type 2: an echogenic mass containing small cysts (Figure 7.1-2)
Type 3: a homogeneously echogenic mass (Figure 7.1-3).

If large, it may cause mediastinal shift or inversion of the diaphragm, and the fetus may have ascites, pleural effusions, or full-blown hydrops (Figure 7.1-4).

Color Doppler can be used to determine that the blood supply to the mass arises from the pulmonary artery (Figure 7.1-5). This can be of value in distinguishing a homogeneously echogenic cystic adenomatoid malformation from a pulmonary sequestration.

Differentiation of a cystic adenomatoid malformation from a diaphragmatic hernia is made by based on the following observations:

Extent and location of the mass: a cystic adenomatoid malformation is solely intrathoracic, whereas a diaphragmatic hernia extends from below to above the diaphragm.

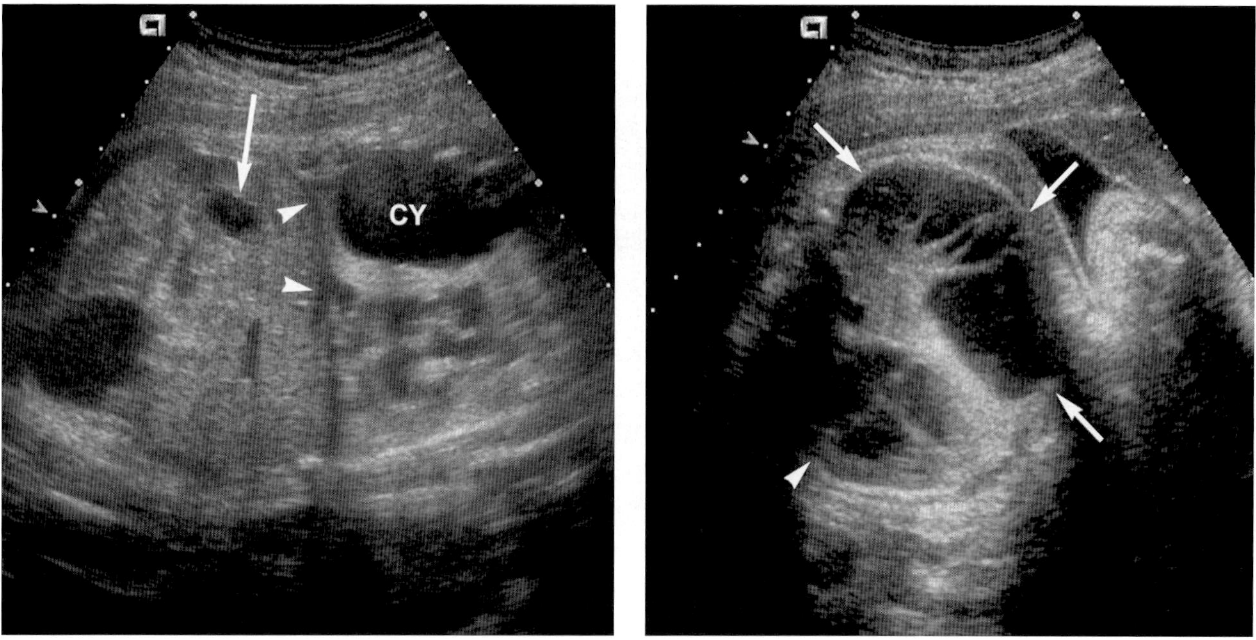

FIGURE 7.1-1. **Type 1 cystic adenomatoid malformation of the lung. A:** Longitudinal view through the fetal thorax and abdomen shows a large cystic lesion (CY) lying within the left hemithorax, superior to the diaphragm *(arrowheads)*. The stomach *(arrow)* is below the diaphragm. **B:** Transverse view through the fetal thorax demonstrates that the cystic lesion *(arrows)* is multiseptate and displaces the heart *(arrowhead)* to the right.

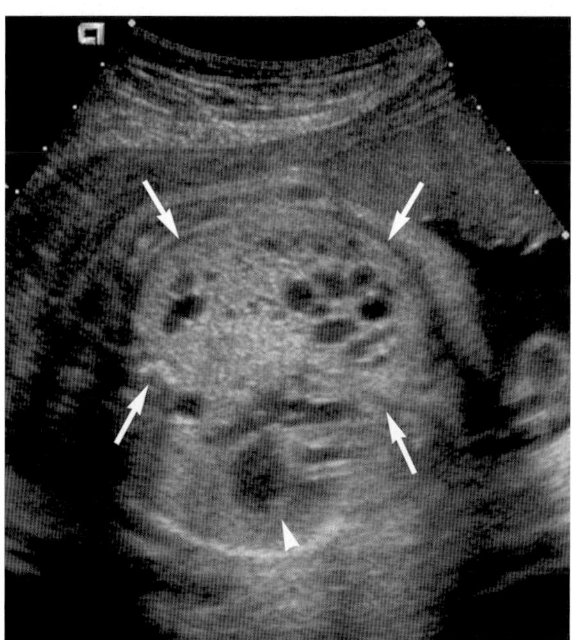

FIGURE 7.1-2. **Type 2 cystic adenomatoid malformation of the lung.** Transverse view through the fetal thorax demonstrates a large mass *(arrows)* in the left hemithorax containing multiple small cysts and displacing the heart *(arrowhead)* to the right.

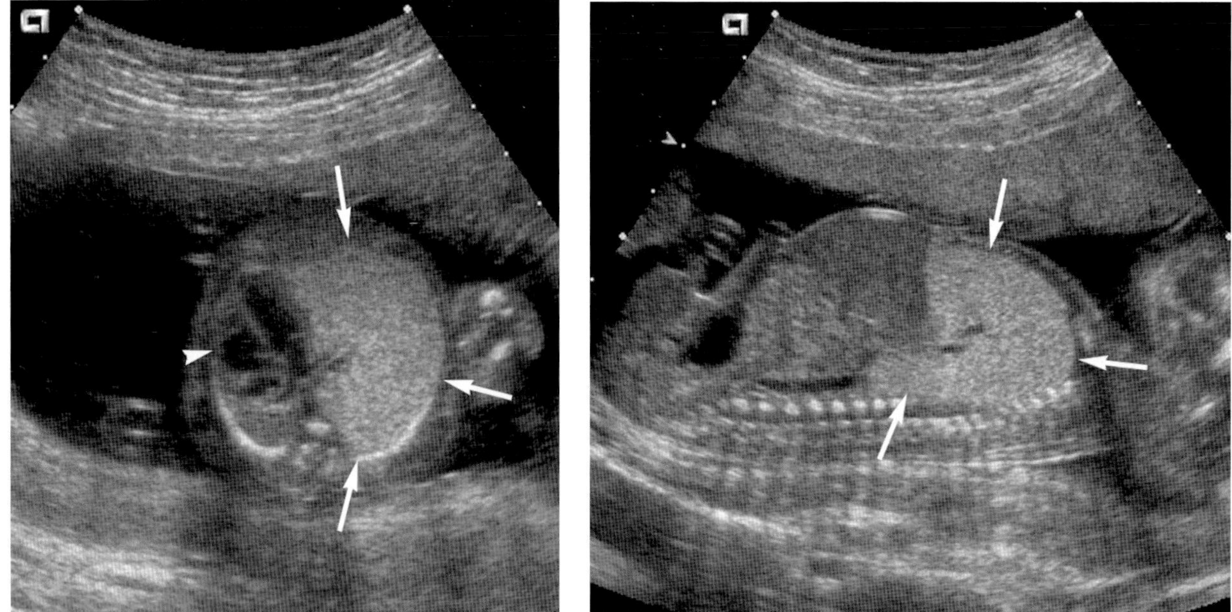

FIGURE 7.1-3. Type 3 cystic adenomatoid malformation of the lung. A: Transverse view through the fetal thorax demonstrates an echogenic mass *(arrows)* in the left hemithorax displacing the heart *(arrowhead)* to the right. **B:** Sagittal view through the fetal left hemithorax demonstrates the echogenic mass *(arrows)*.

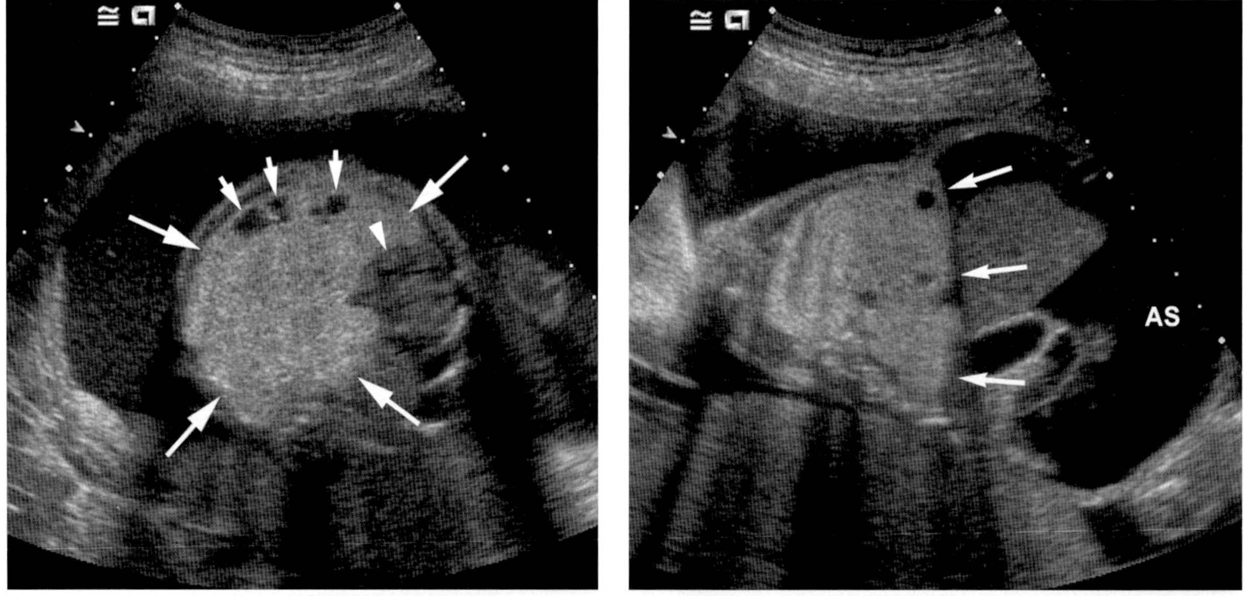

FIGURE 7.1-4. Cystic adenomatoid malformation of the lung causing ascites. A: Transverse view of the thorax demonstrates a large right-sided mass *(long arrows)* deviating the heart *(arrowhead)* to the left. The mass is mainly echogenic, with several cysts that are large enough to be sonographically identifiable *(short arrows)*. **B:** Sagittal view through the fetal abdomen and thorax demonstrates inversion of the diaphragm *(arrows)* by the mass. There is a large amount of ascites (AS) in the fetal abdomen.

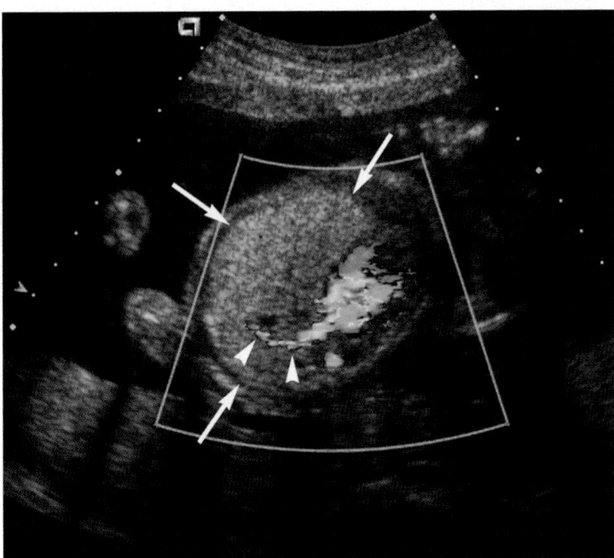

FIGURE 7.1-5. Cystic adenomatoid malformation with color Doppler. Transverse view of the thorax with color Doppler demonstrates that the cystic adenomatoid malformation *(arrows)* in Figure 7.1-4 receives its blood supply from a branch of the pulmonary artery *(arrowheads)*.

Location of the stomach: the stomach is intra-abdominal with a cystic adenomatoid malformation and is usually intrathoracic with a diaphragmatic hernia.

Fetal diaphragmatic motion: the diaphragm moves normally with a cystic adenomatoid malformation and generally displays paradoxical motion with a diaphragmatic hernia (i.e., abdominal structures on the side with the intact diaphragm move inferiorly with inspiration, while structures on the affected side move superiorly).

7.2. PULMONARY SEQUESTRATION

Description and Clinical Features

A sequestration is a lobe or segment of lung with systemic blood supply (i.e., arterial supply from the aorta) and no communication with the tracheobronchial tree. A sequestration may be located either within the pleura that surrounds the normal lung (intrapulmonary sequestration) or be covered by its own pleura (extralobar sequestration). It is generally unilateral and is most often located in the left lower thorax but can also be situated just below the left hemidiaphragm. Like cystic adenomatoid malformations, sequestrations diagnosed *in utero* sometimes decrease in size as pregnancy progresses.

Sonography

A sequestration appears on ultrasound as a homogeneously echogenic mass located either within the thorax (Figure 7.2-1) or just below the diaphragm (Figure 7.2-2). Color Doppler can help to identify the arterial blood supply arising from the aorta (Figure 7.2-1). This finding helps to distinguish a sequestration from a type 3 (microcystic) cystic adenomatoid malformation of the lung, which receives its blood supply from the pulmonary artery.

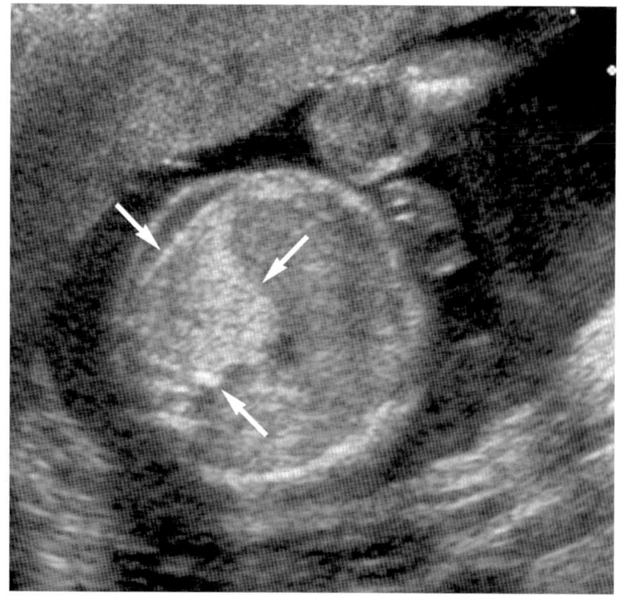

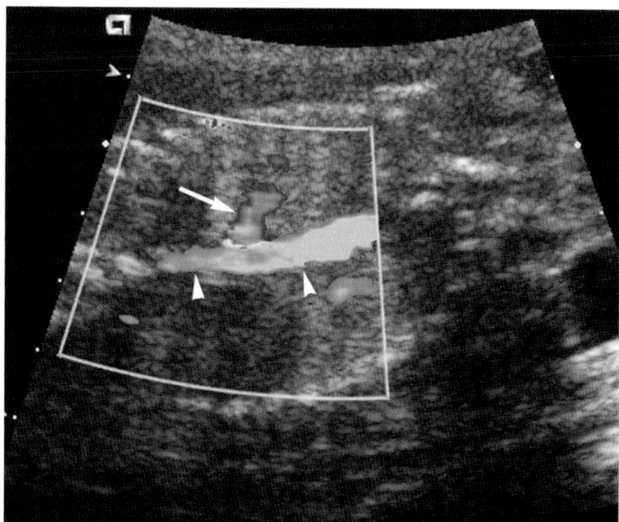

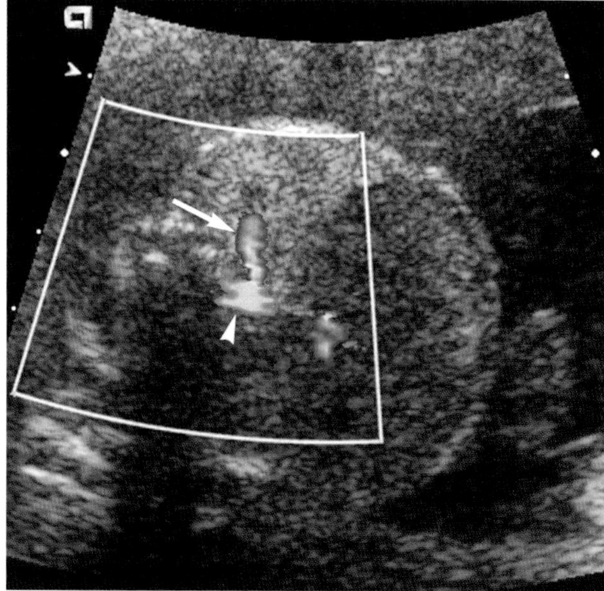

FIGURE 7.2-1. Pulmonary sequestration at the lung base. A: Transverse view of the fetal thorax reveals a homogeneously echogenic mass *(arrows)* in the posterior aspect of the left lower hemithorax. Coronal **(B)** and transverse **(C)** views with color Doppler demonstrate that the feeding vessel *(arrows)* to the mass is a branch of the descending thoracic aorta *(arrowheads)*.

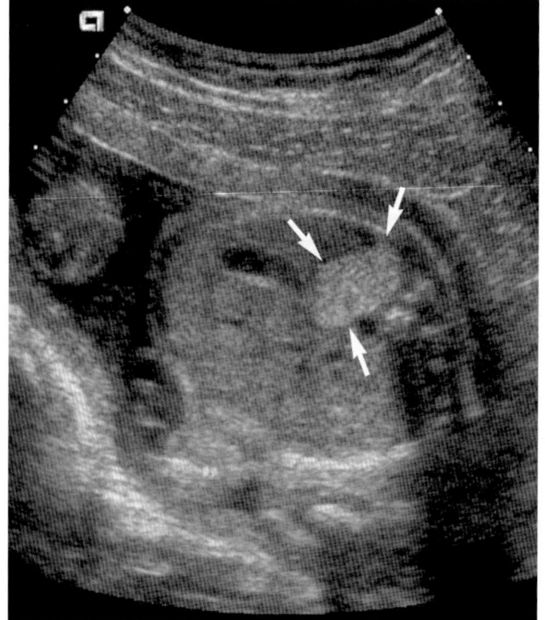

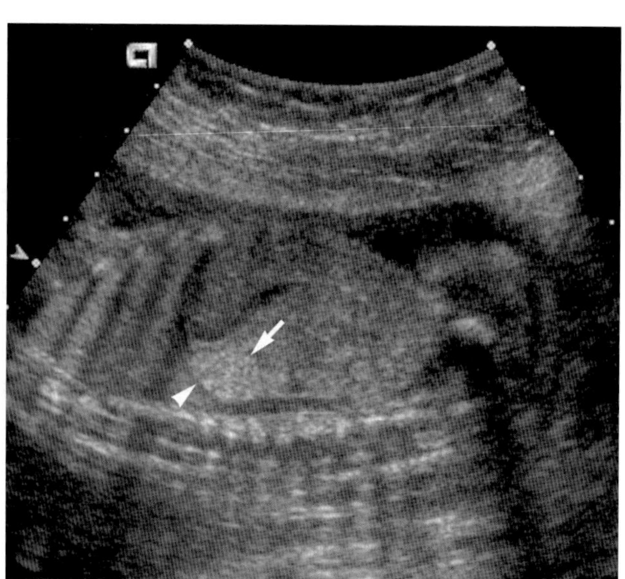

7.3. DIAPHRAGMATIC HERNIA

Description and Clinical Features

Diaphragmatic hernia refers to herniation of the intra-abdominal contents into the thorax through an opening in the diaphragm. Herniation usually occurs through one of the naturally occurring openings in the diaphragm, the anteriorly located foramen of Morgagni or the posteriorly located foramen of Bochdalek, and may be right or left sided. The most common variety is a left Bochdalek (posterior) hernia. Approximately 10%–20% of diaphragmatic hernias are right sided. In rare cases, there are bilateral Bochdalek hernias. Morgagni hernias are also rare.

The nature of the herniated tissue depends, in part, on the location of the hernia. With a left posterior hernia, the stomach is typically intrathoracic, and the bowel and/or liver may also lie within the thorax. With a right-sided hernia, the liver is generally intrathoracic, and there is often ascites in the thorax.

Prognosis with a diaphragmatic hernia is guarded because the neonate often has pulmonary hypertension and/or pulmonary hypoplasia. Associated anomalies are also common and contribute to the poor prognosis. With a left posterior hernia, *in utero* adverse prognostic features include the small size of the right lung and herniation of a portion of the liver into the thorax. *In utero* therapy, via tracheal occlusion to expand the lungs, has been attempted to improve fetal outcome, but the results have been disappointing.

Sonography

With a left diaphragmatic hernia, ultrasound demonstrates a left-sided thoracic mass that is generally heterogeneous and shifts the mediastinum to the right. Sonographic findings that permit differentiation of a left diaphragmatic hernia from a completely intrathoracic mass (e.g., cystic adenomatoid malformation) include the following:

- Presence of an intrathoracic stomach: seen as a smooth-walled intrathoracic fluid collection, with no stomach identified in the abdomen (Figure 7.3-1).
- Demonstration of an opening in the diaphragm, best seen on a sagittal view through the fetal thorax and abdomen as a disruption of the diaphragm through which material extends from the abdomen into the thorax.
- Observation of peristalsis within the thorax.
- Paradoxical motion of the intra-abdominal contents with fetal respiratory motion, such that abdominal structures on the right side (the side with the intact diaphragm) move inferiorly with inspiration while left-sided structures move superiorly toward the thorax or into it (Figure 7.3-1).

When a left diaphragmatic hernia has been diagnosed, sonographic features that predict a poor prognosis include the following:

- Presence of the liver within the thorax: Intrathoracic liver appears as a homogeneous mass in the thorax that is continuous with the intra-abdominal liver across the diaphragmatic defect. Continuity with the rest of the liver can be confirmed by demonstrating connecting hepatic vessels via color Doppler (Figure 7.3-2).
- Small size of the right lung: Because the heart is usually deviated to the right with a left diaphragmatic hernia, the right lung is generally located behind the heart. An index sometimes used for evaluating the size of the right lung is the lung/head ratio: the product of the anteroposterior and transverse diameters of the lung

FIGURE 7.2-2. Subdiaphragmatic pulmonary sequestration. A: Transverse view through the upper abdomen reveals a homogeneously echogenic mass *(arrows)* situated left posteriorly. **B:** Sagittal view demonstrates the mass *(arrow)* just below the left hemidiaphragm *(arrowhead).*

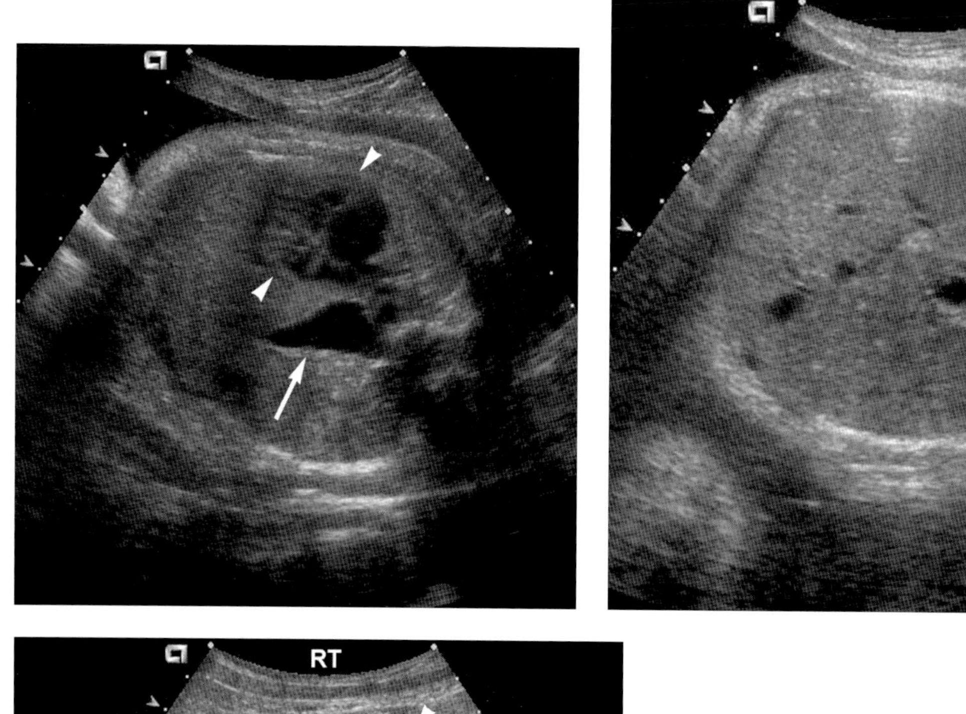

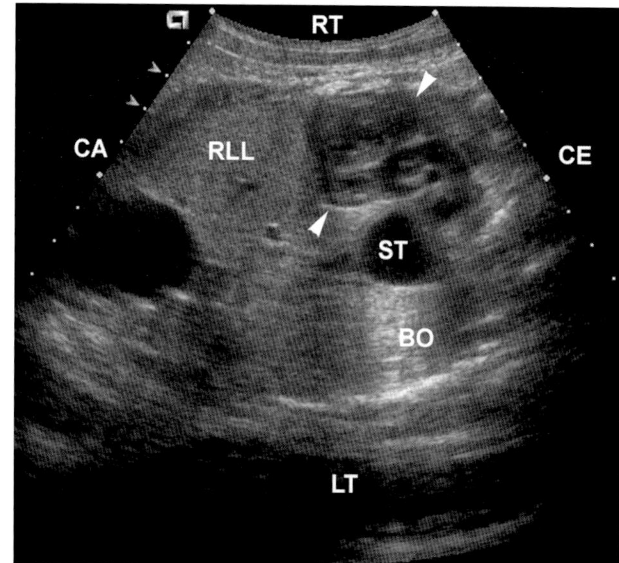

FIGURE 7.3-1. **Left diaphragmatic hernia. A:** Transverse view of the fetal thorax demonstrates a fluid-filled structure *(arrow)* in the thorax deviating the heart *(arrowheads)* to the right. **B:** There is no stomach identified on the transverse view of the upper abdomen, confirming that the fluid-filled structure in the thorax is the stomach. **C:** Coronal view of the thorax and abdomen (CE, cephalad; CA, caudad; RT, right; LT, left) demonstrates the stomach (ST) and bowel (BO) in the left hemithorax deviating the heart *(arrowheads)* to the right. The right lobe of the liver (RLL) lies within the abdomen. On real-time sonography, there was paradoxical motion during fetal respiration, such that the right lobe of the liver moved caudally and the stomach and herniated bowel moved in a cephalad direction during inspiration.

divided by the head circumference (all measured in millimeters) (Figure 7.3-3). At 24–26 weeks, a lung/head ratio less than 1.0 is associated with a dismal prognosis, a ratio between 1.0 and 1.4 with a moderate prognosis, and a ratio more than 1.4 with an excellent prognosis.

Presence of hydrops or other anomalies.

The most common sonographic finding with a right diaphragmatic hernia is deviation of the heart to the left by a solid homogeneous intrathoracic mass, representing the liver (Figure 7.3-4). Fluid is often present in the thorax. A right diaphragmatic hernia is more likely to be missed on ultrasound than a left diaphragmatic hernia because the liver and lung have similar sonographic appearances *in utero*. Leftward deviation of the heart may be the key observation indicating that an abnormality is present. The diagnosis of a right diaphragmatic hernia is then established by demonstrating an intrathoracic liver using gray-scale sonography and Doppler ultrasound.

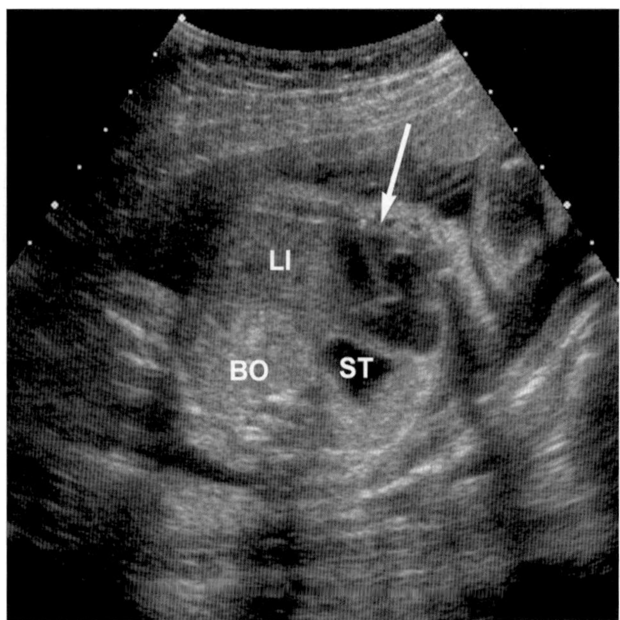

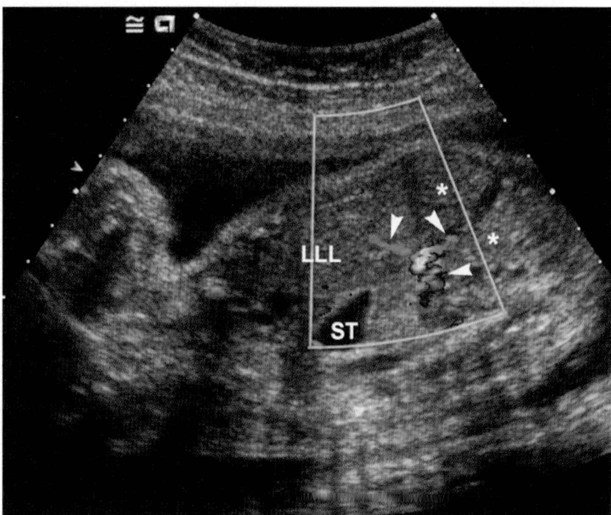

FIGURE 7.3-2. Left diaphragmatic hernia with an intrathoracic liver confirmed by color Doppler. A: Transverse view of the fetal thorax demonstrates a left diaphragmatic hernia with the heart *(arrow)* deviated to the right. The herniated tissue in the left hemithorax includes more echogenic tissue posteriorly, representing the bowel (BO), and somewhat less echogenic tissue anteriorly, representing liver (LI). The stomach (ST) lies in the thorax as well, displaced into the right hemithorax by the herniated bowel and liver. **B:** Sagittal view of the thorax and abdomen with color Doppler confirms that the left lobe of the liver (LLL) is herniated, as common vessels *(arrowheads)* extend from the intra-abdominal portions of the liver *(*)* into the thorax. The stomach (ST) is again seen within the thorax.

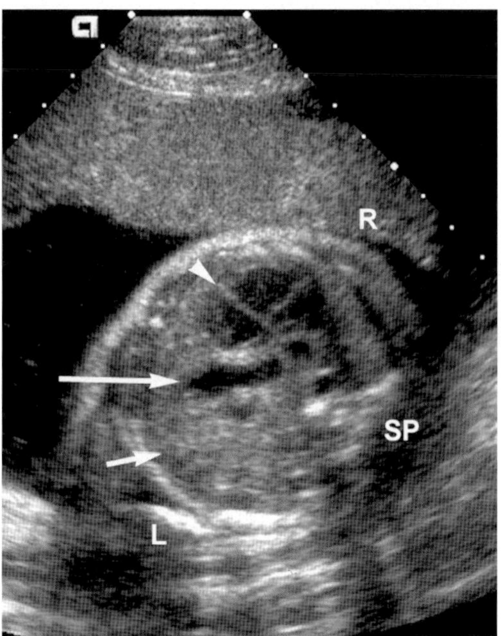

FIGURE 7.3-3. Left diaphragmatic hernia with a measurement of the lung-head ratio. A: Transverse view of the fetal thorax (L, left side; R, right side; SP, spine) demonstrates the heart *(arrowhead)* deviated to the right by the intrathoracic stomach *(long arrow)* and bowel *(short arrow)*.

(continued)

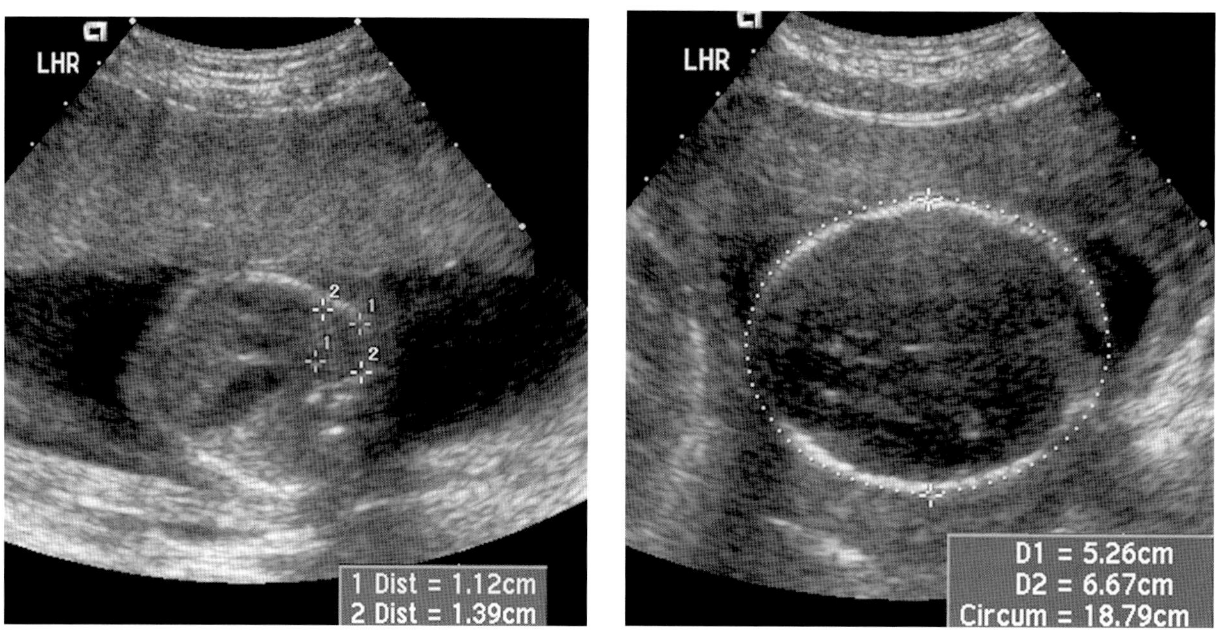

FIGURE 7.3-3. ***(continued)*** **B:** The right lung (calipers, 1.12 × 1.39 cm) lies posterior to the heart. **C:** Axial view of the fetal head demonstrates an elliptical caliper measuring the circumference to be 18.79 cm. The lung/head ratio, calculated using the measurements in millimeters, is (11.2 × 13.9)/187.9 or 0.83.

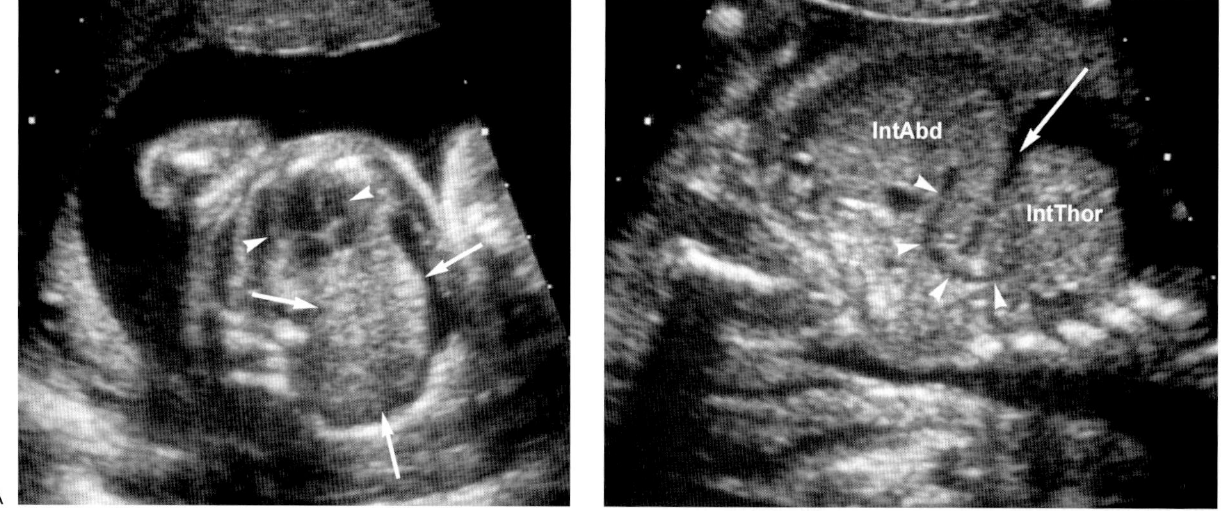

FIGURE 7.3-4. Right diaphragmatic hernia. A: Transverse view of the fetal thorax demonstrates a solid structure *(arrows)* in the right hemithorax deviating the heart *(arrowheads)* to the left. **B:** Right parasagittal view reveals that the intrathoracic (IntThor) structure is a portion of the liver with a vessel *(arrowheads)* connecting it to the intra-abdominal (IntAbd) portion of the liver. The diaphragm *(arrow)* is hypoechoic and can be seen indenting the liver where it herniates through the diaphragmatic defect.

7.4. TRACHEAL ATRESIA

Description and Clinical Features

If the trachea is atretic, pulmonary secretions remain trapped behind the atresia in the lungs. This leads to distention of the lungs. Tracheal atresia is likely to be fatal at birth if not diagnosed prenatally because the neonate will be unable to breathe, and attempts at establishing an airway may be futile.

Sonography

With tracheal atresia, both lungs are large and echogenic (Figure 7.4-1) owing to excessive fluid within the lungs and multiple interfaces between fluid and soft tissues. The heart appears relatively small within the thorax, and both hemidiaphragms are inverted owing to hyperexpansion of the lungs. The bronchi may be dilated, identifiable as distended fluid-filled tubular structures within the lungs. The fetus may be hydropic, likely due to increased intrathoracic pressure leading to decreased venous return to the heart.

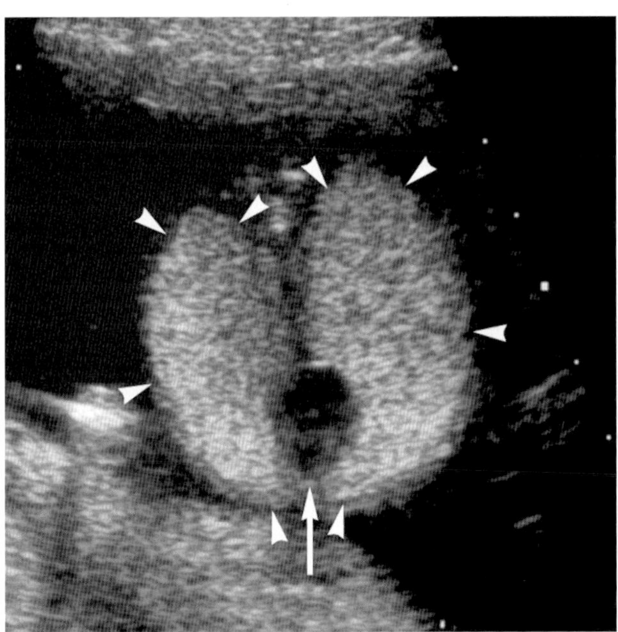

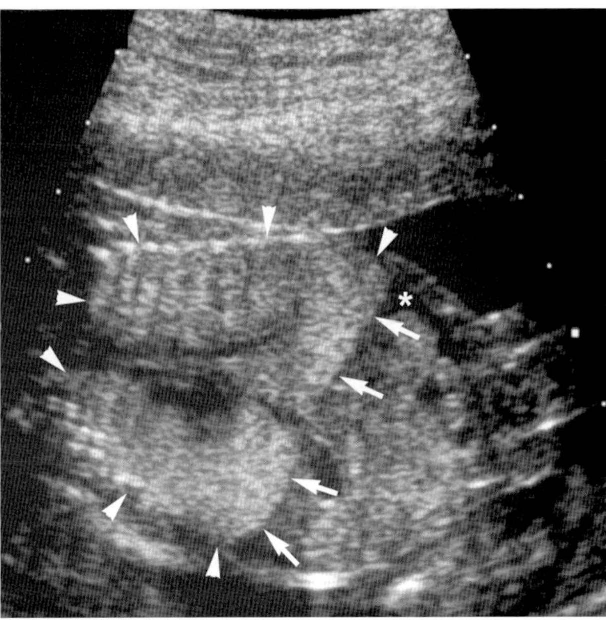

FIGURE 7.4-1. Tracheal atresia. A: Transverse view of the fetal thorax reveals the lungs *(arrowheads)* to be large and hyperechoic. The heart *(arrow)* is compressed by the enlarged lungs. **B:** Coronal view demonstrates large echogenic lungs *(arrowheads)* inverting the hemidiaphragms *(arrows)*. There is a moderate amount of ascites *(*)*, likely due to high intrathoracic pressure obstructing venous return.

7.5. UNILATERAL PULMONARY AGENESIS

Description and Clinical Features

Complete agenesis of a lung is a rare anomaly. It is often associated with other abnormalities, especially involving the contralateral lung, heart, and skeleton. The prognosis depends on the presence and severity of coexisting anomalies.

Sonography

The major sonographic finding with unilateral pulmonary agenesis is marked deviation of the heart to the extreme left or right lateral aspect of the thorax (Figure 7.5-1). To make

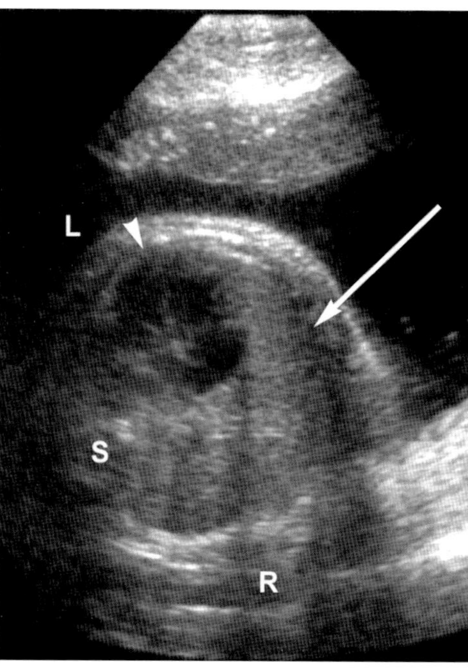

FIGURE 7.5-1. Unilateral pulmonary agenesis. Transverse view of the fetal thorax demonstrates that the heart *(arrowhead)* is deviated to the extreme left side (L) of the thorax (R, right side; S, spine). The right lung is seen *(arrow)*, but no left lung is identified.

the diagnosis of unilateral pulmonary agenesis, other entities that cause mediastinal shift, including thoracic masses and bronchial atresia, must be excluded. With unilateral pulmonary agenesis, the tissue adjacent to the heart has the echogenicity of normal lung. With intrathoracic masses and bronchial atresia, conversely, a heterogeneous mass or a hyperechoic lung is seen in the hemithorax opposite the heart.

7.6. TERATOMAS OF THE NECK AND MEDIASTINUM

Description and Clinical Features

Tumors of the fetal neck and mediastinum are most often teratomas, which derive from germ cells and are composed of multiple tissue types. The prognosis is related to the size of the tumor, the degree of vascularity, and the extent of tumor invasion into or compression of surrounding structures. These tumors tend to grow rapidly during gestation. If they are hypervascular, they can cause high-output congestive heart failure and hydrops in the fetus.

Sonography

A mediastinal teratoma appears as a complex mass in the midline and anterior chest. The mass is typically predominantly solid with some small cystic areas. Large mediastinal tumors may extend up into the neck. Teratomas may also arise primarily in the neck and extend into the mediastinum (Figure 7.6-1) or intracranially.

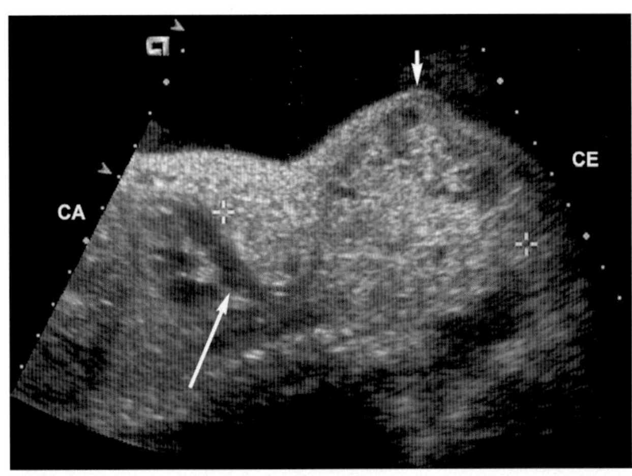

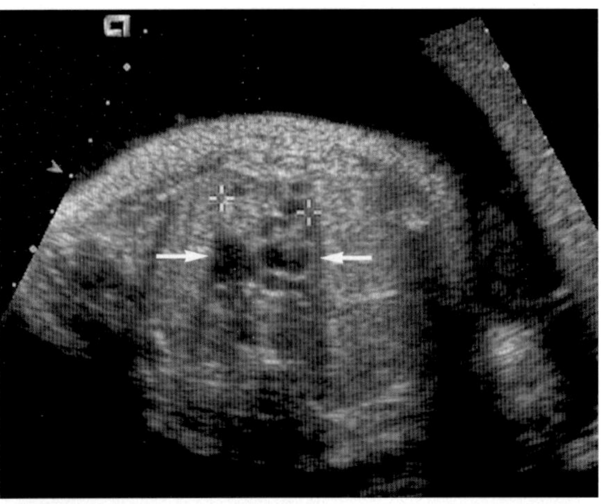

A B

FIGURE 7.6-1. Teratoma involving the neck and thorax. A: Sagittal view (CA, caudal; CE, cephalad) demonstrates a large echogenic mass *(calipers)* whose cephalad end is within the fetal neck, bulging it anteriorly *(short arrow)*, and whose caudal end is within the mediastinum adjacent to one of the great vessels *(long arrow)*. **B:** Transverse view of the thorax demonstrates the mass *(calipers)* in the mediastinum, anterior to the great vessels *(arrows)*.

7.7. THICKENED NUCHAL TRANSLUCENCY (11–14 WEEKS GESTATION)

Description and Clinical Features

The thickness of the tissue posterior to the cervical spine at 11–14 weeks has been found to have important prognostic significance. Abnormal thickening without a frank fluid collection is likely due to soft-tissue edema and has been associated with an increased likelihood of chromosomal anomalies, cardiac abnormalities, a variety of syndromes, and spontaneous miscarriage. Specific chromosomal anomalies associated with nuchal thickening include 45X (Turner syndrome) and trisomy 21 (Down syndrome) as well as trisomy 13 and trisomy 18.

If the nuchal translucency is thickened in a 11–14-week fetus, the parents should be counseled about the risk of aneuploidy and offered karyotype testing via amniocentesis or chorionic villus sampling. If the karyotype proves to be normal (or the parents elect not to undergo karyotype testing), a repeat sonogram should be performed at approximately 18 weeks to assess for cardiac or other structural anomalies.

Sonography

On ultrasound in the latter part of the first trimester, there is a sonolucent region (nuchal translucency or nuchal lucency) between the spine and posterior skin (Figure 7.7-1). The nuchal translucency can routinely be identified from the mid to late first trimester onward, and its upper limit of normal in thickness is approximately 2.2 mm at 11 weeks gestation, increasing to 2.8 mm at 14 weeks. The measurement is obtained from a midline sagittal view of the fetus, including only the hypoechoic zone, by placing the posterior cursor inside the echogenic skin. Care must be taken to distinguish the posterior skin surface from the amnion (Figure 7.7-2).

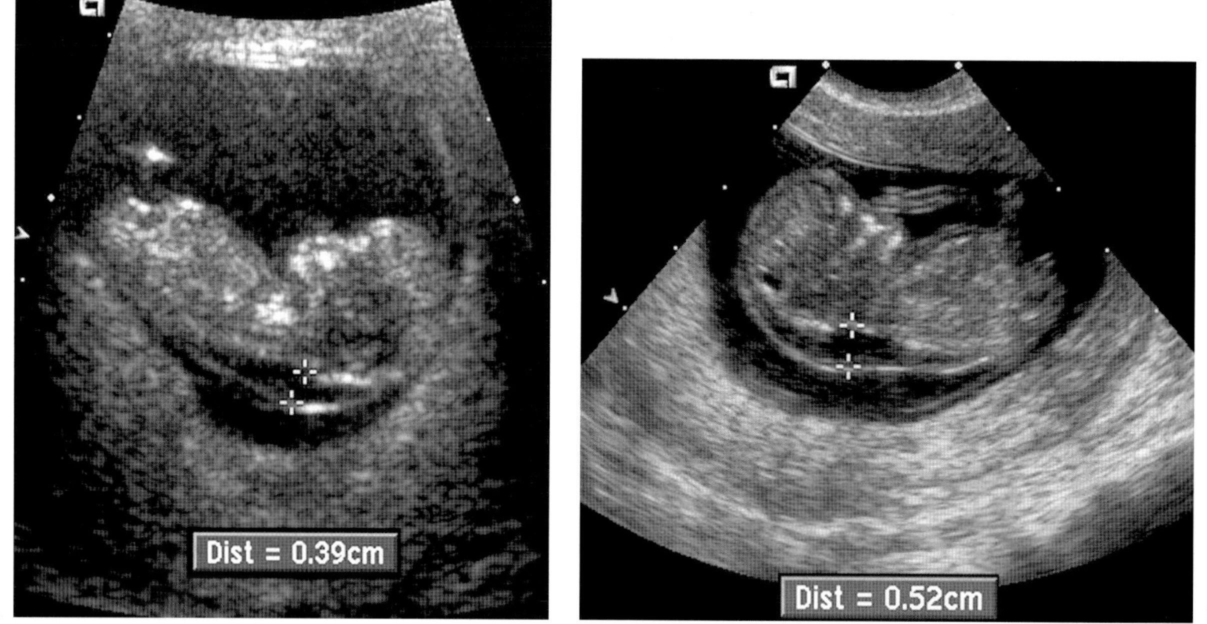

FIGURE 7.7-1. Thickened nuchal translucency. Sagittal views demonstrate thickened nuchal translucencies in two fetuses: nuchal translucency of 3.9 mm *(calipers)* in a fetus with normal chromosomes **(A)** and nuchal translucency of 5.2 mm *(calipers)* in a fetus with trisomy 18 **(B)**.

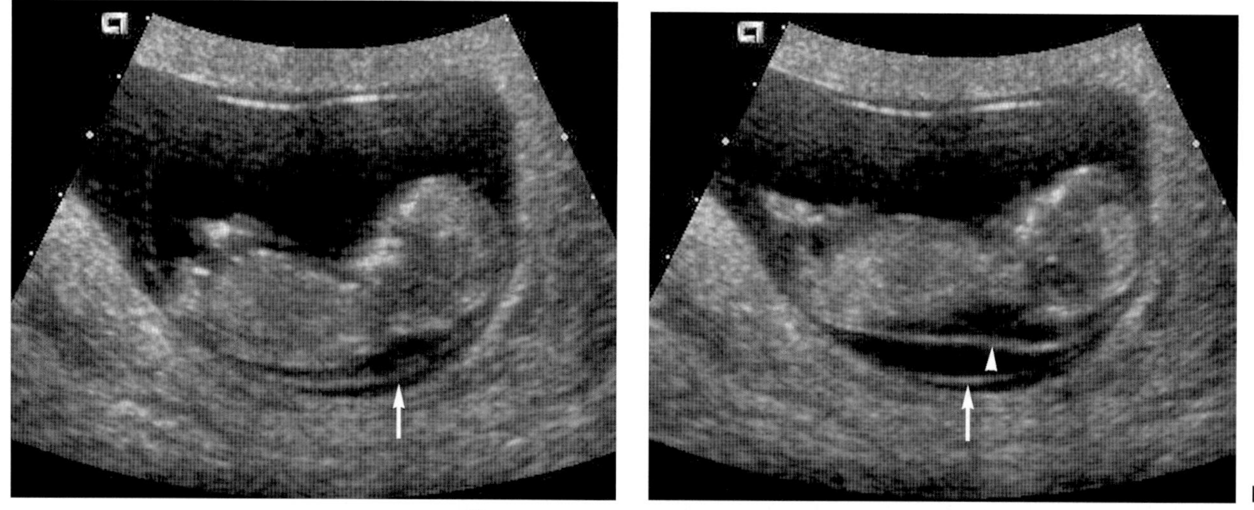

FIGURE 7.7-2. Thickened nuchal translucency potentially mistaken for the amnion. **A:** The fetus is lying supine, and there is a linear structure *(arrow)* behind the fetal neck. On this image, it is unclear whether this linear structure represents the amnion or the skin surface, and hence the nuchal translucency cannot be reliably measured. **B:** Shortly thereafter, the fetus jumped up, separating the skin surface *(arrowhead)* from the amnion *(arrow)*, revealing the nuchal translucency to be abnormally thick.

7.8. THICKENED NUCHAL FOLD (16–20 WEEKS GESTATION)

Description and Clinical Features

Neonates with trisomy 21 (Down syndrome) often have thickening of the soft tissues in the posterior neck. This has a prenatal analog because thickening of these soft tissues (the nuchal fold) at approximately 16–20 weeks gestation has been found to be associated with a ten- to 25-fold increased risk of trisomy 21. When a thickened nuchal fold is found in a 16–20-week fetus, the parents should be counseled about the risk of aneuploidy and offered karyotype testing via amniocentesis.

Sonography

The nuchal fold should be routinely measured on all sonograms performed between 16 and 20 weeks gestation. It is measured on a transverse view of the fetal head in a plane that is close to axial but angled slightly coronally to include the cerebellum and occipital bone. The measurement is taken from just outside the occipital bone to the outer skin surface (Figure 7.8-1). A nuchal fold measurement of 6 mm or larger is abnormal and should prompt a careful sonographic search for other anomalies, especially those associated with trisomy 21.

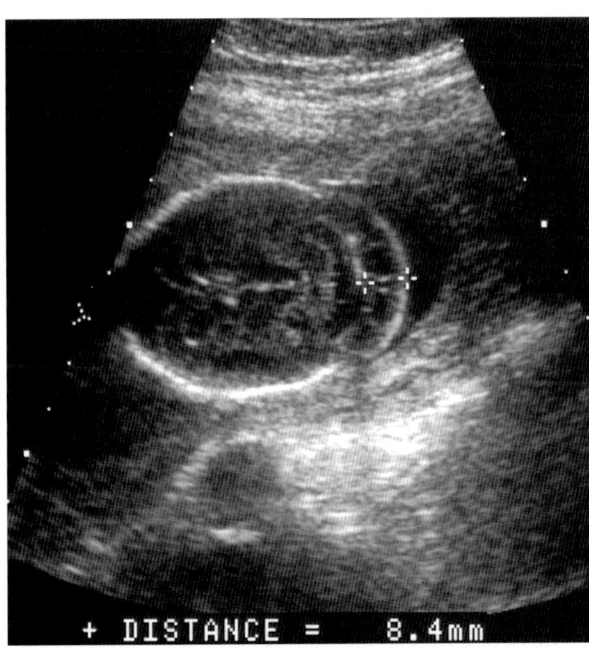

FIGURE 7.8-1. Thickened nuchal fold. Angled axial view through the fetal head, taken in a plane that includes the cerebellum and occipital bone, demonstrates an abnormally thickened nuchal fold measuring 8.4 mm in thickness *(calipers)*.

7.9. CYSTIC HYGROMA AND LYMPHANGIECTASIA

Description and Clinical Features

A cystic hygroma is a uni- or multilocular subcutaneous mass filled with lymphatic fluid. It most commonly occurs in the posterior neck, although it can be seen elsewhere in the body.

A cystic hygroma results from a localized area of lymphatic dysplasia, with dilation of, or leakage from, lymphatic vessels. If the subcutaneous lymphatic dysplasia is widespread, fluid collections and/or subcutaneous edema will encompass the entire fetal body (generalized lymphangiectasia). Even when generalized, the largest fluid collections are typically in the posterior neck.

Fetuses with Turner syndrome (45X karyotype), trisomy 21 (Down syndrome), trisomy 13, and trisomy 18 are at elevated risk of cystic hygromas or generalized lym-

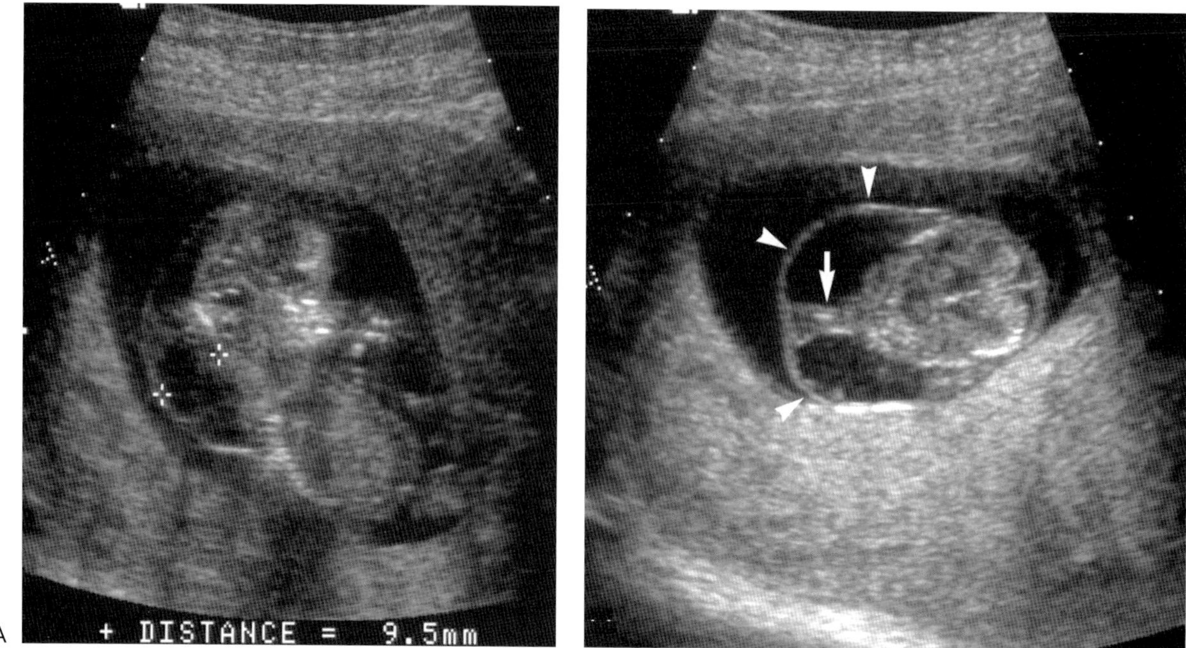

FIGURE 7.9-1. Nuchal cystic hygroma in the first trimester. A: In this 12-week fetus, a sagittal view demonstrates a 9.5-mm complex cystic mass *(calipers)* behind the fetal head and neck. **B:** Transverse view demonstrates a largely cystic mass *(arrowheads)* with septation *(arrow)*. The fetus was found to have Turner syndrome (45X).

phangiectasia. In view of this, the sonographic finding of cystic hygroma or generalized lymphangiectasia should prompt genetic counseling. Regardless of the fetal karyotype, fetuses with severe generalized lymphangiectasia have high mortality rates.

Sonography

A cystic hygroma appears sonographically as a cystic mass in the subcutaneous tissues, generally in the posterior neck (Figure 7.9-1 and 7.9-2). In some cases, one or more septations are present. Cystic hygromas can also occur elsewhere in the body (Figure 7.9-3).

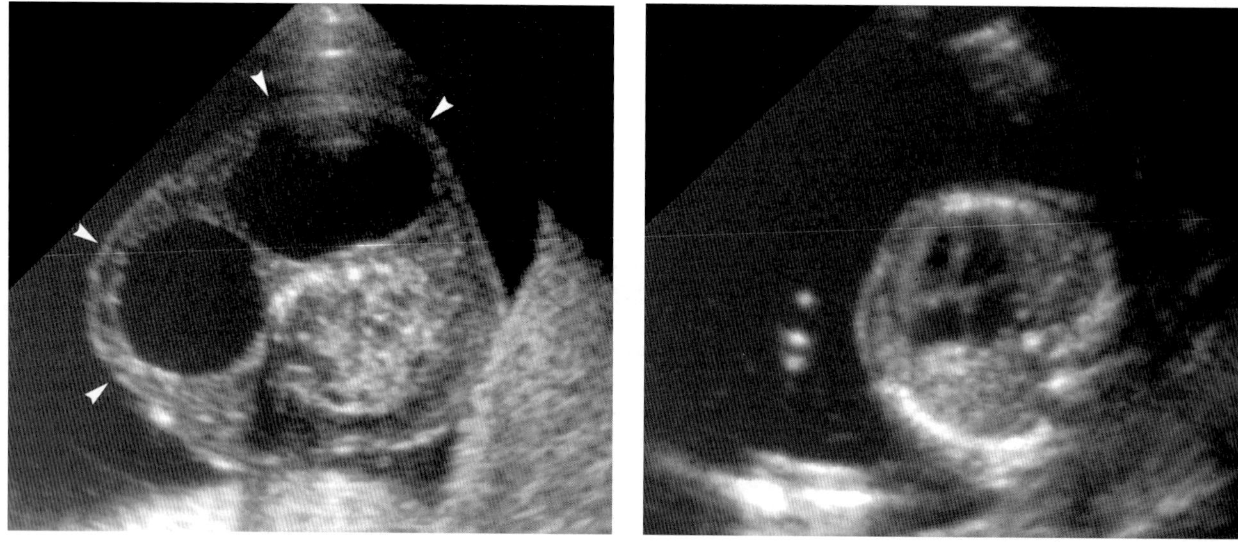

FIGURE 7.9-2. Nuchal cystic hygroma in the second trimester. A: Transverse view through the fetal neck demonstrates a large septate cystic mass *(arrowheads)* posteriorly. The mass was localized to this region, with the thorax **(B)** and abdomen **(C)** appearing normal.

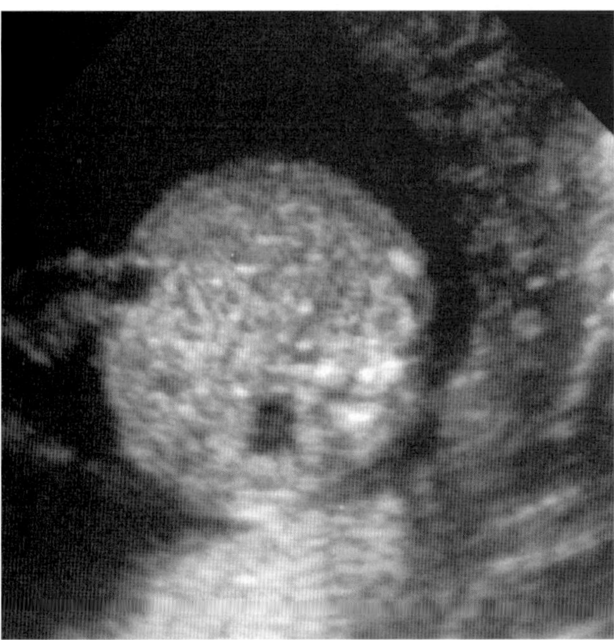

C

FIGURE 7.9-2C. ***(continued).***

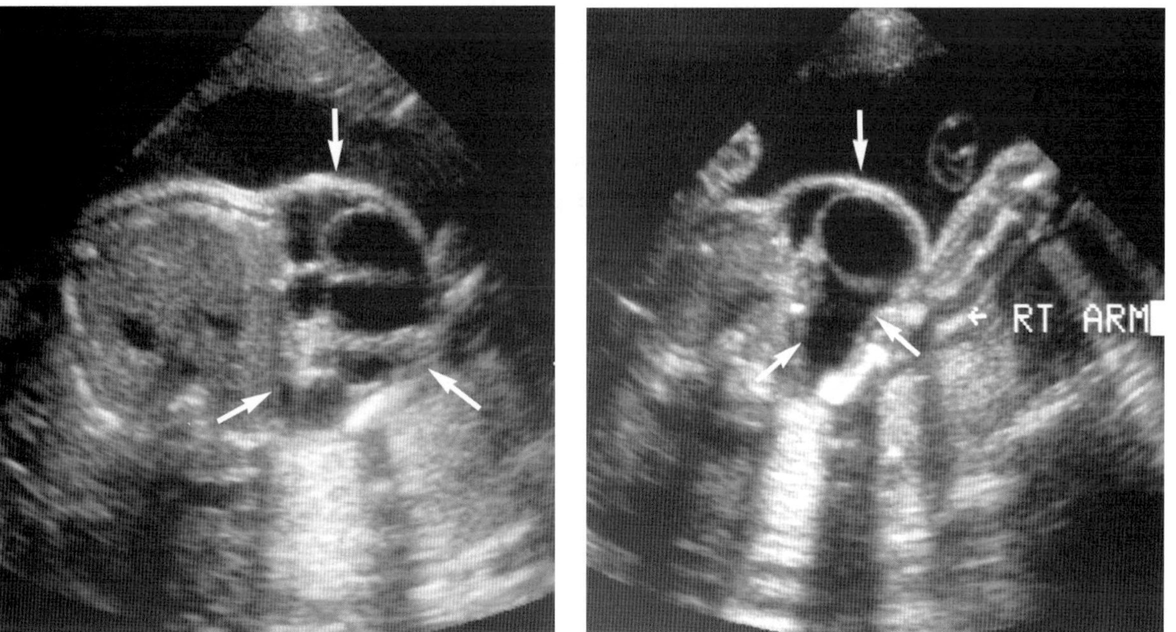

A B

FIGURE 7.9-3. Cystic hygroma involving the lateral thoracic and abdominal walls. A: Transverse view of the fetal abdomen reveals a multiseptate cystic mass (arrows) involving the right lateral abdominal wall. **B:** Transverse view of the fetal thorax reveals that the multiseptate cystic mass *(arrows)* extends up to the right axilla.

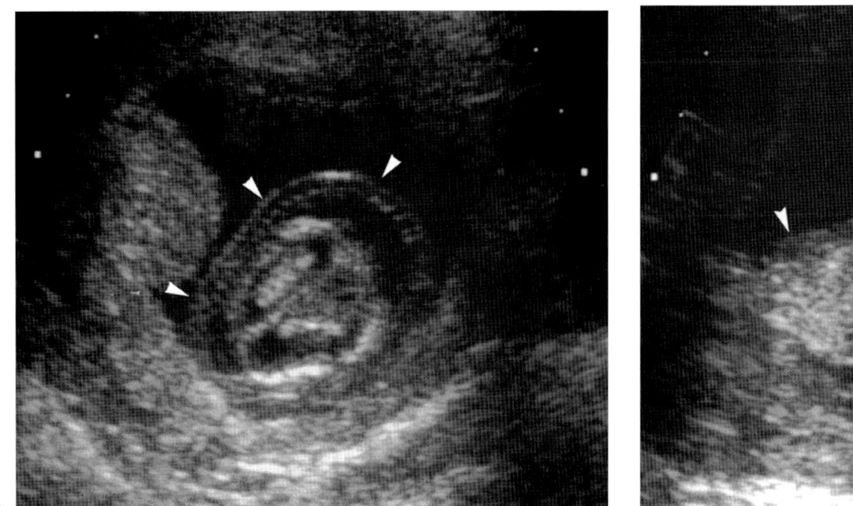

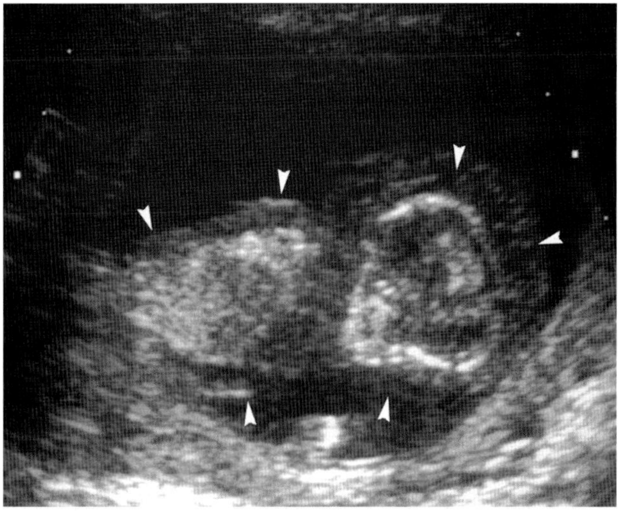

FIGURE 7.9-4. Lymphangiectasia. A: Transverse view of the head of this 14-week fetus demonstrates marked thickening of the subcutaneous tissues *(arrowheads)*, representing subcutaneous edema. **B:** Sagittal view reveals generalized subcutaneous edema *(arrowheads)* around the entire fetus. The fetus died 2 weeks later and was found to have trisomy 18.

With generalized lymphangiectasia, the entire fetus is surrounded by a hypoechoic halo, representing subcutaneous edema (Figure 7.9-4). There may be well-defined cystic spaces interspersed within the diffuse edema. In some cases, ascites, pleural effusions, or pericardial effusions may be present as well.

7.10. PLEURAL EFFUSION

Description and Clinical Features

Pleural effusion may occur as an isolated thoracic abnormality or as a component of generalized hydrops. Isolated pleural effusions, which may be unilateral or bilateral, are thought to be due, in most cases, to lymphatic duct dysplasia. This entity is often referred to as primary chylothorax because the pleural fluid is milky (chylous) in the neonate owing to the presence in lymphatic fluid of chylomicrons, which are microscopic particles of fat derived from ingested milk. In the fetus, the pleural fluid is serous and straw colored.

Some cases of isolated pleural effusions are transient, with the effusion disappearing without intervention. In other cases, *in utero* thoracentesis or pleuroamniotic shunting may be useful to permit lung expansion or improve hydrops.

Sonography

A pleural effusion appears as an anechoic rim around a fetal lung. Effusions may be unilateral or bilateral and, if bilateral, may be symmetric (Figure 7.10-1) or asymmetric (Figure 7.10-2). They may be transient, appearing at one time and then resolving spontaneously by the time of a follow-up sonogram (Figure 7.10-3). If the effusion is large, the lung appears as a small nubbin of tissue adjacent to the mediastinum.

When the effusion is due to thoracic lymphatic dysplasia (primary chylothorax), there is often skin thickening around the thorax (Figure 7.10-1). Unlike generalized lymphangiectasia or hydrops, the fluid and skin thickening in fetuses with primary chylothorax are restricted to the thorax.

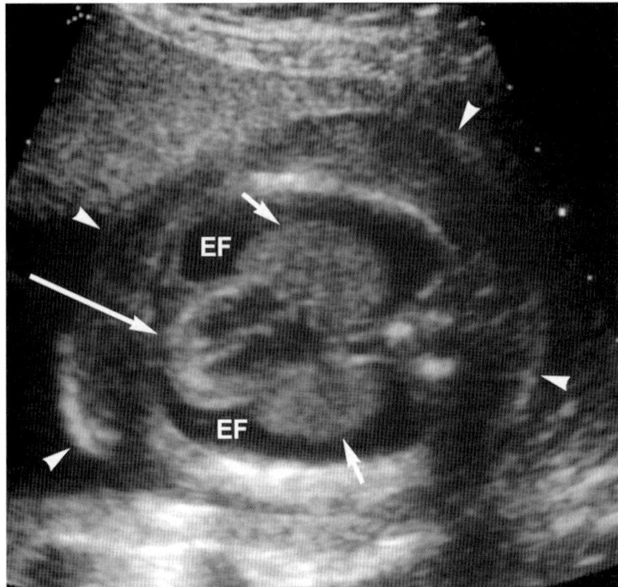

FIGURE 7.10-1. Bilateral pleural effusions. Transverse view through the thorax demonstrates moderate-size bilateral pleural effusions (EF) surrounding the lungs *(short arrows)* and heart *(long arrow)*. There is subcutaneous edema *(arrowheads)* around the thorax.

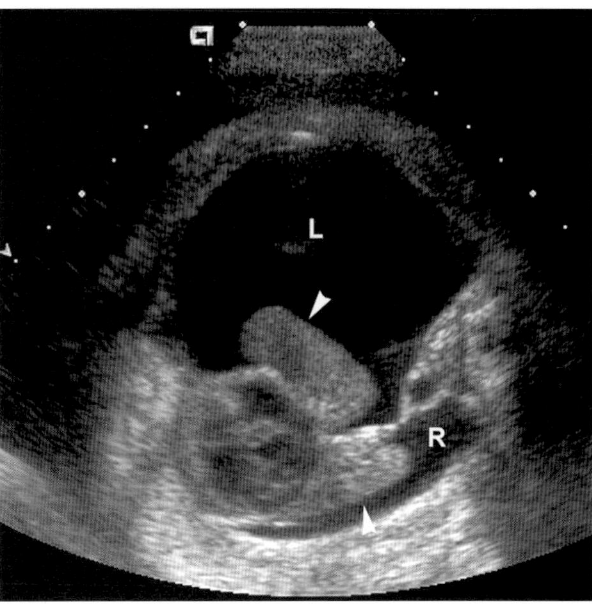

FIGURE 7.10-2. Asymmetric pleural effusions. Transverse view through the thorax reveals a large left pleural effusion (L) and a small right pleural effusion (R) surrounding the lungs *(arrowheads)*.

A
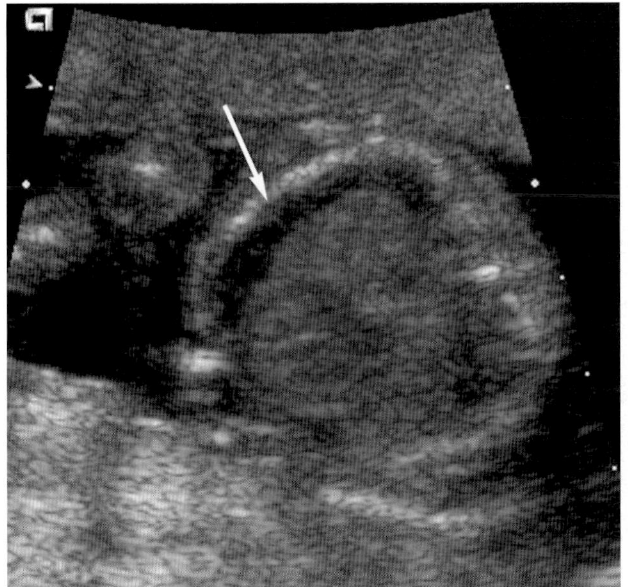

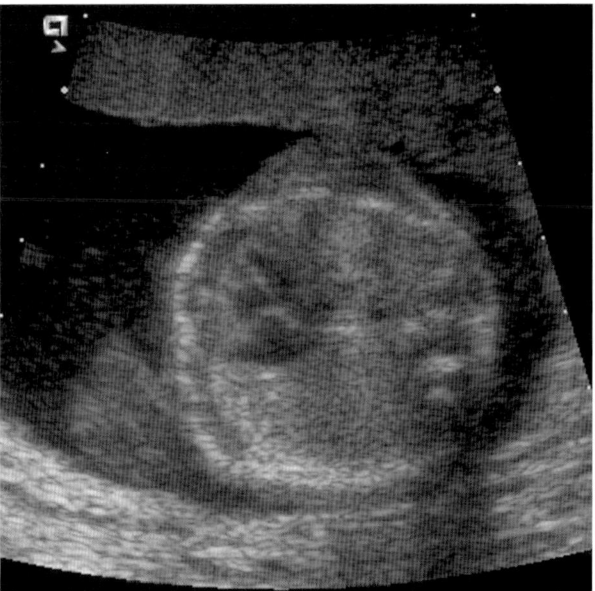
B

FIGURE 7.10-3. Spontaneously resolving pleural effusions. A: Transverse view through the thorax demonstrates a left pleural *effusion (arrow)* at 18 weeks gestation. **B:** The effusion is no longer present at 20 weeks.

7.11. HYDROPS

Description and Clinical Features

Hydrops is most commonly defined as the presence of at least two of the following abnormal intrafetal fluid collections: pleural effusion(s), pericardial effusion, ascites, and subcutaneous edema. A partial list of causes includes the following:

- Immune hydrops: hydrops due to fetal anemia resulting from maternal antibodies crossing the placenta and destroying fetal red blood cells (e.g., Rh incompatibility)
- Nonimmune hydrops
  - Fetal structural anomaly
    - Cardiac (e.g., hypoplastic ventricle, atrioventricular canal)
    - Lymphatic dysplasia
    - Cystic adenomatoid malformation
    - Diaphragmatic hernia
  - Fetal arrhythmia (e.g., supraventricular tachycardia)
  - Fetal chromosomal anomaly [e.g., Turner syndrome (45X); trisomy 13, 18, 21]
  - Fetal anemia (nonimmune, e.g., thalassemia)
  - Fetal infection (e.g., cytomegalovirus, toxoplasmosis)
  - Placental chorioangioma
  - Idiopathic

In utero treatment options are available for a number of causes of hydrops, including fetal anemia (immune or nonimmune), arrhythmias, and toxoplasmosis. Most other causes of hydrops, including idiopathic nonimmune hydrops, carry a poor prognosis.

Sonography

Ultrasound plays an important role in diagnosing hydrops, determining its cause, and guiding treatment. The sonographic diagnosis of hydrops follows directly from its defin-

A

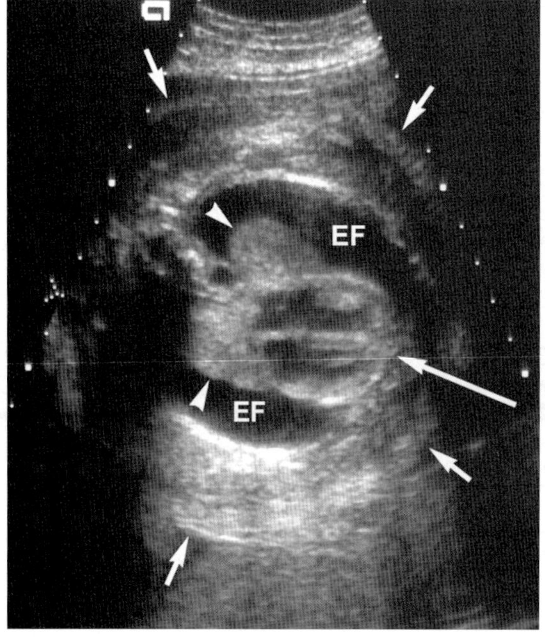

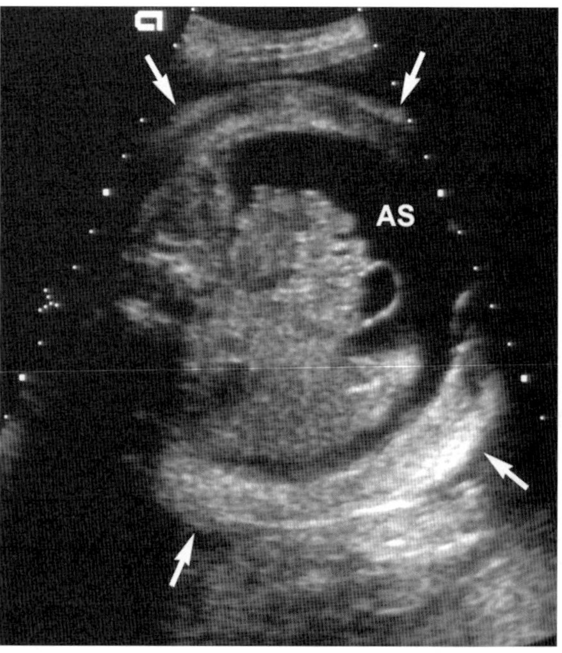

B

FIGURE7.11-1. Idiopathic nonimmune hydrops. A: Transverse view of the thorax demonstrates bilateral pleural effusions (EF) outlining the lungs *(arrowheads)* and heart *(long arrow)*. There is subcutaneous edema *(short arrows)* around the thorax. **B:** Transverse view of the abdomen demonstrates ascites (AS) and subcutaneous edema *(arrows)*.

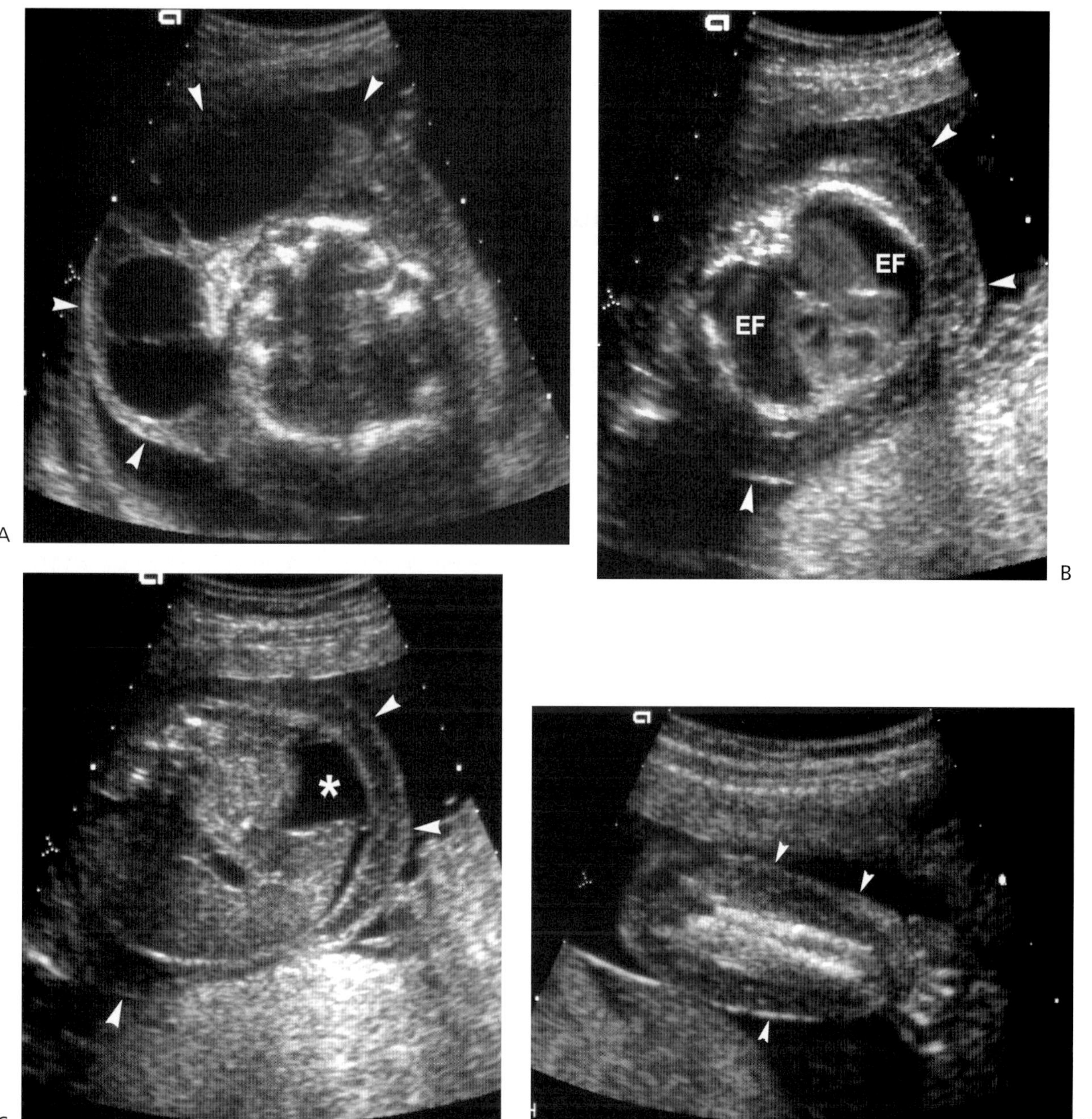

FIGURE 7.11-2. Hydrops with a cystic hygroma. A: Transverse view of the neck demonstrates a large cystic hygroma posteriorly *(arrowheads).* **B:** Transverse view of the thorax demonstrates subcutaneous edema *(arrowheads)* and bilateral pleural effusions (EF). **C:** Transverse view of the abdomen demonstrates subcutaneous edema *(arrowheads)* and ascites *(*).* **D:** Longitudinal view of a forearm demonstrates subcutaneous edema *(arrowheads).*

ition: visualization of at least two of the following: pleural effusion(s), pericardial effusion, ascites, and subcutaneous edema (Figures 7.11-1 and 7.11-2). When subcutaneous edema is present, there are often coexisting focal uni- or multilocular fluid collections (cystic hygromas) in the soft tissues, especially in the posterior nuchal region (Figure 7.11-2). In addition to these fetal findings, the placenta is often thick and polyhydramnios may be present.

When hydrops is diagnosed by sonography, an attempt should be made to determine its cause. In particular, a careful fetal anatomic survey should be performed, with particular attention to the fetal heart and thorax, the fetal cardiac rate and rhythm should be assessed, and the placenta should be examined for chorioangiomas. When appropriate, ultrasound-guided amniocentesis (to evaluate for aneuploidy or infection) or percutaneous umbilical blood sampling (to assess for anemia or aneuploidy) can be carried out. If the fetus is found to be anemic, it can be treated by means of ultrasound-guided blood transfusion.

SUGGESTED READINGS

1. Benacerraf BR, Adzick NS. Fetal diaphragmatic hernia: ultrasound diagnosis and clinical outcome in 19 cases. *Am J Obstet Gynecol* 1987;156:573–576.
2. Benacerraf BR, Neuberg D, Bromley B, et al. Sonographic scoring index for prenatal detection of chromosomal abnormalities. *J Ultrasound Med* 1992;11:449–458.
3. Bromley B, Parad R, Estroff JA, et al. Fetal lung masses: prenatal course and outcome. *J Ultrasound Med* 1995;14:927–936.
4. Challis DE, Ryan G, Jefferies A. Fetal hydrops. In: Rumack CM, Wilson SR, Charboneau JW, eds. *Diagnostic ultrasound*, 2nd ed. St. Louis: Mosby, 1998:1303–1322.
5. Comstock CH, Kirk JS. The fetal chest and abdomen. In: Rumack CM, Wilson SR, Charboneau JW, eds. *Diagnostic ultrasound*, 2nd ed. St. Louis: Mosby, 1998:1069–1092.
6. Goldstein RB. Ultrasound evaluation of the fetal thorax. In: Callen PW, ed. *Ultrasonography in obstetrics and gynecology*, 4th ed. Philadelphia: WB Saunders, 2000:427–455.
7. Guibaud L, Filiatrault D, Garel L, et al. Fetal congenital diaphragmatic hernia: accuracy of sonography in diagnosis and prediction of the outcome after birth. *AJR Am J Roentgenol* 1996;166: 1195–1202.
8. Hagay Z, Reece EA, Roberts A, et al. Isolated fetal pleural effusion: a prenatal management dilemma. *Obstet Gynecol* 1993;81:147–152.
9. Hiippala A, Eronen M, Taipale P, et al. Fetal nuchal translucency and normal chromosomes: a long-term follow-up study. *Ultrasound Obstet Gynecol* 2001;18:18–22.
10. Jeanty P, Goncalves LF. Neck and chest fetal anomalies. In: Fleischer AC, Manning FA, Jeanty P, et al., eds. *Sonography in obstetrics & gynecology: principles and practice*, 6th ed. New York: McGraw-Hill, 2001:389–407.
11. Kuller JA, Yankowitz J, Goldberg JD, et al. Outcome of antenatally diagnosed cystic adenomatoid malformations. *Am J Obstet Gynecol* 1992;167:1038–1041
12. Michailidis GD, Economides DL. Nuchal translucency measurement and pregnancy outcome in karyotypically normal fetuses. *Ultrasound Obstet Gynecol* 2001;17:102–105.
13. Pandya PP, Kondylios A, Hilbert L, et al. Chromosomal defects and outcome in 1015 fetuses with increased nuchal translucency. *Ultrasound Obstet Gynecol* 1995;5:15–19.
14. Scott JN, Trevenen CL, Wiseman DA, et al. Tracheal atresia: ultrasonographic and pathologic correlation. *J Ultrasound Med* 1999;18:375–377.
15. Sherer DM, Manning FA. First-trimester nuchal translucency screening for fetal aneuploidy. In: Fleischer AC, Manning FA, Jeanty P, et al., eds. *Sonography in obstetrics & gynecology: principles and practice*, 6th ed. New York: McGraw-Hill, 2001:89–112.
16. Souka AP, Krampl E, Bakalis S, et al. Outcome of pregnancy in chromosomally normal fetuses with increased nuchal translucency in the first trimester. *Ultrasound Obstet Gynecol* 2001;18:9–17.
17. Taipale P, Hiilesmaa V, Salonen R, et al. Increased nuchal translucency as a marker for fetal chromosomal defects. *N Engl J Med* 1997;337:1654–1658.
18. van Vugt JMG, van Zalen-Sprock RM, Kostense PJ. First-trimester nuchal translucency: a risk analysis on fetal chromosome abnormality. *Radiology* 1996;200:537–540.

8

HEART

8.1. OVERVIEW OF CONGENITAL HEART DISEASE

Congenital heart disease affects between 1 and 8 per 1,000 livebirths and 27 per 1,000 stillbirths. The risk of congenital heart disease increases if one parent has congenital heart disease or if the couple has had a previous child with congenital heart disease. Risks are also increased with a variety of genetic syndromes, both dominant and recessive, and with aneuploidy. Approximately 5% of infants born with cardiac anomalies have a positive family history of congenital heart disease, whereas approximately 12% have abnormal chromosomes.

Cardiac anomalies detected prenatally tend to be more severe than those missed on prenatal ultrasound. Thus, the survival rate of only 17% for cardiac defects detected prenatally is much worse than the survival rate of approximately 80% for anomalies undetected before birth. Approximately one-fourth of infants born with congenital heart disease have other anomalies as well.

8.2. HYPOPLASTIC LEFT HEART SYNDROME AND AORTIC STENOSIS

Description and Clinical Features

Hypoplastic left heart syndrome is a group of cardiac malformations characterized by a small or absent left ventricle. Hypoplasia of the left ventricle occurs as a result of abnormalities that limit the flow of blood through the left side of the heart, including stenosis or atresia of the foramen ovale, mitral valve, or aortic valve.

Aortic stenosis or atresia most commonly results from an abnormal aortic valve, but occasionally the obstruction occurs in the subaortic region of the left ventricular outflow tract or beyond the valve. Not all cases of aortic stenosis or atresia lead to hypoplasia of the left ventricle. In particular, in some cases of aortic stenosis or atresia, a ventricular septal defect is present, allowing some blood to flow through the left ventricle, preventing the development of a hypoplastic left ventricle. Even in cases of aortic stenosis or atresia without a ventricular septal defect, the left ventricle may not become hypoplastic but may instead develop myocardial fibroelastosis, becoming progressively less contractile.

In general, the prognosis for a hypoplastic left ventricle is poor. Fetuses may develop hydrops *in utero* and may die before birth. The prognosis for aortic stenosis is related to the degree of function of the left ventricle.

Sonography

A hypoplastic left ventricle can be diagnosed on a four-chamber view of the heart by demonstrating a small left ventricle (Figure 8.2-1), often with poor contractility. The size of the left ventricular chamber is variable. In some cases, no left ventricle can be identified (Figure 8.2-2). In others, the left ventricle is only somewhat smaller than the right (Figure 8.2-1). With myocardial fibroelastosis, the left ventricular myocardium becomes

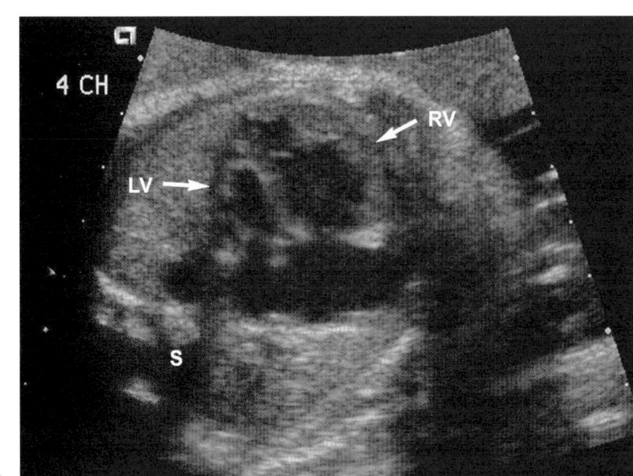

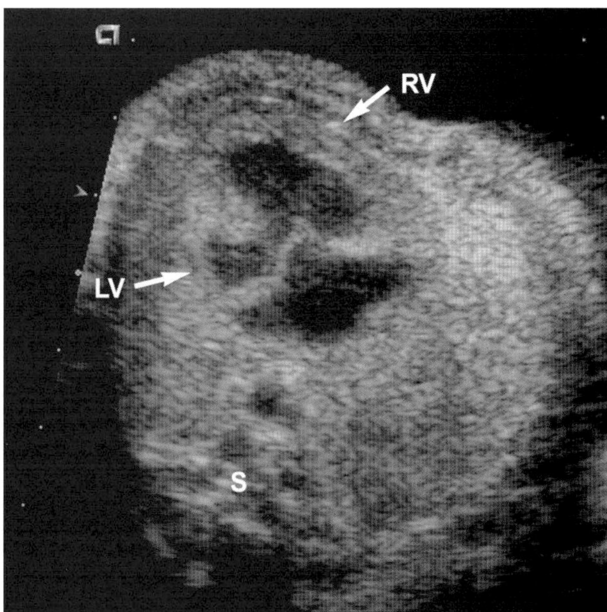

FIGURE 8.2-1. **Hypoplastic left ventricle. A and B:** Transverse images of a fetal thorax at the level of the four-chamber view of the heart in two different fetuses with hypoplastic left ventricles demonstrate small left ventricles *(LV arrow)* and larger right ventricles *(RV arrow)*. S, spine; 4CH, four-chamber heart.

echogenic and poorly contractile (Figure 8.2-3), and the left ventricular size may be normal or even enlarged.

Aortic stenosis is characterized by narrowing of the aortic valve and decreased movement of the valve leaflets. The narrowed aortic valve can be visualized on a long axis view of the left ventricle and left ventricular outflow tract (Figure 8.2-4). The width of the valve can be measured and compared with norms for gestational age. The stenotic valve is often brightly echogenic. The ascending aorta may be enlarged due to poststenotic dilation.

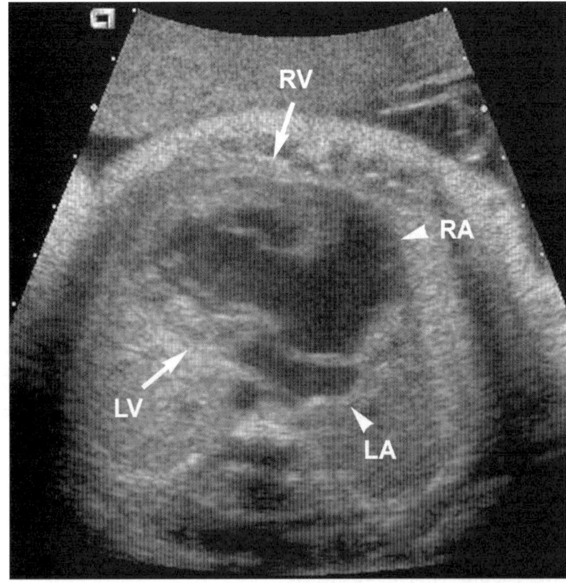

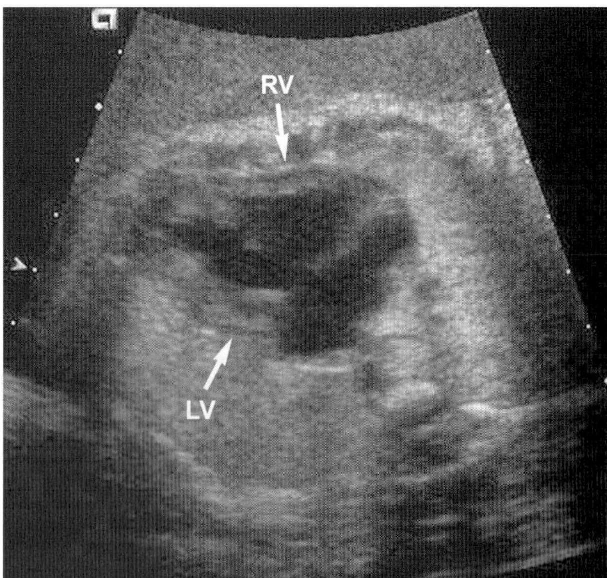

FIGURE 8.2-2. **Hypoplastic left ventricle with no left ventricular chamber. A:** Transverse image of the thorax demonstrates a heart with a large right ventricle *(RV arrow)* and no appreciable left ventricular chamber *(LV arrow)* (*LA arrow*, left atrium; *RA arrow*, right atrium). **B:** Transverse image of the heart in another fetus with a large right ventricle *(RV arrow)* and no left ventricular chamber *(LV arrow)*.

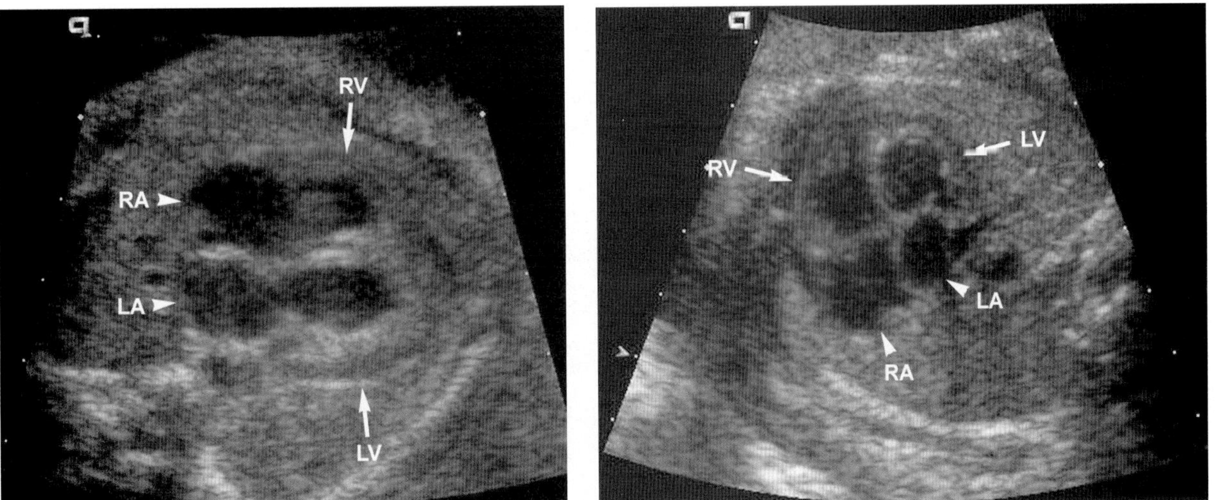

FIGURE 8.2-3. Left ventricular myocardial fibroelastosis. A and B: Four-chamber views of the heart in two different fetuses developing hypoplastic left ventricles demonstrate echogenic left ventricular walls *(LV arrow)* with poor left ventricular contractility. (*RV arrow*, right ventricle; *LA arrowhead*, left atrium; *RA arrowhead*, right atrium).

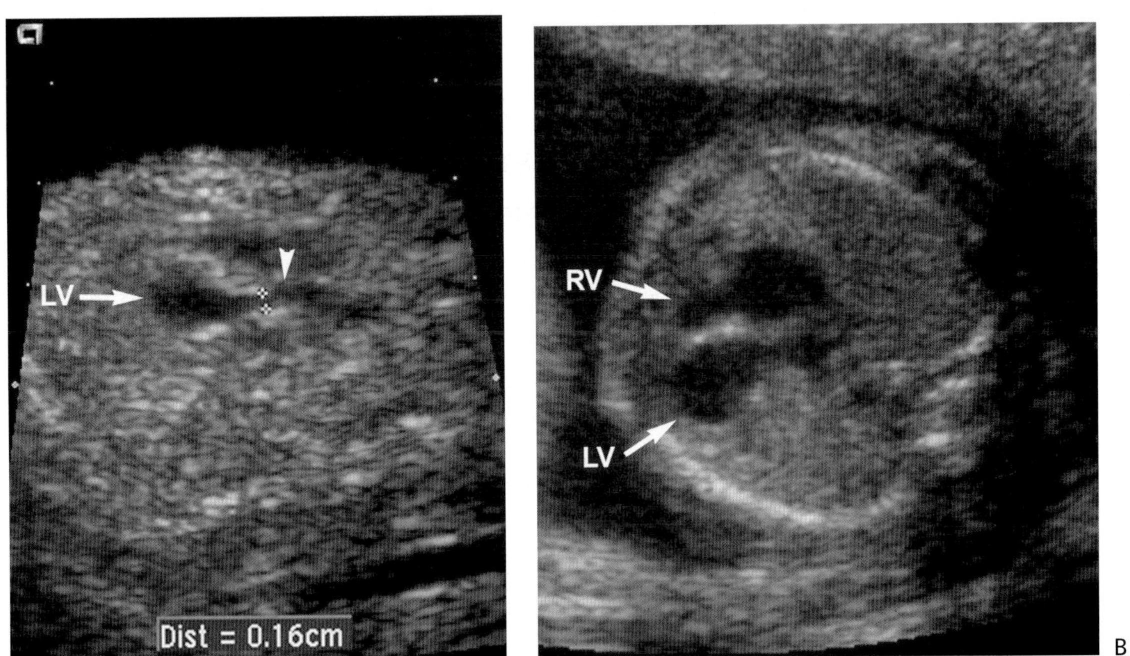

FIGURE 8.2-4. Aortic stenosis with hypoplastic left ventricle. A: Longitudinal image of left ventricular *(LV arrow)* outflow tract to the aorta *(arrowhead)*. The aortic valve *(calipers)* is narrowed. **B:** Four-chamber image of the heart demonstrates a mildly dilated left ventricle *(LV arrow)* with a calcified wall. (*RV arrow*, right ventricle). *(continued)*

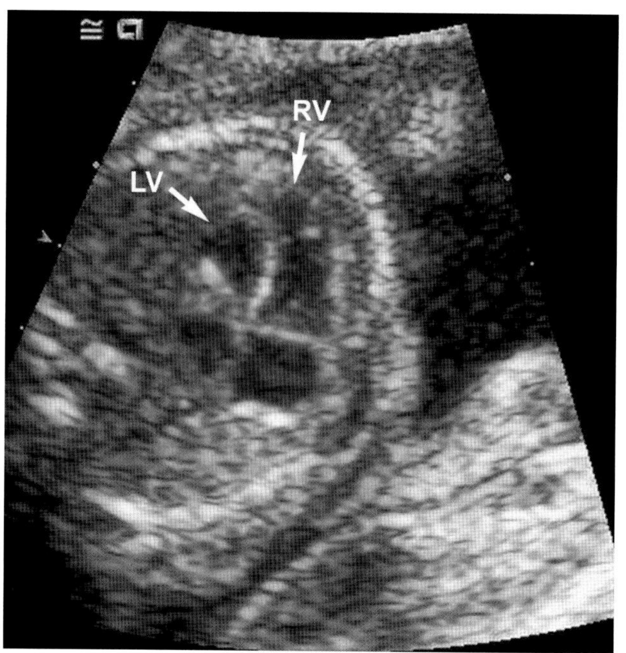

FIGURE 8.2-4. ***(continued)*** **C:** Four-chamber view taken 1 week after that in **(B)** demonstrates a decrease in size of the left ventricle *(LV arrow)*, now smaller than the right ventricle *(RV arrow)*. The left ventricle had almost no contractility.

8.3. HYPOPLASTIC RIGHT VENTRICLE AND PULMONIC STENOSIS

Description and Clinical Features

A hypoplastic right ventricle, which is less common than a hypoplastic left heart, is characterized by a small or absent right cardiac ventricle. This most often results from pulmonic stenosis or atresia with an intact ventricular septum, but can also result from stenosis or atresia of the tricuspid valve. With all these, there is obstruction of blood flow either into the right ventricle or out of the right ventricle, leading to shunting of blood across the foramen ovale to the left side of the heart. The left ventricle may be enlarged and hypertrophic. A hypoplastic right ventricle may cause fetal cardiac failure and hydrops.

Pulmonic stenosis is characterized by an abnormal pulmonic valve that obstructs the blood flow through the right ventricular outflow tract. The stenosis may be an isolated abnormality of the heart or a component of a more complex congenital cardiac malformation such as tetralogy of Fallot or Uhl anomaly. With isolated pulmonic stenosis, the right ventricle may be small or large, depending on the degree of shunting of blood across the foramen ovale and the extent of tricuspid regurgitation.

Sonography

A hypoplastic right ventricle is best diagnosed on a four-chamber view of the heart when the right ventricle is smaller than the left ventricle (Figures 8.3-1 and 8.3-2). In rare cases, no right ventricle can be found. In the latter case, the distinction between hypoplastic right ventricle and hypoplastic left ventricle may not be possible with prenatal sonography.

With pulmonic stenosis, there is narrowing at the level of the pulmonic valve (Figure 8.3-3). Measurement of the pulmonic valve can be compared with norms for gestational age to assess the degree of narrowing. Poststenotic dilation of the pulmonic artery may be

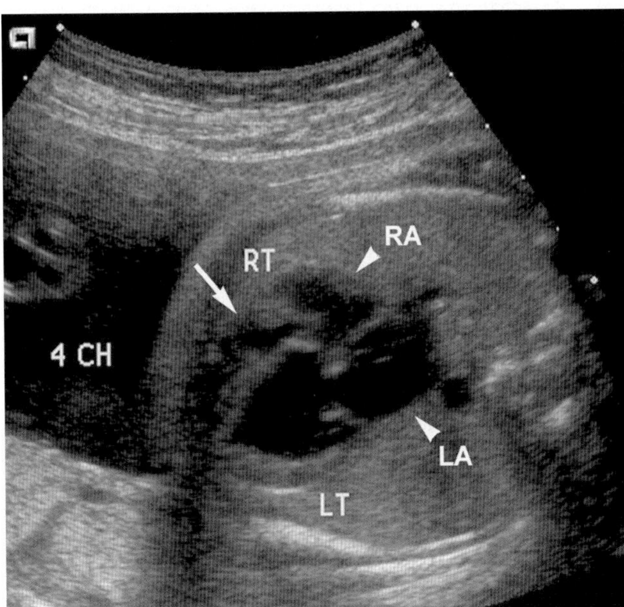

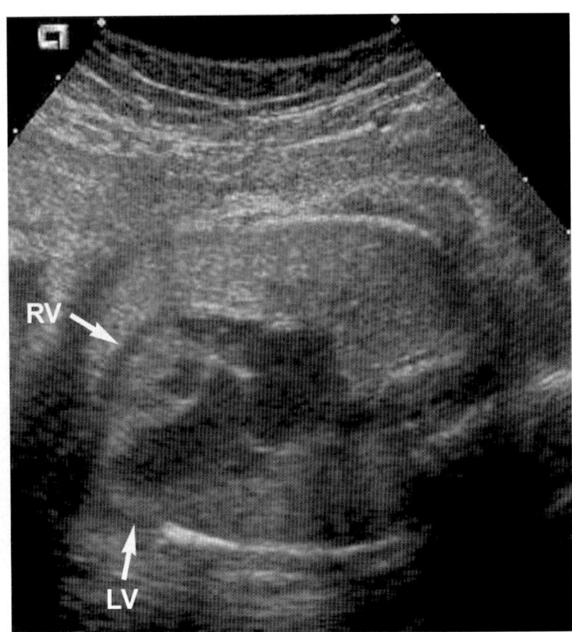

FIGURE 8.3-1. Hypoplastic right ventricle. A: Transverse image of a fetal thorax at the level of a four-chamber view (4 CH) of the heart demonstrates a small right ventricle *(RT arrow)* and a large left ventricle (LT) (*RA arrowhead*, right atrium; *LA arrowhead*, left atrium). **B:** Four-chamber view of another fetus shows a thick-walled right ventricle *(RV arrow)* with a very small chamber and an enlarged left ventricle *(LV arrow)*.

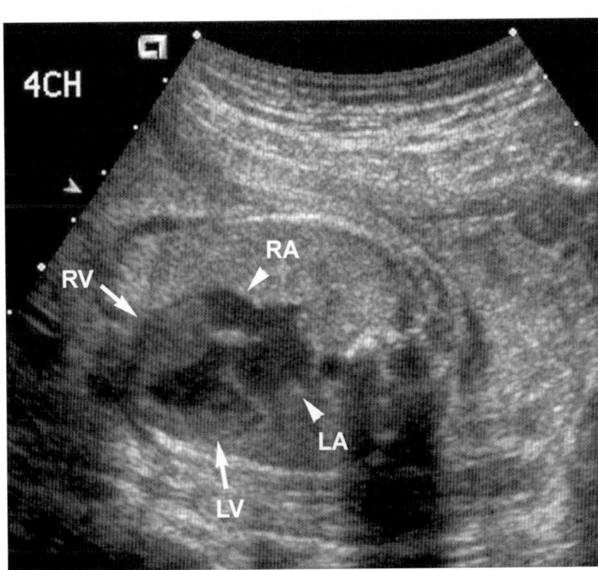

FIGURE 8.3-2. Hypoplastic right ventricle with no right ventricular chamber. Four-chamber view of the heart (4CH) demonstrates a thick-walled right ventricle *(RV arrow)* with no appreciable chamber (*LV arrow*, left ventricle; *RA arrowhead*, right atrium; *LA arrowhead*, left atrium).

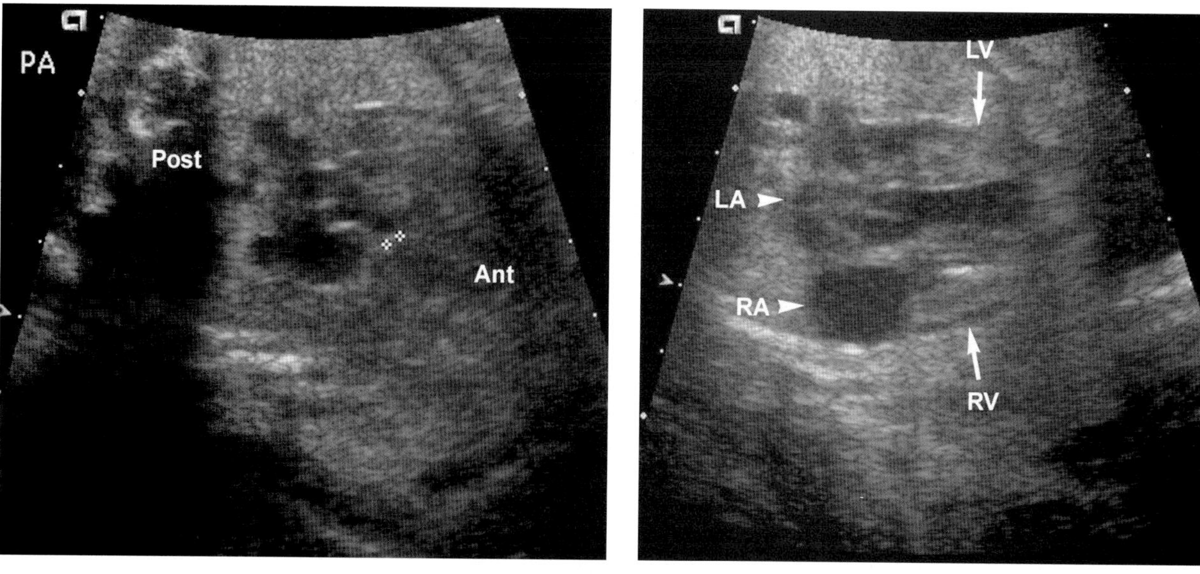

FIGURE 8.3-3. Pulmonic stenosis causing a hypoplastic right ventricle. A: Oblique view of the right ventricular outflow tract demonstrates a very small pulmonary artery (PA) at the level of the pulmonic valve *(calipers)* (Ant, anterior; Post, posterior). **B:** Four-chamber image of the heart in the same patient demonstrates a small right ventricle *(RV arrow)* and large, thick-walled left ventricle *(LV arrow)* (*RA arrowhead*, right atrium; *LA arrowhead*, left atrium).

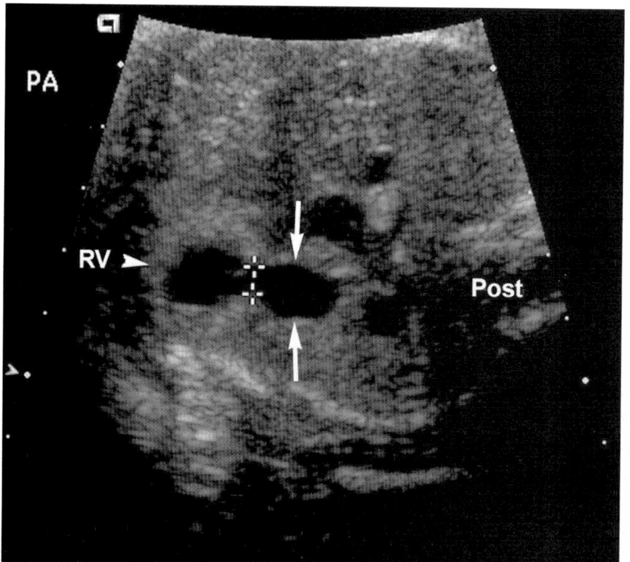

FIGURE 8.3-4. Pulmonic stenosis with poststenotic dilation of the pulmonary artery. Oblique image of right ventricular *(RV arrow)* outflow tract demonstrates a narrow pulmonic valve *(calipers)* with poststenotic dilation of the pulmonary artery (PA) *(arrows)* (Post, posterior).

seen in some cases of isolated pulmonic stenosis (Figure 8.3-4). With pulmonic atresia, the pulmonic valve and right ventricular outflow tract may not be visible. Careful assessment for accompanying cardiac anomalies is warranted, especially looking for abnormalities of the tricuspid valve and ventricular septum.

8.4. EBSTEIN ANOMALY

Description and Clinical Features

Ebstein anomaly is an anomaly that results from the malformation and malposition of the tricuspid valve. The valve is displaced into the right ventricle so that a portion of the right ventricle is contiguous with the right atrium. The tricuspid valve is dysplastic and incompetent, leading to tricuspid regurgitation and enlargement of the right atrium. During atrial systole, blood flows from the right atrium toward the apex of the right ventricle. During ventricular systole, the blood regurgitates from the portion of the right ventricle distal to the tricuspid valve back across the dysplastic tricuspid valve into the right atrium. Hydrops may develop *in utero* owing to fetal cardiac failure.

The prognosis for this cardiac anomaly is poor, with 80% of infants dying in the perinatal period. The prognosis is particularly poor if hydrops develops *in utero* or when there is pulmonary hypoplasia as a result of compression of the lungs by the enlarged heart. Long-term survivors of Ebstein anomaly often have persistent cardiac arrhythmias.

Sonography

With Ebstein anomaly, the four-chamber view of the heart is abnormal. The heart is markedly enlarged, and the right atrium is especially dilated (Figures 8.4-1 and 8.4-2). The tricuspid valve can be seen displaced toward the apex of the right ventricle, located within the right ventricle (Figures 8.4-1 and 8.4-2) rather than at the atrioventricular junction. Tricuspid regurgitation can be demonstrated with color or spectral Doppler (Figure 8.4-3).

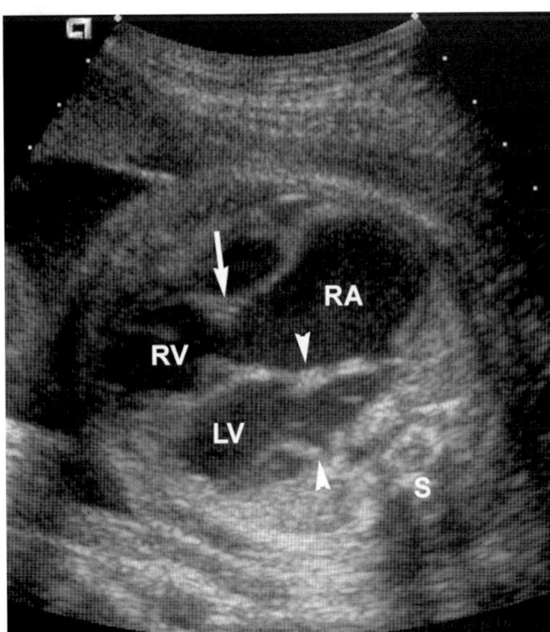

FIGURE 8.4-1. Ebstein anomaly. Transverse image of the thorax with a four-chamber view of heart demonstrates a markedly enlarged right atrium (RA) and mildly enlarged right and left ventricles (RV and LV). The tricuspid valve *(arrow)* is displaced into the right ventricle below the level of the normally positioned mitral valve *(arrowheads)* (S, spine).

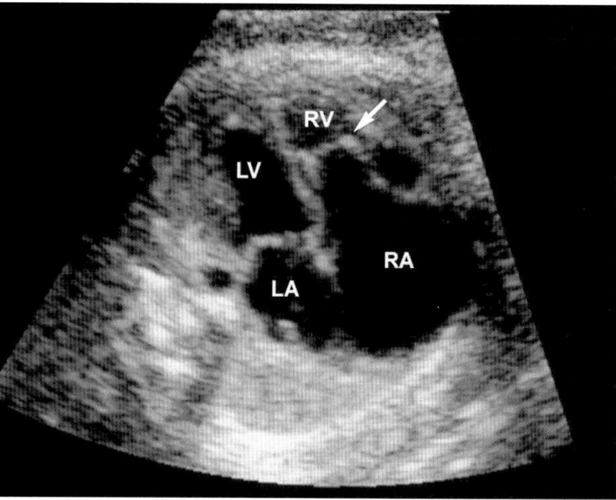

FIGURE 8.4-2. Ebstein anomaly. Four-chamber image of the heart demonstrates an enlarged right atrium (RA) and displacement of the tricuspid valve *(arrow)* into the right ventricle, leaving a small right ventricular chamber (RV) (LA, left atrium; LV, left ventricle).

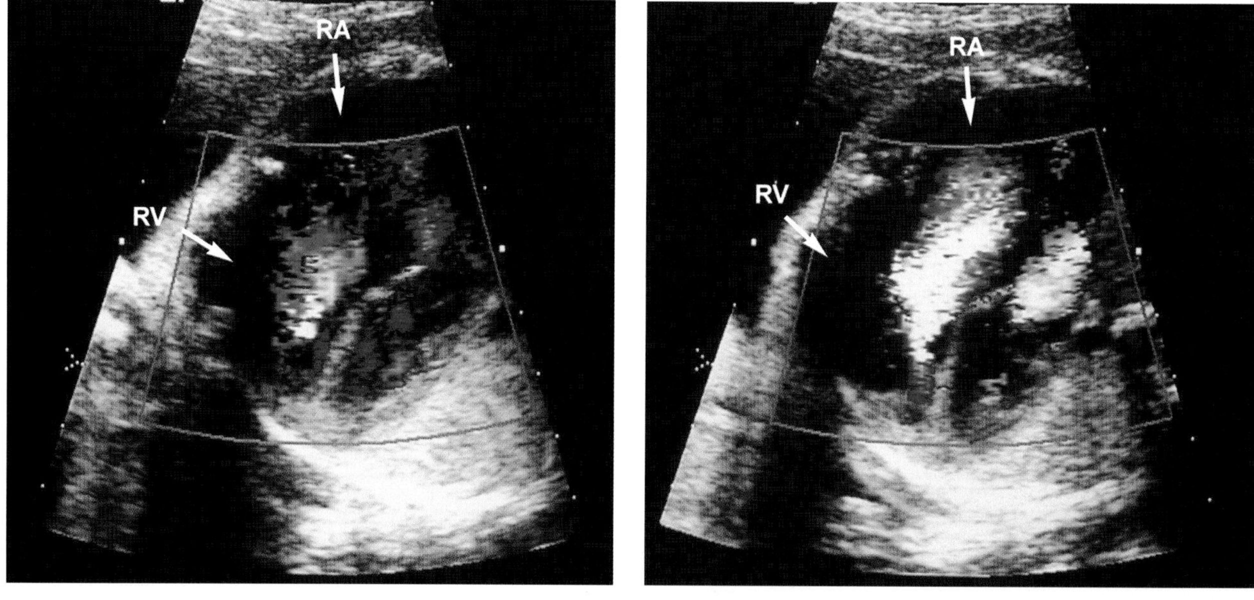

FIGURE 8.4-3. Color Doppler of Ebstein anomaly with tricuspid regurgitation. Color Doppler images of a four-chamber view of heart demonstrates forward flow (blue on color Doppler) from the right atrium *(RA arrow)* to the right ventricle *(RV arrow)* during atrial systole **(A)** and reversed flow (red on color Doppler) back into the right atrium *(RA arrow)* from the right ventricle *(RV arrow)* during ventricular systole **(B)**.

8.5. VENTRICULAR SEPTAL DEFECT

Description and Clinical Features

An opening in the muscular or membranous portion of the interventricular septum is called a ventricular septal defect. These defects may be small and clinically insignificant or quite large, causing significant shunting of blood across the defect. Some of the small defects close spontaneously after birth. Defects in the membranous portion of the septum are more common than those in the muscular septum and tend to be smaller.

Ventricular septal defects may be isolated anomalies or part of a more complex cardiac malformation. Isolated defects have an excellent prognosis.

Sonography

Many ventricular septal defects can be diagnosed on a four-chamber view of the fetal heart (Figure 8.5-1). The diagnosis is made when a gap is seen in the septum between the right and left ventricles. Other defects will only be seen on a long axis view of the left ventricle and left ventricular outflow tract (Figure 8.5-2). On this view, smaller defects in the membranous portion of the septum, not visible on the four-chamber view, may be seen. Small membranous defects, however, are often not visible at all by ultrasound.

Because a ventricular septal defect may be a component of a complex cardiac anomaly, careful assessment of ventricular and atrial chamber sizes, atrioventricular valves, ventricular outflow tracts, and the atrial septum is warranted.

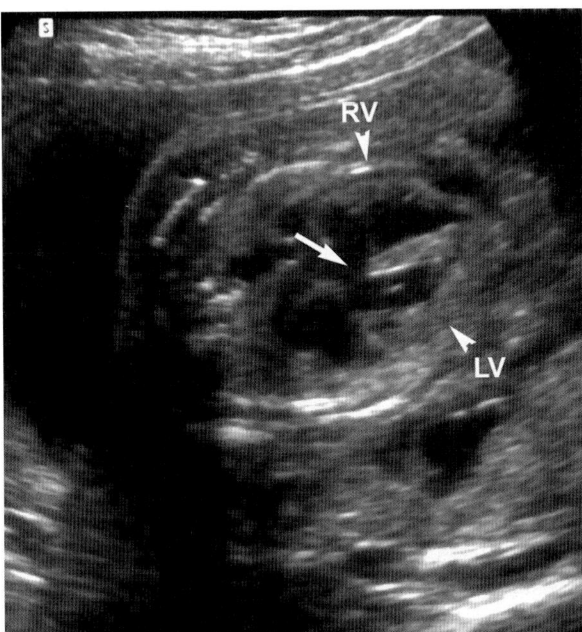

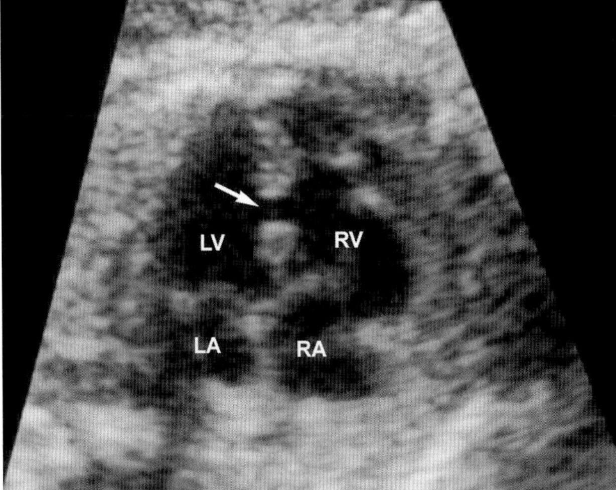

FIGURE 8.5-1. Ventricular septal defects. A: Four-chamber image of a heart demonstrates a large defect *(arrow)* in the upper septum between the right and left ventricles (RV and LV). **B:** Four-chamber view of the heart demonstrates a defect *(arrow)* in the muscular ventricular septum between the right and left ventricles (RV and LV) (LA, left atrium; RA, right atrium).

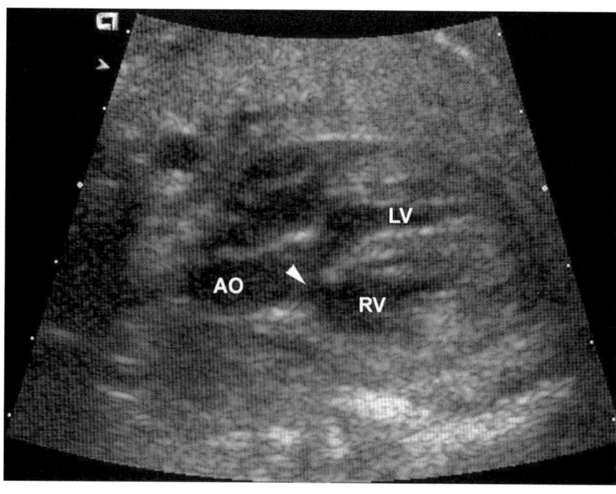

FIGURE 8.5-2. **Ventricular septal defect.** Long axis image of the left ventricle (LV) and its aortic outflow tract (AO) demonstrates a defect in the upper interventricular septum *(arrowhead)* (RV, right ventricle).

8.6. ATRIOVENTRICULAR CANAL

Description and Clinical Features

Atrioventricular canal is a severe cardiac anomaly characterized by a large defect in the central portion of the heart. This part of the heart is sometimes referred to as the "endocardial cushion," and hence atrioventricular canal is sometimes termed "endocardial cushion defect." The defect involves both atrioventricular valves and both the atrial and ventricular septa, such that the atria and ventricles communicate across septal defects and there is a large communication between the atria and ventricles across the defect in the atrioventricular valves. Anomalous formation of the ventricular outflow tracts is common. Fetuses with this cardiac anomaly have other structural anomalies or aneuploidy, particularly trisomy 21. The prognosis is usually poor.

Sonography

On the four-chamber view of the heart, atrioventricular canal is evident as a large defect in the middle of heart, with absence of portions of the atrial and ventricular septa and abnormal atrioventricular valves (Figures 8.6-1, 8.6-2, and 8.6-3). The atrioventricular valves may appear as one large valve between the atria and ventricles. Because of the association of atrioventricular canal with aneuploidy and other cardiac and noncardiac anomalies, a careful fetal anatomic survey should be performed to search for other anomalies.

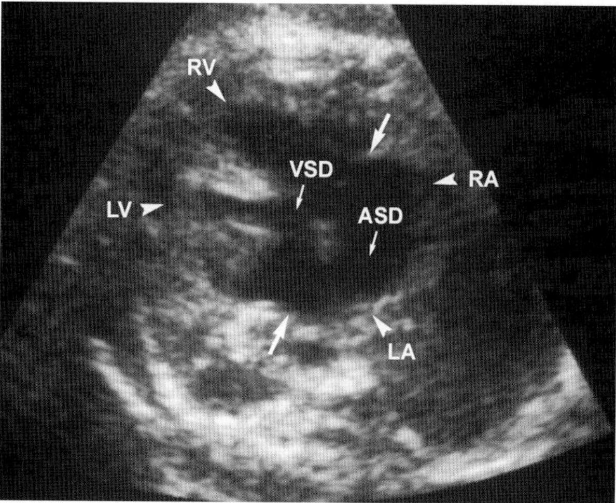

FIGURE 8.6-1. Atrioventricular canal. Four-chamber view of the heart demonstrates a large defect in the middle of the heart involving the ventricular septum (VSD, *small arrow*), atrial septum (ASD, *small arrow*) and both atrioventricular valves *(between large arrows)* (*RV arrowhead*, right ventricle; *LV arrowhead*, left ventricle; *RA arrowhead*, right atrium; *LA arrowhead*, left atrium).

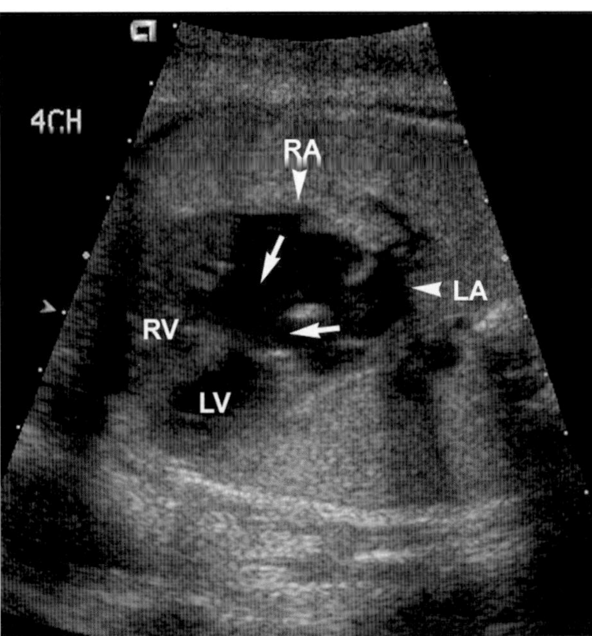

FIGURE 8.6-2. Atrioventricular canal in a 25-week fetus. Four-chamber image of the heart (4CH) demonstrates a large defect in the middle of the heart representing a common atrioventricular valve *(arrows)*, with communication between both atria and both ventricles (RV, right ventricle; LV, left ventricle; *RA arrowhead*, right atrium; *LA arrowhead*, left atrium).

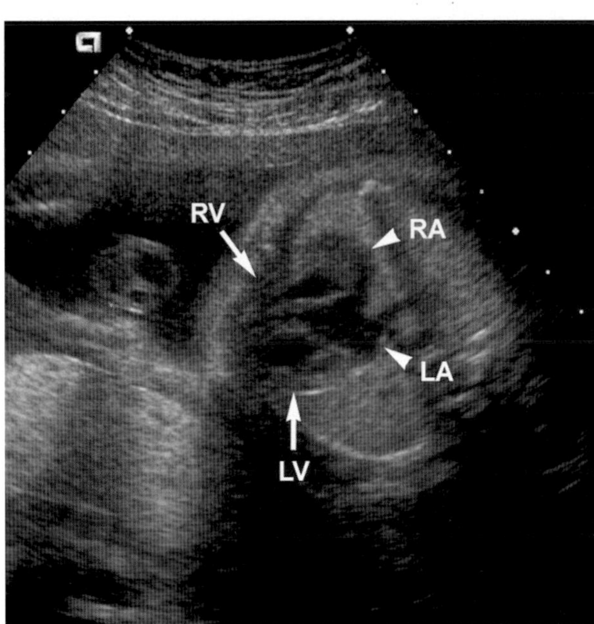

FIGURE 8.6-3. Atrioventricular canal in an 18-week fetus. Four-chamber view of the heart demonstrates a large defect between the four chambers. (*RV arrow*, right ventricle; *LV arrow*, left ventricle; *RA arrowhead*, right atrium; *LA arrowhead*, left atrium).

8.7. TETRALOGY OF FALLOT

Description and Clinical Features

Tetralogy of Fallot is a complex cardiac anomaly comprising four cardiac abnormalities in the neonate: pulmonic stenosis, ventricular septal defect, overriding aorta, and right ventricular hypertrophy. In the fetus with tetralogy of Fallot, only the first three components of this anomaly are present. In general, the prognosis is good for this cardiac malformation because corrective surgery can be performed after birth. Rarely will the fetus have hydrops due to cardiac failure.

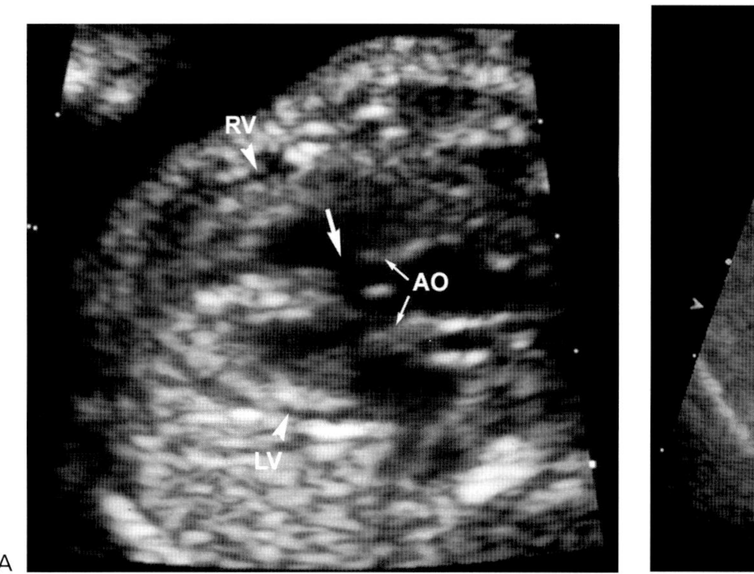

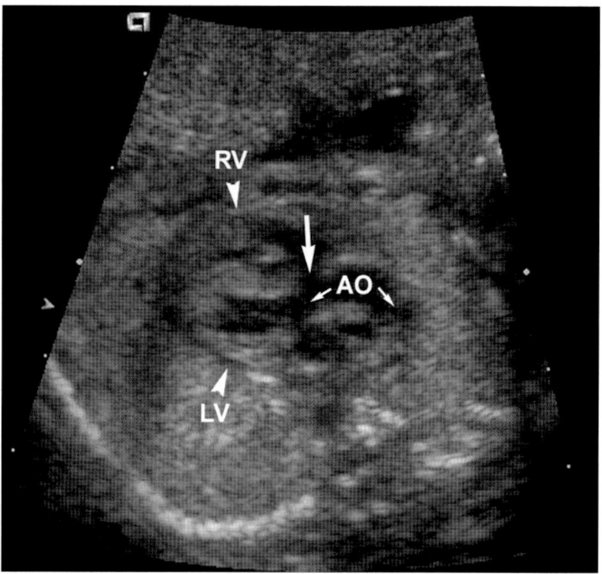

FIGURE 8.7-1. Overriding aorta with tetralogy of Fallot. A and B: Oblique views of two different cases demonstrate an overriding aorta (AO, *small arrows*) and a ventricular septal defect *(large arrow)* (*RV arrowhead*, right ventricle; *LV arrowhead*, left ventricle).

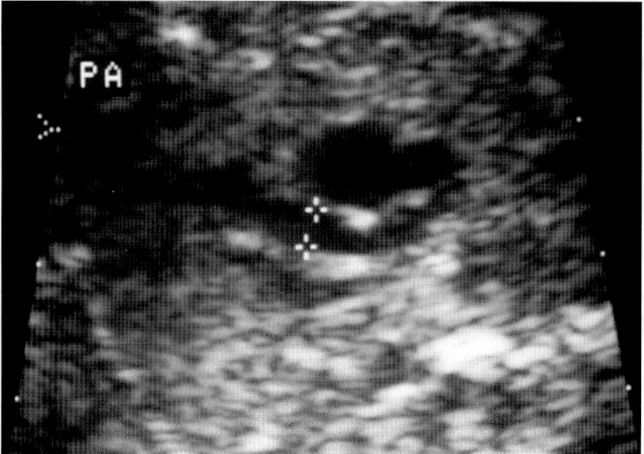

FIGURE 8.7-2. Pulmonic stenosis with tetralogy of Fallot. Oblique image of the right ventricular outflow tract of same patient as in Figure 8.7-1A demonstrates a small pulmonary artery *(PA calipers)*.

Sonography

Fetuses with tetralogy of Fallot may have a normal four-chamber view of the heart, and the diagnosis may be missed if the ventricular outflow tracts are not evaluated. Tetralogy of Fallot is best diagnosed on a long axis view of the left ventricular outflow tract where the ventricular septal defect and overriding aorta are visible (Figure 8.7-1). The aorta is widened at the level of the aortic valve, such that the ascending aorta extends over the ventricular septal defect to overlie part of the right ventricle. Narrowing of the pulmonic valve can be demonstrated on either a transverse or longitudinal view of the right ventricular outflow tract (Figure 8.7-2).

8.8. TRANSPOSITION OF THE GREAT VESSELS

Description and Clinical Features

Transposition of the great vessels is characterized by reversed ventricular outflow tracts, with the pulmonary artery arising from the left ventricle and the aorta arising from the right ventricle. The anomaly is often accompanied by a ventricular septal defect. It has a good prognosis because corrective surgery can be performed after birth.

Sonography

With transposition of the great vessels, the pulmonary artery and aorta arise from the base of the heart in parallel, as opposed to the crossed configuration of the normal heart. Because of this, the diagnosis is best made on a long axis view of the left ventricle, which demonstrates both great vessels extending cephalad in parallel, the aorta anterior to the pulmonary artery (Figures 8.8-1 and 8.8-2). The four-chamber view is usually normal unless a ventricular septal defect is present.

A

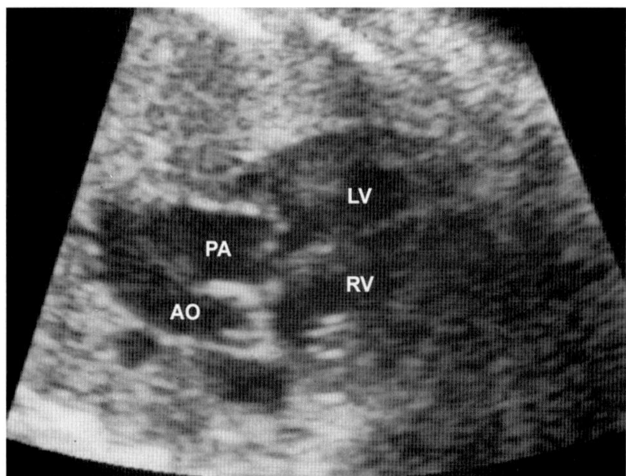

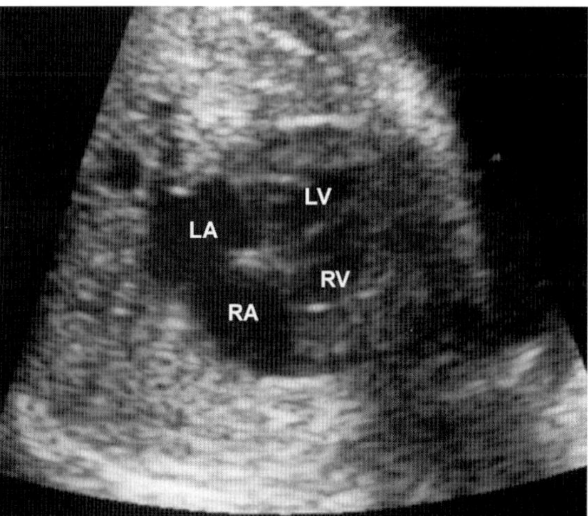

B

FIGURE 8.8-1. Transposition of the great vessels. A: Oblique view of the heart demonstrates both ventricular outflow tracts arising in parallel, with the pulmonary artery (PA) arising from the left ventricle (LV) and the aorta (AO) arising from the right ventricle (RV). **B:** The four-chamber view of the heart is normal (RV, right ventricle; LV, left ventricle; RA, right atrium; LA, left atrium).

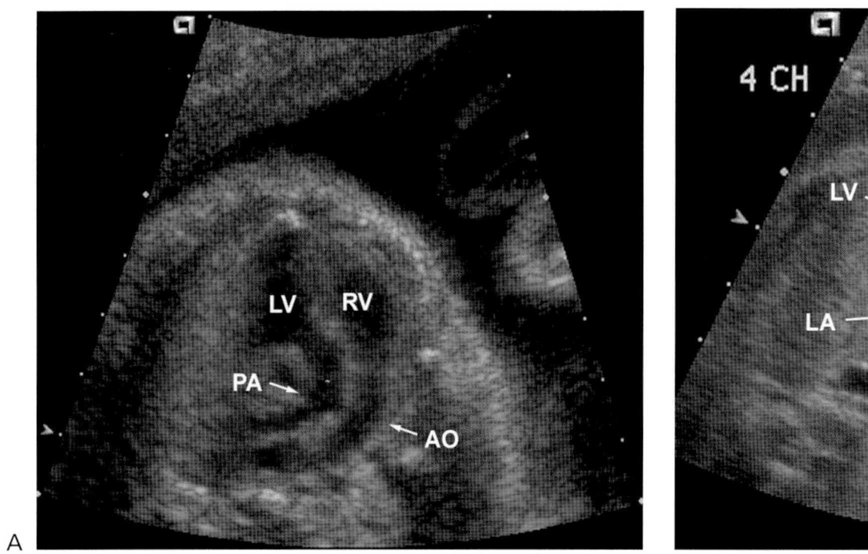

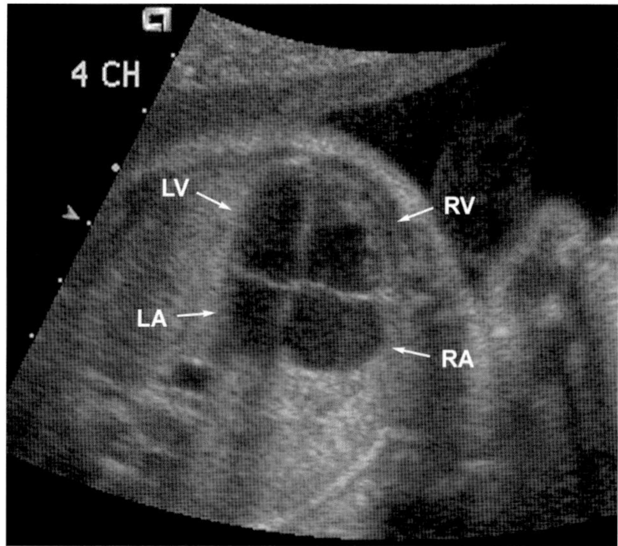

FIGURE 8.8-2. Transposition of the great vessels. A: Image of the outflow tracts demonstrates the aorta *(AO small arrow)* arising from the right ventricle (RV) and the pulmonary artery *(PA small arrow)* arising from the left ventricle (LV). **B:** The four-chamber view of the heart is normal (*RV small arrow*, right ventricle; *LV small arrow*, left ventricle; *RA small arrow*, right atrium; *LA small arrow*, left atrium).

8.9. TRUNCUS ARTERIOSUS

Description and Clinical Features

With truncus arteriosus, a single large vessel arises from both ventricles, giving branches that supply pulmonary, coronary, and systemic arteries. Truncus arteriosus is classified based on the type of branching of the truncus into the different arteries. This anomaly is

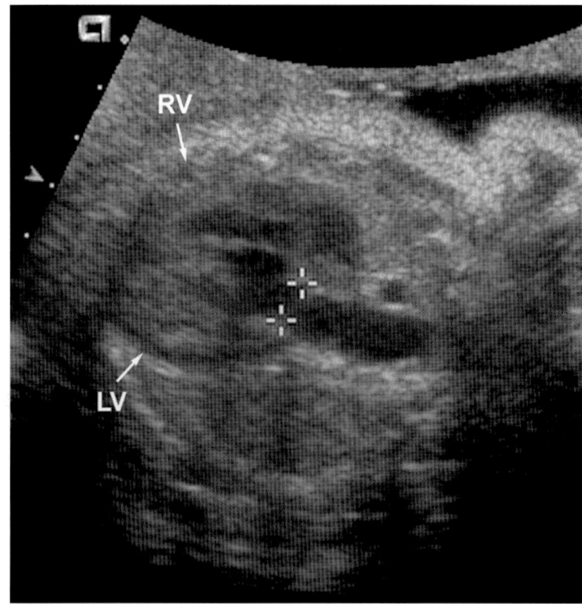

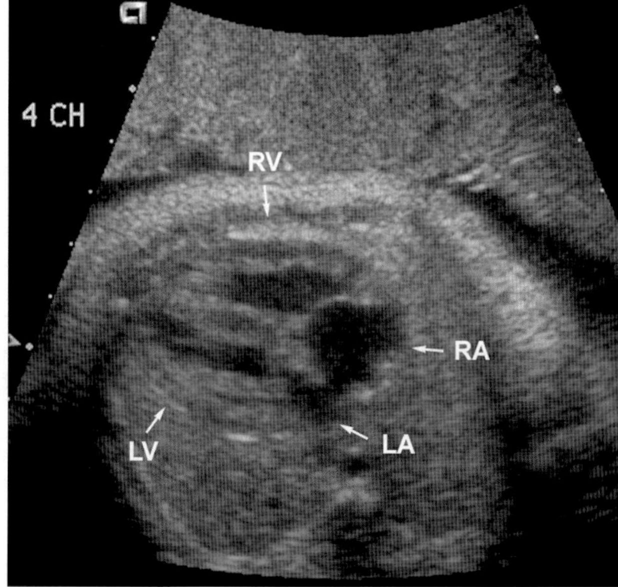

FIGURE 8.9-1. Truncus arteriosus. A: Oblique sonogram demonstrates a single large vessel *(calipers)* arising from both the right *(RV arrow)* and left *(LV arrow)* ventricles. **B:** The heart appears normal on the four-chamber view (*RV arrow*, right ventricle; *LV arrow*, left ventricle; *RA arrow*, right atrium; *LA arrow*, left atrium).

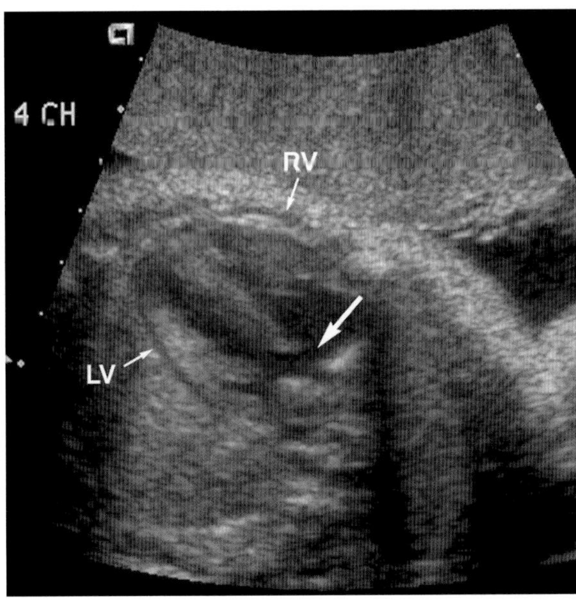

FIGURE 8.9-1. ***(continued)*** **C:** A ventricular septal defect *(arrow)* is present between the right *(RV small arrow)* and left *(LV small arrow)* ventricles.

typically a component of a complex congenital cardiac malformation, often involving hypoplasia of the left or right ventricle, a large ventricular septal defect, or an atrioventricular canal. The prognosis depends on the extent of the entire cardiac anomaly and, in general, is poor.

Sonography

When truncus arteriosus is present, a single large vessel is seen arising from the heart (Figure 8.9-1). Because of the association of truncus arteriosus with other anomalies of the heart, careful assessment of the cardiac ventricles and ventricular septum should be performed.

8.10. MYOCARDIAL TUMORS

Description and Clinical Features

Tumors of the myocardium are most often rhabdomyomas, which, when multiple, are usually a manifestation of tuberous sclerosis. Rhabdomyomas arise in the myocardium and tend to grow during gestation. Cardiac failure with hydrops may result either from obstruction of blood flow by the rhabdomyoma or from poor cardiac contractility owing to the replacement of normal myocardium by tumor. The prognosis is worse if hydrops is present prenatally.

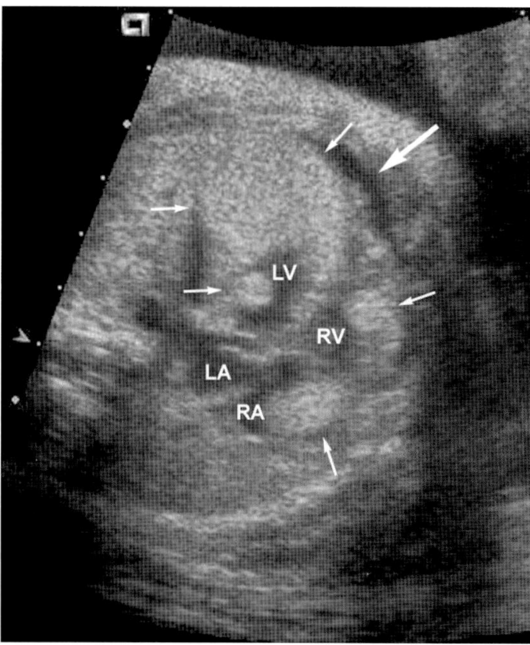

FIGURE 8.10-1. Multiple rhabdomyomas. Four-chamber view of the heart demonstrates multiple homogeneous masses *(small arrows)* arising from the myocardium (RV, right ventricle; LV, left ventricle; RA, right atrium; LA, left atrium). A small pericardial effusion *(large arrow)* is present.

Sonography

Cardiac rhabdomyomas are usually round or oval echogenic masses arising from the myocardium. They may be single or multiple (Figure 8.10-1). When hydrops is present, pericardial fluid may outline the myocardial tumors.

8.11. ARRHYTHMIAS

Description and Clinical Features

A variety of abnormal cardiac rhythms may be encountered in the fetus, including premature atrial contractions, bradycardia, atrioventricular heart block, and a number of tachyarrhythmias (e.g., supraventricular tachycardia, atrial flutter, and atrial fibrillation). In general, the prognosis is related to whether hydrops develops *in utero*. For some cardiac arrhythmias, antiarrhythmic drugs that cross the placenta can be given to the mother to correct the fetal arrhythmia.

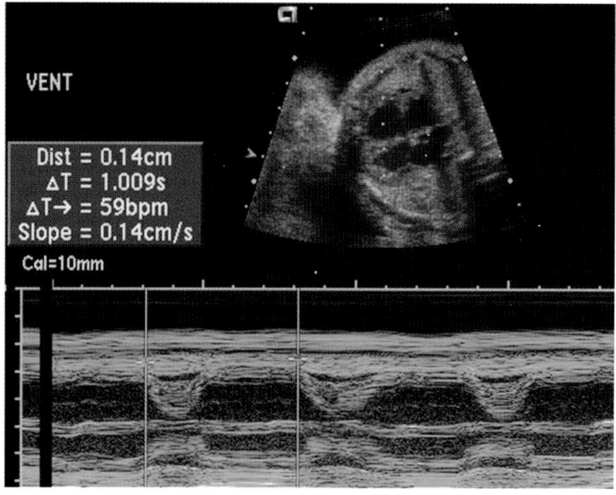

FIGURE 8.11-1. Bradycardia. M-mode images through both ventricles of the heart demonstrate a slow heart rate of 59 beats per minute *(calipers)*.

Premature atrial contractions occur commonly and are typically benign and self-limited. Fetuses with premature atrial contractions rarely develop hydrops or require medication *in utero* or after birth.

Sonography

An abnormal cardiac rhythm can be seen with real-time sonography. M-mode sonography is useful to document and characterize the arrhythmia because it can quantify atrial and ventricular rates. With bradycardia, the heart rate is abnormally slow (Figure 8.11-1). With supraventricular tachycardia, the heart rate is faster than normal, more than 180–200 beats per minute (Figure 8.11-2). With atrioventricular heart block, there is dissociation between the atrial beats and the ventricular beats (Figure 8.11-3). When atrial

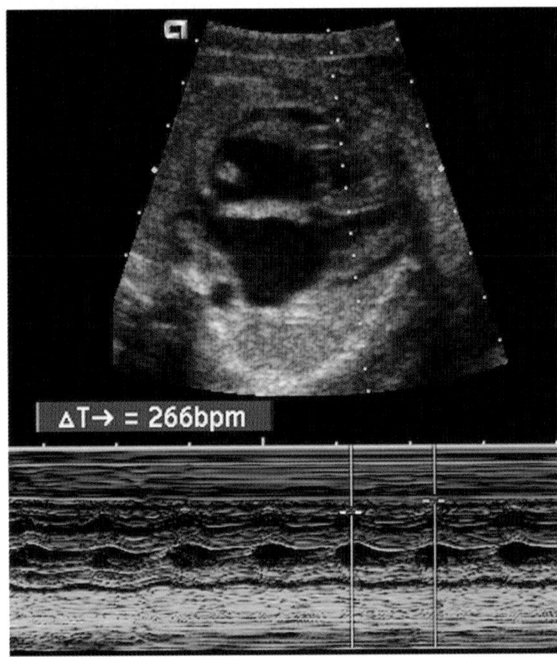

FIGURE 8.11-2. Supraventricular tachycardia. M-mode through both ventricles of the heart demonstrate a fast heart rate of 266 beats per minute *(calipers)*. There is a small pericardial effusion due to hydrops.

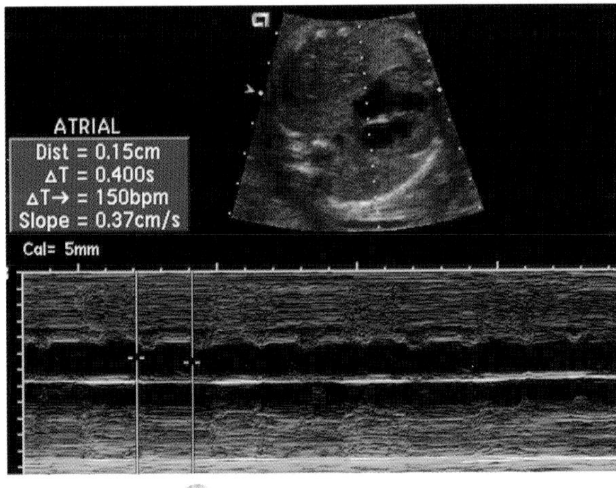

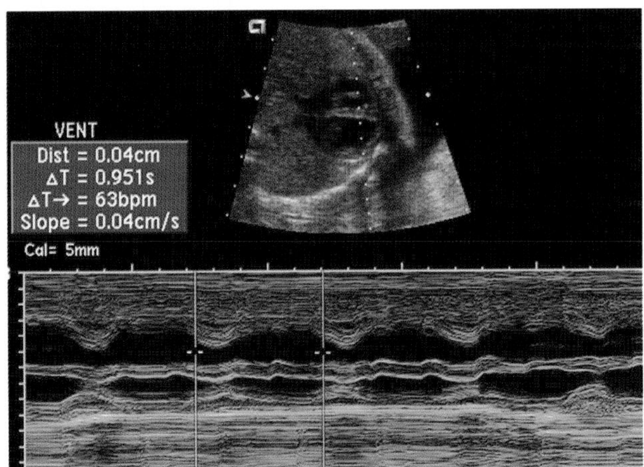

FIGURE 8.11-3. Atrioventricular heart block. M-mode through both atria demonstrates an atrial rate of 150 beats per minute *(calipers)* **(A)** and through both ventricles demonstrates a rate of 63 beats per minute *(calipers)*, due to atrioventricular heart block **(B)**.

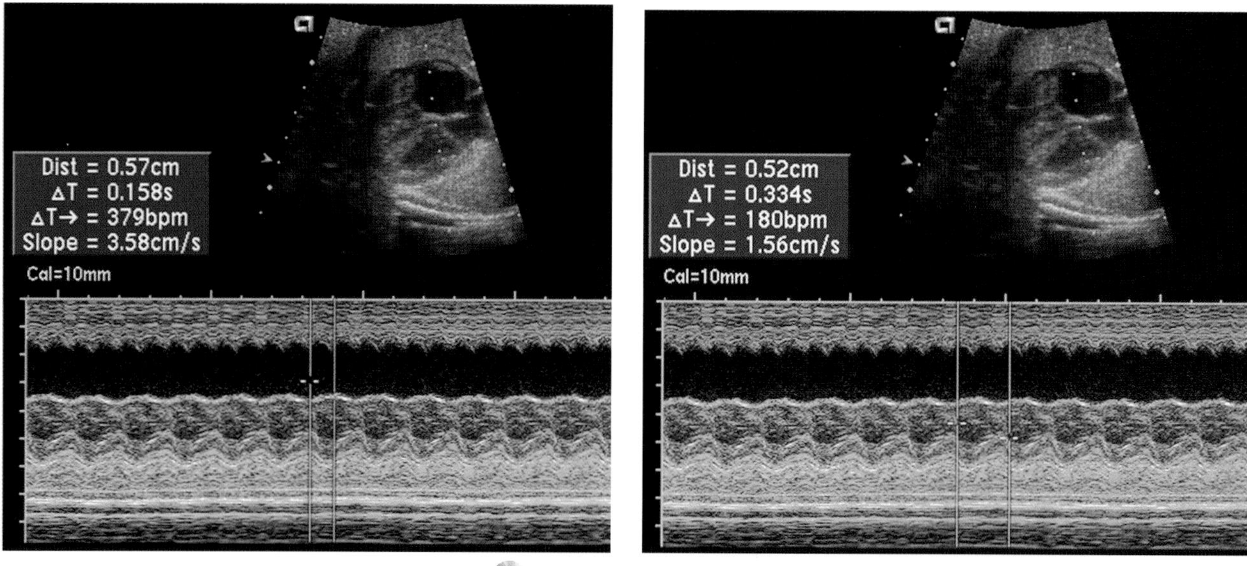

FIGURE 8.11-4. Atrial flutter with two-to-one conduction. M-mode through the right atrium and left ventricle demonstrates a very fast atrial rate of 379 beats per minute *(calipers)* **(A)** and a slower ventricular rate of 180 beats per minute *(calipers)* **(B)**.

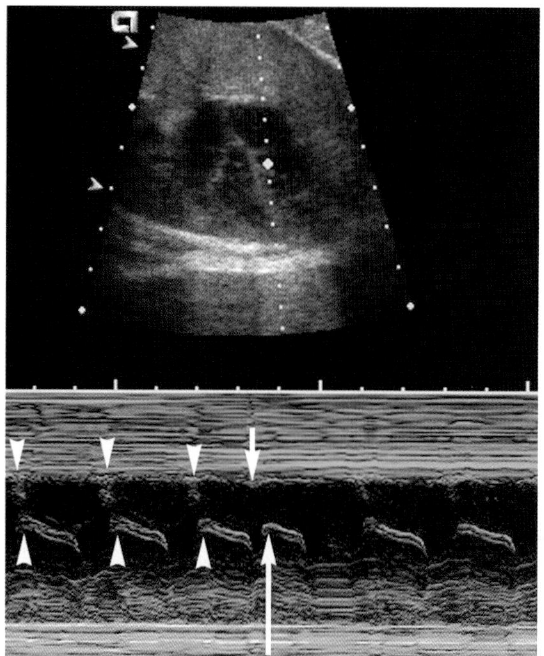

FIGURE 8.11-5. Premature atrial contraction. M-mode through the left atrium and ventricle with atrial beats on top and ventricular beats below demonstrates regular cardiac rhythm *(arrowheads)*, interrupted by a premature atrial *(short arrow)* and ventricular beat *(long arrow)*. The premature beat is followed by a pause in cardiac contractions before the normal rhythm resumes.

flutter is present, the atrial rate is very fast, usually more than 300 beats per minute, and the rate is faster still (more than 400 bpm) with atrial fibrillation. The ventricular rate may be equally fast but is often slower than the atrial rate owing to incomplete conduction, such as three-to-one or two-to-one conduction (Figure 8.11-4).

Premature atrial contractions cause irregularity of the fetal heart rate characterized by early beating of the atria and ventricles followed by a pause before the normal rhythm resumes. This can be observed in real time or documented by M-mode sonography (Figure 8.11-5).

8.12. ECTOPIA CORDIS

Description and Clinical Features

Ectopia cordis is a rare anomaly in which the heart is located outside the fetal thorax, protruding through a defect in the anterior chest wall. In many cases, the heart is structurally abnormal in addition to being abnormally located. Although ectopia cordis may be an isolated anomaly, it is often a component of a syndrome such as pentalogy of Cantrell or amniotic bands. The prognosis is usually dismal.

Sonography

When ectopia cordis is present, the heart is seen within the amniotic cavity connected to the rest of the fetus through a defect in the anterior thoracic wall (Figure 8.12-1). Pentalogy of Cantrell is diagnosed when there is ectopia cordis and an omphalocele.

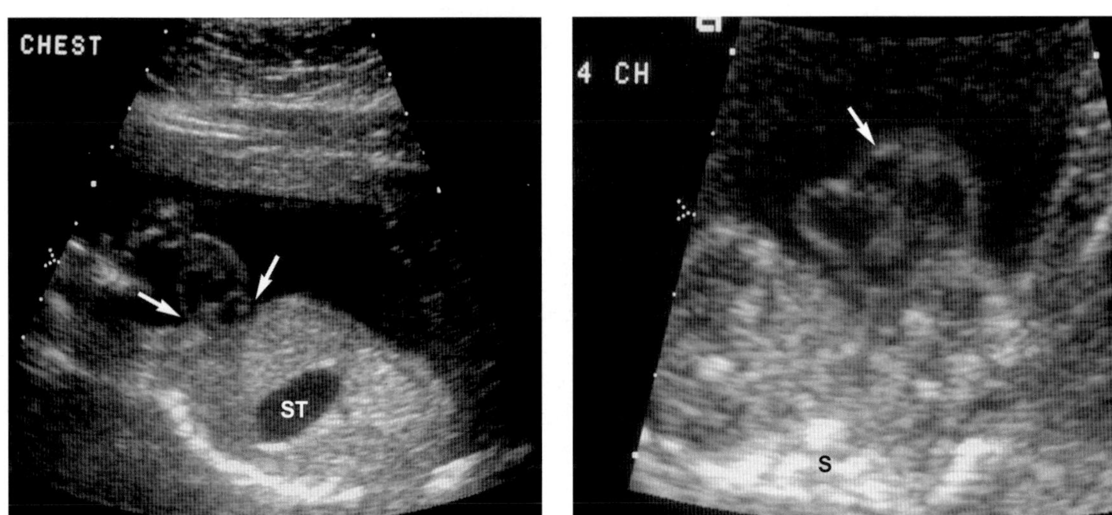

FIGURE 8.12-1. Ectopia cordis. A: Oblique longitudinal image demonstrates a defect in the anterior chest wall *(arrows)* through which the heart has herniated (ST, stomach). **B:** Transverse image of the thorax demonstrates the heart *(arrow)* outside the chest anteriorly (S, spine).

8.13. PERICARDIAL EFFUSION

Description and Clinical Features

Pericardial effusion is the abnormal accumulation of fluid between the visceral and parietal layers of the pericardium. The effusion may be isolated or a component of fetal hydrops. Small isolated effusions are commonly seen and have an excellent prognosis. With a large effusion or one that is a component of hydrops, the prognosis is related to the underlying cause of the pericardial effusion or to the degree of hydrops.

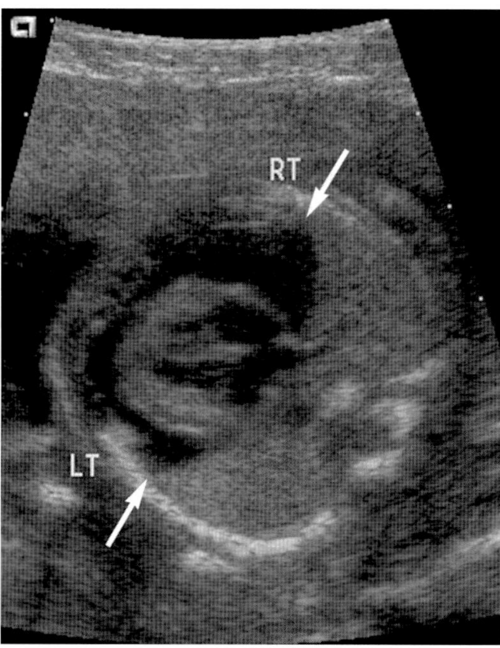

FIGURE 8.13-1. Isolated pericardial effusion. Transverse image through the fetal thorax and a four-chamber view of heart demonstrates a large pericardial effusion *(arrows)* surrounding the heart (LT, left; RT, right).

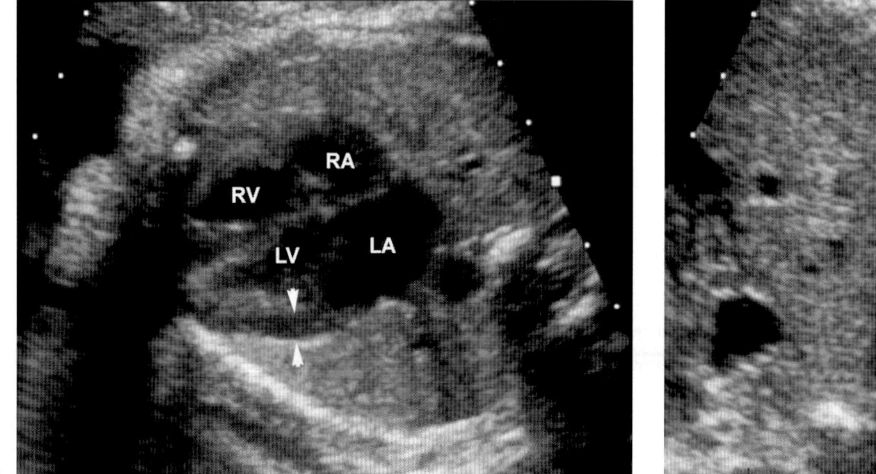

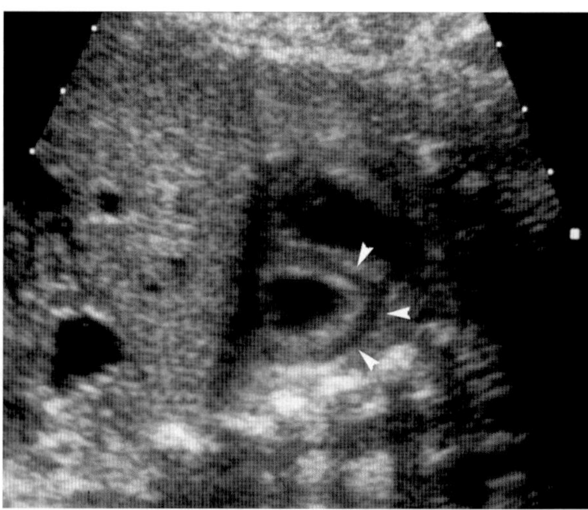

FIGURE 8.13-2. Myocardium mimics pericardial fluid. A: Four-chamber view of the heart in which hypoechoic myocardium of the left ventricular wall *(arrowhead)* might be mistaken for pericardial fluid (RV, right ventricle; LV, left ventricle; RA, right atrium; LA, left atrium). **B:** Short-axis image of the heart shows that the hypoechoic myocardium *(arrowheads)* extends into the interventricular septum, proving that it is not fluid in the pericardial space.

Sonography

With ultrasound, a pericardial effusion is seen as a rim of fluid around the fetal heart (Figure 8.13-1). Care must be taken not to mistake the normal hypoechoic myocardium for pericardial fluid (Figure 8.13-2). Pericardial effusions change in shape with cardiac contractility and are completely anechoic. When the pericardial effusion is a component of hydrops, ascites, pleural effusions, and skin thickening may also be seen (Figure 8.13-3).

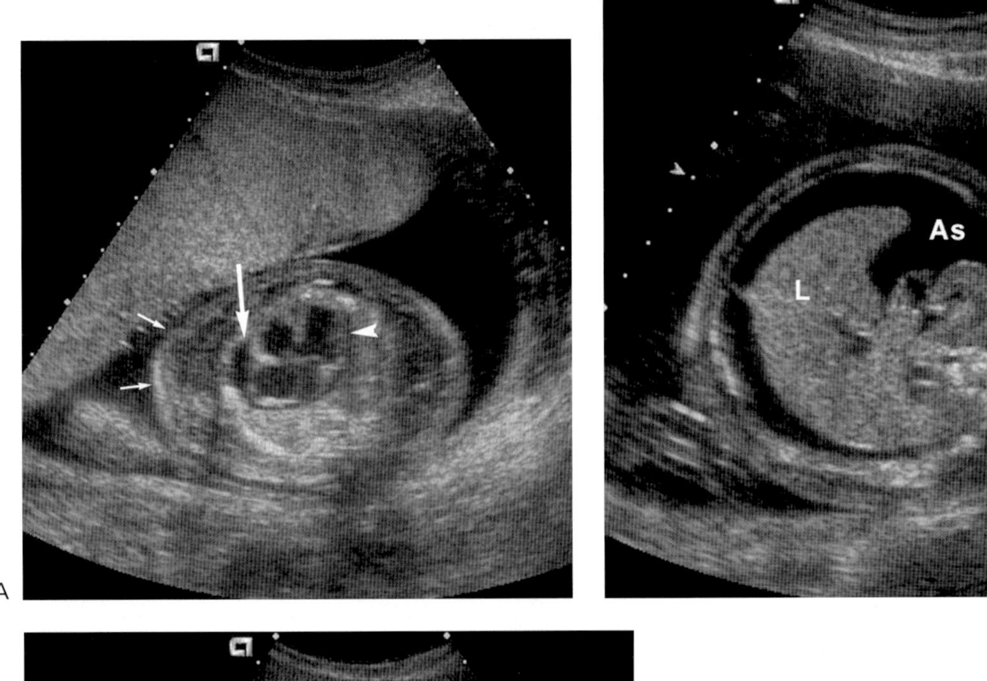

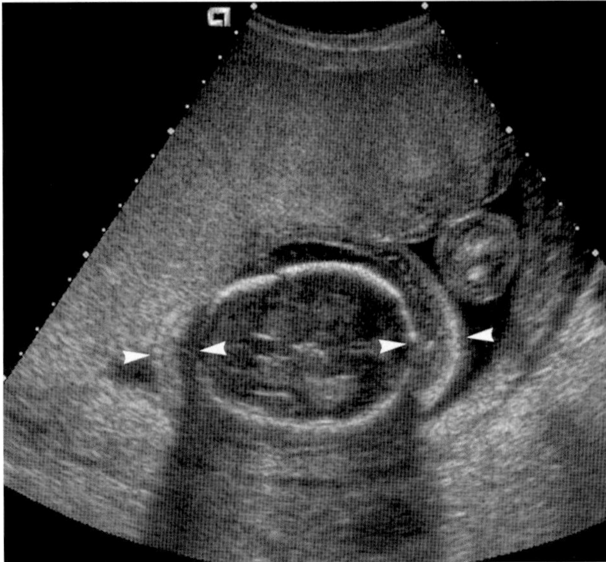

FIGURE 8.13-3. Pericardial effusion with hydrops. A: Transverse image of the fetal thorax demonstrates pericardial fluid *(arrow)* around the heart *(arrowhead)*. Marked skin thickening *(small arrows)* is also apparent. **B:** Transverse image of the fetal abdomen demonstrates a large amount of ascites (As) surrounding the liver (L). **C:** Marked skin thickening *(arrowheads)* surrounds the fetal head.

SUGGESTED READINGS

1. Benacerraf BR, Pober BR, Sanders SP. Accuracy of fetal echocardiography. *Radiology* 1987;165: 847–849.
2. Benson CB, Brown DL, Roberts DJ. Uhl's anomaly of the heart mimicking Ebstein's anomaly *in utero*: case report. *J Ultrasound Med* 1995;14:781–783.
3. Di Salvo DN, Brown DL, Doubilet PM, et al. Clinical significance of isolated fetal pericardial effusion. *J Ultrasound Med* 1994;13:291–293.
4. Frates MC. Sonography of the normal fetal heart: a practical approach. *AJR Am J Roentgenol* 1999; 173:1363–1370.
5. Hess DB, Hess LW, eds. *Fetal echocardiography*. Stamford: Appleton & Lange, 1999.
6. Nyberg DA, Emerson DS. Cardiac malformations. In: Nyberg DA, Mahony BS, Pretorius DH, eds. *Diagnostic ultrasound of fetal anomalies: text and atlas*. Chicago: Year Book Medical Publishers, 1990: 300–341.
7. Pilu G, Jeanty P, Perolo A, et al. Prenatal diagnosis of congenital heart disease. In: Fleischer AC, Manning FA, Jeanty P, et al., eds. *Sonography in obstetrics & gynecology: principles and practice*, 6th ed. New York: McGraw-Hill, 2001:157–176.
8. Silverman NH, Schmidt KG. Ultrasound evaluation of the fetal heart. In: Callen PW, ed. *Ultrasonography in obstetrics and gynecology*, 3rd ed. Philadelphia: WB Saunders, 1994:291–332.
9. Stamm ER, Drose JA. The fetal heart. In: Rumack CM, Wilson SR, Charboneau JW, eds. *Diagnostic ultrasound*, 2nd ed. St. Louis: Mosby, 1998:1123–1159.

9

GASTROINTESTINAL TRACT

9.1. ESOPHAGEAL ATRESIA

Description and Clinical Features

Esophageal atresia is a disorder in which the esophagus is obstructed owing to a segment that has complete obliteration of the lumen. It occurs in a variety of subtypes, depending on whether, and at what level, the esophagus and trachea are connected. In the most common subtype, there is a fistulous connection between the trachea and the distal portion of the esophagus.

Esophageal atresia can occur on its own or in conjunction with other structural anomalies. One of the anomaly groupings that includes esophageal atresia is the VATER grouping.

*V*ertebral anomalies
*A*nal atresia
*T*racheoesophageal fistula
*E*sophageal atresia
*R*adial/renal dysplasia

The prognosis is variable, depending in part on the presence or absence of associated anomalies.

Sonography

The sonographic findings of esophageal atresia are little or no fluid in the fetal stomach and polyhydramnios (Figure 9.1-1). If there is no tracheoesophageal fistula (and hence no route by which amniotic fluid can reach the fetal stomach), there will be complete absence of fluid in the fetal stomach and severe polyhydramnios. If there is a distal tracheoesophageal fistula, amniotic fluid can traverse this fistula to reach the fetal stomach. In these cases, the degree of polyhydramnios may be variable and there may be some fluid in the fetal stomach.

The findings of polyhydramnios together with little or no fluid in the fetal stomach can also be present in fetuses with a facial or mouth lesion that obstructs swallowing (e.g., lower facial teratoma). Hence, when the sonogram demonstrates polyhydramnios and little or no fluid in the fetal stomach, the fetal face should be examined before concluding that the diagnosis is esophageal atresia.

When the diagnosis of esophageal atresia is made, the entire fetus should be carefully assessed for the presence of associated anomalies.

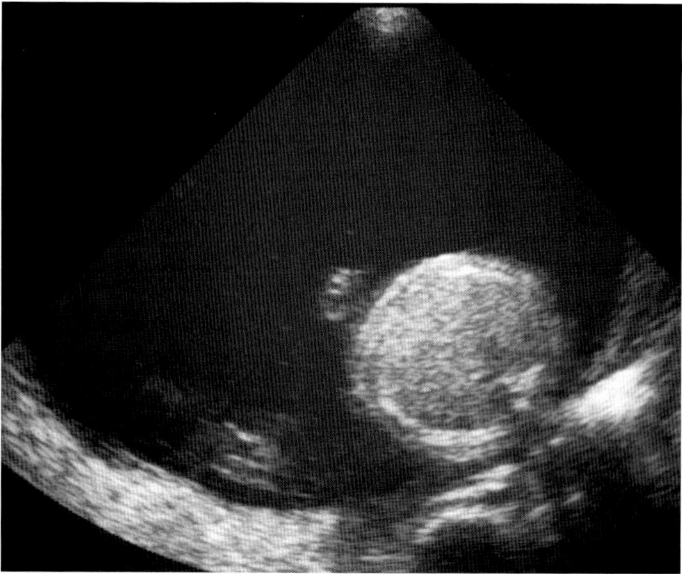

FIGURE 9.1-1. Esophageal atresia. Transverse view of the fetal upper abdomen demonstrates severe polyhydramnios and no identifiable stomach.

9.2. DUODENAL ATRESIA

Description and Clinical Features

Duodenal atresia is a disorder in which the duodenum is obstructed owing to a segment that has complete obliteration of the lumen. The atretic segment is usually just distal to the duodenal bulb.

Duodenal atresia may occur as an isolated anomaly or in association with other anomalies. Approximately one-third of fetuses with duodenal atresia have trisomy 21.

Duodenal atresia is the most common, but not the only, cause of duodenal obstruction. Other causes include annular pancreas, intestinal malrotation with Ladd's bands, and duodenal web.

Sonography

Sonographic diagnosis of duodenal obstruction is made when two findings are present (Figure 9.2-1): (1) dilation of the fetal stomach and duodenum ("double bubble"), appearing sonographically as two prominent fluid-filled structures in the upper abdomen and (2) polyhydramnios. On a sagittal or oblique view of the fetal abdomen, the dilated stomach and duodenum can be seen to be connected to one another. The specific diagnosis of duodenal atresia can be suspected but not established with certainty because other causes of duodenal obstruction have similar sonographic findings (Figure 9.2-2).

Because duodenal atresia is the most common cause of duodenal obstruction and is often associated with other structural or chromosomal anomalies, the entire fetus should be carefully examined whenever duodenal obstruction is suspected (i.e., whenever there is a "double bubble" and polyhydramnios). The parents should also be counseled that the fetus is at substantially increased risk of trisomy 21.

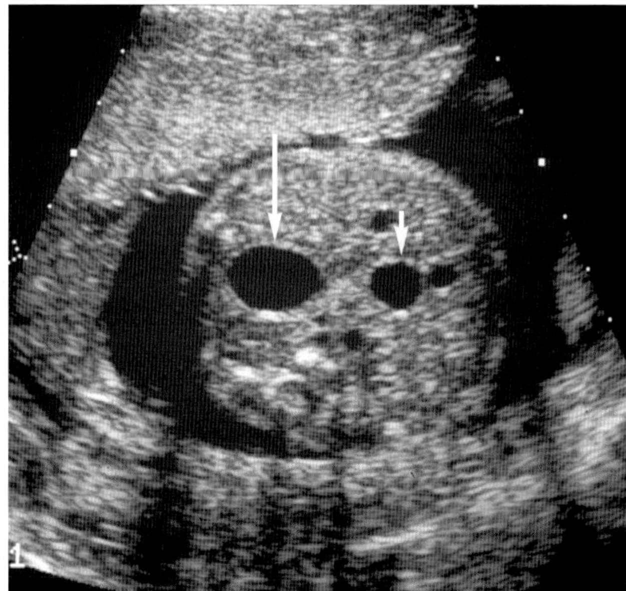
A

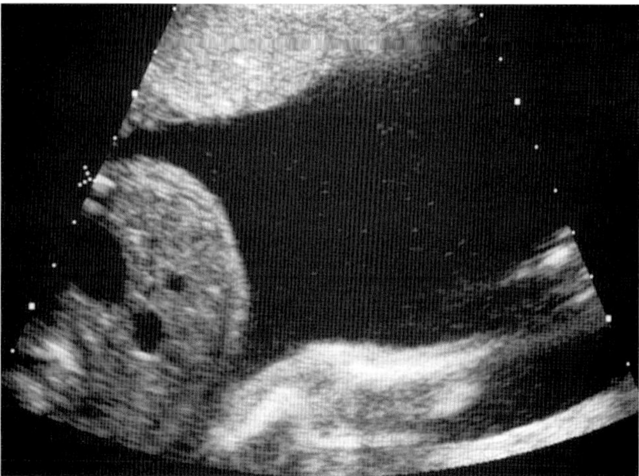
B

FIGURE 9.2-1. Duodenal atresia in a fetus with trisomy 21. A: Transverse view of the fetal upper abdomen demonstrates two fluid-filled structures ("double bubble") representing the dilated stomach *(long arrow)* and duodenum *(short arrow)*. **B:** Amniotic fluid volume is high. Amniocentesis was performed and revealed trisomy 21.

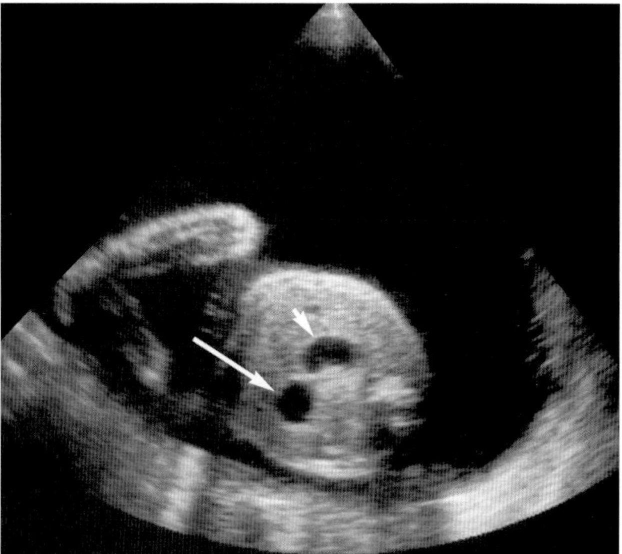

FIGURE 9.2-2. Duodenal obstruction due to annular pancreas. The stomach *(long arrow)* and duodenum *(short arrow)* are distended, and there is polyhydramnios. The baby died shortly after birth, and an annular pancreas was found at autopsy.

9.3. SMALL BOWEL OBSTRUCTION

Description and Clinical Features

Small bowel obstruction can occur at any point (or points) along the small bowel, from the proximal jejunum to the distal ileum. It can result from a number of causes, including atresia, volvulus, and a meconium plug. The latter cause is typically seen in fetuses with cystic fibrosis.

Because amniotic fluid is consumed by fetal swallowing and small bowel absorption, the amniotic fluid volume is usually increased when the fetus has a small bowel obstruction. In general, the more proximal the obstruction is, the more severe the polyhydramnios.

Sonography

The sonographic findings of a small bowel obstruction depend on the level of obstruction but typically include dilated fluid-filled loops of bowel and polyhydramnios. With proximal jejunal obstruction, the sonogram shows a short segment of dilated bowel and moderate-to-severe polyhydramnios (Figure 9.3-1). With a distal ileal obstruction, there will be multiple loops of dilated bowel, and the amniotic fluid volume will be normal or mildly elevated (Figure 9.3-2).

In some cases, the specific cause of obstruction can be diagnosed on the basis of the sonographic findings. For example, the presence of a markedly dilated bowel loop in a "coffee bean" configuration, with less severely dilated bowel proximal to it, is indicative of volvulus (Figure 9.3-3). Frequently, however, the specific cause cannot be determined

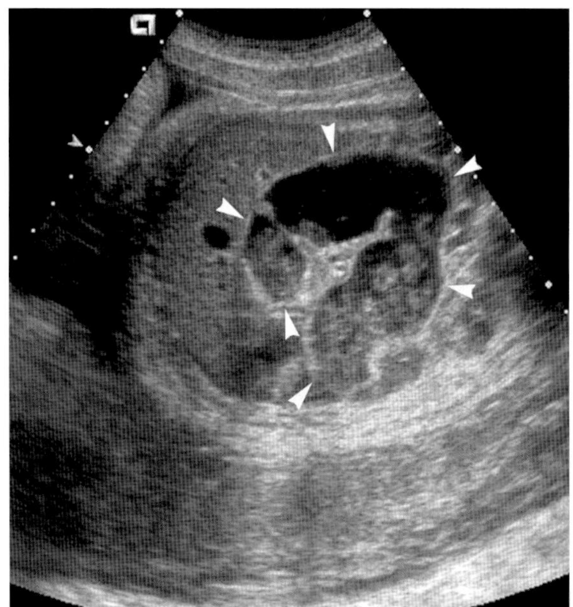

A

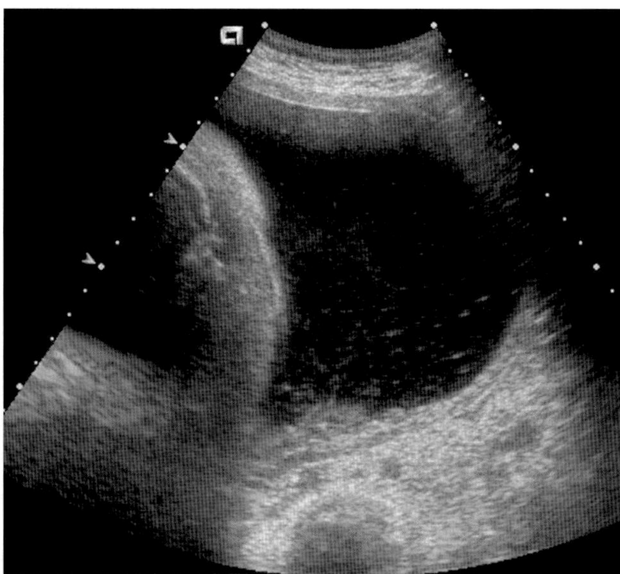

B

FIGURE 9.3-1. **Jejunal atresia. A:** Transverse view through the fetal abdomen reveals a dilated segment of bowel *(arrowheads)* filled with fluid and debris. **B:** The amniotic fluid volume is elevated for the gestational age of 38 weeks.

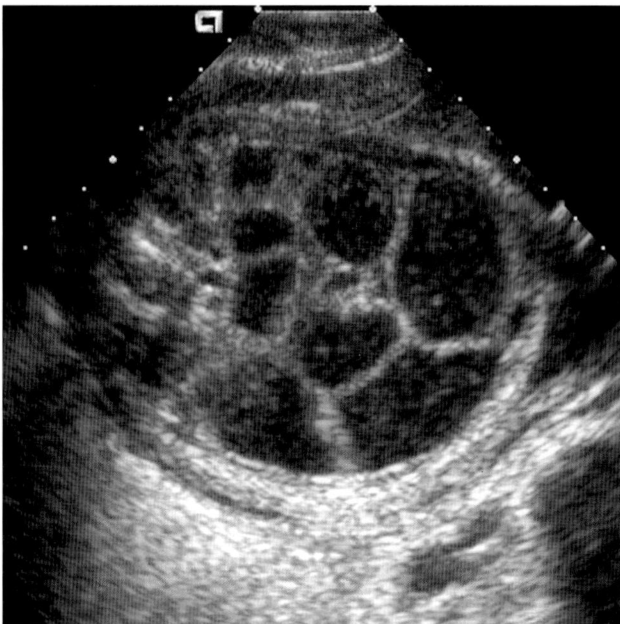

FIGURE 9.3-2. **Ileal atresia.** Transverse view through the fetal abdomen reveals multiple, dilated, fluid-filled loops of bowel. The amniotic fluid volume was normal.

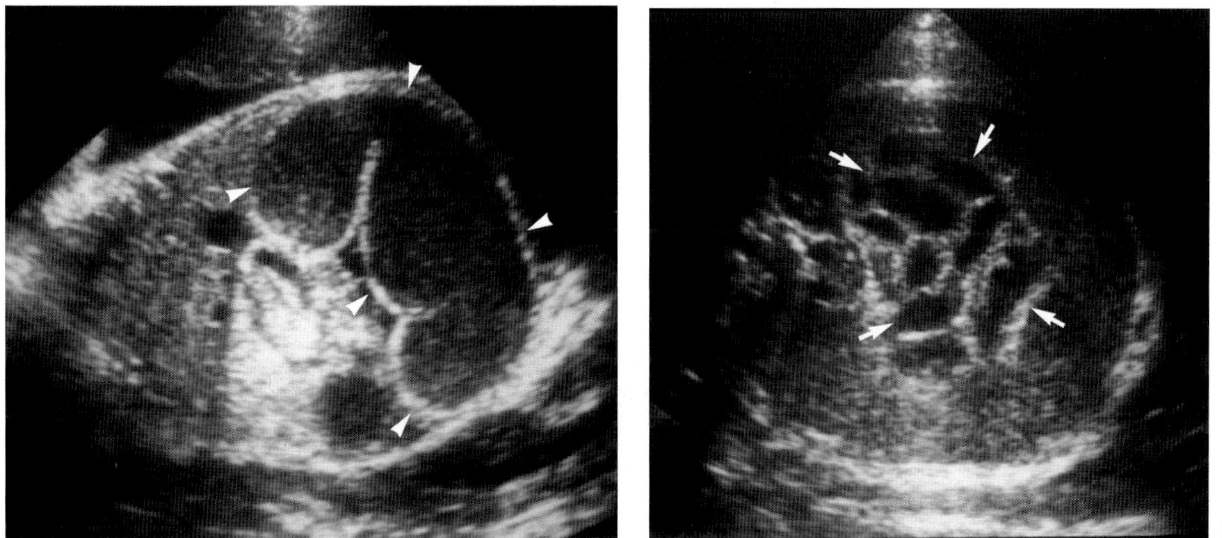

FIGURE 9.3-3. Volvulus. A: Oblique view of the fetal abdomen reveals a markedly dilated loop of bowel *(arrowheads).* **B:** Transverse section of the upper abdomen, superior to above this dilated loop, reveals multiple minimally dilated segments of bowel *(arrows).* Based on this appearance, a diagnosis of volvulus was made prenatally and was confirmed after birth.

by prenatal sonography. Postnatal imaging procedures and other diagnostic tests (e.g., sweat test for cystic fibrosis) or surgery are generally needed to establish the diagnosis and alleviate the obstruction.

9.4. MECONIUM PERITONITIS

Description and Clinical Features

Meconium is normally contained within the lumen of the fetal gastrointestinal tract. If it spills through a perforation in the bowel wall into the peritoneal cavity, it is irritative and elicits an inflammatory response. This inflammatory condition is termed meconium peritonitis.

The fetal response to this chemical peritonitis produces a number of intraperitoneal abnormalities that evolve over time after the meconium leak occurs. There may be abnormal fluid in the peritoneal cavity, either free (ascites) or walled off into a meconium cyst. Subsequently, intraperitoneal calcifications may develop, either on the serosal surface of the bowel or liver or in the wall of a meconium cyst.

Meconium leakage usually occurs just proximal to an area of bowel obstruction because high pressure proximal to the site of obstruction leads to rupture of the bowel wall. For example, meconium peritonitis can occur proximal to an atretic segment of small bowel or proximal to a meconium plug in a fetus with cystic fibrosis. In some cases, the cause of the meconium leak cannot be determined.

Sonography

The sonographic findings of meconium peritonitis are variable, depending in part on the time interval between meconium leakage and the sonogram. If sequential scans are performed, the sonographic findings can track the evolution of the intra-abdominal abnormalities (Figure 9.4-1): initially, free intraperitoneal fluid, subsequently, an irregular, thick-walled intra-abdominal cyst, often with calcification in its wall, and, finally, isolated

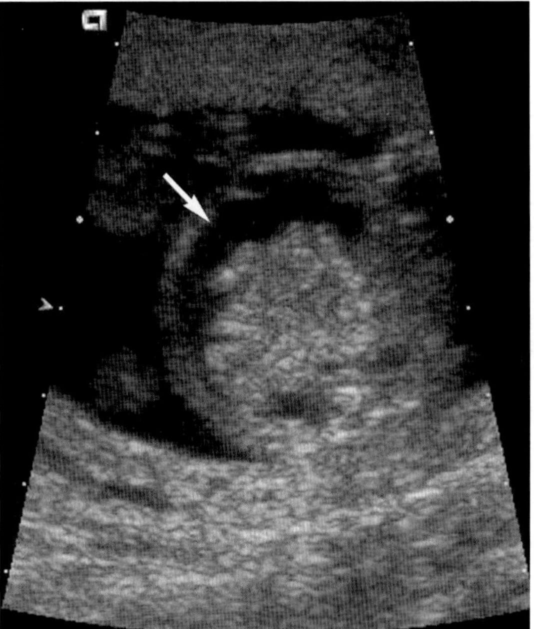

FIGURE 9.4-1. Meconium peritonitis: evolution over several weeks. A: Transverse view of the fetal abdomen at 16 weeks gestation demonstrates a moderate amount of free intraperitoneal fluid *(arrow)*.

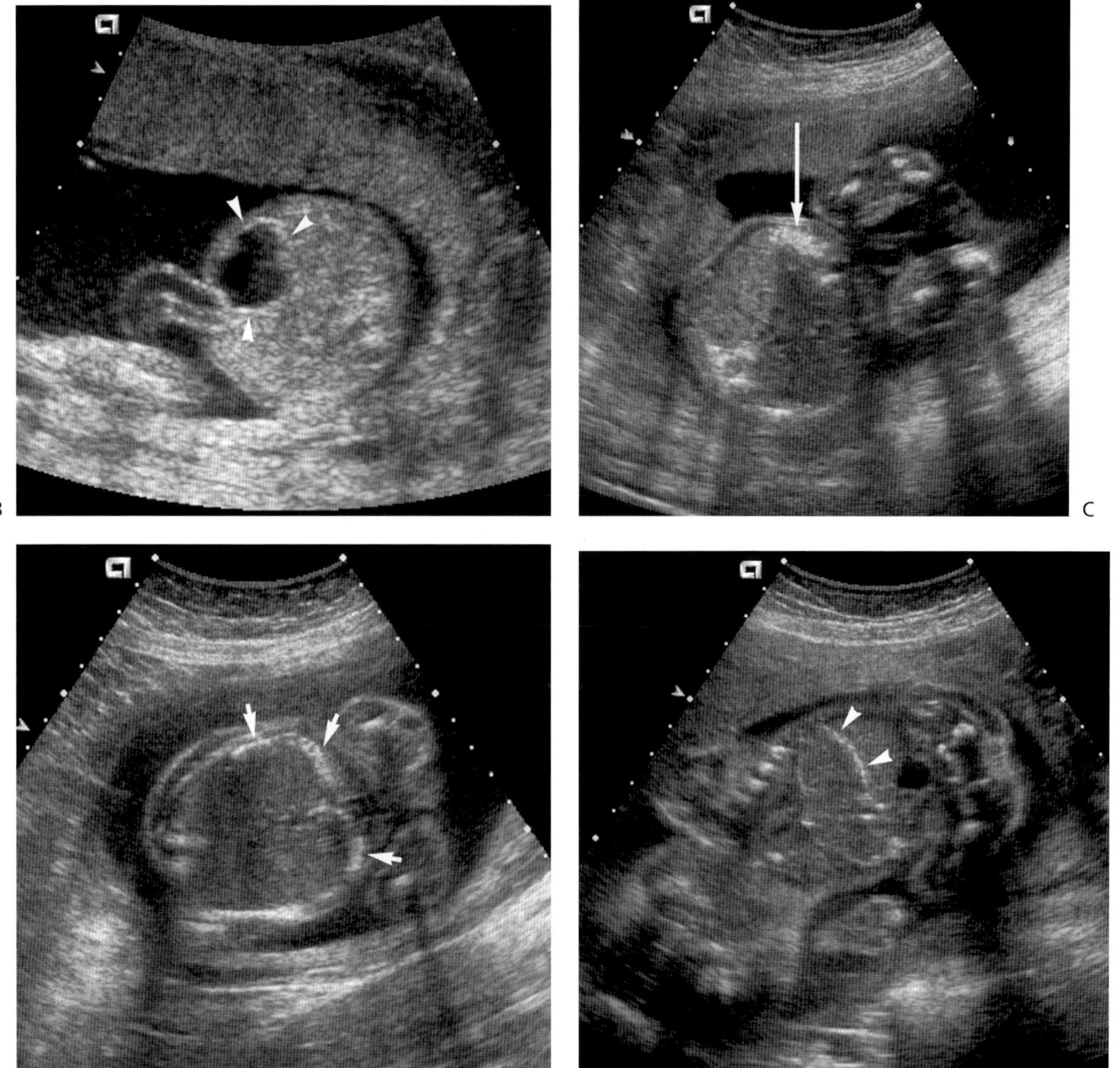

FIGURE 9.4-1. *(continued)* B: Transverse view of the abdomen at 20 weeks gestation demonstrates an intra-abdominal cyst *(arrowheads)* with a thick, irregular wall. **C–E:** Images from a 23-week sonogram demonstrate multiple intra-abdominal calcifications, including a clump of calcification *(arrow)* **(C)**, calcification along the peritoneal surface around the periphery of the abdomen *(arrows)* **(D)**, and calcification along the lower edge of the liver *(arrowheads)* **(E)**.

intraperitoneal calcifications. If only a single scan is performed, the findings can be any of the above (Figures 9.4-2 and 9.4-3).

The diagnosis of meconium peritonitis should be made if ultrasound demonstrates intra-abdominal calcification or a thick-walled, irregular cyst. Meconium peritonitis should be considered in the differential diagnosis of isolated ascites with no other abnormal fluid collections to suggest hydrops.

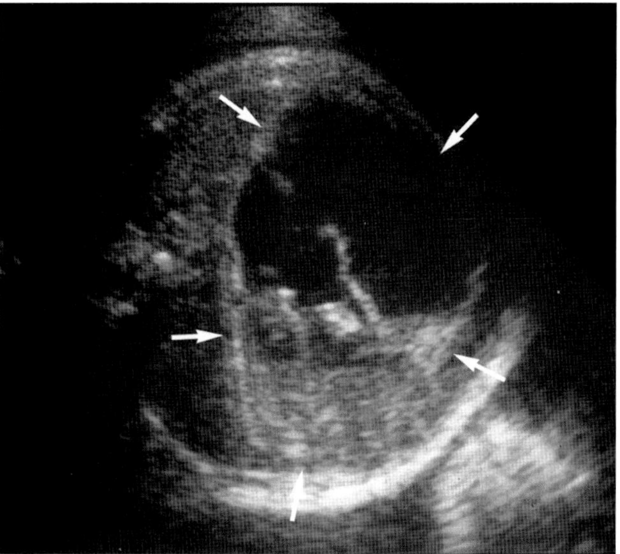

FIGURE 9.4-2. Meconium peritonitis: meconium cyst. Transverse view of the fetal abdomen demonstrates a large, irregular cyst *(arrows)*. Septations and layering debris are noted within the cyst.

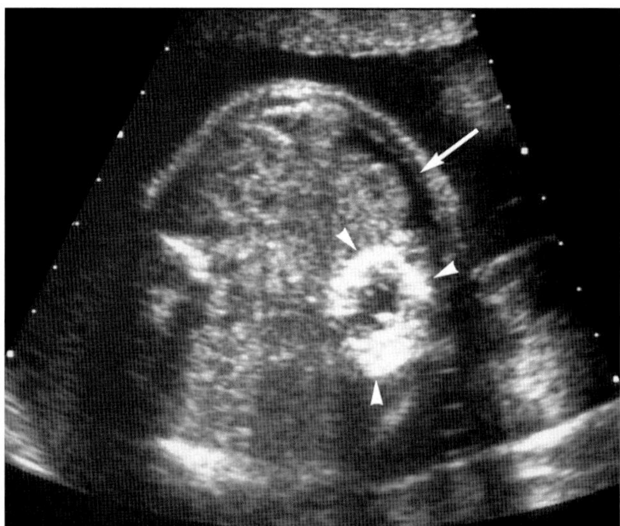

FIGURE 9.4-3. Meconium peritonitis: meconium cyst with a calcified wall. Transverse view of the fetal abdomen reveals a ring of calcification *(arrowheads)* around a small cyst, as well as ascites *(arrow)*.

9.5. CHOLELITHIASIS

Description and Clinical Features

In utero cholelithiasis is uncommon. In most reported cases, there is no predisposing condition, and the fetus is otherwise normal.

Sonography

The presence of one or more echogenic shadowing structures in the fetal gallbladder is the most definitive sonographic evidence for cholelithiasis (Figure 9.5-1). When this finding is present on a prenatal ultrasound, neonatal sonography will generally confirm the presence of gallstones.

Nonshadowing echogenic material in the fetal gallbladder, with or without distal reverberation ("comet-tail") artifact, is a more common prenatal sonographic finding (Figure 9.5-2). When this is observed in the fetus, the postnatal sonogram of the gallbladder is most often normal. This suggests that nonshadowing echogenic material in the gallbladder represents sludge or crystalline material rather than true gallstones.

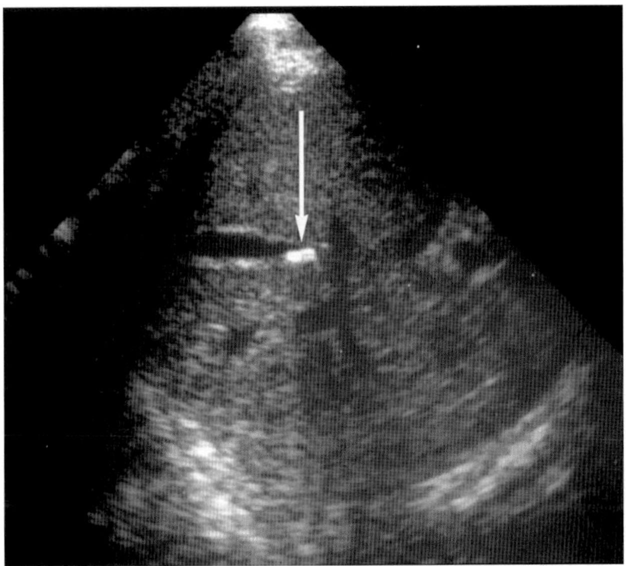

FIGURE 9.5-1. Cholelithiasis. Transverse view of the fetal abdomen demonstrates an echogenic structure in the fetal gallbladder *(arrow)* with distal shadowing. Postnatal ultrasound confirmed the presence of a gallstone.

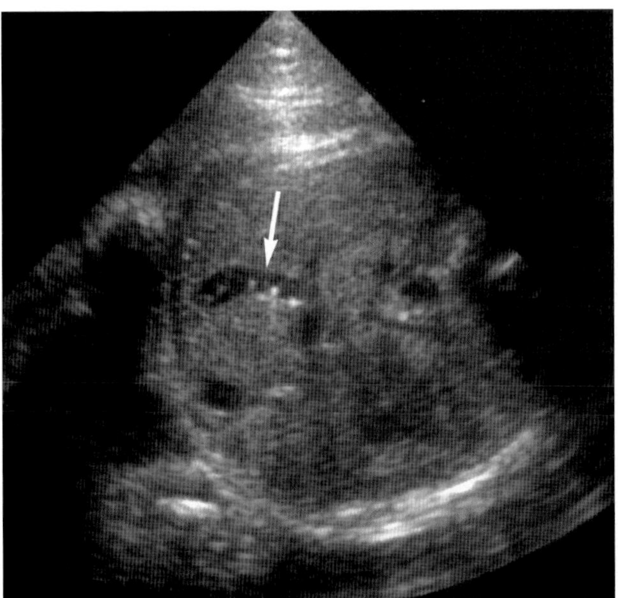

A

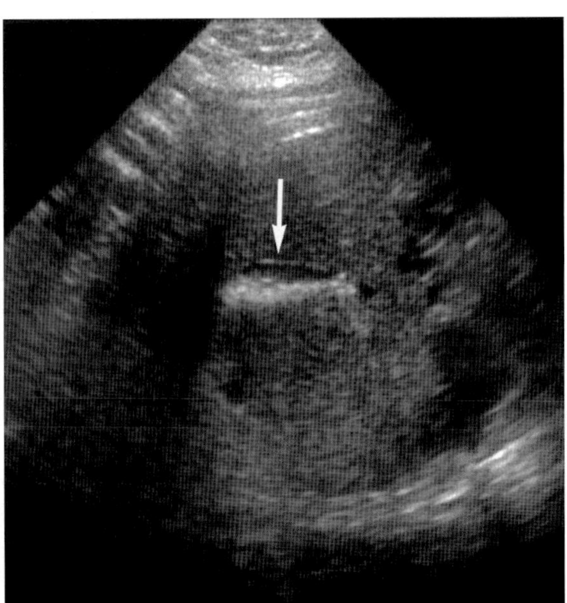

B

FIGURE 9.5-2. Transient echogenic material in the gallbladder. Transverse views of two fetal abdomens demonstrate nonshadowing echogenic material in the fetal gallbladders *(arrows)*, with **(A)** and without **(B)** the "comet-tail" artifact. Postnatal sonograms in both of these fetuses demonstrated normal gallbladders without stones or sludge.

9.6. LIVER MASSES, CYSTS, AND CALCIFICATIONS

Description and Clinical Features

There have been several reports of prenatally diagnosed solid liver masses, including hemangioendotheliomas, hemangiomas, mesenchymal hamartomas, and metastatic neuroblastomas. If large and highly vascular, a liver mass can lead to fetal hydrops on the basis of high-output cardiac failure.

Liver cysts may be isolated or may occur in conjunction with cysts in the kidneys or pancreas. One type of isolated cyst is a choledochal cyst.

Most reported intrahepatic calcifications in the fetus have had no known cause and have not been associated with an adverse outcome. This differs from intrahepatic calcifications in the neonate, which have been found to be associated with infections (e.g., cytomegalovirus), vascular accidents, and a number of other etiologic factors.

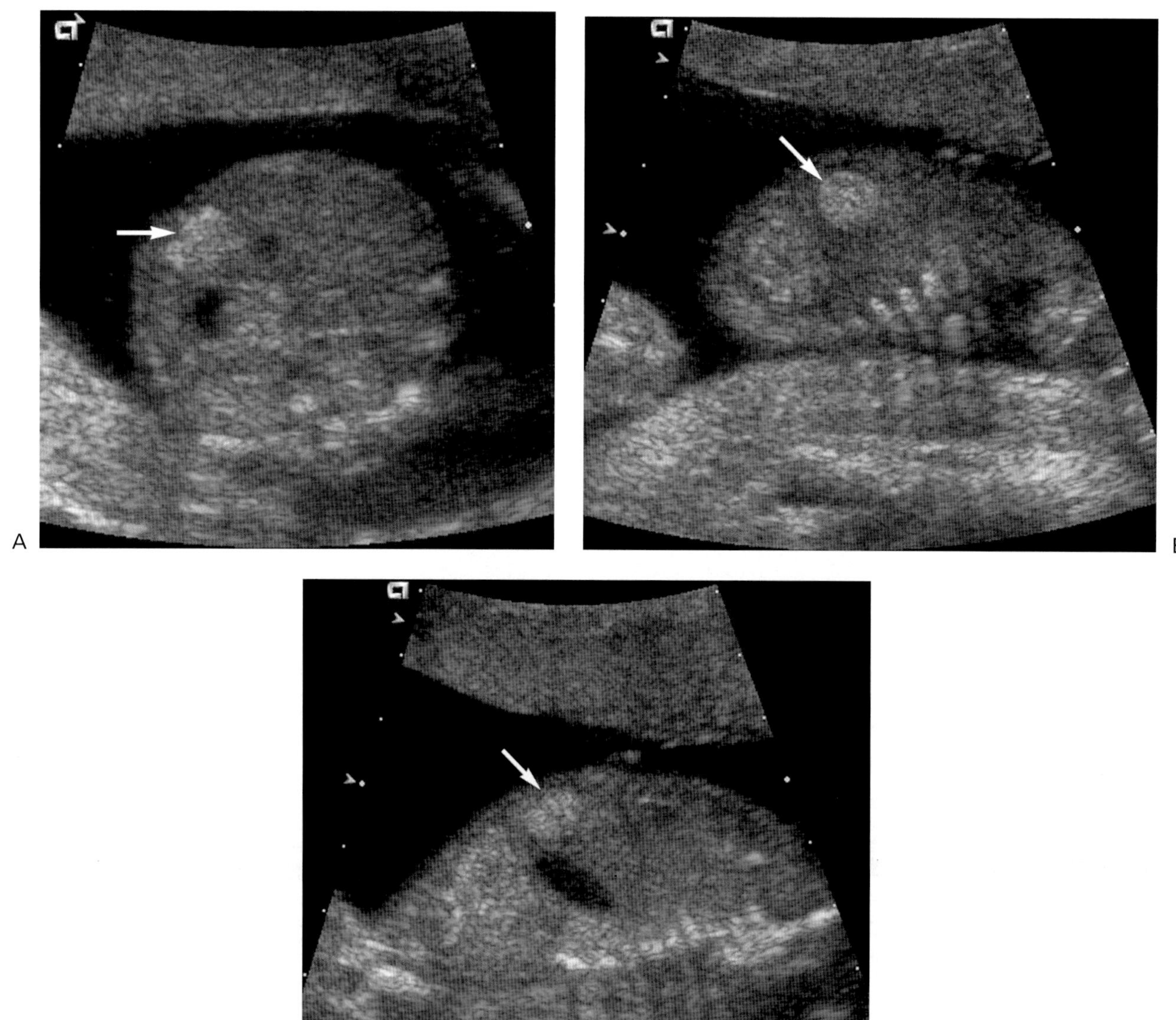

FIGURE 9.6-1. Hepatic mass. Transverse **(A)**, oblique **(B)**, and sagittal **(C)** views through the fetal abdomen demonstrate an echogenic mass *(arrows)* in the fetal liver.

Sonography

Solid liver masses are usually hypoechoic but may also be hyperechoic (Figure 9.6-1) or of mixed echogenicity. They are often hypervascular. When a liver mass is identified on ultrasound, it is important to determine whether the lesion is solitary or multiple and whether other extrahepatic mass lesions (e.g., adrenal neuroblastoma) are present.

A liver lesion is identifiable as a cyst if it is anechoic and smooth-walled and has enhanced through-transmission (Figure 9.6-2). When seen on ultrasound, important observations include the presence of tubular structures connecting into it, which would suggest a choledochal cyst, or coexisting renal and pancreatic cysts.

An intrahepatic calcification appears as a highly echogenic shadowing focus within the liver (Figure 9.6-3). Distinction must be made between calcification within the liver and intraperitoneal calcification, because the latter is indicative of meconium peritonitis.

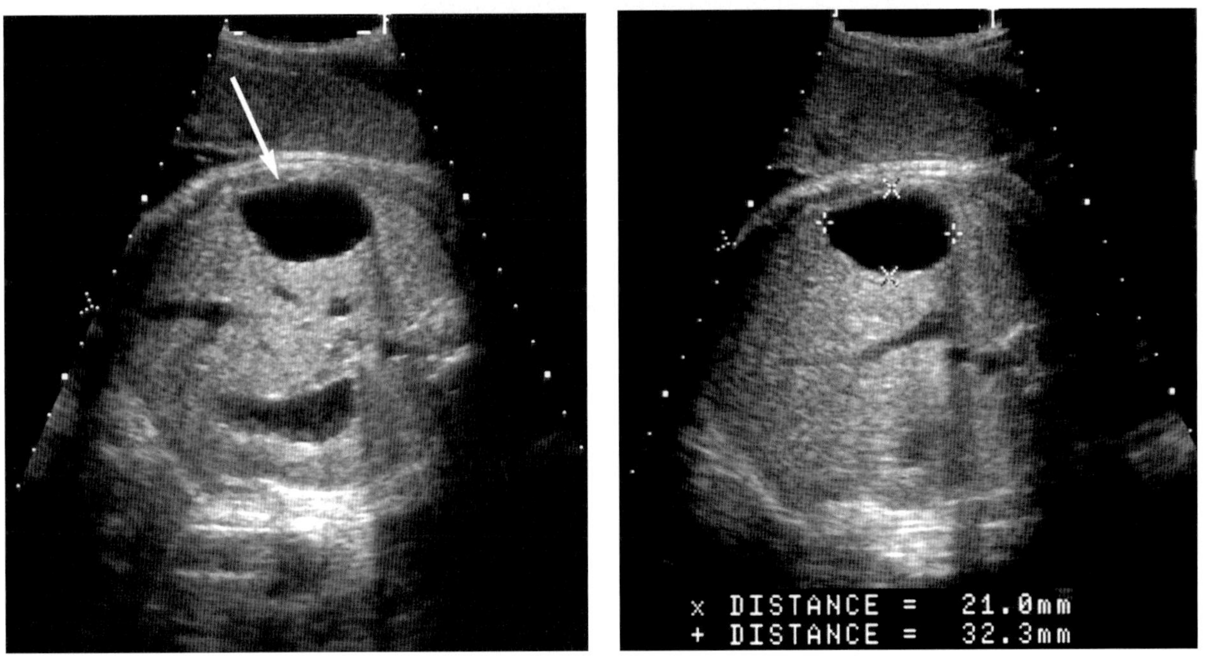

FIGURE 9.6-2. Hepatic cyst. A: Transverse view through the fetal abdomen reveals a simple cyst in the fetal liver *(arrow)*. **B:** Calipers delineate the anteroposterior and transverse diameters of the cyst.

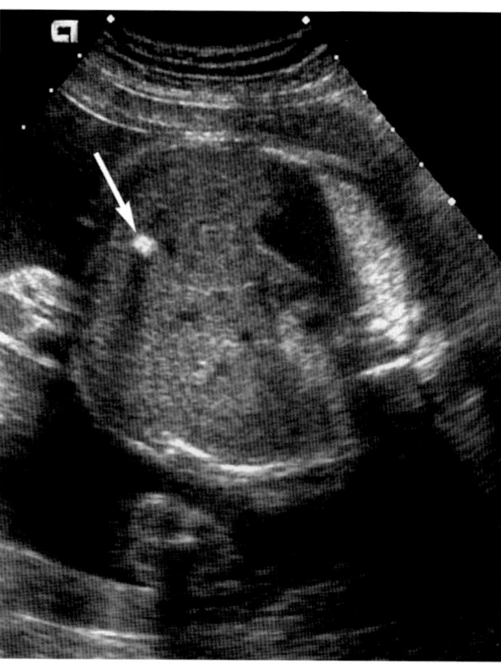

FIGURE 9.6-3. Intrahepatic calcification. Transverse view of the fetal abdomen reveals a calcification *(arrow)* with distal shadowing in the fetal liver.

SUGGESTED READINGS

1. Brown DL, Teele RL, Doubilet PM, et al. Echogenic material in the fetal gallbladder: sonographic and clinical observations. *Radiology* 1992;182:73–76.
2. Foster MA, Nyberg DA, Mahoney BS, et al. Meconium peritonitis: prenatal findings and their clinical significance. *Radiology* 1987;165:661–665.
3. Hertzberg BS. Sonography of the fetal gastrointestinal tract: anatomic variants, diagnostic pitfalls, and abnormalities. *AJR Am J Roentgenol* 1994;162:1175–1182.
4. Hertzberg BS, Kliewer MA, Bowie JD. Sonography of the fetal gastrointestinal system. In: Fleischer AC, Manning FA, Jeanty P, et al., eds. *Sonography in obstetrics & gynecology: principles and practice*, 6th ed. New York: McGraw-Hill, 2001:409–430.
5. Hill LM. Ultrasound of fetal gastrointestinal tract. In: Callen PW, ed. *Ultrasonography in obstetrics and gynecology*, 4th ed. Philadelphia: WB Saunders, 2000:457–487.
6. Stein B, Bromley B, Michlewitz H, et al. Fetal liver calcifications: sonographic appearance and postnatal outcome. *Radiology* 1995;197:489–492.

10

VENTRAL WALL

10.1. OMPHALOCELE

Description and Clinical Features

An omphalocele is a ventral wall defect at the umbilicus through which abdominal contents herniate into the base of the umbilical cord. The herniated contents are contained by a peritoneal membrane, and the vessels of the umbilical cord travel through the omphalocele. Omphaloceles are associated with other anomalies in approximately 80% of cases and with aneuploidy in approximately one-half of cases. The risk of aneuploidy is lower if the omphalocele contains liver than when liver is not herniated.

Sonography

An omphalocele appears as a rounded, well-circumscribed mass protruding from the anterior abdomen (Figure 10.1-1). The omphalocele sac usually contains bowel and may also contain liver (Figure 10.1-2). Rarely, other intra-abdominal organs are herniated into the sac. The vessels of the umbilical cord travel through the mass. Because of the association with other anomalies, a careful fetal survey should be performed after an omphalocele has been identified.

A 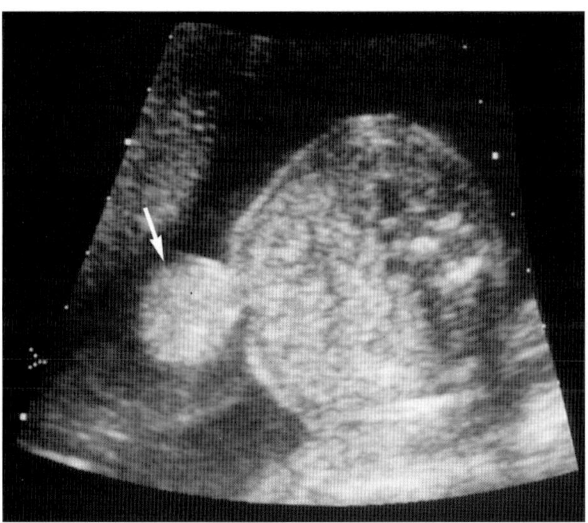

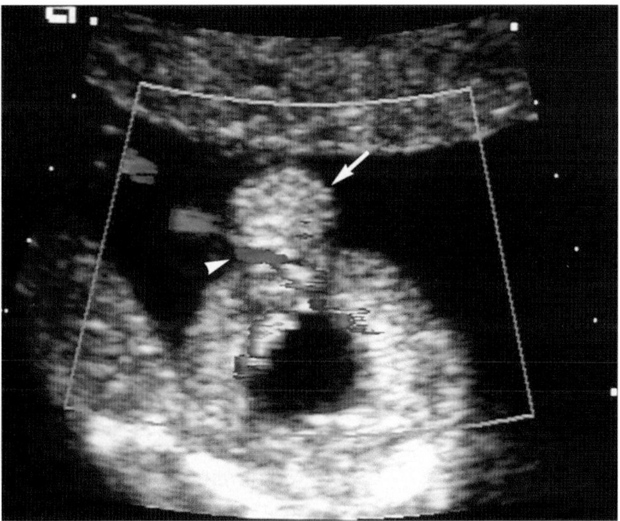 B

FIGURE 10.1-1. Omphalocele containing bowel only. A: Transverse image of the fetal abdomen demonstrates a small mass *(arrow)* protruding anteriorly at the umbilical cord insertion. **B:** Color Doppler image demonstrates the umbilical vein *(arrowhead)* coursing through the omphalocele sac *(arrow)* on one side.

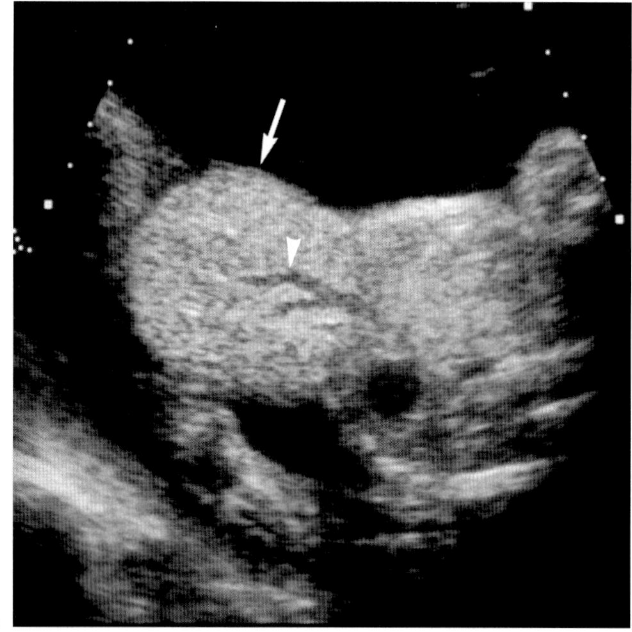
A

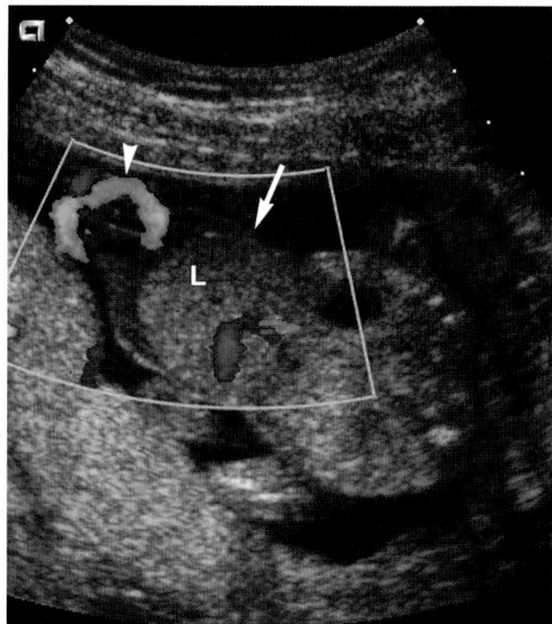

B

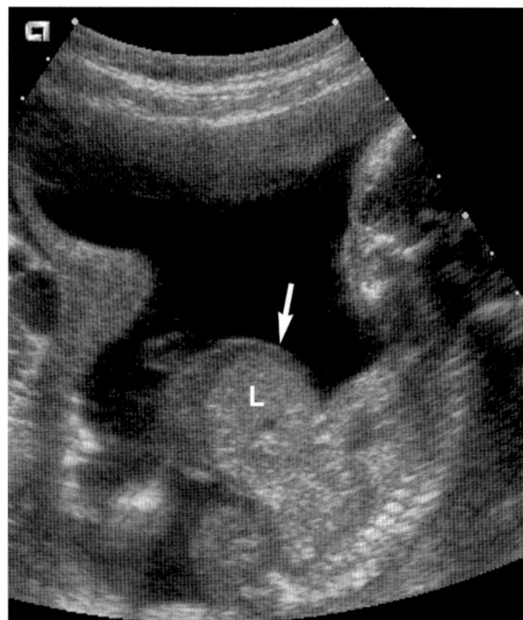

C

FIGURE 10.1-2. **Omphalocele containing liver. A:** Transverse image of the fetal abdomen demonstrates a large, rounded omphalocele *(arrow)* protruding from the anterior abdominal wall. Hepatic vessels *(arrowhead)* are seen in the liver, contained within the omphalocele. **B:** Color Doppler image of a large omphalocele *(arrow)* containing bowel and liver (L). Umbilical vessels *(arrowhead)* are seen inserting into the omphalocele sac. **C:** Sagittal image of the same fetus as in **(B)** demonstrates a large omphalocele *(arrow)* containing liver (L).

10.2. GASTROSCHISIS

Description and Clinical Features

Gastroschisis is a paraumbilical defect in the anterior abdominal wall through which intra-abdominal contents, usually bowel, herniate into the amniotic cavity. Unlike an omphalocele, the herniated tissue is free-floating in the amniotic fluid, not contained by a membrane. The defect is usually to the right of the umbilicus. Gastroschisis tends to affect young mothers more often than older mothers. Aneuploidy is uncommon. Other anomalies are present in approximately 25% of cases, but many of these associated anomalies, such as malrotation, are related to the gastroschisis.

The prognosis for gastroschisis is fairly good. Infants require surgery shortly after birth and many have gastrointestinal and infectious complications after the repair. Long-term gastrointestinal complications, including malabsorption, are common.

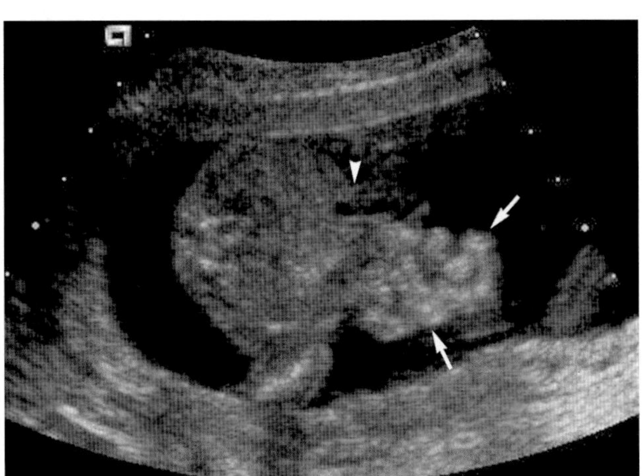

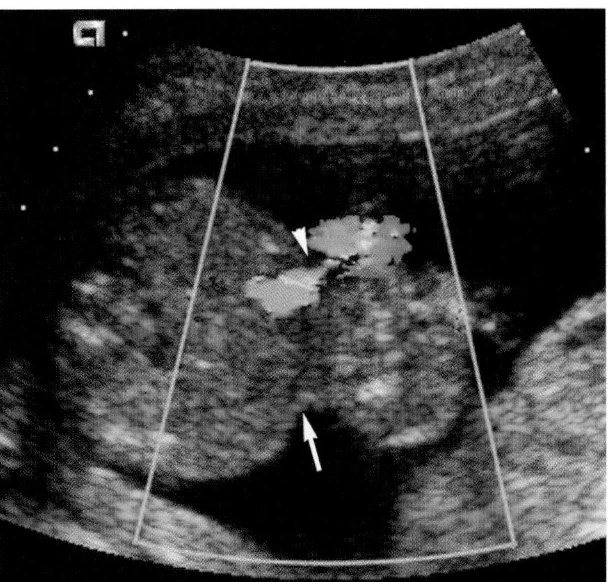

A B

FIGURE 10.2-1. **Gastroschisis. A:** Transverse image of the abdomen demonstrates loops of bowel *(arrows)* protruding from the anterior abdominal wall, adjacent to the cord insertion *(arrowhead)*. **B:** Color Doppler image demonstrates the umbilical cord insertion *(arrowhead)* adjacent to the defect *(arrow)* of gastroschisis.

Sonography

In the second trimester, gastroschisis typically appears as an irregular mass of tissue anterior to the abdomen on one side of the umbilical cord insertion (Figure 10.2-1). The amount of bowel herniated may increase as pregnancy progresses, and the herniated bowel loops may become dilated (Figure 10.2-2). Partial bowel obstruction may cause dilation

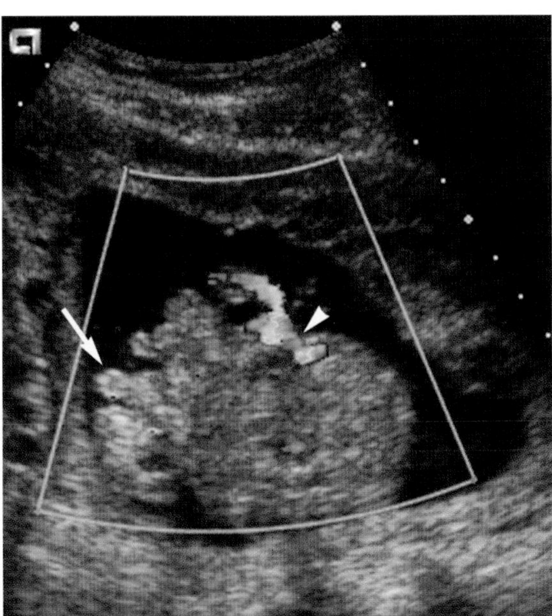

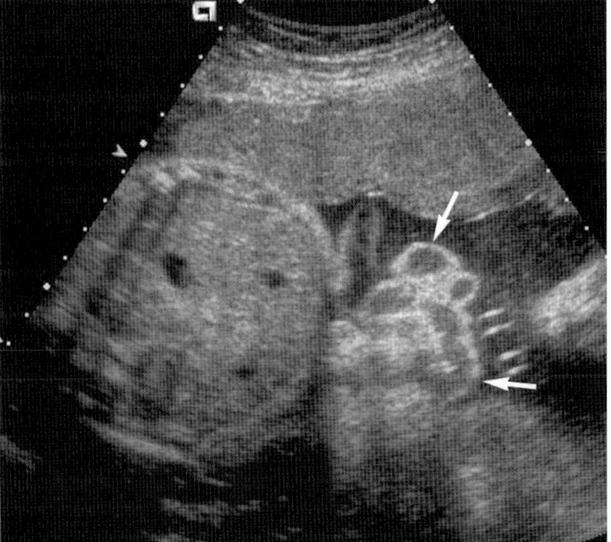

A B

FIGURE 10.2-2. Gastroschisis with progressive bowel dilation. A: Transverse color Doppler image of the abdomen in an 18-week fetus demonstrates nondilated loops of bowel *(arrow)* herniated through the gastroschisis defect. The umbilical cord insertion *(arrowhead)* is intact. **B:** Image of the abdomen in the same fetus at 32 weeks demonstrates dilation of the herniated bowel *(arrows)*.

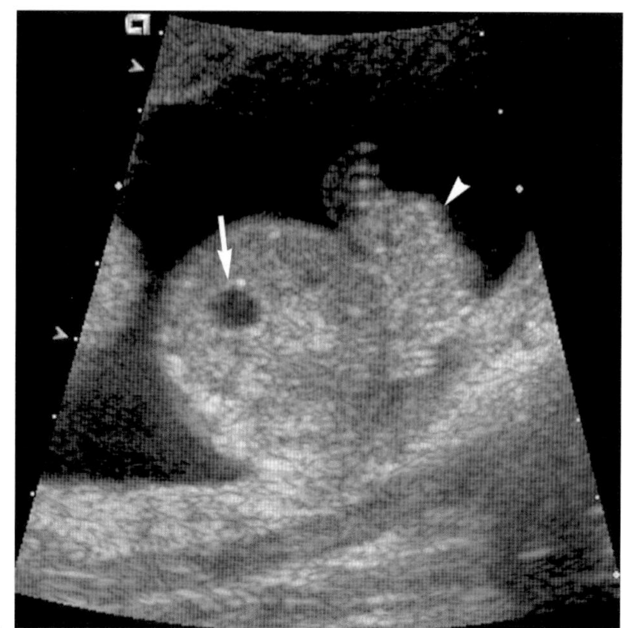

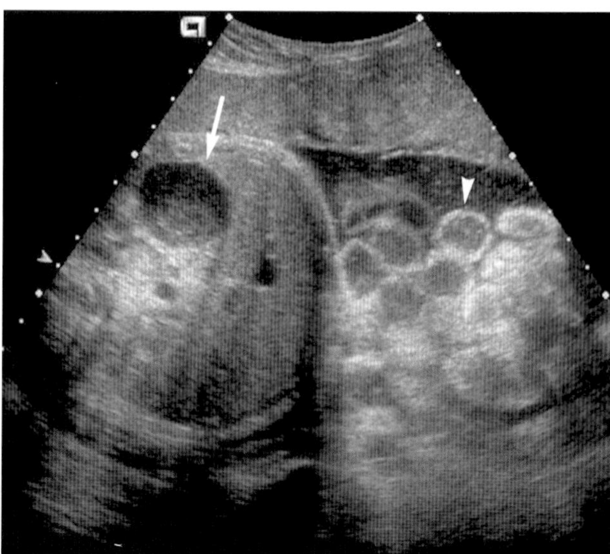

FIGURE 10.2-3. Gastroschisis with progressive dilation of the stomach and bowel. A: Transverse image of the abdomen in a 16-week fetus with gastroschisis. Nondilated bowel *(arrowhead)* is seen herniated into the amniotic cavity. The stomach *(arrow)* is normal size. **B:** Image of the same fetus at 34 weeks demonstrates dilation of the stomach *(arrow)* and the herniated loops of bowel *(arrowhead)*.

of the stomach (Figure 10.2-3) and polyhydramnios. Rarely, the liver or other abdominal organs may herniate through the gastroschisis defect.

10.3. AMNIOTIC BAND SYNDROME

Description and Clinical Features

Amniotic band syndrome is a disorder in which free edges of the amnion adhere to the fetus and entrap fetal parts, leading to a variety of fetal malformations. These deformities include amputations of limbs, abdominal and thoracic wall defects, facial clefts, and encephaloceles. The malformations may be extensive, leading to a marked disruption of the fetal trunk, spine, and head, or the malformations may be localized to a single limb.

Amniotic band syndrome is thought to result from early rupture of the amnion. The prognosis depends on the extent of the malformations.

Sonography

The diagnosis of amniotic band syndrome should be suspected when there are limb amputations or when there are atypical defects in the body wall or cranium. Adherent bands of amnion are sometimes visible crossing the amniotic cavity attached to the fetus. The deformities of the trunk may produce marked distortion of the fetus, with abdominal and/or thoracic contents herniated into the amniotic cavity and deformity of the spine (Figures 10.3-1 and 10.3-2). When the bands involve the head, distortion of the cranium may be seen, often with an encephalocele. The deformities vary considerably from case to case.

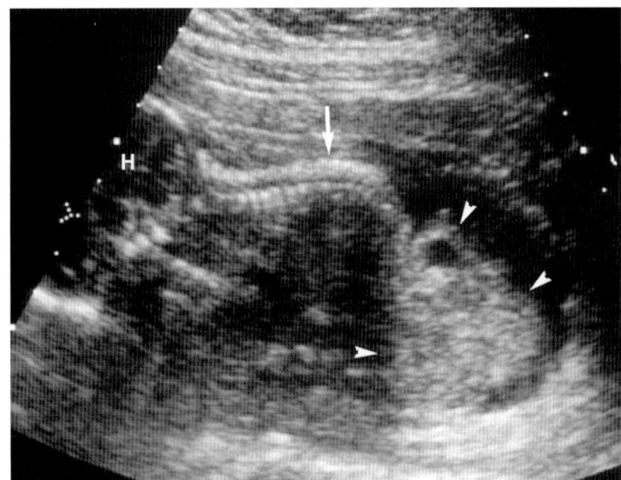

A

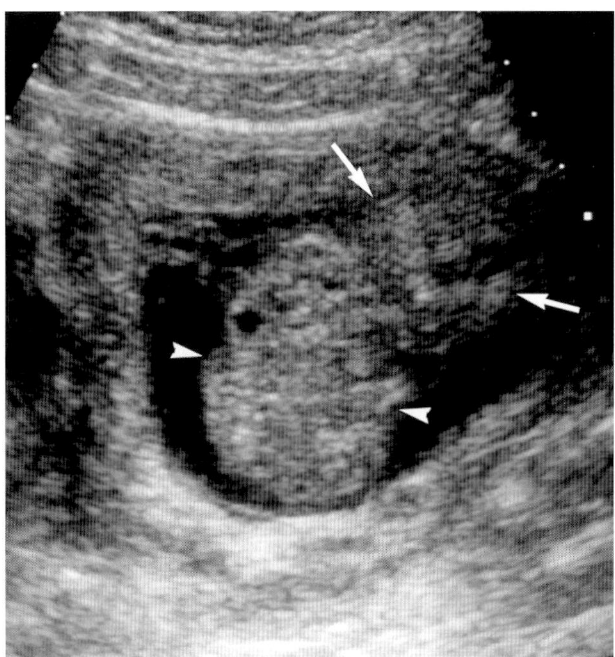

B

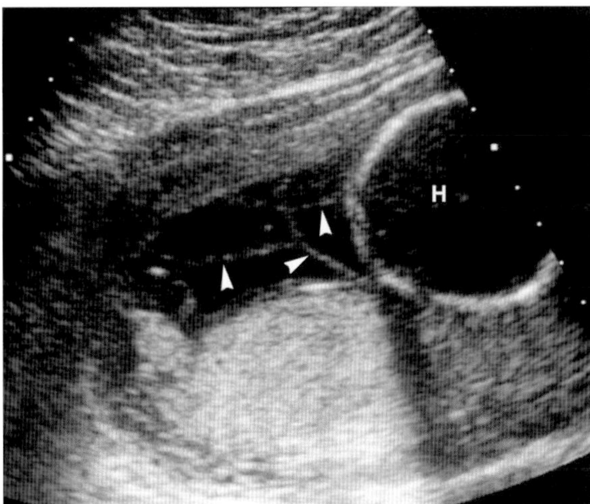

C

FIGURE 10.3-1. Amniotic band syndrome. A: Sagittal image of a fetus demonstrates an intact head (H) and upper spine *(arrow)* and disruption of the anterior and inferior trunk. Abdominal contents *(arrowheads)* float freely within the amniotic cavity. The lower spine is absent. **B:** Transverse image demonstrates most of the abdominal contents *(arrowheads)* floating in the amniotic cavity outside what is left of the fetal trunk *(arrows)*. **C:** Membranes *(arrowheads)* are seen crossing the amniotic cavity adjacent to the fetal head (H).

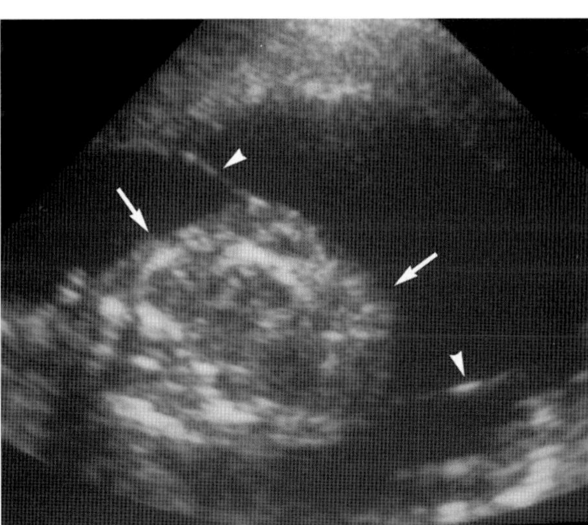

A

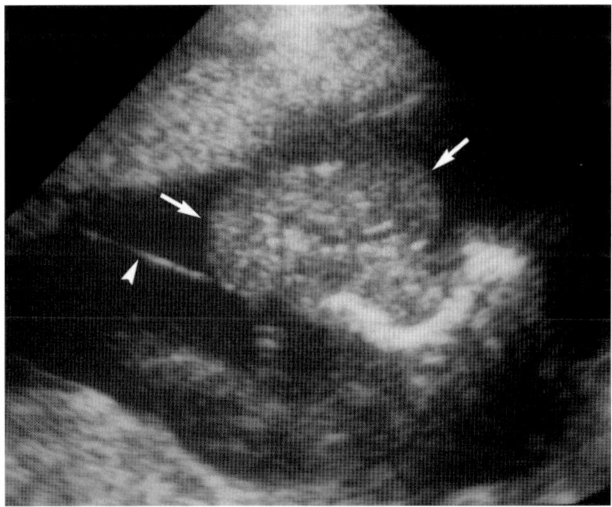

B

FIGURE 10.3-2. Amniotic band syndrome. A: Image of the upper abdomen *(arrows)* demonstrates loss of the normal round contour and disruption of the abdomen by amniotic bands *(arrowheads)* that extend from the edge of the gestational sac to the fetus. **B:** Abdominal organs *(arrows)* are herniated out of the abdomen, disrupted by bands *(arrowhead)* extending across the amniotic cavity.

SUGGESTED READINGS

1. Angtuaco T. Fetal anterior abdominal wall defect. In: Callen PW, ed. *Ultrasonography in obstetrics and gynecology*, 4th ed. Philadelphia: WB Saunders, 2000:489–516.
2. Bair JH, Russ PD, Pretorius DH, et al. Fetal omphalocele and gastroschisis: a review of 24 cases. *AJR Am J Roentgenol* 1986;147:1047–1051.
3. Cullinan JA, Nyberg DA. Fetal abdominal wall defects. In: Rumack CM, Wilson SR, Charboneau JW, eds. *Diagnostic ultrasound*, 2nd ed. St. Louis: Mosby, 1998:1161–1175.
4. Durfee SM, Benson CB, Wilson. J. Postnatal outcome of fetuses with the prenatal diagnosis of gastroschisis. *J Ultrasound Med* 2002;21:269–274.
5. Evans MI. Amniotic bands. *Ultrasound Obstet Gynecol* 1997;10:307–308.
6. Langer JC, Khanna J, Caco C, et al. Prenatal diagnosis of gastroschisis: development of objective sonographic criteria for predicting outcome. *Obstet Gynecol* 1993;81:53–56.
7. Nyberg DA, Fitzsimmons J, Mack L, et al. Chromosomal abnormalities in fetuses with omphalocele: significance of omphalocele contents. *J Ultrasound Med* 1989;8:299–308.

11

GENITOURINARY TRACT

11.1. UNILATERAL AND BILATERAL RENAL AGENESIS

Description and Clinical Features

Renal agenesis, which may be unilateral or bilateral, results from failure of the ureteric bud to develop during early embryogenesis. Unilateral agenesis occurs in approximately three per 10,000 births. When this abnormality is present, the single kidney hypertrophies *in utero* and renal function is normal. There are often associated genital tract anomalies, including bicornuate uterus or other uterine duplication anomalies. Prognosis for unilateral renal agenesis is excellent.

Bilateral renal agenesis is a lethal anomaly occurring in approximately one to four per 10,000 births. This anomaly occurs more frequently in males than females, with a ratio of 2.5:1. Bilateral renal agenesis leads to severe oligohydramnios, leaving no buffer of amniotic fluid between the uterine wall and the fetus. The resulting pressure on the developing fetus causes a number of fetal deformities, including pulmonary hypoplasia, abnormal facies, and limb positional abnormalities (e.g., clubfeet). The combination of bilateral renal agenesis and these related anomalies has been termed Potter syndrome. The fetus with bilateral renal agenesis usually survives until birth and then dies shortly thereafter from pulmonary hypoplasia. Recurrence in subsequent pregnancies is rare.

Sonography

Sonographic diagnosis of unilateral renal agenesis is made on the basis of nonvisualization of one of the fetal kidneys (Figure 11.1-1). Color Doppler can provide supporting evidence for this diagnosis by identifying a renal artery on only one side of the aorta. The solitary kidney is typically compensatorily large for gestational age.

Two potential errors must be avoided in diagnosing unilateral renal agenesis: missing the diagnosis by mistaking an adrenal gland for a kidney and erroneously diagnosing unilateral agenesis when one of the kidneys is in an ectopic location (e.g., pelvic kidney). The first error can result from the fact that the adrenal gland tends to assume a flattened ("lying-down") configuration in the renal fossa (Figure 11.1-2). Mistaking the flattened adrenal for a kidney can be avoided by recognizing that the adrenal gland does not have the internal architecture of a kidney, including renal cortex, pyramids, and central sinus. The second error can be avoided by scanning the fetal pelvis and lower abdomen to be sure that the missing kidney is truly absent rather than ectopically located.

Bilateral renal agenesis can be diagnosed by ultrasound from approximately 16 weeks gestation onward. The diagnosis is established by nonvisualization of the kidneys and urinary bladder in conjunction with severe oligohydramnios (Figure 11.1-3). Other sono-

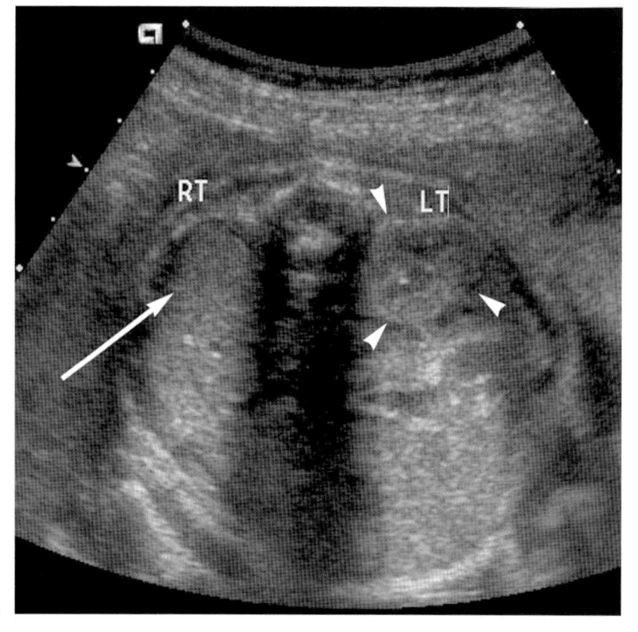

A

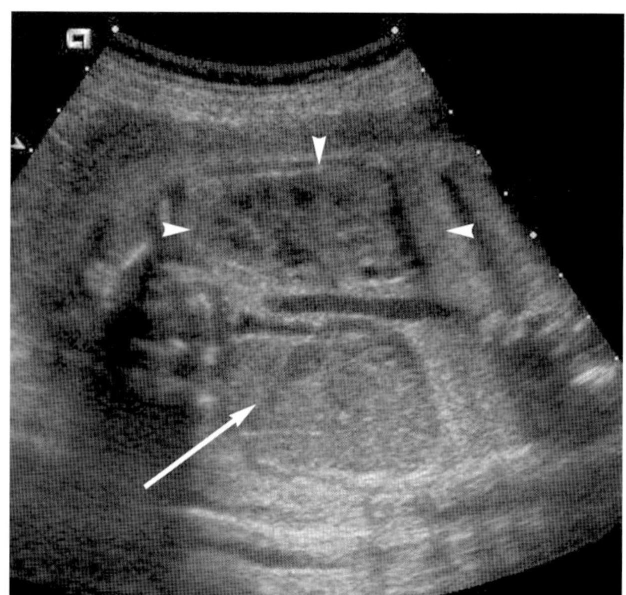

B

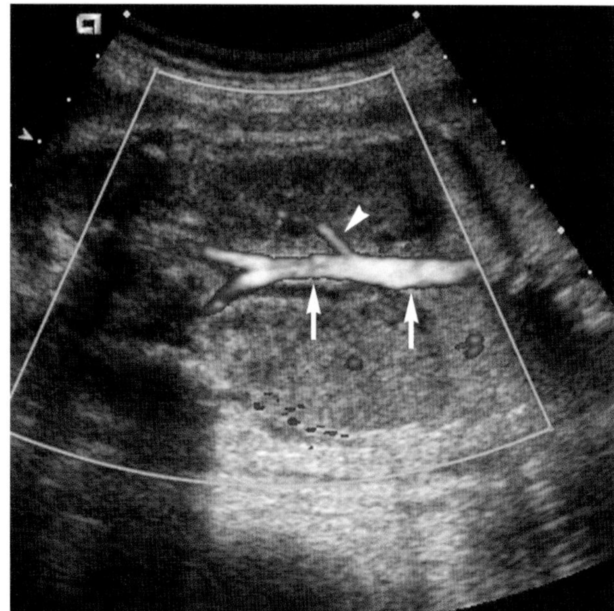

C

FIGURE 11.1-1. Unilateral renal agenesis. A: Transverse view of the fetal abdomen demonstrates a left (LT) kidney *(arrowheads)*. There is no kidney seen in the renal fossa *(arrow)* on the right (RT). **B:** Coronal view of the abdomen demonstrates a kidney on one side *(arrowheads)* and no kidney on the other side *(arrow)*. **C:** Power Doppler demonstrates a renal artery *(arrowhead)* arising from the aorta *(arrows)* to supply the single kidney and no renal artery on the other side.

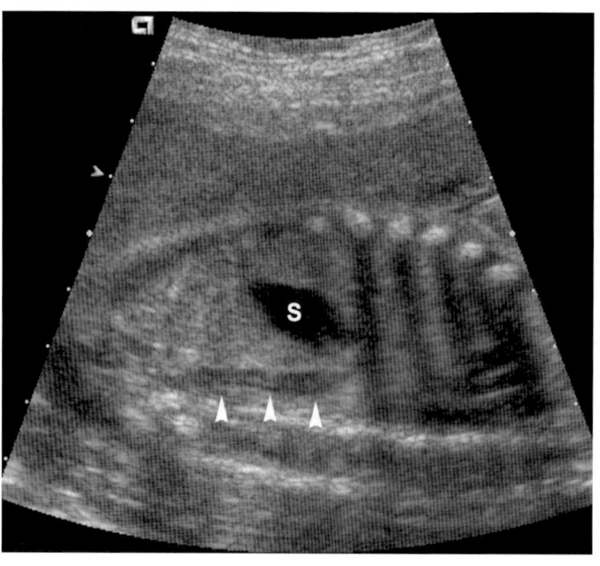

FIGURE 11.1-2. "Lying-down" adrenal gland in a renal fossa with an absent kidney. Left parasagittal view of the abdomen demonstrates the left adrenal gland *(arrowheads)* to be lying in a cephalocaudad orientation behind the stomach (S).

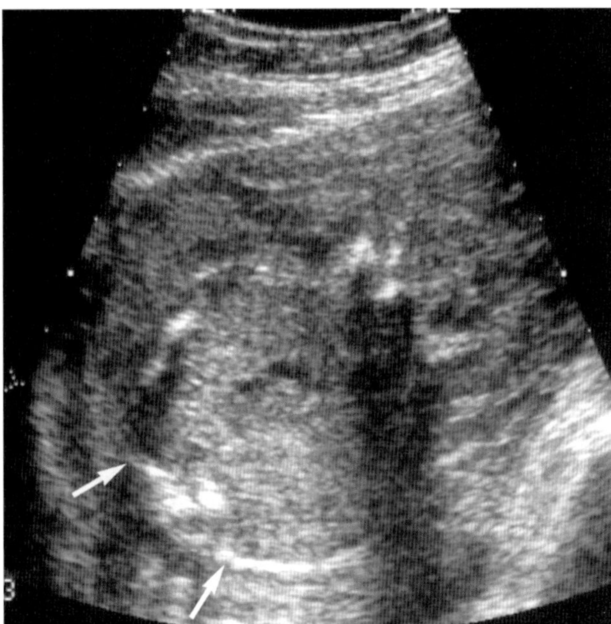

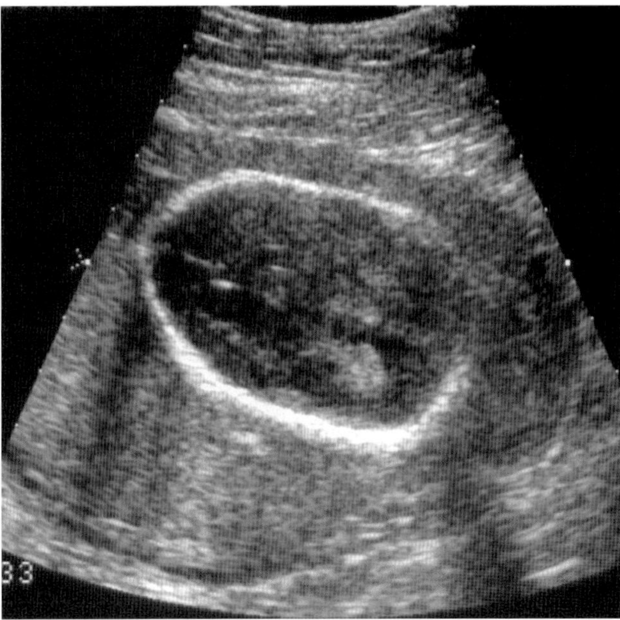

FIGURE 11.1-3. Bilateral renal agenesis. A: Transverse view of the fetal abdomen demonstrates no kidney in either renal fossa *(arrows)*. There is severe oligohydramnios, with no amniotic fluid seen around the abdomen. **B:** Axial view of the fetal head demonstrates it to be somewhat elongated and flattened (dolichocephalic) as a result of pressure from the uterine wall in the absence of amniotic fluid.

graphic findings often seen with bilateral renal agenesis include dolichocephaly and a small thorax, due to uterine compression on the fetus. Because bilateral renal agenesis is a fatal anomaly and the fetus is suboptimally imaged when it is not surrounded by amniotic fluid, the diagnosis of bilateral renal agenesis should be made only after a careful search of the fetal abdomen and pelvis for the kidneys and bladder. As with unilateral renal agenesis, it is important to avoid mistaking a "lying-down" adrenal gland for a kidney on one or both sides of the abdomen.

11.2. HYDRONEPHROSIS

Description and Clinical Features

Hydronephrosis refers to dilation of the fetal renal collecting system. It can result from urinary tract obstruction, vesicoureteral reflux, or deficient musculature in the walls of the urinary tract and abdomen (prune belly syndrome). The most common site of urinary tract obstruction is at the ureteropelvic junction (UPJ). Obstruction may also occur in the ureter, at the ureterovesical junction, or in the urethra.

Sonography

Visualization of a small amount of fluid in the renal pelvis is a normal finding on a second- or third-trimester sonogram. Hydronephrosis is diagnosed when the collecting system is abnormally distended. More specifically, hydronephrosis should be diagnosed when either the renal calyces are dilated (Figure 11.2-1) or the anteroposterior diameter of the renal pelvis (measured on a transverse view through the kidney) is 7 mm or more before 20 weeks, or 10 mm or more after 20 weeks gestation (Figure 11.2-2). Because hydronephrosis can develop at any time during pregnancy, it is prudent to label a kidney with a renal pelvis of 4–6 mm before 20 weeks or 5–9 mm after 20 weeks as possibly or

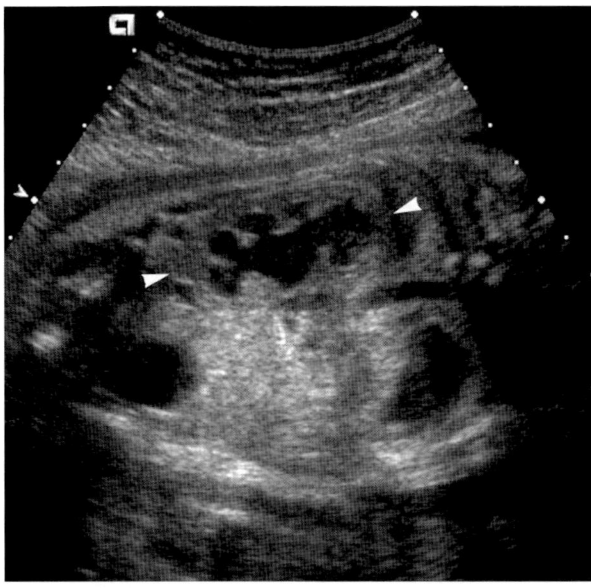

FIGURE 11.2-1. Hydronephrosis diagnosed on the basis of calyceal dilation. Sagittal view of the fetal abdomen demonstrates a kidney *(arrowheads)* with marked calyceal dilation.

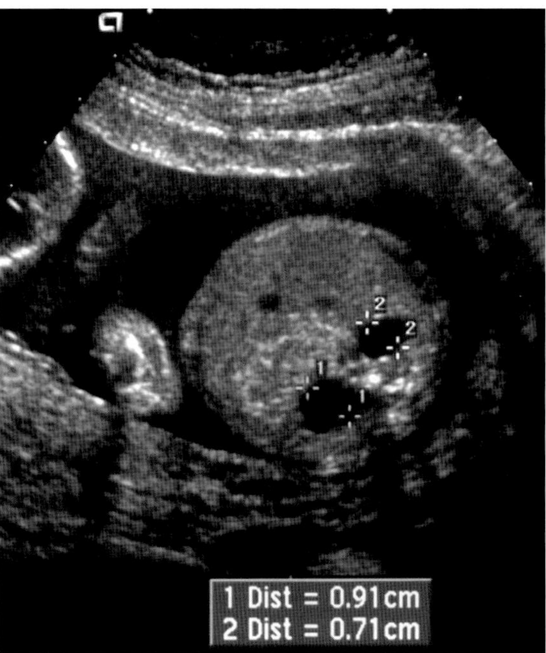

FIGURE 11.2-2. Hydronephrosis diagnosed on the basis of dilation of the renal pelvis. The anteroposterior diameters of the renal pelves *(calipers)*, measured on a transverse view of the abdomen in this 18-week fetus, are 9.1 and 7.1 mm. Both measurements are abnormally large at this gestational age.

borderline hydronephrotic (Figure 11.2-3) and to follow the case either to resolution or to development of definite hydronephrosis.

When hydronephrosis is diagnosed, the contralateral kidney should be evaluated to determine whether the hydronephrosis is unilateral or bilateral. The renal parenchyma should be examined for evidence of dysplasia. Imaging of the ureters and bladder is important to determine the lowest extent of urinary tract dilation. The amniotic fluid volume should be assessed because the fluid volume provides information about urine output and renal function. A careful search should be made for other fetal anomalies because the presence of one fetal anomaly increases the risk of other anomalies and because of the possible association between hydronephrosis and trisomy 21.

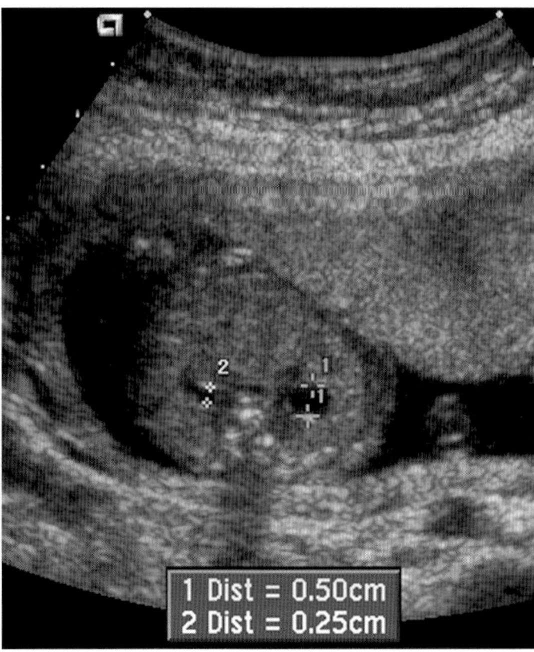

FIGURE 11.2-3. Borderline hydronephrosis. The anteroposterior diameters of the renal pelves *(calipers)*, measured on a transverse view of the abdomen in this 19-week fetus, are 5.0 and 2.5 mm. The former measurement represents borderline hydronephrosis, and the latter is normal.

11.3. URETEROPELVIC JUNCTION OBSTRUCTION

Description and Clinical Features

Uteropelvic junction (UPJ) obstruction, obstruction at the junction between the renal pelvis and the proximal ureter, is the most common cause of hydronephrosis in the neonate. It is bilateral in 30% of cases and occurs more often in males than females. Renal dysplasia is unusual but may occur if there is severe long-standing obstruction.

Sonography

The sonographic diagnosis of UPJ obstruction is made when there is hydronephrosis without hydroureter. It may be either bilateral (Figure 11.3-1) or unilateral (Figure

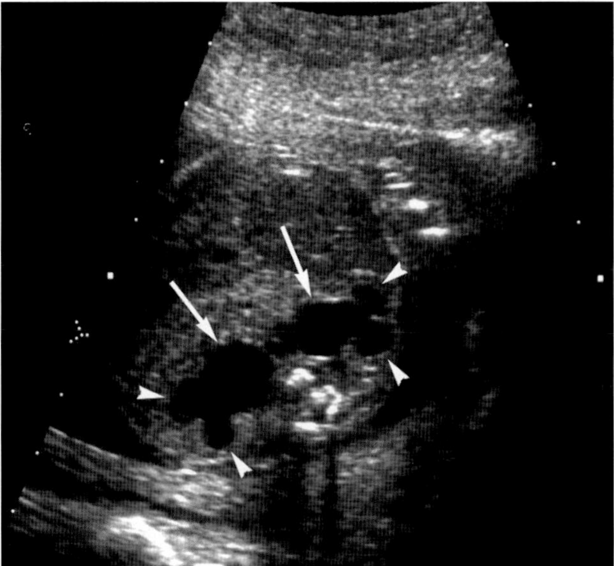

FIGURE 11.3-1. Bilateral ureteropelvic junction obstruction. Transverse view through the fetal abdomen demonstrates dilation of both renal pelves *(arrows)* as well as dilation of the calyces *(arrowheads)* in both kidneys.

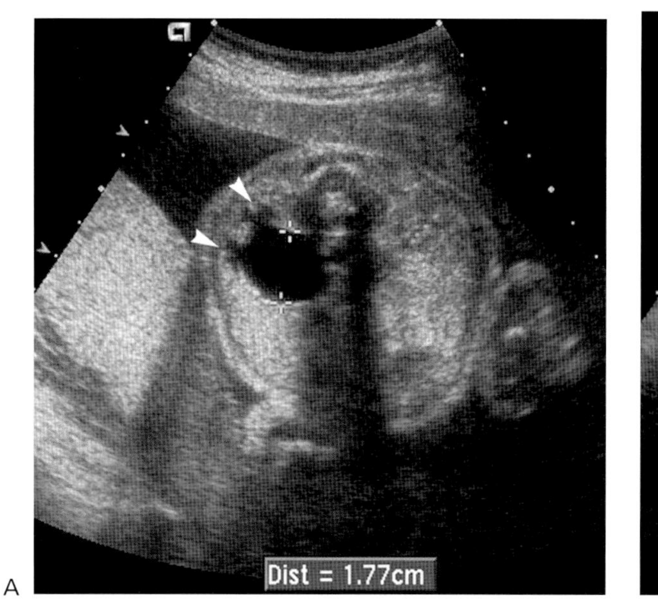

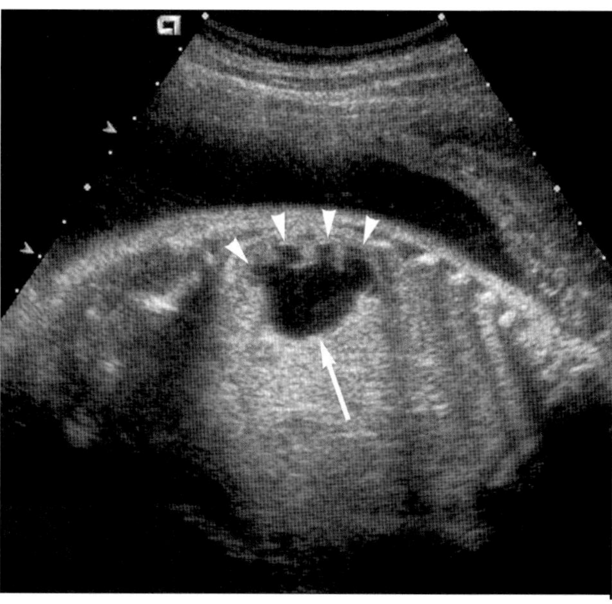

FIGURE 11.3-2. Unilateral ureteropelvic junction obstruction. A: Transverse view through the fetal abdomen demonstrates dilation of the right renal pelvis *(calipers)*, measuring 17.7 mm in anteroposterior diameter, as well as dilation of the calyces *(arrowheads)* in the right kidney. **B:** Longitudinal view through the right side of the fetal abdomen demonstrates dilation of the renal pelvis *(arrow)* and calyces *(arrowheads)*, with no ureteral dilation.

11.3-2). The amniotic fluid volume is usually normal. Development of dysplasia in a kidney with UPJ obstruction is uncommon but should be suspected if the parenchyma is abnormally echogenic or contains cysts.

11.4. VESICOURETERAL REFLUX

Description and Clinical Features

The ureter normally traverses the bladder wall at a shallow angle, leading to a configuration that acts as a valve preventing reflux of urine from the bladder into the ureter. Reflux occurs when the ureter has an abnormally steep, short course through the bladder wall. Reflux is often bilateral and is more common in males than females.

Reflux often resolves spontaneously *in utero* or within the first 1 to 2 years of life. If it is present at birth, the infant is at risk of urinary tract infections until it resolves. Appropriate management after birth, in most cases, is to treat with prophylactic antibiotics until resolution of reflux. Surgical correction is reserved for those cases that are severe at birth or fail to resolve.

Sonography

The prenatal sonographic findings of vesicoureteral reflux are hydronephrosis and hydroureter (Figure 11.4-1). In severe cases, the ureter is markedly dilated and tortuous. Milder cases may be misdiagnosed as UPJ obstruction or missed altogether because the hydronephrosis or hydroureter can be intermittent.

The combination of hydronephrosis and hydroureter is not specific for reflux because the same findings are seen with primary megaureter. The distinction between these two urinary tract abnormalities generally cannot be made *in utero* but must await postnatal voiding cystourethrography and intravenous pyelography.

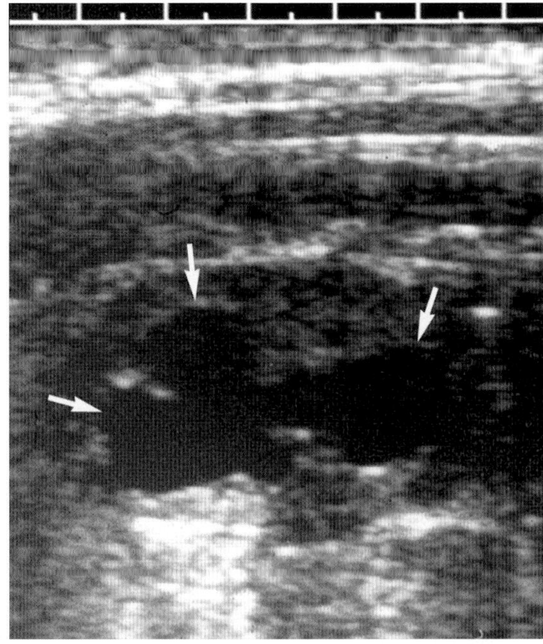

FIGURE 11.4-1. Vesicoureteral reflux. Prenatal sonogram demonstrates dilated calyces *(arrows)* **(A)** and ureter *(arrowheads)* **(B)** on the left. **C:** Postnatal voiding cystourethrogram, performed by catheterizing the bladder (BL) and instilling contrast, demonstrates severe reflux into the dilated left ureter *(long arrow)* and intrarenal collecting system *(white arrowheads)* as well as mild reflux into the right ureter *(short arrow)* and intrarenal collecting system *(black arrowheads)*.

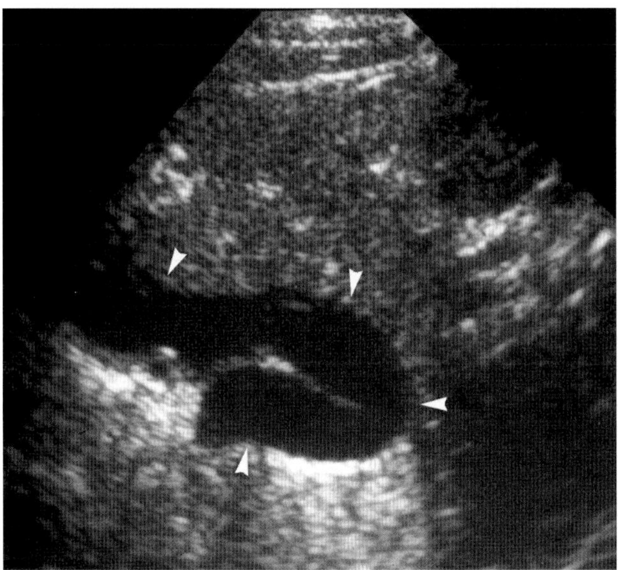

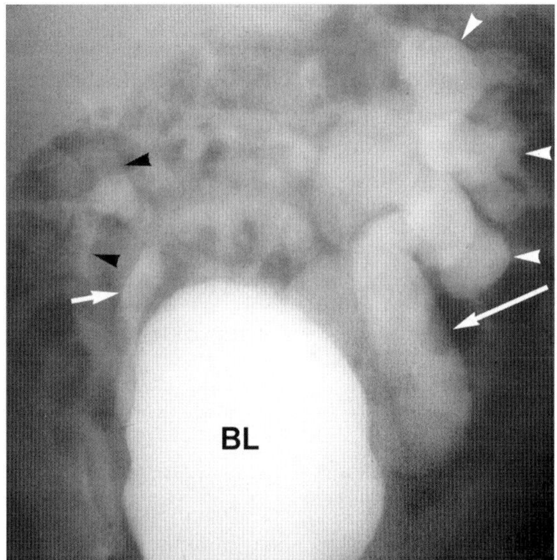

11.5. PRIMARY MEGAURETER (URETEROVESICAL JUNCTION OBSTRUCTION)

Description and Clinical Features

Several congenital abnormalities can interfere with the flow of urine through the ureter. The most common is an aperistaltic distal ureteral segment, which causes a functional obstruction. This abnormality, termed primary megaureter, generally has a good prognosis. In mild cases, no intervention is required, and in more severe cases, it is correctable by surgical resection of the affected segment.

Webs and strictures are less common ureteral abnormalities. Management and prognosis depend largely on the degree of obstruction.

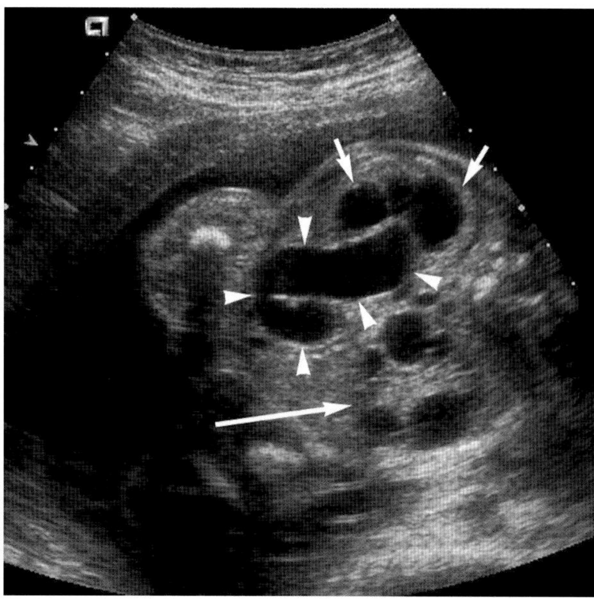

FIGURE 11.5-1. Primary megaureter. Transverse view through the fetal abdomen demonstrates dilated calyces *(short arrows)* and a dilated tortuous hydroureter *(arrowheads),* shown postnatally to represent a primary megaureter. There is a contralateral multicystic dysplastic kidney *(long arrow).*

Sonography

The prenatal sonographic findings of primary megaureter or other causes of ureteral obstruction are hydronephrosis and hydroureter (Figure 11.5-1). When these findings are present, the differential diagnosis also includes vesicoureteral reflux. Definitive diagnosis of the cause of hydronephrosis and hydroureter, as noted in the previous section, is made by postnatal testing.

11.6. POSTERIOR URETHRAL VALVES AND OTHER URETHRAL OBSTRUCTIONS

Description and Clinical Features

The major cause of urethral obstruction is posterior urethral valves, which occurs almost exclusively in males. Other causes include urethral atresia, which occurs in both males and females.

Prognosis is poor if the obstruction is complete, because the fetus is likely to have bilateral renal dysplasia and pulmonary hypoplasia. The latter occurs for the same reason that it does in fetuses with bilateral renal agenesis: lack of urine output leads to severe oligohydramnios and thereby to pressure of the uterine wall on the fetal thorax, which restricts pulmonary growth. Renal dysplasia occurs because the kidneys develop in the setting of high output pressure. In some cases, prognosis can be improved by prenatal treatment, either by percutaneously placing a shunt catheter from the fetal bladder to the amniotic fluid space or by creating bilateral ureterostomies via hysterotomy and fetal surgery.

Sonography

With urethral obstruction, there is oligohydramnios and the fetal urinary bladder is dilated and may have a thick wall. If the site of obstruction is distal to the vesicourethral junction, as it is with posterior urethral valves, a portion of the urethra will be dilated and appear as a projection from the bladder base (Figure 11.6-1). In most cases, bilateral hydronephrosis and hydroureters are seen, unless the kidneys have stopped producing urine because of dysplasia or high pressure has led to calyceal rupture, thereby decompressing the collecting system. In the former case, the kidneys are usually small and the renal parenchyma is cystic or echogenic (Figure 11.6-2). In the latter, fluid is seen in the perinephric space or abdomen (Figure 11.6-3).

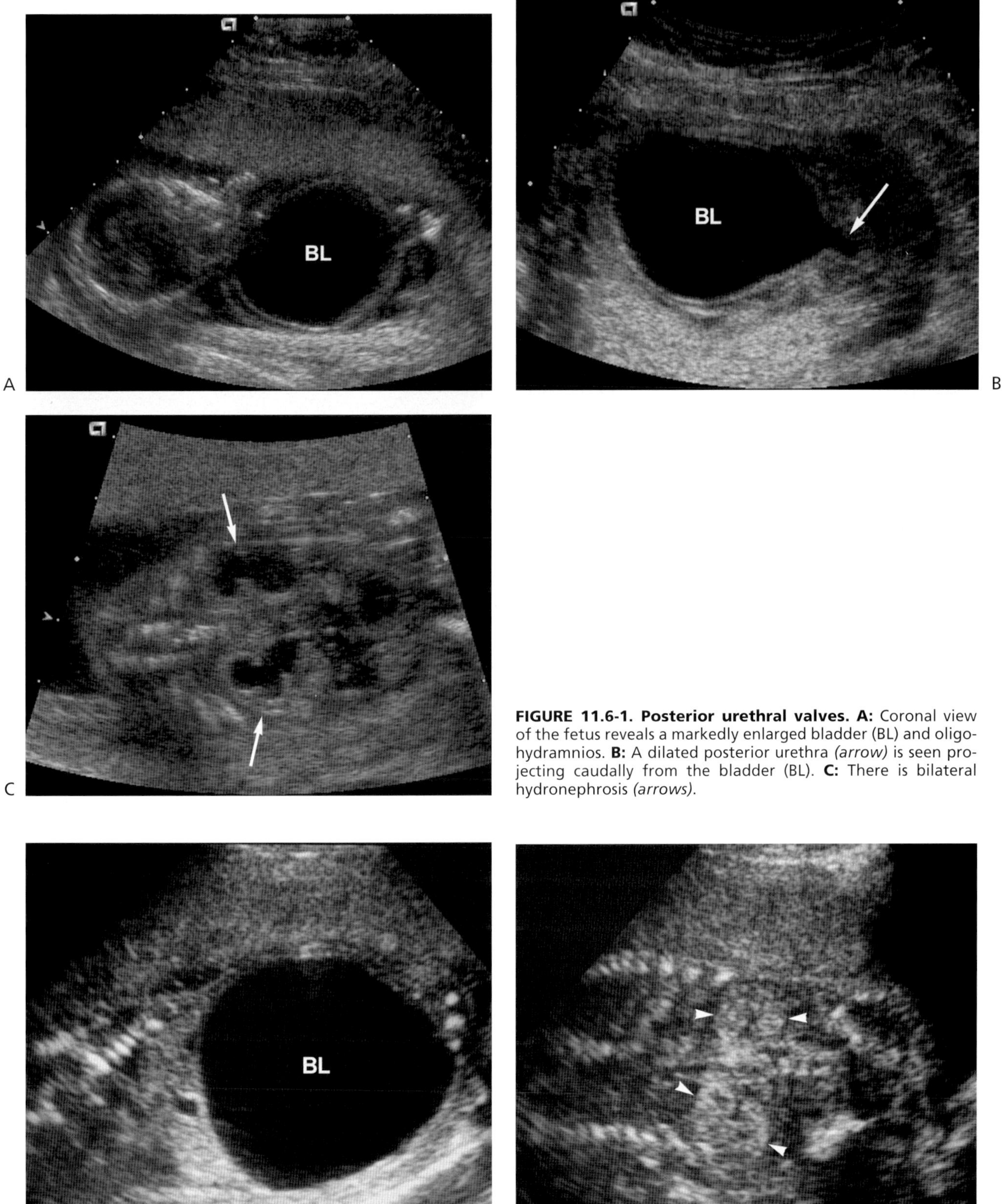

FIGURE 11.6-1. Posterior urethral valves. A: Coronal view of the fetus reveals a markedly enlarged bladder (BL) and oligohydramnios. **B:** A dilated posterior urethra *(arrow)* is seen projecting caudally from the bladder (BL). **C:** There is bilateral hydronephrosis *(arrows)*.

A BL B

FIGURE 11.6-2. Urethral obstruction with renal parenchymal dysplasia. A: The bladder (BL) is markedly enlarged, filling most of the fetal abdomen, and there is severe oligohydramnios. **B:** The kidneys *(arrowheads)* are echogenic and nonhydronephrotic, consistent with renal parenchymal dysplasia and lack of urine production.

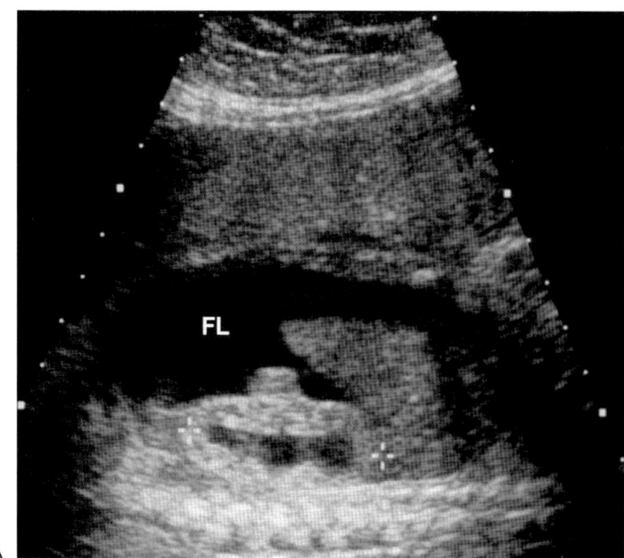

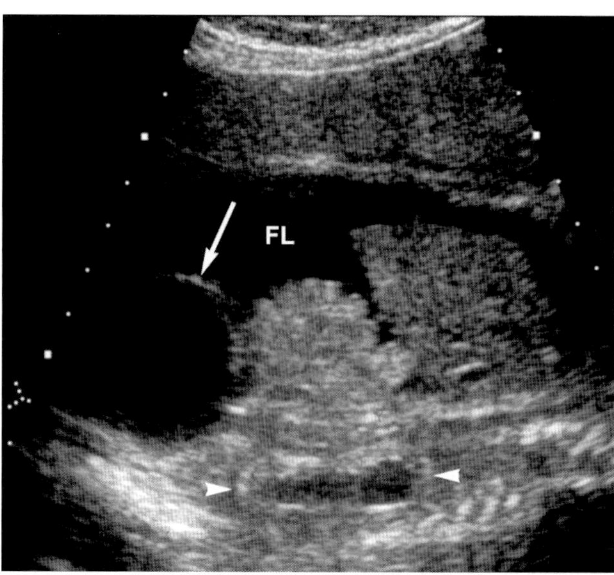

FIGURE 11.6-3. Urethral obstruction with urine ascites. A: Sagittal view through the right side of the fetal abdomen demonstrates a hydronephrotic right kidney *(calipers)*. There is a large amount of fluid (FL) in the fetal abdomen. **B:** Sagittal view through the left side of the fetal abdomen demonstrates a hydronephrotic left kidney *(arrowheads)* and fluid (FL) within the abdomen. The bladder *(arrow)* is distended.

11.7. MULTICYSTIC DYSPLASTIC KIDNEY AND RENAL DYSPLASIA FROM OBSTRUCTION

Description and Clinical Features

A multicystic dysplastic kidney is a nonfunctioning kidney consisting of noncommunicating cysts of various sizes, replacing the normal renal parenchyma. This anomaly is usually unilateral, but in 40% of cases, the contralateral kidney is abnormal, with UPJ obstruction being the most common contralateral abnormality. In rare cases, multicystic dysplastic kidneys occur bilaterally.

If the multicystic dysplastic kidney is unilateral and the contralateral kidney is normal, the renal function will be normal and the prognosis is excellent. The multicystic dysplastic kidney may cause problems by compressing adjacent organs, but surgical removal is not usually needed because the abnormal kidney generally atrophies spontaneously after birth.

The prognosis is worse if the contralateral kidney has a significant abnormality that reduces its function. The outcome is especially bad with bilateral multicystic dysplastic kidneys, which is a fatal condition that is functionally equivalent to bilateral renal agenesis.

A multicystic dysplastic kidney is thought to be caused by complete obstruction or atresia at the level of the renal pelvis or proximal ureter before 10 weeks gestation. The obstructed outflow from the developing kidney is hypothesized to lead to dysplastic, cyst-filled renal parenchyma.

Renal dysplasia can also develop with urinary tract obstruction that begins after 10 weeks or is an incomplete obstruction. In these cases, with prolonged obstruction at any level (UPJ, ureterovesical junction, or bladder outlet), one or both kidneys become hydronephrotic initially, then develop parenchymal dysplasia characterized by microscopic (as opposed to macroscopic) cysts and cortical thinning.

Sonography

A multicystic dysplastic kidney appears as a mass in the renal fossa composed of multiple cysts of various sizes (Figure 11.7-1). The cysts can be quite large, and the multicystic dys-

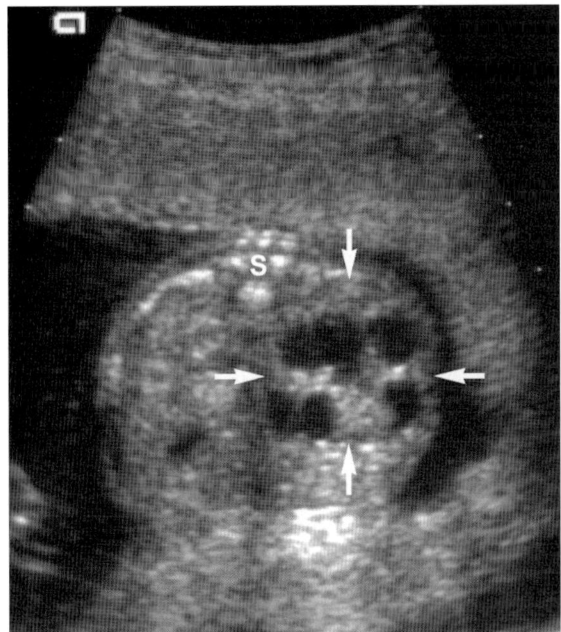

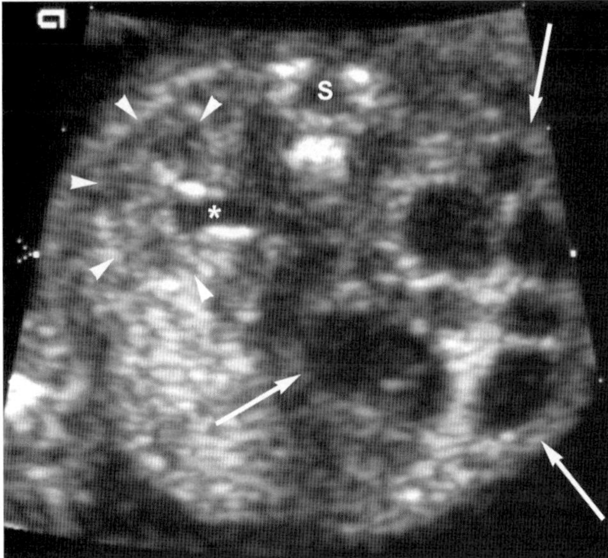

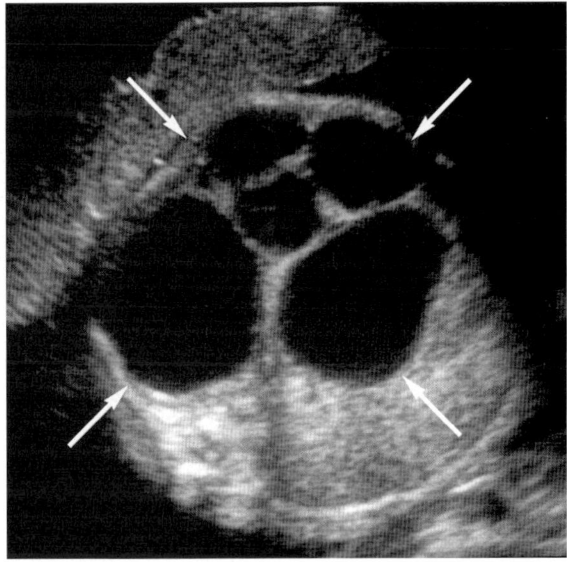

FIGURE 11.7-1. Unilateral multicystic dysplastic kidney increasing in size. A: Transverse view through the fetal abdomen at 19 weeks gestation demonstrates a mass *(arrows)* with multiple cysts located adjacent to the spine (S) in the expected location of a kidney, representing a multicystic dysplastic kidney. No normal renal tissue is seen on this side. **B:** Another transverse view in this 19-week fetus shows the multicystic dysplastic kidney *(arrows)* beside the spine (S) and demonstrates that the contralateral kidney *(arrowheads)* is normal, with a small amount of fluid in its renal pelvis *(*)*. **C:** On a follow-up scan at 33 weeks gestation, the multicystic dysplastic kidney *(arrows)* has increased markedly in size, occupying a substantially greater proportion of the fetal abdomen. From Benson CB, Doubilet PM. Fetal genitourinary system. In: Fleischer AC, Manning FA, Jeanty P, Romero R, eds. *Sonography in obstetrics and gynecology: principles and practice,* 6th ed. New York: McGraw-Hill, 2000, p. 237–244, with permission.)

plastic kidney is often much larger than a normal kidney. If multiple scans are performed during the pregnancy, the multicystic dysplastic kidney may be seen to increase or decrease in size. The amniotic fluid volume is usually normal. If there is oligohydramnios, the contralateral kidney should be carefully examined, searching for another multicystic dysplastic kidney (Figure 11.7-2) or for obstruction, dysplasia, or agenesis.

When dysplasia occurs as a result of obstruction after 10 weeks gestation, the dysplastic kidney initially maintains a more reniform shape and does not usually have the large cysts characteristic of a multicystic dysplastic kidney. The earliest sonographic findings of dysplasia in a hydronephrotic kidney are parenchymal cysts or a thin, echogenic renal cortex. As the dysplasia worsens and urine output from the involved kidney decreases, the hydronephrosis will diminish or resolve, leaving a shrunken echogenic kidney. Ultimately, little or no renal tissue may remain (Figure 11.7-3).

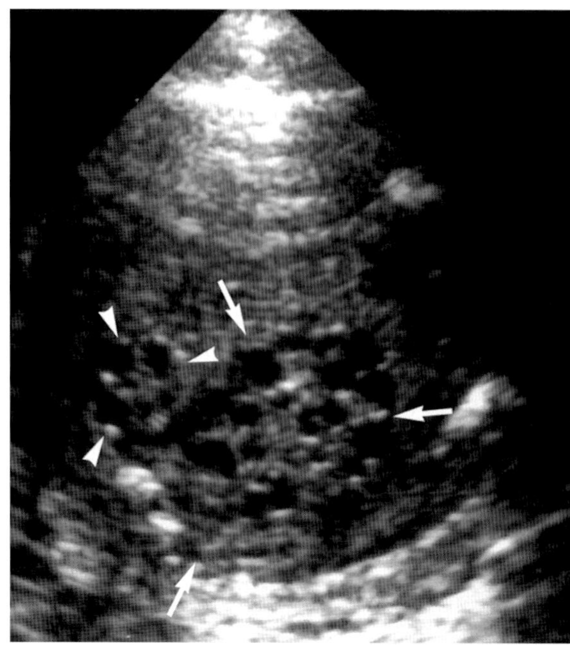

FIGURE 11.7-2. Bilateral multicystic dysplastic kidneys. Transverse view of the fetal abdomen demonstrates bilateral multicystic dysplastic kidneys, large on one side *(arrows)* and small on the other *(arrowheads)*. There is severe oligohydramnios.

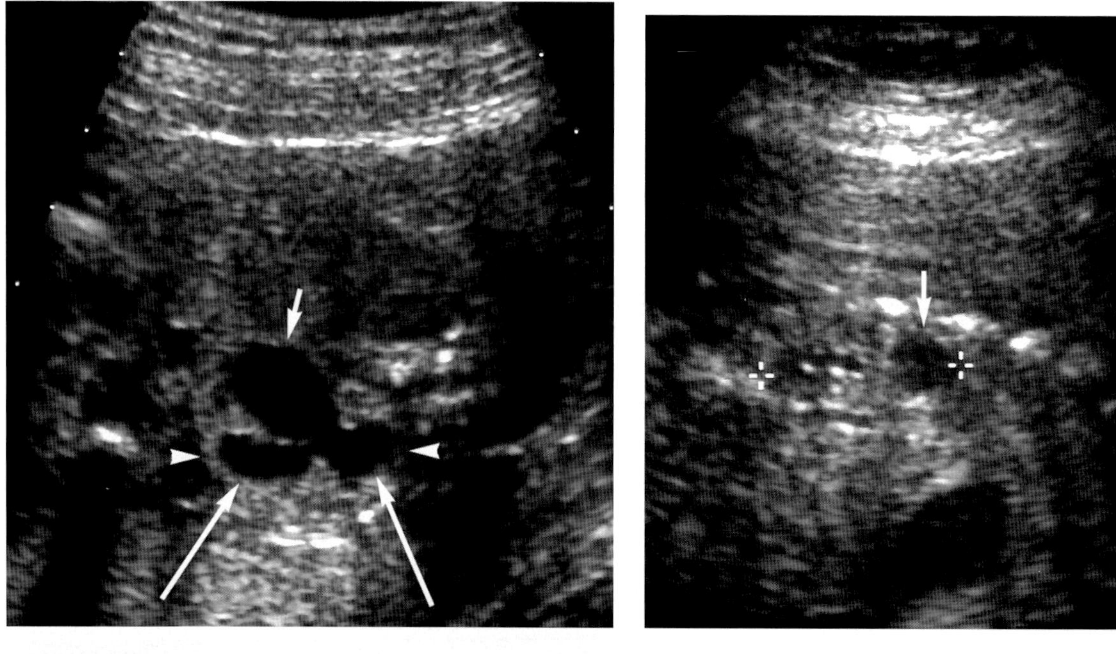

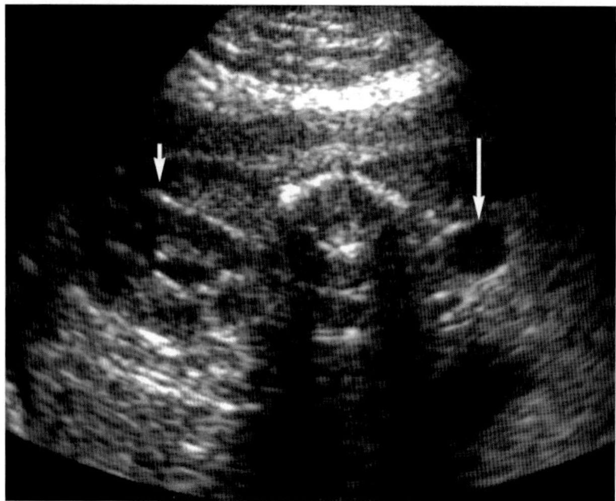

FIGURE 11.7-3. Renal dysplasia secondary to ureteropelvic junction obstruction. A: Transverse view of the fetal abdomen at 18 weeks demonstrate a hydronephrotic left kidney *(arrowheads)* with dilated calyces *(long arrows)* and renal pelvis *(short arrow)*. The renal parenchyma surrounding the dilated collecting system is thin and echogenic. **B:** At 29 weeks, the left kidney *(calipers)* is small and irregular in echogenicity with a cyst at the upper pole *(arrow)*. **C:** At 33 weeks, all that remains of the previously obstructed kidney is a small cyst *(long arrow)*. The contralateral kidney is normal *(short arrow)*.

11.8. AUTOSOMAL RECESSIVE POLYCYSTIC KIDNEY DISEASE

Description and Clinical Features

Autosomal recessive polycystic kidney disease, otherwise known as infantile polycystic kidney disease, is an inherited disorder characterized by cystic dilation of the renal tubules. In some cases, there is hepatic fibrosis as well.

The prognosis is poor because the renal abnormality leads to impaired or absent renal function. The time of onset of renal failure varies. In some cases, renal failure begins *in utero*, and the fetus may develop pulmonary hypoplasia as a result of severe oligohydramnios (similar to fetuses with bilateral renal agenesis). In this setting, the neonate is likely to die at birth of pulmonary hypoplasia. In other cases, renal failure does not occur until the first few years of life. In these latter cases, the children may have hepatic fibrosis before renal failure occurs.

A

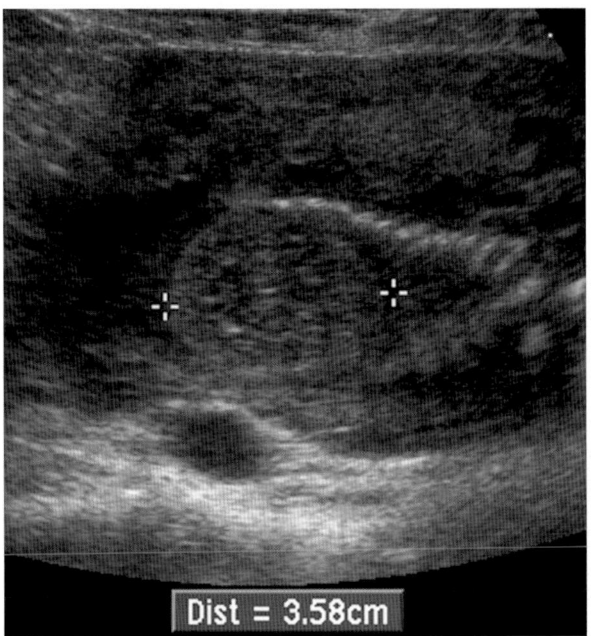

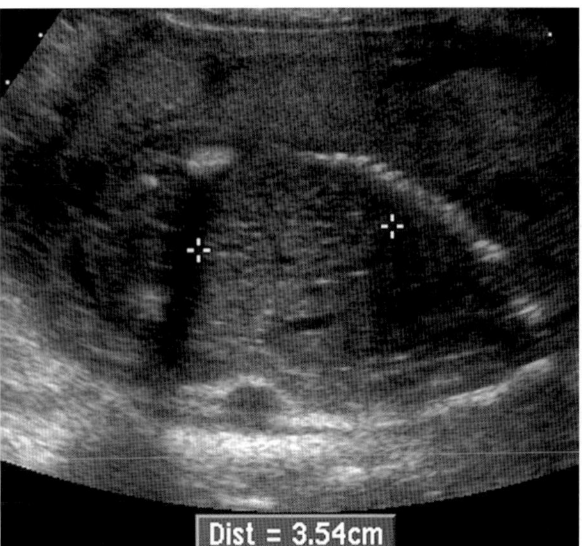

B

C

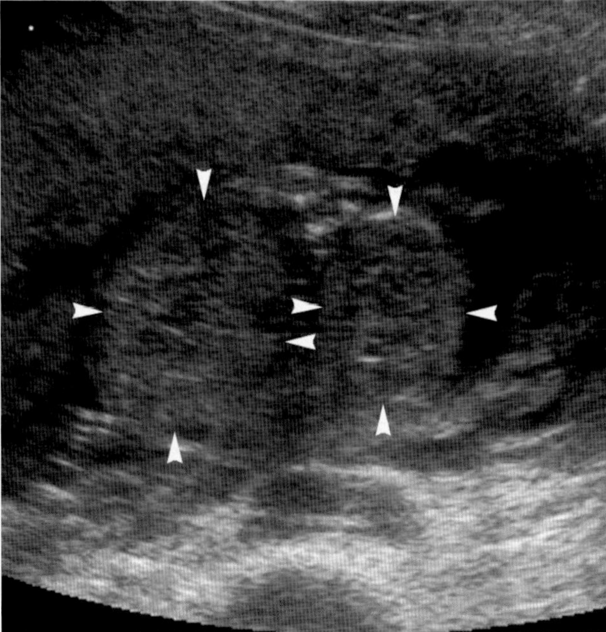

FIGURE 11.8-1. Autosomal recessive polycystic kidney disease in the second trimester. Right **(A)** and left **(B)** sagittal views in an 18-week fetus demonstrate the kidneys *(calipers)* to be enlarged and increased in echogenicity. **C:** The kidneys *(arrowheads)* are enlarged and echogenic on the transverse view. There is oligohydramnios.

Sonography

The sonographic appearance of autosomal recessive polycystic kidney disease *in utero* depends on the time and severity of onset. When the onset is prenatal, ultrasound typically demonstrates bilaterally enlarged echogenic kidneys with enhanced through-transmission and, if the prenatal disease is severe enough to cause renal failure, severe oligohydramnios and absence of the bladder. This appearance may first be seen in the second (Figure 11.8-1) or third (Figure 11.8-2) trimester of pregnancy. In cases with postnatal onset, the appearance of the kidneys *in utero* may be normal.

There are other causes of echogenic kidneys. Enlarged echogenic kidneys may be seen with a number of pathologic entities, including autosomal dominant polycystic kidney disease, a disease that usually presents in early adulthood but may, in rare cases, manifest itself prenatally. Echogenic normal-size kidneys may be a normal variant. When the kidneys appear echogenic on a prenatal sonogram, it is important to look for fluid in the urinary bladder and evaluate the amniotic fluid volume. Postnatal tests of renal function may be needed to distinguish a pathologic condition from a normal variant.

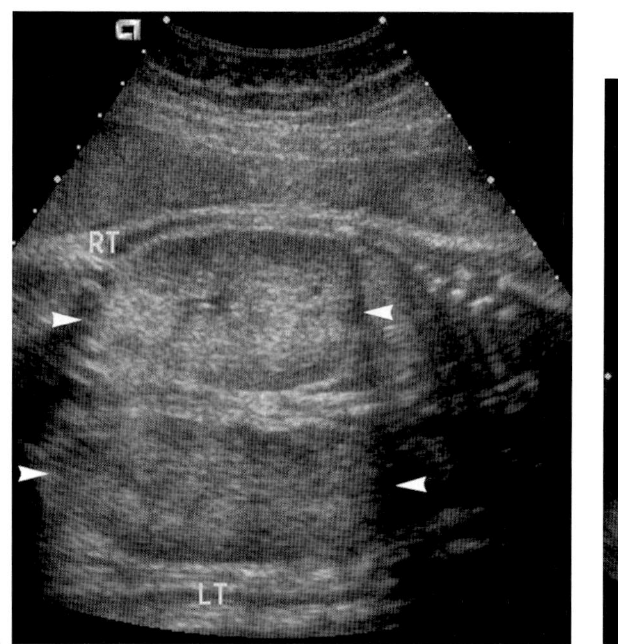

A

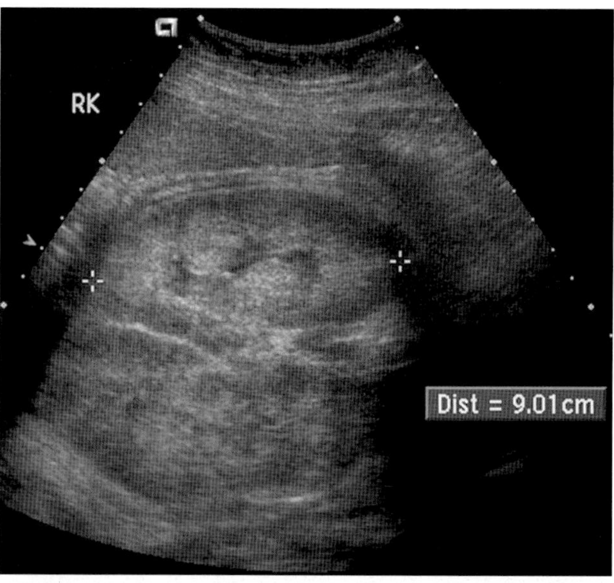

B

FIGURE 11.8-2. Autosomal recessive polycystic kidney disease in the third trimester. A: The right (RT) and left (LT) kidneys *(arrowheads)* are enlarged and increased in echogenicity at 33 weeks. **B:** The right kidney (RK) measures approximately 9 cm in length *(calipers)*. There is severe oligohydramnios.

11.9. RENAL ECTOPIA

Description and Clinical Features

Renal ectopia refers to the presence of one or both kidneys in an abnormal location. This anomaly occurs in approximately one per 1,200 births. The most common location of an ectopic kidney is in the pelvis. Less common forms of ectopia include horseshoe kidney, in which the lower poles of the two kidneys fuse and extend across the midline of the lower abdomen, and cross-fused ectopia, in which one kidney is fused to the lower pole of the contralateral kidney. Ectopic kidneys are at increased risk of urinary obstruction.

Sonography

A pelvic kidney is diagnosed when one renal fossa is empty, and there is a mass in the pelvis that has the sonographic characteristics of a kidney: reniform shape and echogenic cortex with hypoechoic pyramids (Figure 11.9-1). With cross-fused ectopia, one renal fossa will be empty and the contralateral kidney will be very long and have an unusual shape at its lower pole. A horseshoe kidney is diagnosed when renal parenchyma is seen extending across the midline in front of the fetal spine (Figure 11.9-2). In any of these cases, if there is urinary obstruction, one or both kidneys will be hydronephrotic, and there may be parenchymal dysplasia.

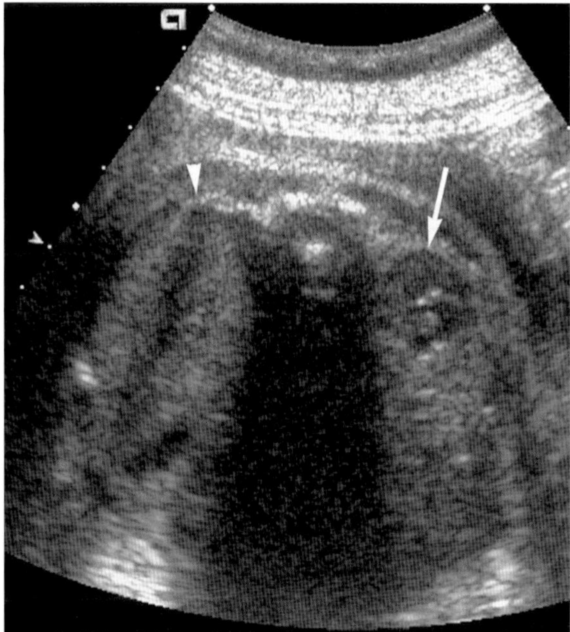

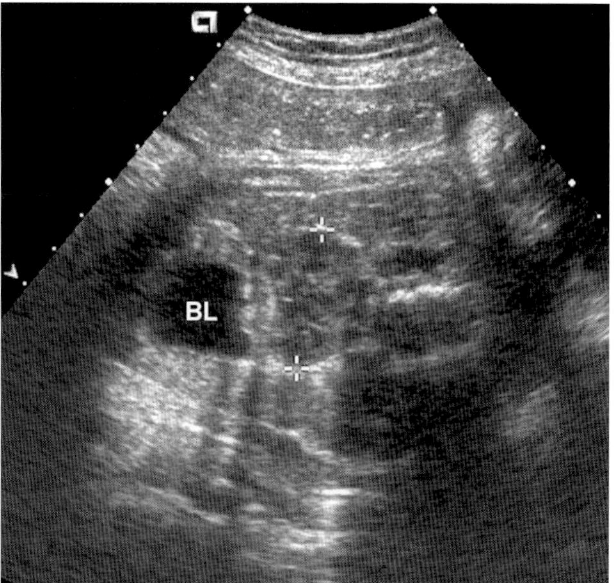

FIGURE 11.9-1. Pelvic kidney. A: Transverse view of the fetal abdomen reveals a normal kidney *(arrow)* on one side of the spine and no kidney on the other side *(arrowhead)*. **B:** A kidney *(calipers)* is seen in the pelvis just cephalad to the bladder (BL).

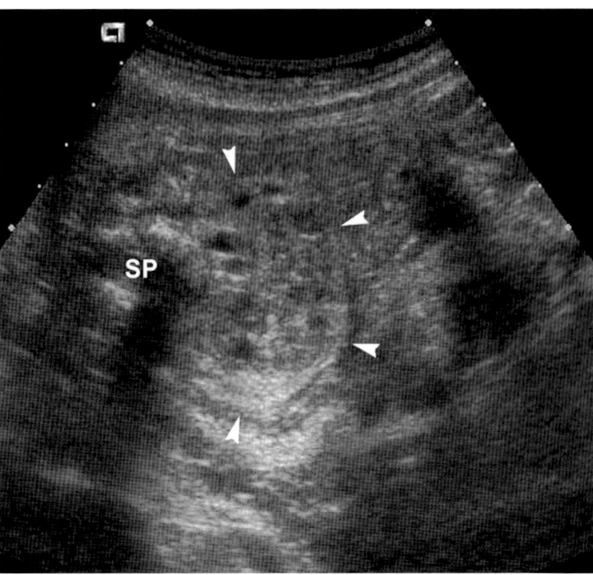

FIGURE 11.9-2. Horseshoe kidney. Transverse view of the fetal abdomen reveals a single horseshoe-shaped kidney *(arrowheads)* extending across the midline anterior to the spine (SP).

11.10. MESOBLASTIC NEPHROMA

Description and Clinical Features

Mesoblastic nephroma is the most common solid fetal renal mass. This lesion, which occurs infrequently, is a hamartoma of the kidney. Wilms' tumor, another solid renal tumor that occurs prenatally or in childhood, is less common than mesoblastic nephroma in the fetus.

Sonography

Mesoblastic nephroma appears sonographically as a solid, fairly homogeneous, mass replacing some (Figure 11.10-1) or all (Figure 11.10-2) of a fetal kidney. Definitive diag-

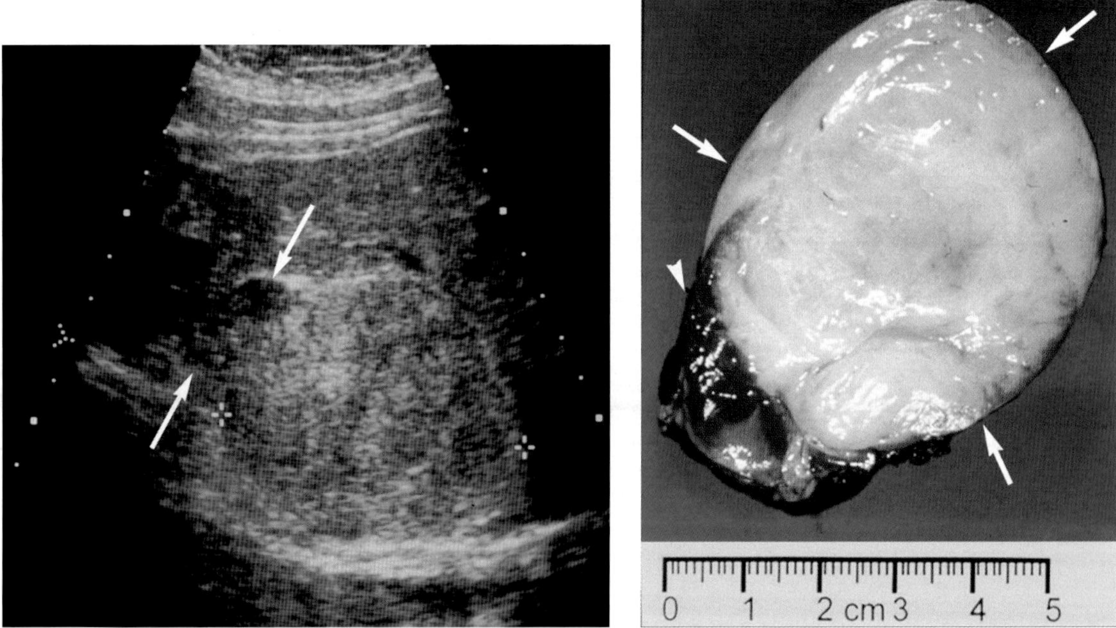

FIGURE 11.10-1. Mesoblastic nephroma occupying most of the fetal kidney. A: There is a large heterogeneous solid renal mass *(calipers)*, with only a small amount of normal renal tissue identified *(arrows)*. **B:** Postnatal surgical specimen confirms the presence of a large mass *(arrows)*, which proved to be a mesoblastic nephroma, above a small amount of normal kidney *(arrowhead)*.

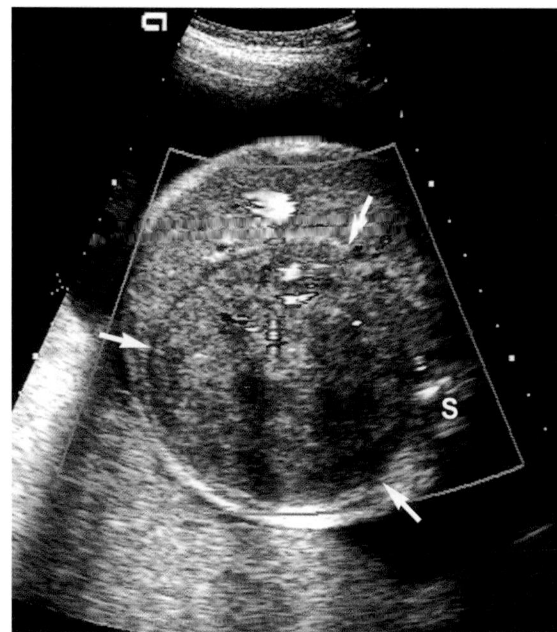

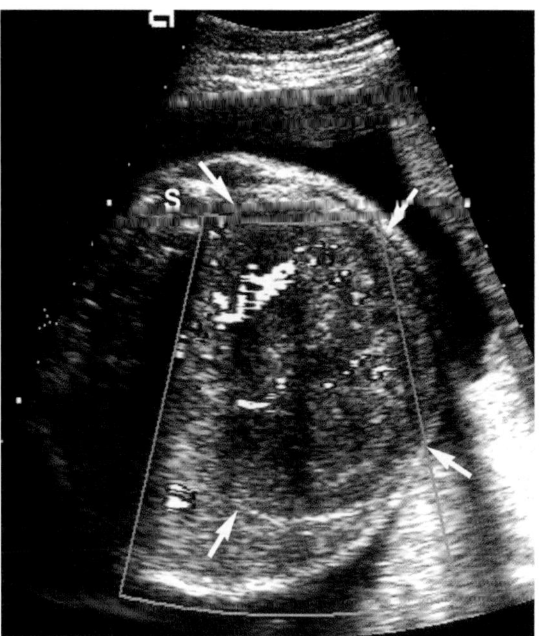

A B

FIGURE 11.10-2. Mesoblastic nephroma replacing the entire fetal kidney. A and B: Transverse views of the fetal abdomen demonstrate a large mass *(arrows)* in the expected location of a kidney, anterolateral to the spine (S). Color Doppler reveals the mass to be moderately vascular.

nosis of mesoblastic nephroma is made by postnatal surgery because its prenatal sonographic appearance is indistinguishable from that of a Wilms' tumor.

11.11. DUPLICATED COLLECTING SYSTEM AND ECTOPIC URETEROCELE

Description and Clinical Features

Duplication of the renal collecting system is a common abnormality that is usually unilateral and affects females more often than males. The lower extent of duplication is variable. In some cases, there is duplication of the proximal ureter, with convergence of the two segments into a single distal ureter on that side. In other cases, there is complete duplication of the ureter, with each implanting separately into the bladder. When this occurs, the lower pole ureter usually implants in the normal location and is prone to reflux, whereas the upper pole ureter commonly implants at a site caudal and medial to normal and may be obstructed. When the upper pole ureter implants ectopically into the bladder, its distal end may bulge into the bladder lumen, forming an ectopic ureterocele.

Sonography

Duplication should be suspected when ultrasound demonstrates hydronephrosis that is significantly different in severity in the two poles of the kidney or hydronephrosis that affects only the upper pole (Figure 11.11-1). There may be a hydroureter extending from the upper and/or lower poles. If an ectopic ureterocele is present, it appears as a cystic structure inside the bladder (Figures 11.11-1 and 11.11-2).

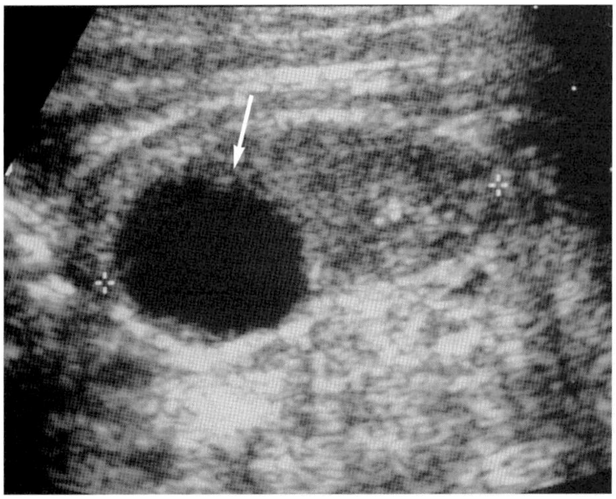

FIGURE 11.11-1. Duplicated collecting system with an upper pole hydroureter and ectopic ureterocele. There is severe hydronephrosis *(arrow)* involving the upper pole of a fetal kidney *(calipers)* **(A)** and a hydroureter *(arrowheads)* extending from this pole **(B)**. **C:** There is a round, thin-walled, fluid-filled structure *(arrow)* in the fetal bladder (BL), representing an ectopic ureterocele.

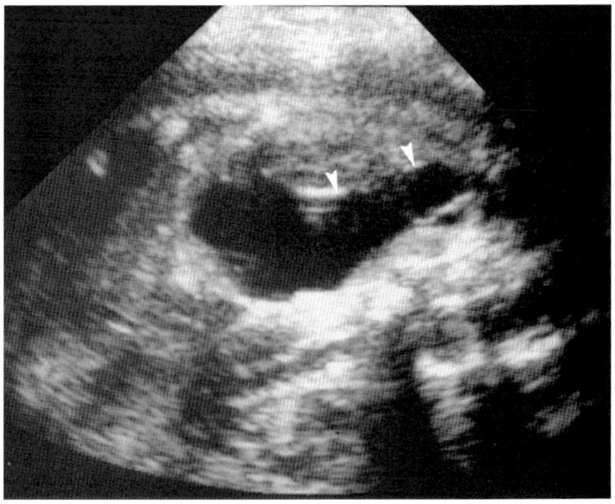

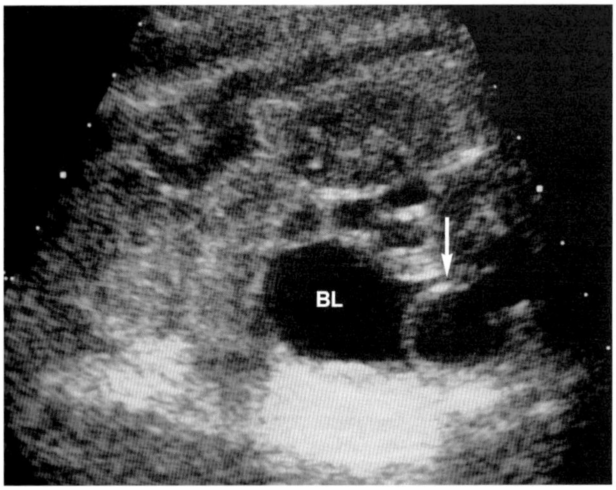

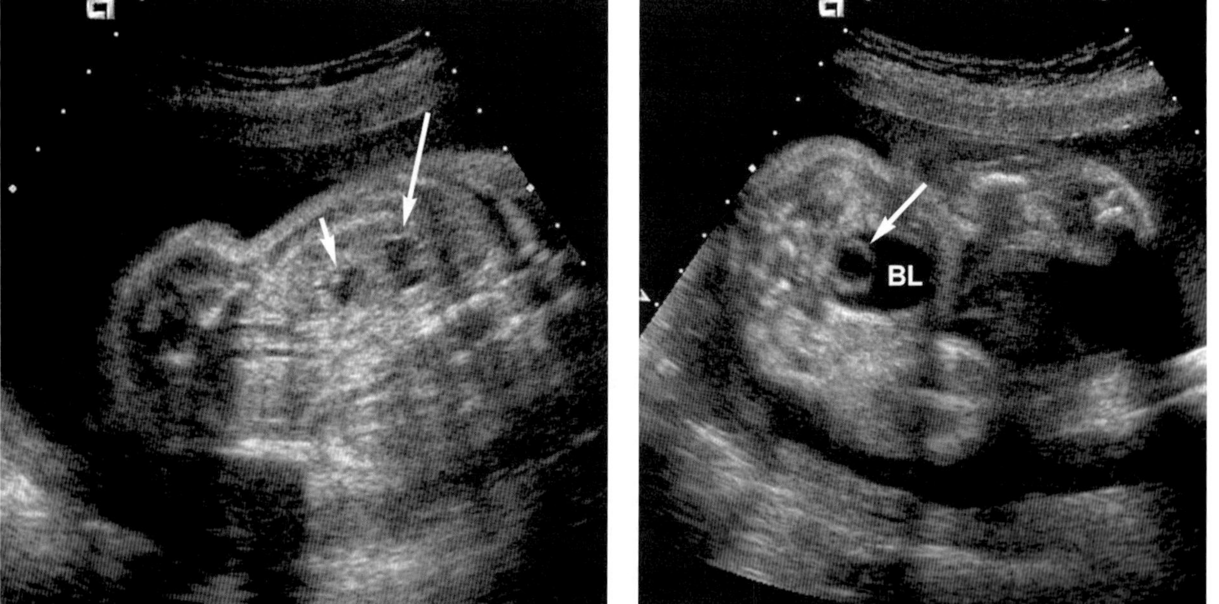

FIGURE 11.11-2. Duplicated collecting system with an ectopic ureterocele. A: There is dilation of the intrarenal collecting systems, slightly more in the upper pole *(long arrow)* than the lower pole *(short arrow)*. **B:** There is a round, thin-walled, fluid-filled structure *(arrow)* in the fetal bladder (BL) representing an ectopic ureterocele.

11.12. OVARIAN CYSTS

Description and Clinical Features

Follicular cysts may occasionally develop in the ovary of a female fetus, probably as a result of stimulation by placental and maternal hormones. Other ovarian cystic lesions, including teratomas and cystadenomas, occur but are far less common. Ovarian cysts are subject to a number of complications *in utero*, including hemorrhage, torsion, and compression of adjacent organs. Most cysts resolve after birth because levels of hormones derived from the mother and placenta drop.

Sonography

Most ovarian cysts appear on ultrasound as simple or septated cysts in the lower fetal abdomen or pelvis (Figure 11.12-1). If a cyst is simple on one sonogram and has inter-

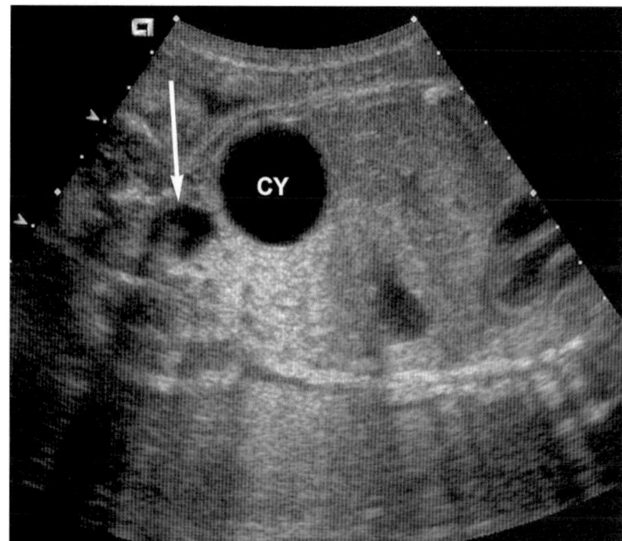

A

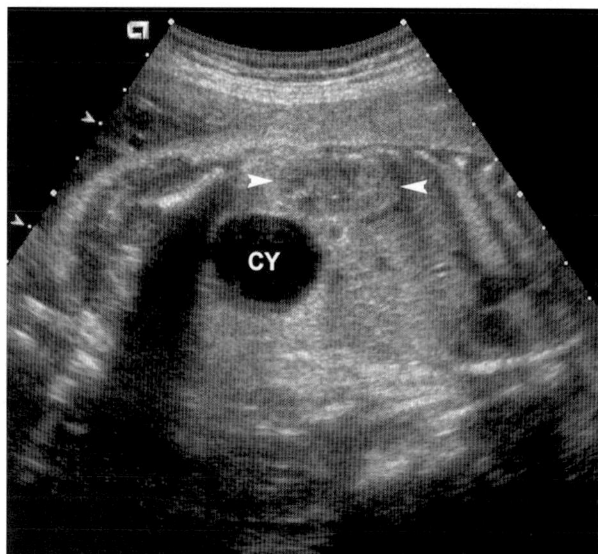

B

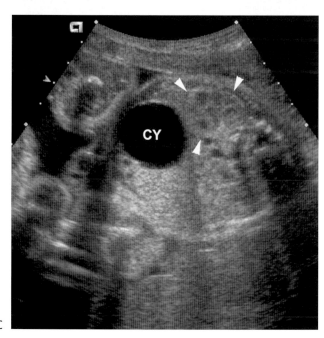

C

FIGURE 11.12-1. Simple ovarian cyst. A: Longitudinal view of the fetal abdomen and pelvis demonstrates a cyst (CY) located just cephalad to the bladder *(arrow)*. Longitudinal **(B)** and transverse **(C)** views demonstrate that the cyst (CY) is separate from the adjacent kidney *(arrowheads)*.

nal echogenic material on a subsequent scan, the likely diagnosis is torsion or hemorrhage (Figure 11.12-2). If a cyst appears complex on the initial sonogram, the differential diagnosis should include teratoma and cystadenoma, in addition to torsion or hemorrhagic cyst.

The diagnosis of ovarian cyst cannot be made with certainty, however, when a cyst is seen in the lower abdomen or pelvis. Other lesions with a similar appearance include mesenteric cysts, omental cysts, gastrointestinal duplication cysts, and hydrometrocolpos.

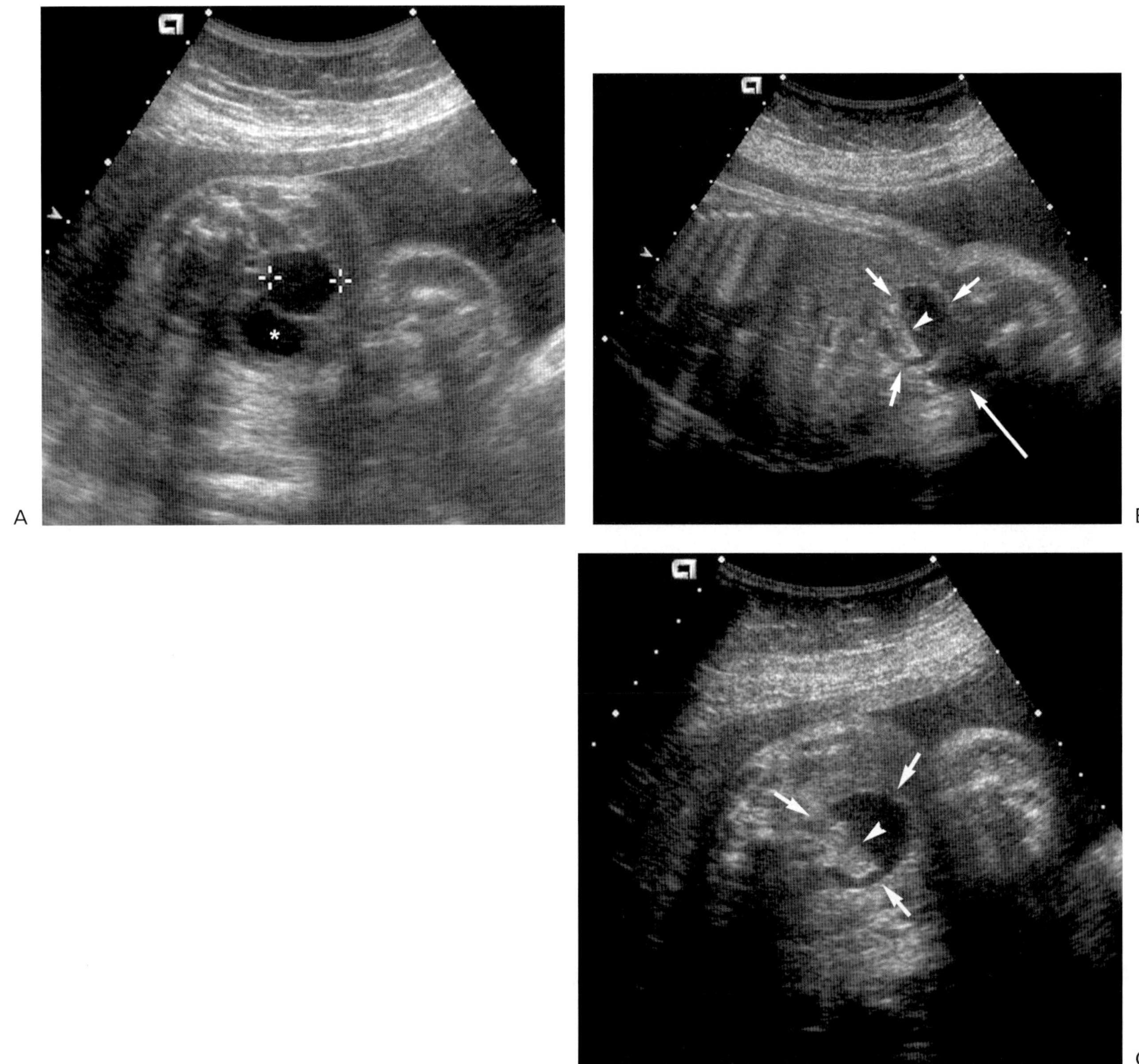

FIGURE 11.12-2. Complex ovarian cyst. A: Transverse view of the fetal pelvis at 29 weeks gestation demonstrates a simple cyst *(calipers)* adjacent to the bladder *(*)*. **B:** Longitudinal view of the fetal abdomen and pelvis 1 week later demonstrates that the cyst *(small arrows)*, located beside the bladder *(long arrow)*, now contains internal debris *(arrowhead)*. **C:** Transverse view of the fetal pelvis, done at the same time as **(B)**, demonstrates the cyst *(arrows)* with internal debris *(arrowhead)*. The change from a simple to a complex cyst indicates that it has undergone hemorrhage or torsion.

11.13. CLOACAL AND BLADDER EXSTROPHY

Description and Clinical Features

Cloacal and bladder exstrophy are two forms of infraumbilical ventral wall defects, a group of anomalies that also includes more minor abnormalities such as epispadius. With bladder exstrophy, the ventral wall defect involves the lower anterior abdominal and bladder walls, so that the bladder mucosa is exposed. Cloacal exstrophy is a more severe anomaly, in which the defect includes the anterior abdominal wall, bladder, and colon. This anomaly, which occurs more frequently in males than females, arises from maldevelopment of the cloaca, an early embryologic structure from which the rectum, bladder, and genitalia develop.

In some cases of bladder or cloacal exstrophy, the defect appears as a cleft in the abdominal wall below the umbilicus. In other cases, there is eversion of the bladder and/or rectum, resulting in a soft-tissue mass protruding anteriorly from the lower abdomen.

Sonography

The sonographic appearance of bladder and cloacal exstrophy depends on the nature and severity of the anomaly. When the bladder, with or without the colon, is everted, a lower anterior abdominal soft-tissue mass is seen on ultrasound (Figures 11.13-1 and 11.13-2). This can be distinguished from an omphalocele or gastroschisis by noting that it is located below the umbilical cord insertion site and no fluid-filled bladder is seen. When there is a cleft without eversion of the bladder or colon, the sole sonographic abnormality may be nonvisualization of the bladder. For this reason, the differential diagnosis should include bladder or cloacal exstrophy whenever there is persistent nonvisualization of the bladder in the presence of normal kidneys and normal amniotic fluid volume. In some cases of exstrophy, however, fluid can be seen in the urinary bladder despite its opening to the amniotic cavity, so that a prenatal diagnosis may not be possible.

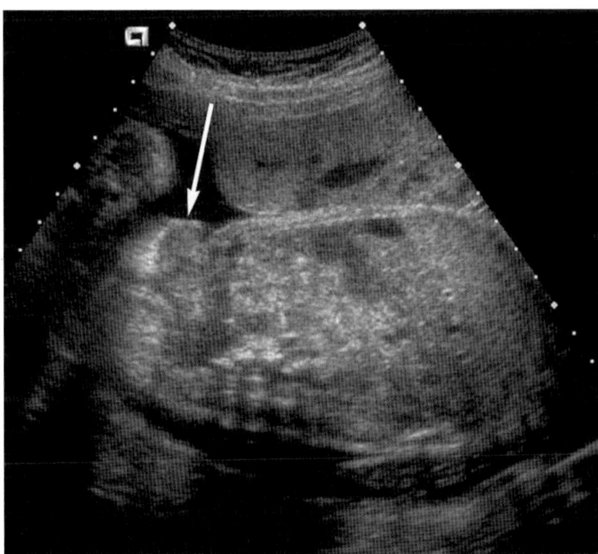

FIGURE 11.13-1. Bladder exstrophy. Longitudinal view of the fetal abdomen and pelvis reveals a soft-tissue mass *(arrow)* extending from the anterior wall of the pelvis. No fetal bladder is identified.

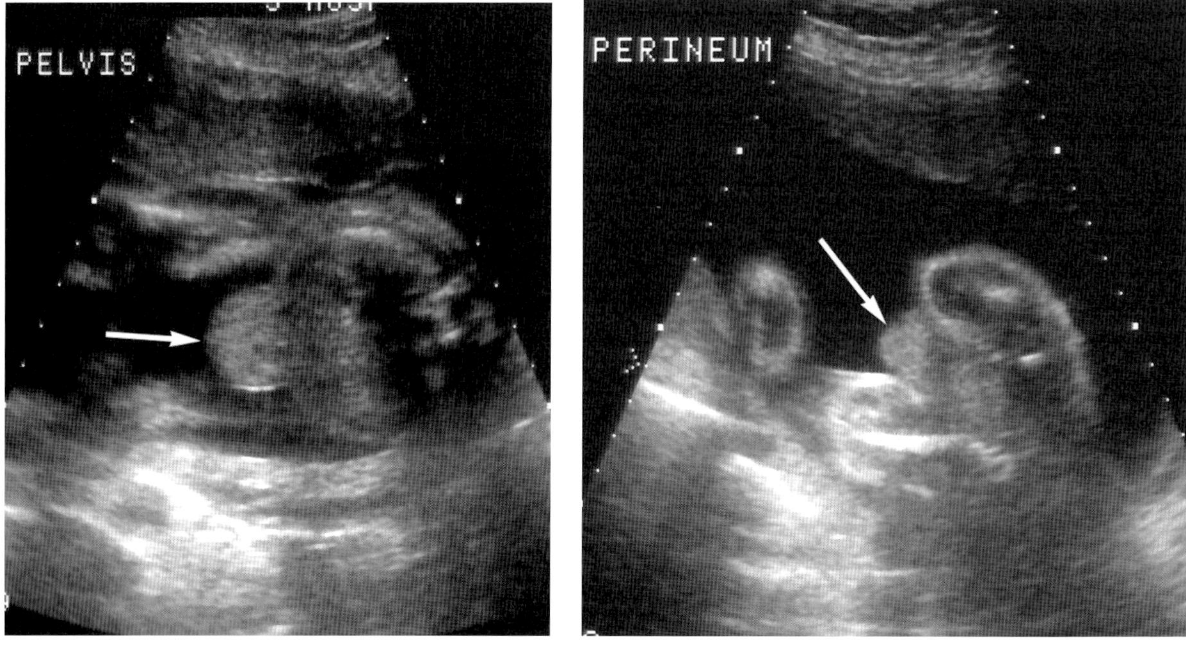

FIGURE 11.13-2. Bladder exstrophy. A: Transverse view of the fetal pelvis demonstrates a homogeneous soft-tissue mass *(arrow)* extending from the anterior wall. **B:** The mass *(arrow)* extends down to the perineum.

SUGGESTED READINGS

1. Arger PH, Coleman BG, Mintz MC, et al. Routine fetal genitourinary tract screening. *Radiology* 1985;156:485–489.
2. Benson CB, Doubilet PM. The fetal genitourinary system. In: Fleischer AC, Manning FA, Jeanty P, et al., eds. *Sonography in obstetrics & gynecology: principles and practice*, 6th ed. New York: McGraw-Hill, 2001:431–444.
3. Blane CE, Barr M, DePeitro MA, et al. Renal obstructive dysplasias: ultrasound diagnosis and therapeutic implications. *Pediatr Radiol* 1991;21:274–277.
4. Bosman G, Reuss A, Nijman JM, et al. Prenatal diagnosis, management and outcome of fetal uretero-pelvic junction obstruction. *Ultrasound Med Biol* 1991;17:117–120.
5. Cooper C, Mahony BS, Bowie JD, et al. Prenatal ultrasound diagnosis of ambiguous genitalia. *J Ultrasound Med* 1985;4:433–436.
6. Estroff JA, Mandell J, Benacerraf BR. Increased renal parenchymal echogenicity in the fetus: importance and clinical outcome. *Radiology* 1991;181:135–139.
7. Feldman DM, DeCambre M, Kong E, et al. Evaluation and follow-up of fetal hydronephrosis. *J Ultrasound Med* 2001;20:1065–1069.
8. Filly RA, Feldstein VA. Fetal genitourinary tract. In: Callen PW, ed. *Ultrasonography in obstetrics and gynecology*, 4th ed. Philadelphia: WB Saunders, 2000:517–550.
9. Fong KW, Ryan G. The fetal urogenital tract. In: Rumack CM, Wilson SR, Charboneau JW, eds. *Diagnostic ultrasound*, 2nd ed. St. Louis: Mosby, 1998:1093–1121.
10. Giulian BB. Prenatal ultrasonographic diagnosis of fetal renal tumors. *Radiology* 1984;152:69–70.
11. Hayden SA, Russ PD, Pretorius DH, et al. Posterior urethral obstruction: prenatal sonography in fourteen cases. *J Ultrasound Med* 1988;7:371–375.
12. Jeanty P, Romero R, Kepple D, et al. Prenatal diagnoses in unilateral empty renal fossa. *J Ultrasound Med* 1990;9:651–654.
13. King KL, Kofinas AD, Simon NV, et al. Antenatal ultrasound diagnosis of fetal horseshoe kidney. *J Ultrasound Med* 1991;10:643–644.
14. Mahony BS, Filly RA, Callen PW, et al. Fetal renal dysplasia: sonographic evaluation. *Radiology* 1984;152:143–146.
15. Meizner I, Bar-Ziv J, Katz M. Prenatal ultrasonic diagnosis of the extreme form of prune belly syndrome. *J Clin Ultrasound* 1985;13:581–583.
16. Meizner I, Levy A, Katz M, et al. Fetal ovarian cysts: prenatal ultrasonographic detection and postnatal evaluation and treatment. *Am J Obstet Gynecol* 1991;164:874–878.

17. Paduano L, Giglio L, Bembi B, et al. Clinical outcome of fetal uropathy. I. Predictive value of prenatal echography positive for obstructive uropathy. *J Urol* 1991;146:1094–1096
18. Paltiel HJ, Lebowitz RL. Neonatal hydronephrosis due to primary vesicoureteral reflux: trends in diagnosis and treatment. *Radiology* 1989;170:787–789.
19. Potter EL. Bilateral absence of kidneys and ureters: a report of 50 cases. *Obstet Gynecol* 1965;25:3–12.
20. Pretorius DH, Lee ME, Manco-Johnson ML, et al. Diagnosis of autosomal dominant polycystic kidney disease in utero and the young infant. *J Ultrasound Med* 1987;6:249–255.
21. Raghavendra BN, Young BK, Greco MA, et al. Use of furosemide in pregnancies complicated by oligohydramnios. *Radiology* 1987;165:455–458.
22. Sairam S, Al-Habib A, Sasson S, et al. Natural history of fetal hydronephrosis diagnosed on mid-trimester ultrasound. *Ultrasound Obstet Gynecol* 2001;17:191–196.
23. Sherer DM, Menashe M, Lebensart P, et al. Sonographic diagnosis of unilateral fetal renal duplication with associated ectopic ureterocele. *J Clin Ultrasound* 1989;17:371–373.
24. Stephens JD. Prenatal diagnosis of testicular feminisation. *Lancet* 1984;2:1038.

12

SKELETAL SYSTEM

12.1. SKELETAL DYSPLASIA

Description and Clinical Features

Skeletal dysplasias, also called osteochondral dysplasias, result from abnormal formation and remodeling of bone, which lead to diffuse skeletal deformity and shortening. Skeletal dysplasias are characterized based on the severity of the deformities and the ability of an affected infant to survive. Forms of skeletal dysplasia that are lethal include thanatophoric dysplasia, osteogenesis imperfecta type II, achondrogenesis, and hypophosphatasia. With these skeletal dysplasias, the thorax fails to develop large enough for adequate lung growth, and neonates typically die at birth from pulmonary hypoplasia. In these cases, the entire skeleton is affected, with poor cranial ossification and bowing, fractures, and deformities of the long bones. The long bones are typically very short.

Less severe skeletal dysplasias, such as heterozygous achondroplasia and osteogenesis imperfecta types I, III, and IV, may be compatible with life. Affected infants may have moderate shortening of the long bones and poor mineralization of osseous structures.

Sonography

The diagnosis of a skeletal dysplasia is made when the long bones are markedly short, measuring more than four standard deviations below the mean for gestational age. Additional findings include poor mineralization of bones, particularly the skull, long-bone fractures and bowing, and a narrow thorax. Determination of the specific type of skeletal dysplasia may be possible with careful sonographic assessment of the degree of long-bone shortening, degree of cranial ossification, and the shape of the cranium.

Thanatophoric dysplasia is one of the more common lethal skeletal dysplasias. This dysplasia is characterized by marked shortening of the long bones, bowing of the long bones, a narrow thorax, and cloverleaf deformity of the skull (Figure 12.1-1).

Osteogenesis imperfecta type II is an autosomal recessive skeletal dysplasia characterized by fractures and deformities of the ribs and long bones, a small thorax, poor mineralization of the cranium, and a soft skull (Figure 12.1-2). The cranium may be compressible with gentle pressure from the ultrasound transducer.

Achondrogenesis is an autosomal recessive lethal skeletal dysplasia in which there is almost complete absence of ossification except for the calvarium. The vertebral bodies fail to ossify, and the long bones are markedly shortened and poorly ossified (Figure 12.1-3).

Hypophosphatasia is an autosomal dominant metabolic disorder that causes poor ossification and shortening of the long bones. The skull is typically poorly ossified.

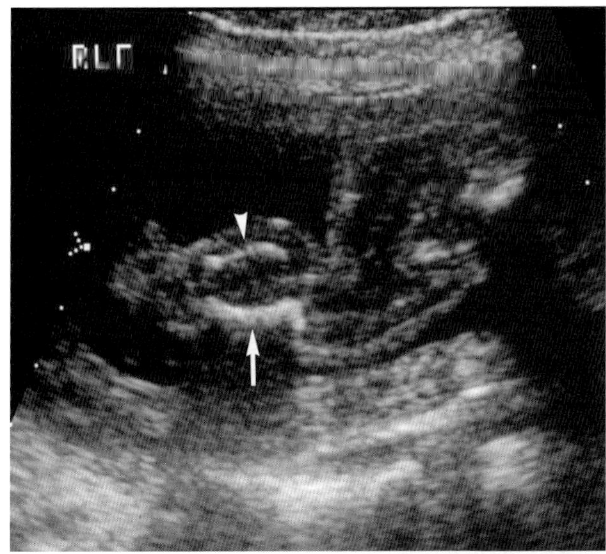

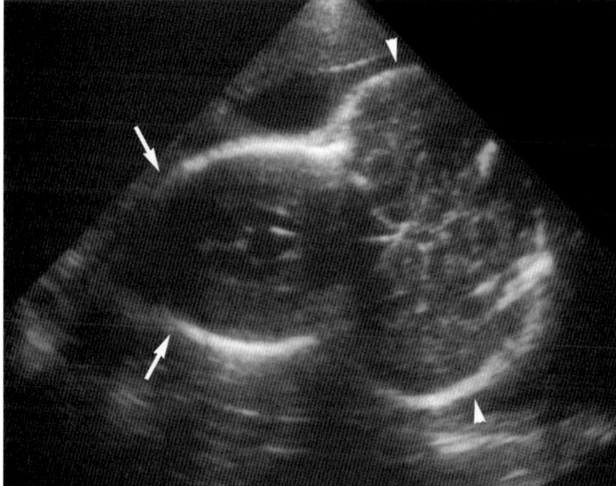

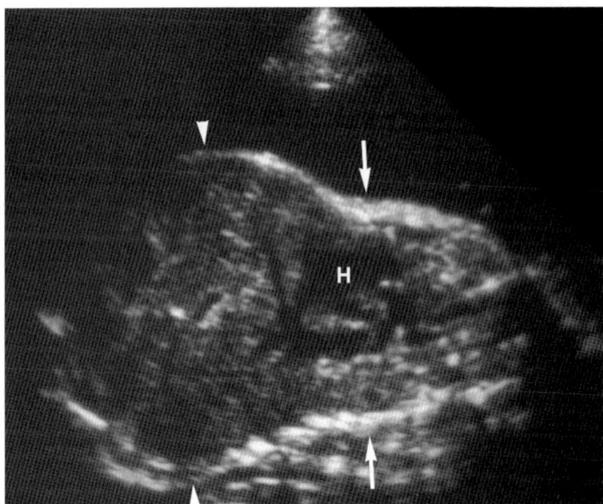

FIGURE 12.1-1. Thanatophoric dysplasia. A: Sonogram of a lower leg demonstrates bowing of both the tibia *(arrow)* and fibula *(arrowhead)*. Both long bones are markedly short for gestational age. **B:** Image of the cranium of another fetus with thanatophoric dysplasia demonstrates a cloverleaf skull, with frontal bossing *(arrows)* and lateral protrusion in the region of the temporal lobes *(arrowheads)*. **C:** Longitudinal image of the same fetus as in **(B)** shows a narrow thorax *(arrows)* in comparison with a larger abdomen *(arrowheads)*. The heart (H) fills much of thorax. (From Benson CB, Lavery MJ, Platt L. *Atlas of obstetrical ultrasound.* Philadelphia: J.B. Lippincott, 1988, with permission.)

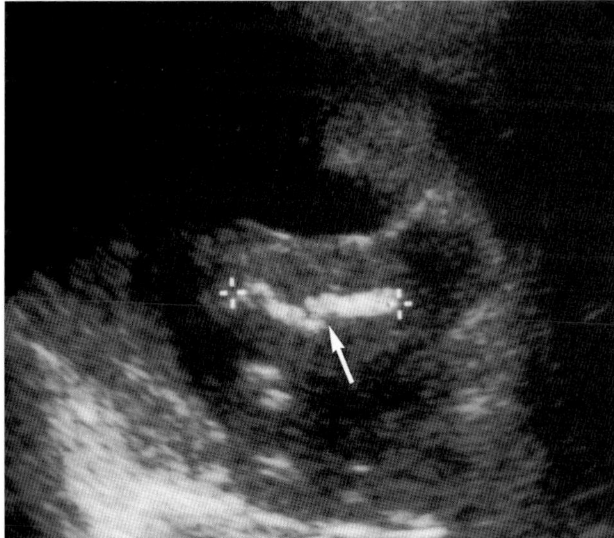

FIGURE 12.1-2. Osteogenesis imperfecta type II. A: Sonogram of a femur *(calipers)* with a mid shaft fracture *(arrow)*. *(continued)*

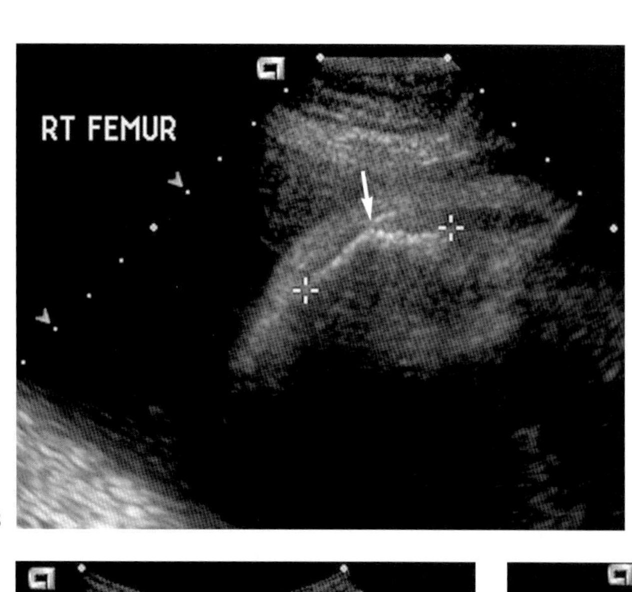

B

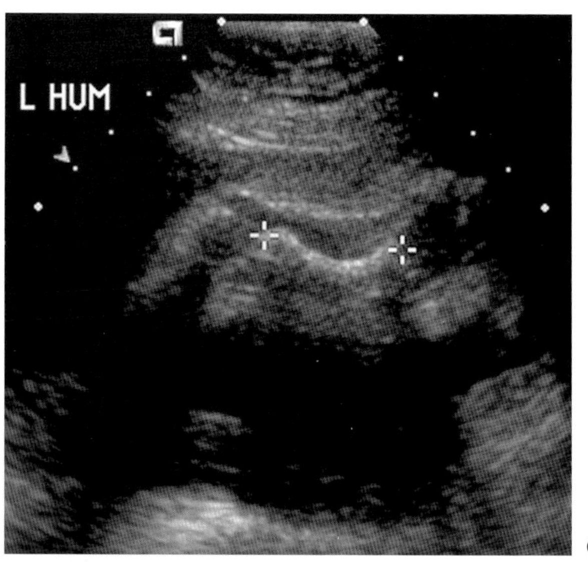

C

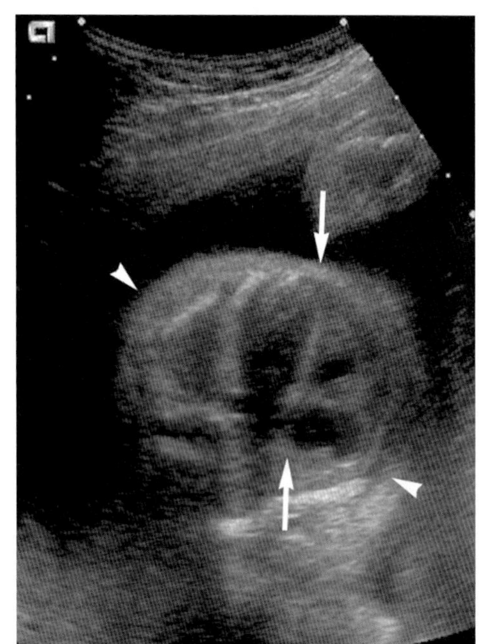
D

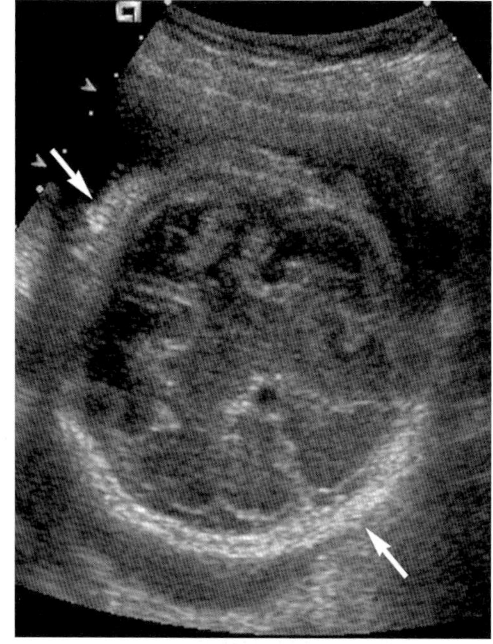
E

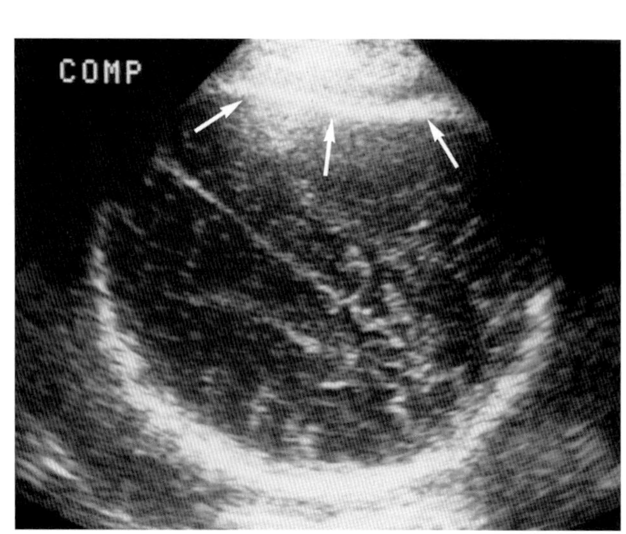

F

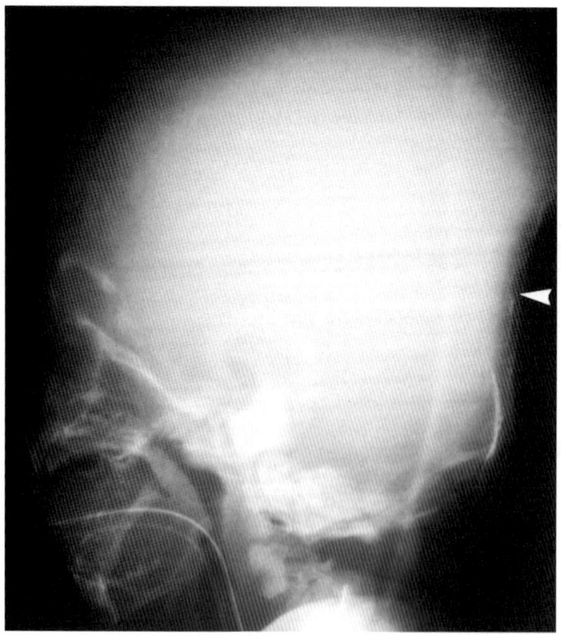
G

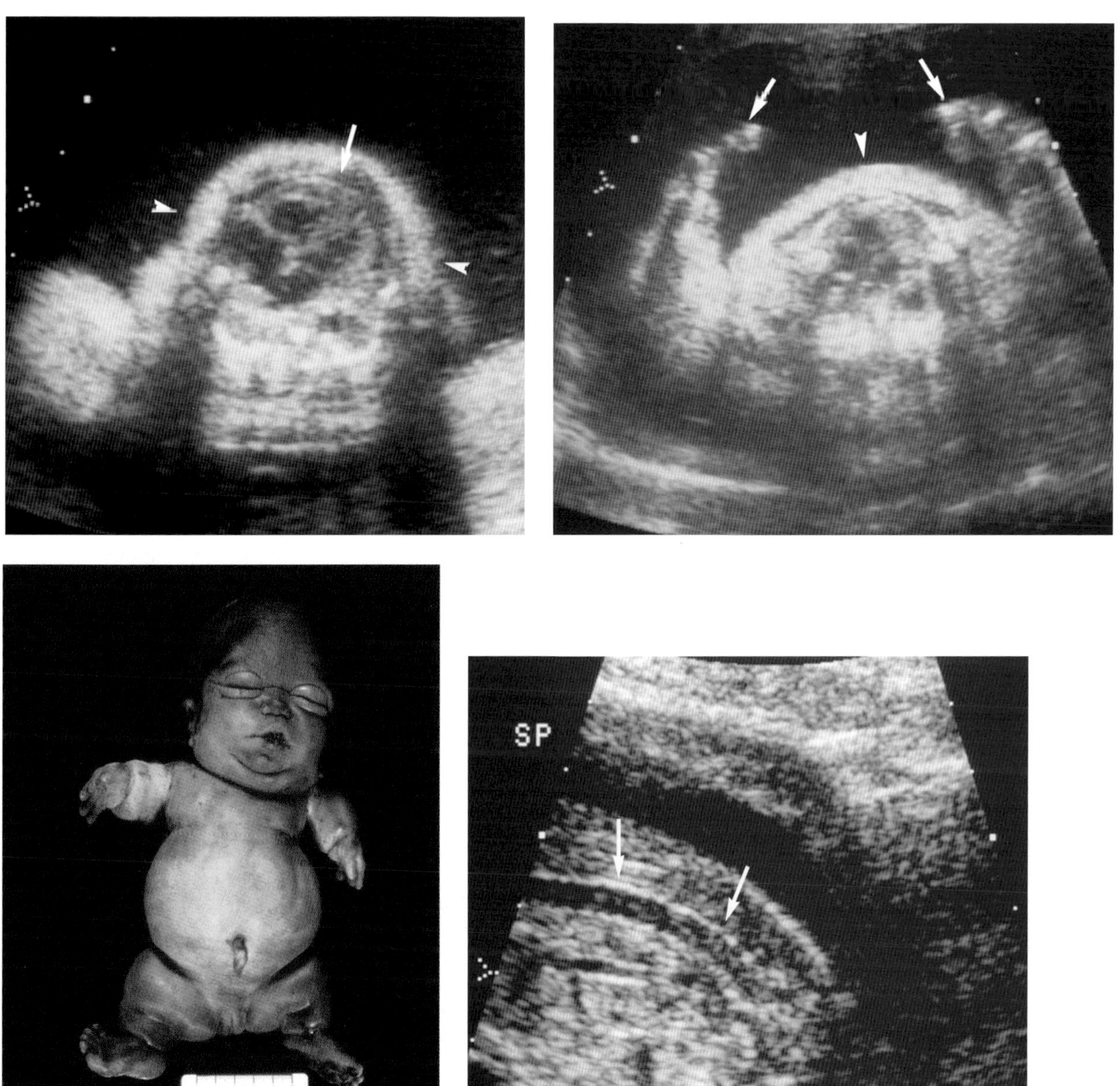

FIGURE 12.1-3. Achondrogenesis. A: Transverse image of a very narrow thorax *(arrowheads)* shows the four-chamber heart *(arrow)* filling the thorax. **B:** Transverse image of the thorax *(arrowhead)* demonstrates very short upper extremities *(arrows)* on both sides. **C:** Photograph of neonate shows a very small thorax and very short upper and lower extremities. **D:** Sonogram of the spine (SP, *arrows*) in another fetus with achondrogenesis demonstrates very poor ossification of the vertebrae.

FIGURE 12.1-2 *(continued)* B: Sonogram of right (RT) femur (calipers) with a fracture deformity *(arrow)* in another fetus with osteogenesis imperfecta type II. **C:** The left humerus (L HUM, *calipers*) is bowed. **D:** The heart *(arrows)* fills most of the narrow thorax *(arrowheads)*. **E:** The cranium *(arrows)* is poorly ossified, making the intracranial anatomy easily visible. **F:** The cranium in a term fetus with osteogenesis imperfecta demonstrates how easily the soft skull compresses *(arrows)* with external pressure (COMP, compression). **G:** X-ray of the skull in the same neonate as in **(F)** demonstrates very poor ossification and indentation *(arrowhead)* of the soft skull from external pressure.

12.2. SKELETAL DYSOSTOSES

Description and Clinical Features

Abnormal formation of one bone or a group of bones is called a skeletal dysostosis. Some skeletal dysostoses have a recognizable pattern of deformities and are part of a known syndrome, such as Nager acrofacial dysostosis, Poland syndrome, and proximal focal femoral deficiency. Nonskeletal anomalies are common in many of these syndromes. Other dysostoses are isolated bony deformities with no known cause and the absence of other fetal anomalies. The prognosis for skeletal dysostoses is related to the degree of severity of other anomalies and the extent of osseous deformities. Deformities of the head, spine, and thorax are associated with a worse prognosis than deformities isolated to the extremities.

Sonography

The sonographic appearance of a skeletal dysostosis depends on the bony structures involved. For example, with Nager acrofacial dysostosis, the upper extremities are markedly shortened, with the absence of one or more of the long bones. The hands are present but incompletely formed. A hypoplastic mandible, external ear deformities, and auditory canal atresia are also present (Figure 12.2-1). Proximal focal femoral deficiency is characterized by the absence of the proximal femur. The finding is unilateral in 90% of cases. The diagnosis is made when there is extreme shortening of one femur with a normal contralateral femur. Other skeletal anomalies may be present, most commonly in the affected lower extremity (Figure 12.2-2).

A

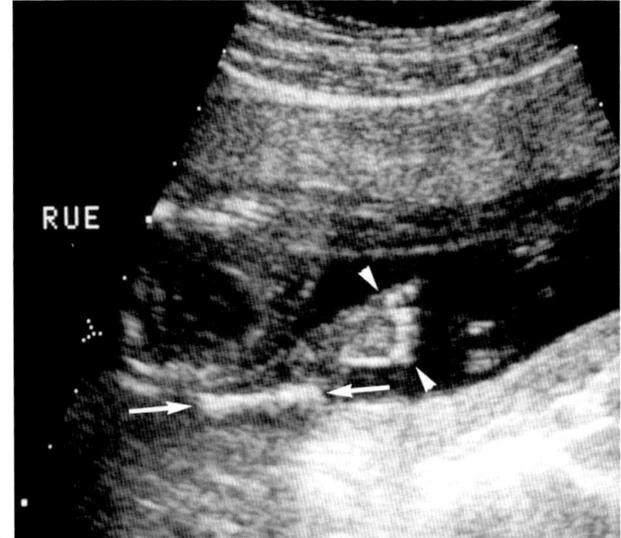

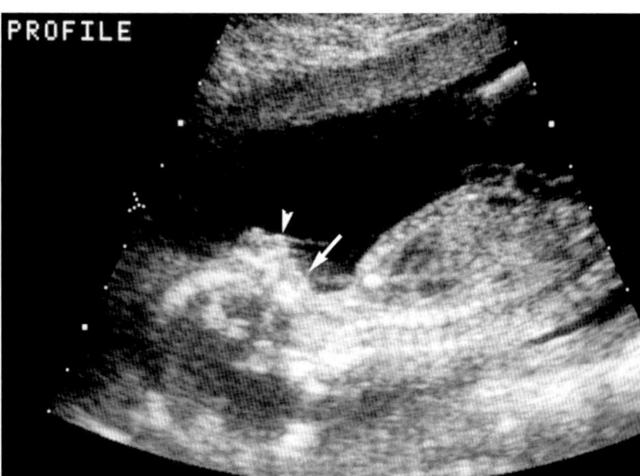

B

FIGURE 12.2-1. Nager acrofacial dysostosis. A: Right upper extremity (RUE) is abnormally formed, with the absence of the bones of the forearm such that the hand *(arrowheads)* is contiguous with a short humerus *(arrows)*. **B:** The mandible *(arrow)* is markedly hypoplastic beneath the normally formed maxilla *(arrowhead)*, visible on a profile of the face.

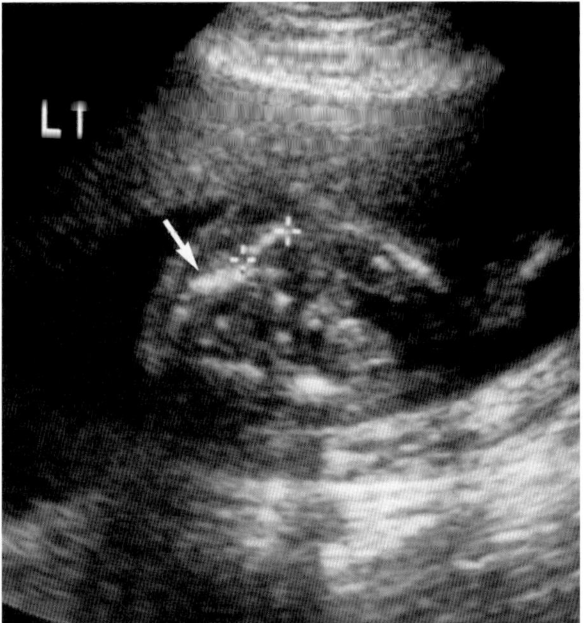

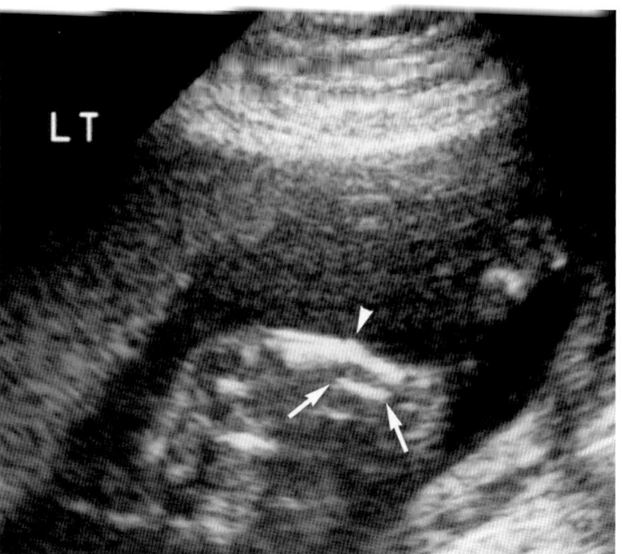

A B

FIGURE 12.2-2. Proximal focal femoral deficiency with abnormal lower extremity long bones. A: The femur *(calipers)*, seen adjacent to the iliac crest *(arrow)*, is very short. The contralateral femur was normal. **B:** The fibula *(arrows)* on the side of the short femur is hypoplastic, and the tibia is bent in the mid *shaft (arrowhead)*.

12.3. LIMB AMPUTATIONS

Description and Clinical Features

Absence of part or all of an extremity can result from amniotic bands that entangle fetal parts during the first or second trimester. These defects are not usually associated with other anomalies.

Sonography

The sonographic appearance of a limb amputation is characterized by the absence of part (Figure 12.3-1) or all (Figure 12.3-2) of an arm or leg.

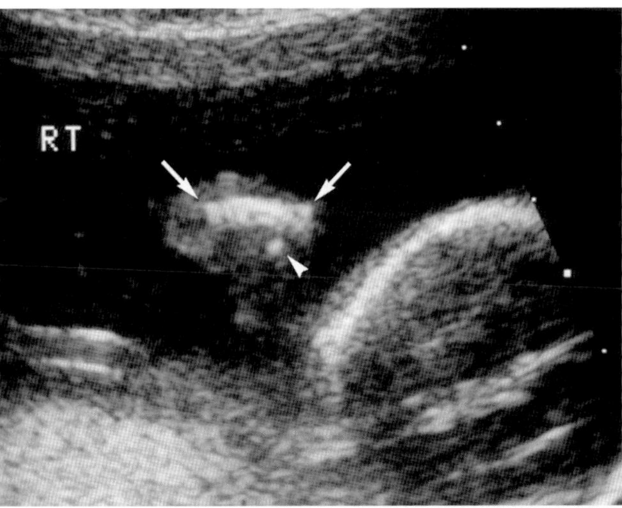

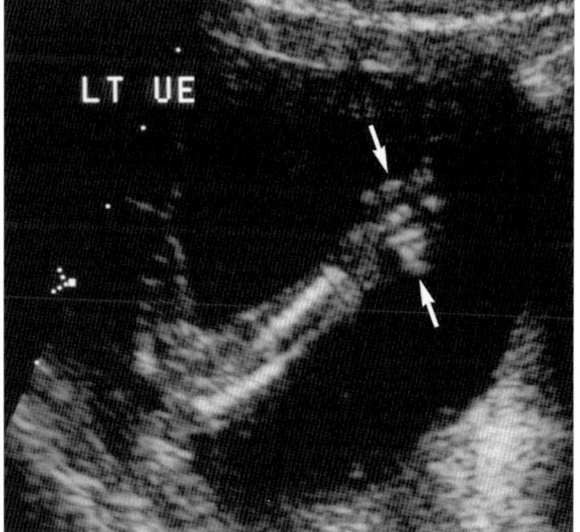

A B

FIGURE 12.3-1. Absence of part of an upper extremity. A: Image of the right (RT) forearm demonstrates a shortened ulna *(arrows)*, a very small part of the radius *(arrowhead)*, and no hand. **B:** The left (LT UE) forearm is normal with a hand *(arrows)* seen distal to a normal radius and ulna.

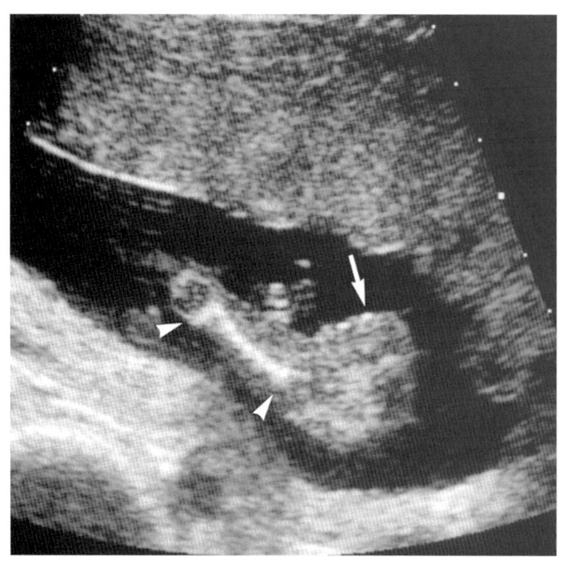
A

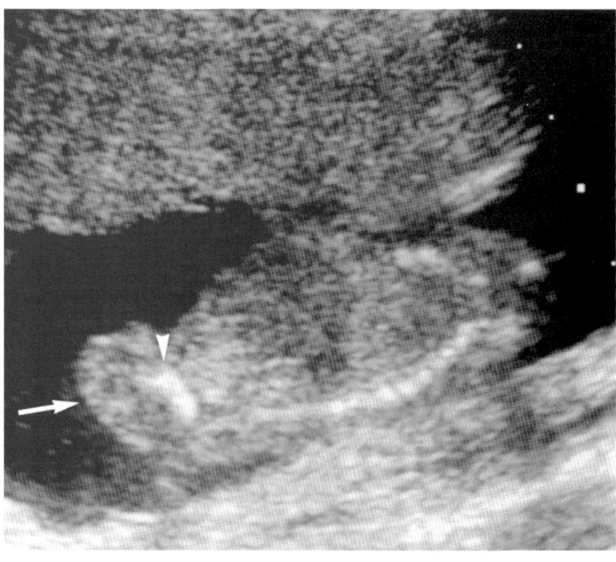
B

FIGURE 12.3-2. Absent lower extremity. A: Transverse image of the lower pelvis demonstrates a normal femur *(arrowheads)* on one side and the absence of the lower extremity *(arrow)* on the other side. **B:** Longitudinal image demonstrates the absence of the lower extremity *(arrow)* below the iliac crest *(arrowhead)*.

12.4. RADIAL RAY DEFECTS

Description and Clinical Features

Radial ray defects are characterized by aplasia or hypoplasia of the radius. The process may be unilateral or bilateral. The radial defect is often part of a syndrome, such as Cornelia de Lange, Fanconi, Holt-Oram, radial aplasia-thrombocytopenia, or VATER syndrome. Many of these syndromes have among their components congenital heart defects. Radial ray defects may also be found in fetuses with aneuploidy, particularly trisomies 13 and 18.

Sonography

With a radial ray defect, the forearm is deformed, with absence or hypoplasia of the radius and the hand rotated toward the forearm (Figure 12.4-1). Because of the association with other anomalies, including cardiac defects and aneuploidy, careful assessment of the other fetal organs is warranted when a radial ray defect is diagnosed.

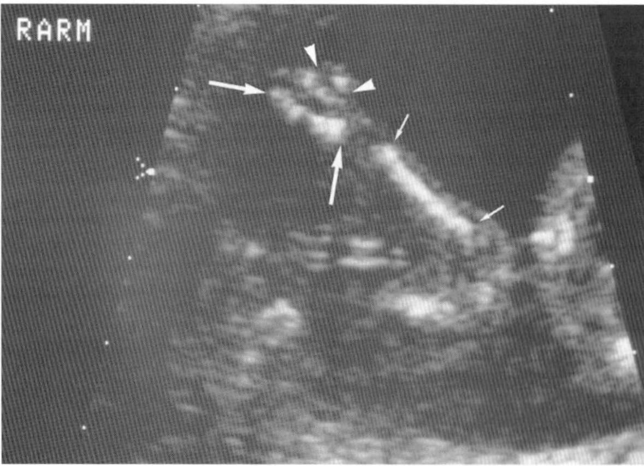

FIGURE 12.4-1. Absent radius. Image of the right arm (RARM) demonstrates no radius adjacent to the ulna *(large arrows)*. The hand *(arrowheads)* is positioned adjacent to the shaft of the ulna. The humerus *(small arrows)* is normal.

12.5. POLYDACTYLY

Description and Clinical Features

Polydactyly is defined as one or more extra digits in a hand or foot. The extra digit may be adjacent to the thumb or big toe (sometimes termed preaxial) or adjacent to the little finger or little toe (sometimes termed postaxial). The extra digit may have three, two, one, or no bony phalanges. It may be as large as a normal digit or quite small. Polydactyly may be an isolated finding or a component of a variety of syndromes, including short rib polydactyly, chondroectodermal dysplasia, asphyxiating thoracic dystrophy, and Meckel-Gruber. It is also a feature of trisomy 13.

Sonography

Polydactyly is diagnosed when one or more extra digits are seen on the hand or foot (Figure 12.5-1). In some cases, ossified phalanges can be seen in the digit (Figure 12.5-2). In others, no phalanges are present, and the digit appears as a soft-tissue structure arising from one side of the hand or foot.

A

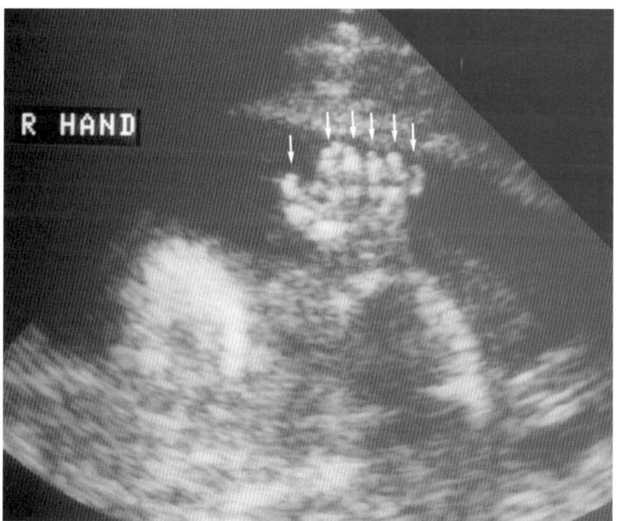

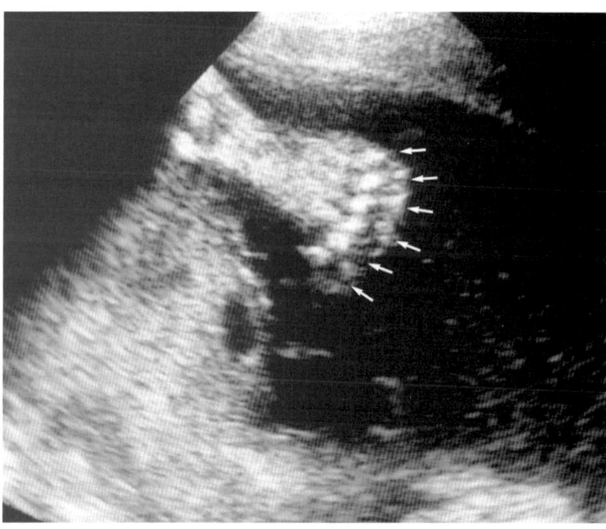

B

FIGURE 12.5-1. Polydactyly. Images of a hand (R HAND) with six digits *(small arrows)* **(A)** and a foot with six phalanges *(small arrows)* **(B)**, forming six toes.

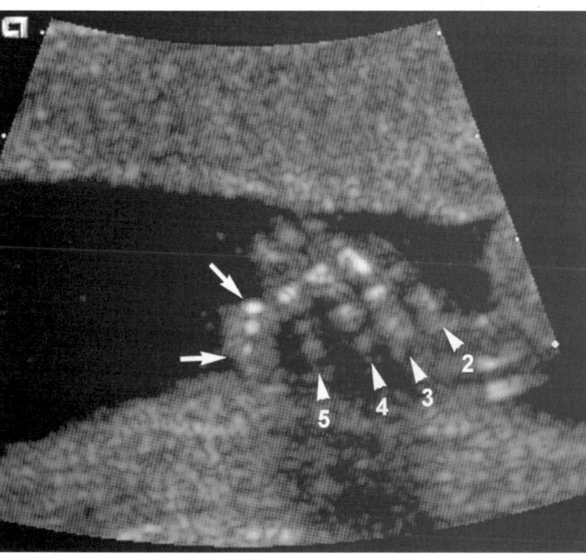

FIGURE 12.5-2. Polydactyly with small phalanges in an extra digit. Image of second to fifth fingers (2, 3, 4, and 5, *arrowheads*) of a hand demonstrates an extra digit *(arrows)* with small phalanges adjacent to the fifth digit.

12.6. CLINODACTYLY

Description and Clinical Features

Clinodactyly is defined as abnormal mediolateral curvature of a finger, often resulting in overlapping of the digits. The defect most commonly affects the index or fifth finger and is commonly associated with aneuploidy. In particular, overlapping of the index finger over the middle finger in a hand persistently clenched is a characteristic feature of trisomy 18. Inward curvature of the fifth finger, as a result of a deformed middle phalanx, is seen with trisomy 21.

Sonography

The sonographic diagnosis of clinodactyly is made by careful assessment of the fetal hands. The overlapping digits can be seen (Figure 12.6-1), particularly with adequate or increased amniotic fluid.

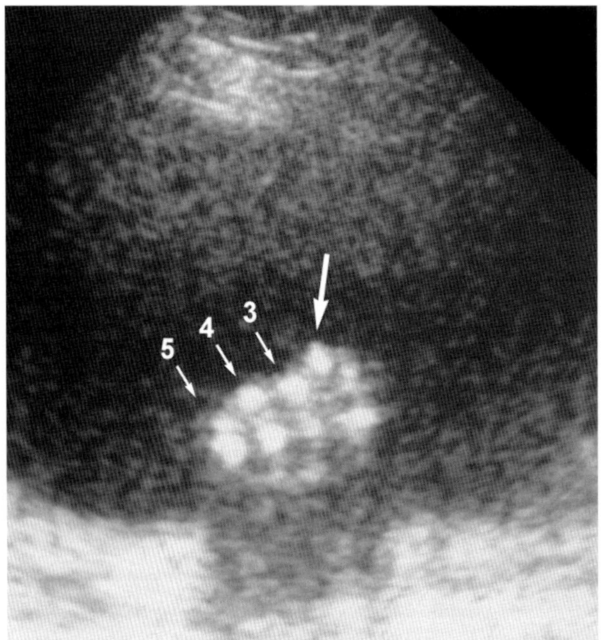

A

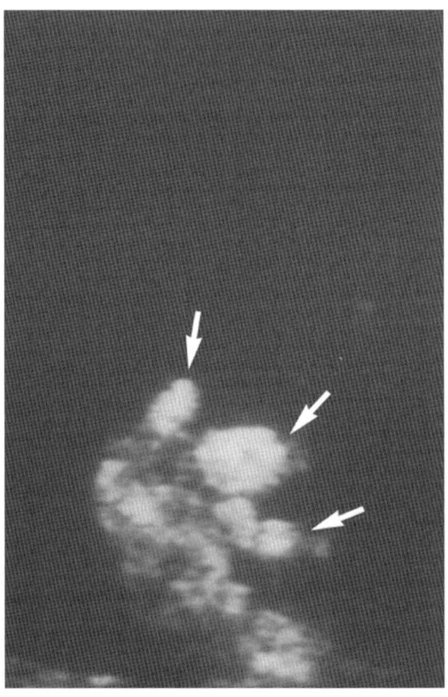

B

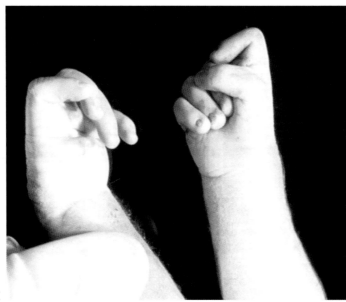

C

FIGURE 12.6-1. Clinodactyly. **A:** Image of a hand surrounded by polyhydramnios demonstrates the index finger *(large arrow)* overlapping the third digit (3, *small arrow*). The fourth and fifth fingers (4 and 5, *small arrows*) are aligned normally. **B:** Image of a hand surrounded by severe polyhydramnios in a fetus with trisomy 18 demonstrates abnormal positioning and curvature of the fingers *(arrows)*. **C:** Photograph of neonatal hands of the fetus shown in **(B)** demonstrates abnormal positioning and curvature of the fingers of both hands.

12.7. CLUBFOOT

Description and Clinical Features

Clubfoot is a malformation of the bones of the foot. There are several variants, but most often the foot is inverted and medially rotated, so that the dorsum of the foot faces inward. Clubfoot is associated with a variety of syndromes and chromosomal defects. It can also result from a restrictive uterine environment, such as with prolonged oligohydramnios or uterine anomalies that restrict fetal space.

Sonography

The diagnosis of clubfoot is made when the bones of the foot, particularly the metatarsals, lie in the same plane as the tibia and fibula (Figure 12.7-1). On some views, the entire foot is seen in the same plane as the bones of the lower leg.

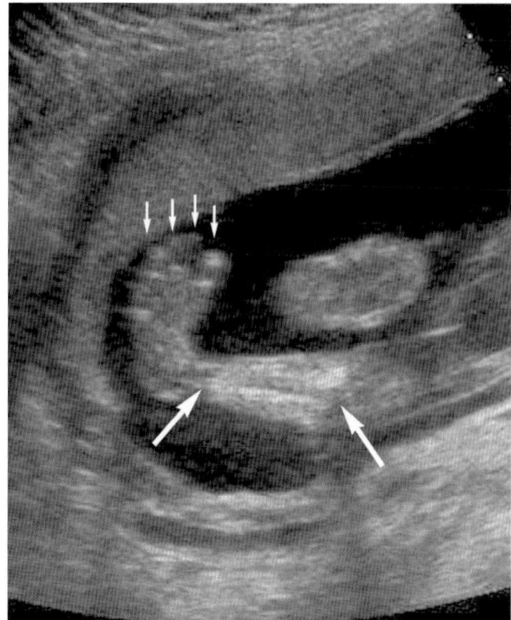

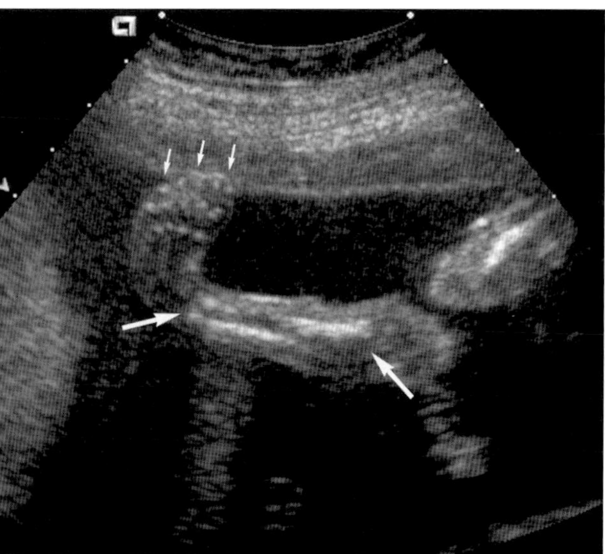

FIGURE 12.7-1. Clubfeet. A and B: Images of the lower legs of two fetuses with clubfeet demonstrate the bones of the feet *(small arrows)* lying in the same plane as the tibia and fibula *(large arrows)*.

12.8. ROCKERBOTTOM FOOT

Description and Clinical Features

Rockerbottom foot is a malformation of the foot in which the bottom of the foot is convex, protruding downward. This anomaly is usually bilateral and is commonly associated with other anomalies, particularly trisomy 18 and some of the skeletal dysplasias.

Sonography

With a rockerbottom foot, the bottom of the foot appears curved convex downward (Figure 12.8-1). In addition, the foot may protrude posteriorly at the heel.

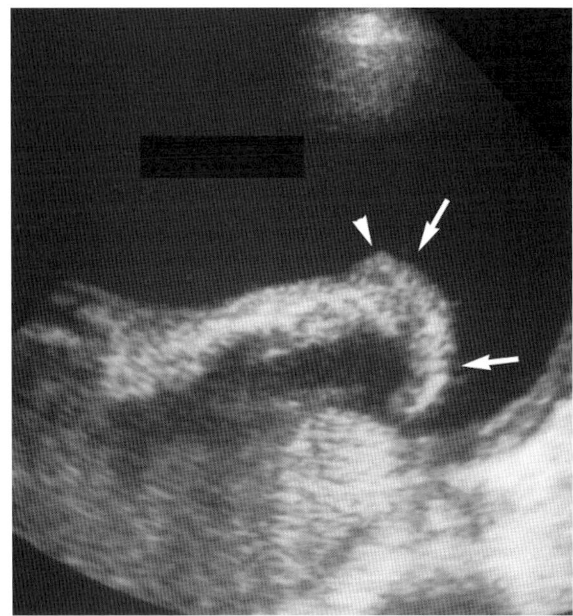
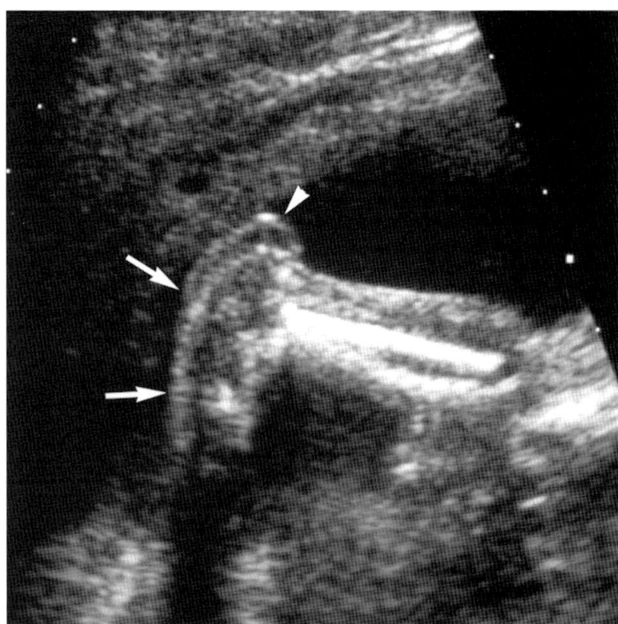

FIGURE 12.8-1. Rockerbottom feet. A and B: Images of the lower legs and feet of two fetuses with rockerbottom feet demonstrate downward convex curvature of the bottom of the foot *(arrows)* and protrusion of the heel *(arrowhead)* posteriorly.

SUGGESTED READINGS

1. Benson CB, Pober BR, Hirsh MP, et al. Sonography of Nager acrofacial dysostosis syndrome *in utero*. *J Ultrasound Med* 1988;7:163–167.
2. Bowerman RA. Anomalies of the fetal skeleton: sonographic findings. *AJR Am J Roentgenol* 1995; 164: 973–979.
3. Budorick N. The fetal musculoskeletal system. In: Callen PW, ed. *Ultrasonography in obstetrics and gynecology*, 4th ed. Philadelphia: WB Saunders, 2000:331–377.
4. Glanc P, Chitayat D, Azouz EM. The fetal musculoskeletal system. In: Rumack CM, Wilson SR, Charboneau JW, eds. *Diagnostic ultrasound*, 2nd ed. St. Louis: Mosby, 1998:1201–1232.
5. Jeanty P, Kleinman G. Proximal femoral focal deficiency. *J Ultrasound Med* 1989;8:639–642.
6. Kurtz AB, Needleman L, Wapner RJ, et al. Usefulness of a short femur in the *in utero* detection of skeletal dysplasias. *Radiology* 1990;177:197–200.
7. Maymon E, Romero R, Ghezzi F, et al. Fetal skeletal anomalies. In: Fleischer AC, Manning FA, Jeanty P, et al., eds. *Sonography in obstetrics & gynecology: principles and practice*, 6th ed. New York: McGraw-Hill, 2001:445–506.
8. Meizner I. Fetal skeletal malformation revisited: steps in the diagnostic approach. *Ultrasound Obstet Gynecol* 1997;10:303–306.
9. Rijhsinghani A, Yankowitz J, Kanis AB, et al. Antenatal sonographic diagnosis of club foot with particular attention to the implications and outcomes of isolated club foot. *Ultrasound Obstet. Gynecol* 1998;11:103–106.
10. Seymour R, Jones A. Strawberry-shaped skull in fetal thanatophoric dysplasia. *Ultrasound Obstet Gynecol* 1994;4:434–436.
11. Tadmor OP, Kreisberg GA, Achiron R, et al. Limb amputation in amniotic band syndrome: serial ultrasonographic and Doppler observations. *Ultrasound Obstet Gynecol* 1997;10:312–315.

13

CHROMOSOMAL ANOMALIES

13.1. TRISOMY 13 (PATAU SYNDROME)

Description and Clinical Features

Trisomy 13 is a chromosomal anomaly in which the fetus has an extra chromosome 13 (i.e., it has three, instead of the normal two, chromosomes 13). It is a rare anomaly, occurring in approximately one per 5,000 births. The incidence increases with advancing maternal age. Fetuses with trisomy 13 generally have severe structural anomalies involving multiple organ systems. Most die in the neonatal period, and the few long-term survivors are severely neurologically impaired.

Sonography

Many of the common structural anomalies in fetuses with trisomy 13 can be identified by ultrasound. Among these are the following:

- Central nervous system
  - Holoprosencephaly
  - Ventriculomegaly
  - Microcephaly
  - Agenesis of the corpus callosum
- Face
  - Microphthalmia
  - Hypotelorism
- Extremities
  - Radial aplasia
  - Polydactyly
  - Flexion deformity of fingers
- Diaphragmatic defects (hernia/eventration)
- Omphalocele
- Cardiac anomalies
- Echogenic enlarged kidneys

When a constellation of anomalies, including several of the above, is detected by ultrasound (Figures 13.1-1, 13.1-2, and 13.1-3), the diagnosis of trisomy 13 should be considered and amniocentesis should be offered. Furthermore, several anomalies that occur in trisomy 13 are associated with an increased incidence of aneuploidy even when seen as an isolated finding (e.g., holoprosencephaly, microcephaly, microphthalmia, omphalocele) and thus are indications for amniocentesis.

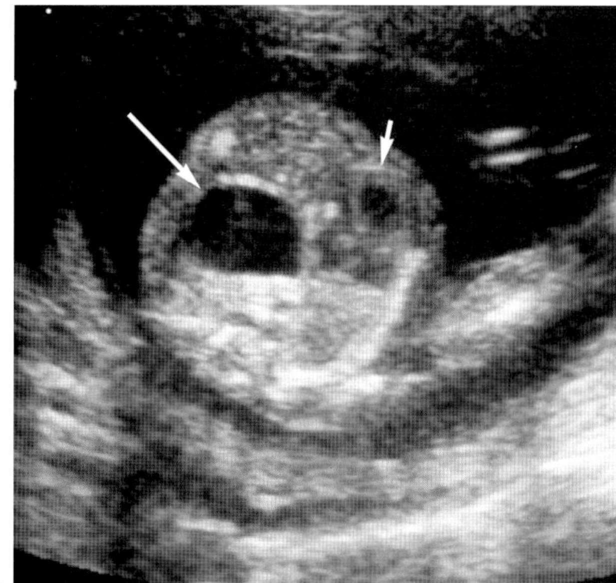

FIGURE 13.1-1. Trisomy 13 with diaphragmatic hernia, micrognathia, and abnormal kidneys. A: Transverse view through the fetal thorax demonstrates a left-sided diaphragmatic hernia with an intrathoracic fetal stomach *(long arrow)* deviating the heart *(short arrow)* to the right. **B:** Sagittal midline view of the face demonstrates an abnormally small jaw *(arrow)*, representing micrognathia. **C:** Coronal view of the abdomen shows both kidneys *(arrowheads)* to be hydronephrotic and hyperechoic.

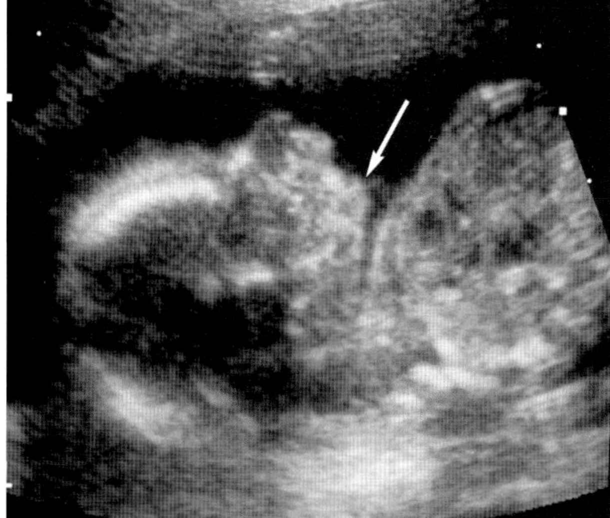

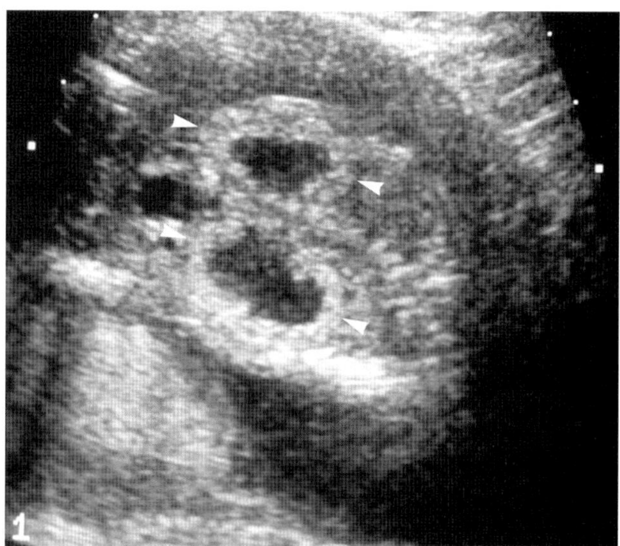

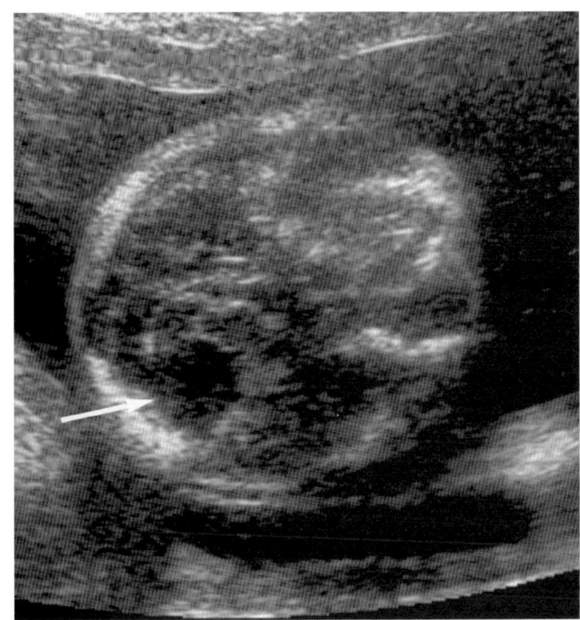
A

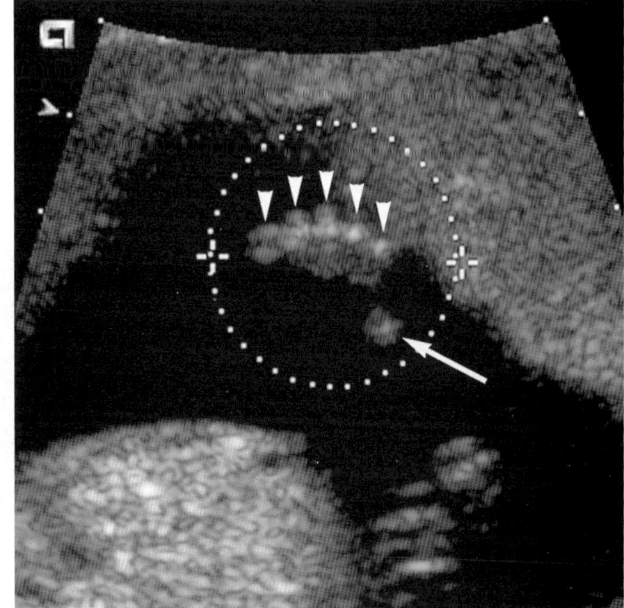
B

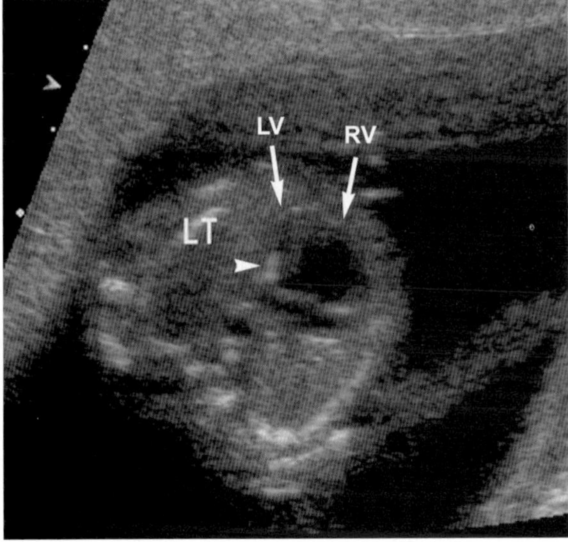

C

FIGURE 13.1-2. Trisomy 13 with a Dandy-Walker malformation, polydactyly, and hypoplastic left heart. A: Transverse view through the head demonstrates a cyst *(arrow)* in the posterior fossa replacing most of the cerebellar vermis, representing a Dandy-Walker malformation. **B:** The left fetal hand has six digits, including the thumb *(arrow)* and five other fingers *(arrowheads)*, representing polydactyly. **C:** The left ventricle *(LV arrow)* is hypoplastic and has echogenic foci *(arrowhead)*. The right ventricle *(RV arrow)* appears enlarged.

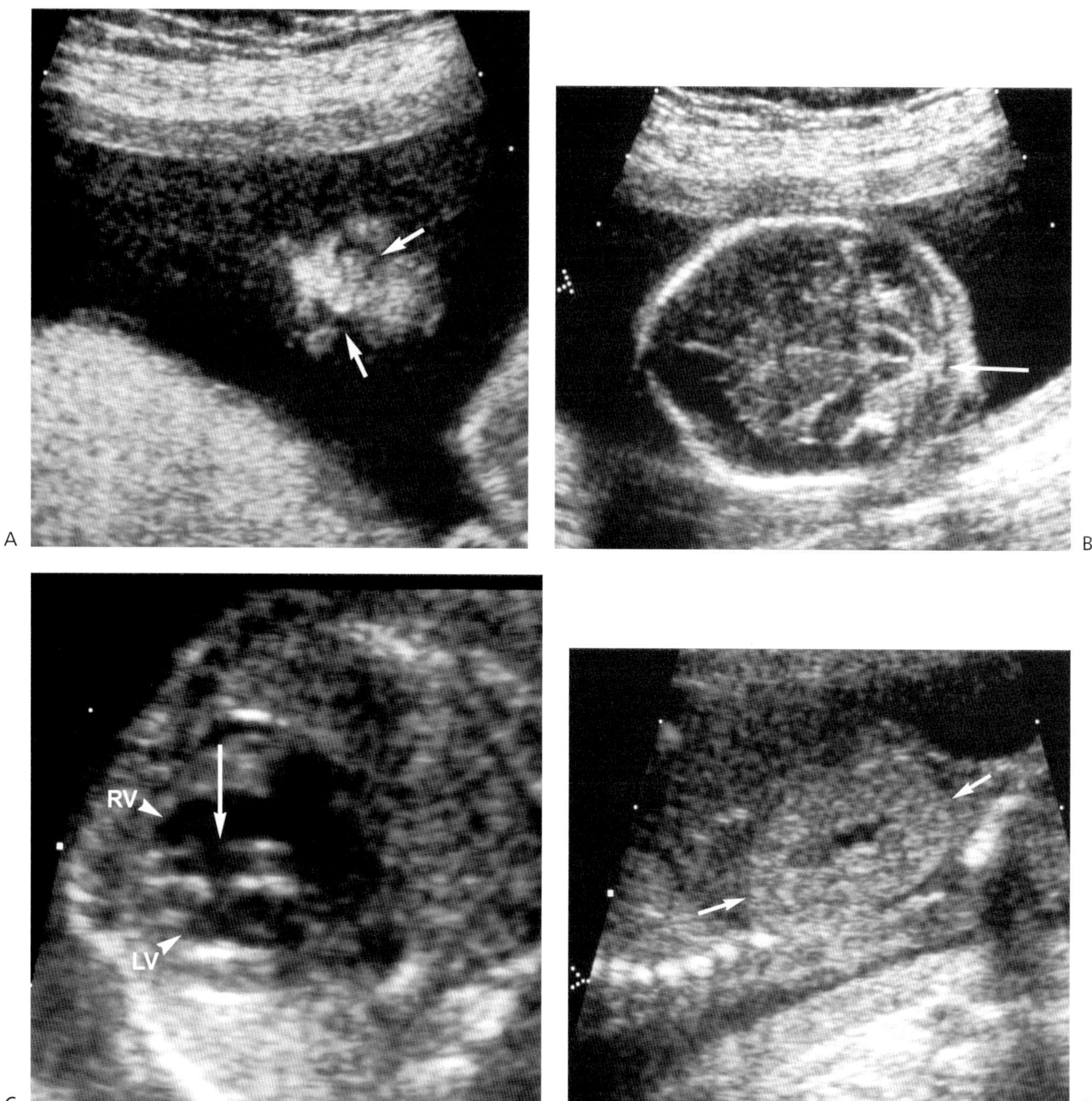

FIGURE 13.1-3. Trisomy 13 with cleft lip, cerebellar hypoplasia, ventricular septal defect, and abnormal kidneys. A: Coronal view through the lower face reveals bilateral clefts *(arrows)* in the upper lip extending to the nostrils. **B:** Axial view of the head demonstrates a small posterior fossa with a hypoplastic cerebellum *(arrow)* and no fluid in the cisterna magna. **C:** Four-chamber view of the heart demonstrates an opening *(arrow)* in the ventricular septum, forming a communication between the left ventricle *(LV arrowhead)* and right ventricle *(RV arrowhead)*. **D:** Longitudinal view of a kidney *(arrows)* demonstrates it to be enlarged and echogenic.

13.2. TRISOMY 18 (EDWARDS SYNDROME)

Description and Clinical Features

Trisomy 18 is a chromosomal anomaly in which the fetus has an extra chromosome 18 (i.e., it has three, instead of the normal two, chromosomes 18). It is a rare anomaly, occurring in approximately three per 10,000 births. Like other trisomies, the incidence increases with advancing maternal age. Fetuses with trisomy 18 generally have severe structural anomalies involving multiple organ systems. Most die within the first year of life, and the few long-term survivors are severely neurologically impaired.

Sonography

Many of the structural anomalies in fetuses with trisomy 18 can be identified by ultrasound. Among these are the following:

- Central nervous system
  - Agenesis of the corpus callosum
  - Choroid plexus cysts
  - Hypoplastic cerebellum with enlarged cisterna magna
- Face
  - Micrognathia
  - Hypotelorism
  - Microphthalmia
- Extremities
  - Clenched handed with overlapping index finger
  - Clubfoot
  - Rockerbottom foot
- Omphalocele
- Diaphragmatic hernia
- Cardiac anomalies
- Renal anomalies
- Intrauterine growth restriction

When a constellation of anomalies, including several of the above, is detected by ultrasound (Figures 13.2-1 and 13.2-2), the diagnosis of trisomy 18 should be considered and amniocentesis should be offered. Furthermore, several anomalies that occur in trisomy 18 are associated with an increased incidence of aneuploidy even when seen as an isolated finding (e.g., microphthalmia, clenched hand with overlapping index finger, rockerbottom foot, omphalocele, diaphragmatic hernia) and thus are indications for amniocentesis.

Fetuses with trisomy 18 have an increased incidence of choroid plexus cysts in the second trimester. There is some disagreement about whether amniocentesis should be offered when ultrasound demonstrates choroid plexus cysts and no other structural anomalies. It is generally agreed, however, that amniocentesis should be offered when the fetus is found to have choroid plexus cysts together with another anomaly (Figure 13.2-3), especially one of the anomalies listed above.

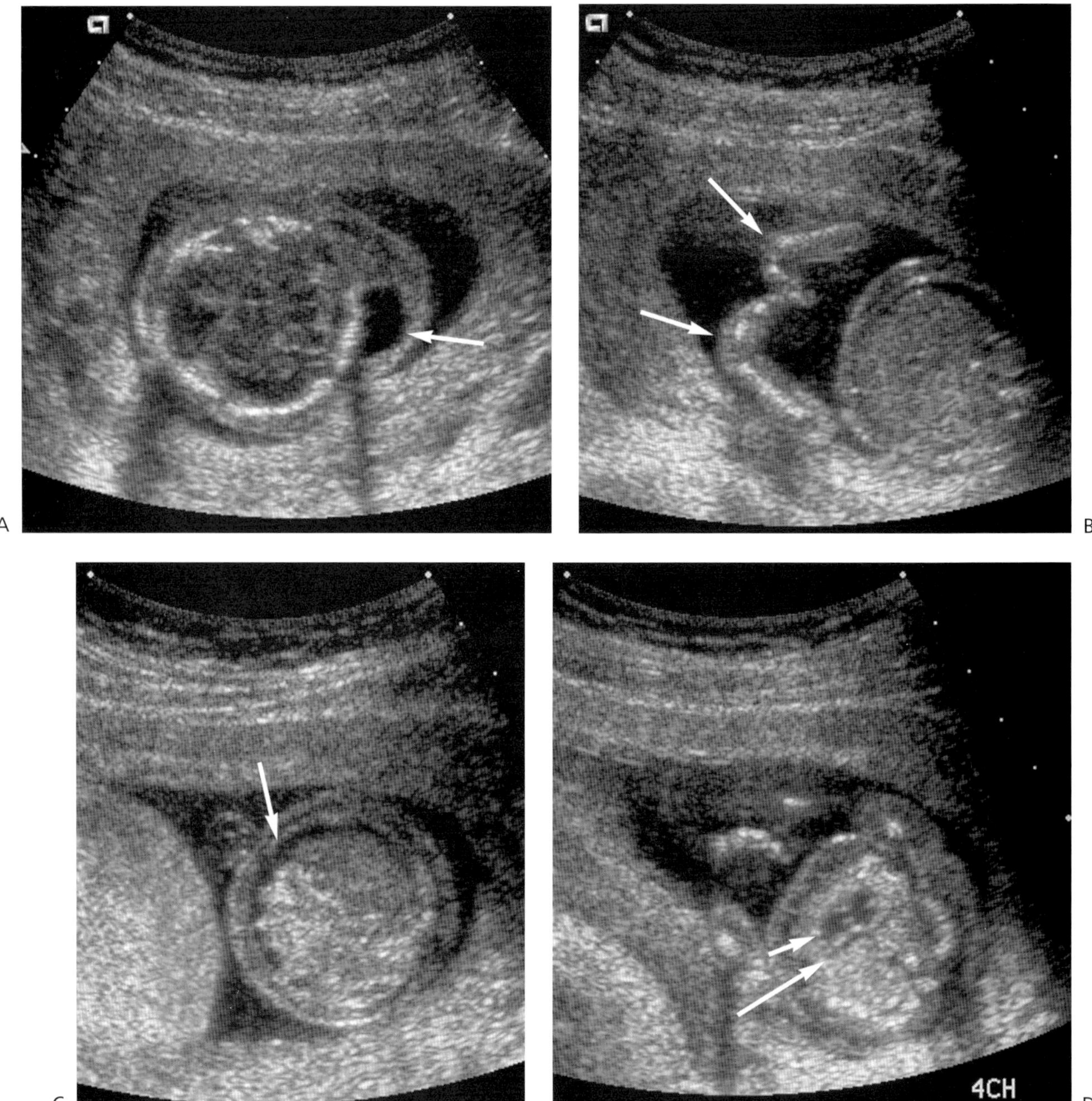

FIGURE 13.2-1. Trisomy 18 with a cystic hygroma, abnormal upper extremities, ascites, and hypoplastic left ventricle. A: Axial view of the head demonstrates a cystic hygroma *(arrow)* in the occipital and posterior nuchal areas. **B:** The wrists are held in persistent flexion. **C:** Transverse view of the abdomen demonstrates ascites *(arrow)*. **D:** Four-chamber view of the heart demonstrates a hypoplastic left ventricle *(long arrow)* with a normal right ventricle *(short arrow)*.

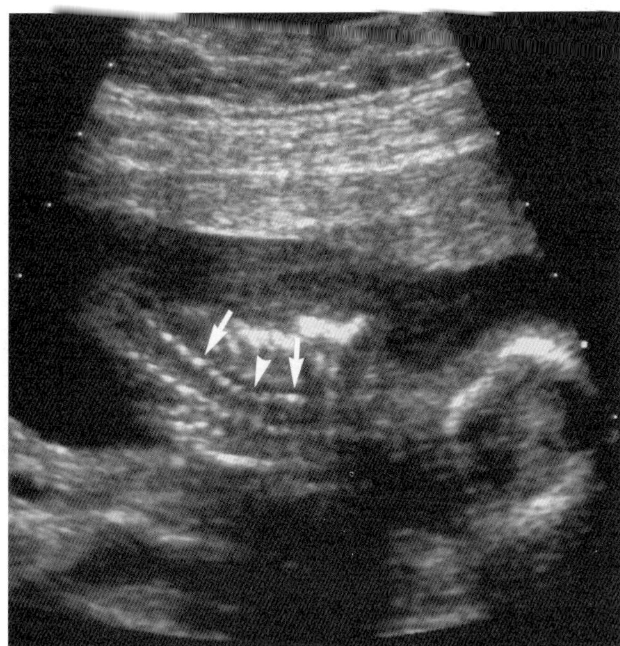
A

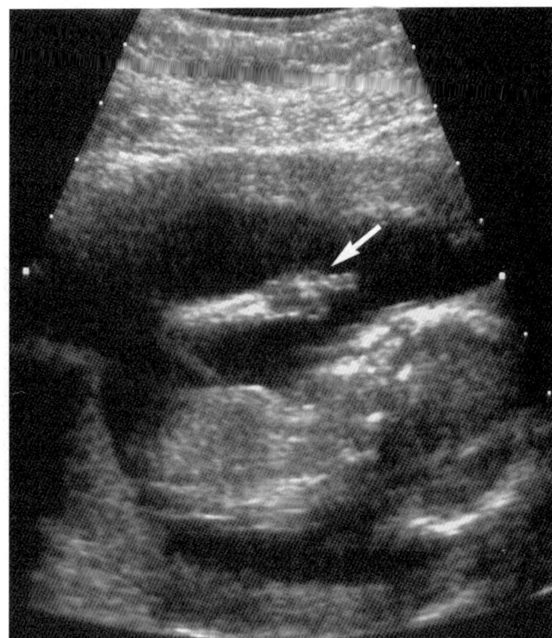
B

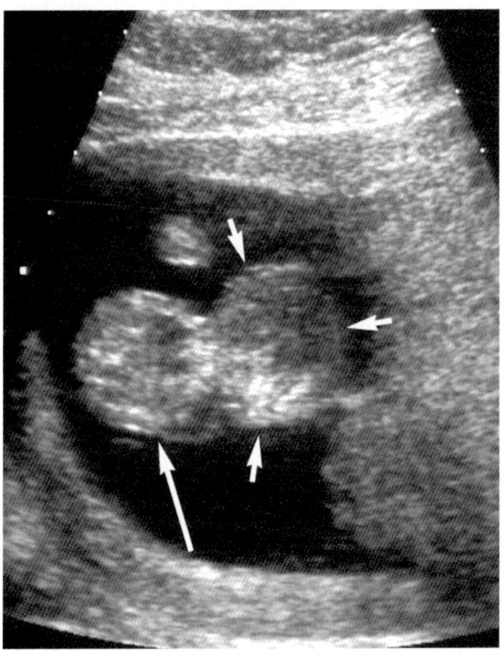
C

FIGURE 13.2-2. Trisomy 18 with scoliosis, abnormal finger positioning, and omphalocele. A: Coronal view of the spine reveals scoliosis, with the lower thoracic spine *(arrows)* bent laterally *(arrowhead)*. **B:** There is abnormal positioning of the fingers of a hand *(arrow)*. **C:** Transverse view of the abdomen demonstrates a large omphalocele *(short arrows)* protruding from the anterior wall of the abdomen *(long arrow)*.

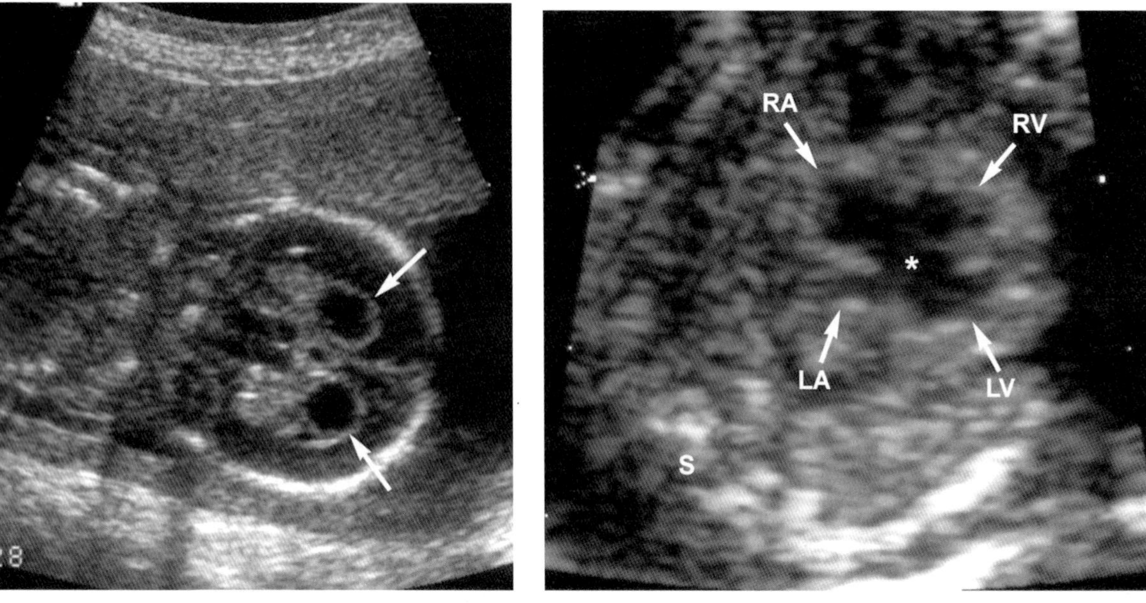

FIGURE 13.2-3. Choroid plexus cysts in a 17-week fetus with trisomy 18. A: Image of the fetal head demonstrates bilateral choroid plexus cysts *(arrows)*. **B:** Transverse view of the fetal chest, with the spine (S) posterior, demonstrates an abnormal four-chamber view of the fetal heart (*RV arrow*, right ventricle; *LV arrow*, left ventricle; *RA arrow*, right atrium; *LA arrow*, left atrium). There is a large opening *(*)* in the midportion of the heart where the ventricular and atrial septa and the atrioventricular valves are expected to lie, establishing the diagnosis of atrioventricular canal.

13.3. TRISOMY 21 (DOWN SYNDROME)

Description and Clinical Features

Trisomy 21 is a chromosomal anomaly in which the fetus has an extra chromosome 21 (i.e., it has three, instead of the normal two, chromosomes 21). It is the most common chromosomal anomaly in newborns, occurring in one per 700 births. Like other trisomies, the incidence of trisomy 21 increases with advancing maternal age.

Fetuses with trisomy 21 have increased incidence of cardiac defects, duodenal atresia, and other structural anomalies. Trisomy 21 is not usually fatal unless there is a life-threatening cardiac structural defect. Children and adults with trisomy 21 have subnormal intelligence.

Sonography

Many of the structural anomalies in fetuses with trisomy 21 can be identified by ultrasound (Figures 13.3-1 and 13.3-2). Among these are the following:

- Cerebral ventriculomegaly
- Cardiac
  - Atrioventricular canal
  - Ventricular septal defect
  - Tetralogy of Fallot
- Neck
  - Nuchal translucency >2.2–2.8 mm at 11–14 weeks
  - Nuchal fold ≥6 mm at 16–20 weeks
- Duodenal atresia

In addition to the above, there are a number of sonographic findings in the second trimester that appear to be weakly associated with trisomy 21 (and, for some of the findings, other forms of aneuploidy). These "minor markers" of aneuploidy include a short

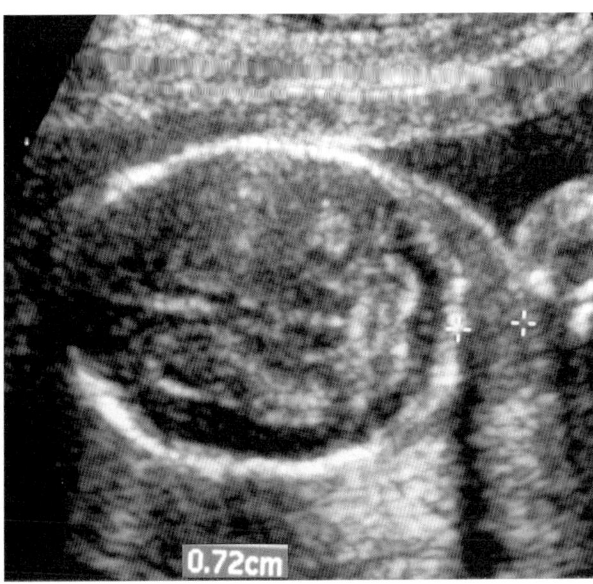

FIGURE 13.3-1. Thick nuchal fold in a fetus with trisomy 21. Angled axial view of the fetal head demonstrates a thick nuchal fold *(calipers)* measuring 7.2 mm.

femur and humerus, echogenic bowel (bowel at least as echogenic as bone), echogenic intracardiac focus, and renal pyelectasis. (*Note:* choroid plexus cysts, another "minor marker" of aneuploidy, are associated with trisomy 18 only). There is some disagreement about whether amniocentesis should be offered when ultrasound demonstrates a single minor marker and no other abnormality. It is generally agreed, however, that the finding of two or more minor markers or one minor marker in conjunction with another significant fetal abnormality (Figure 13.3-3) warrants amniocentesis.

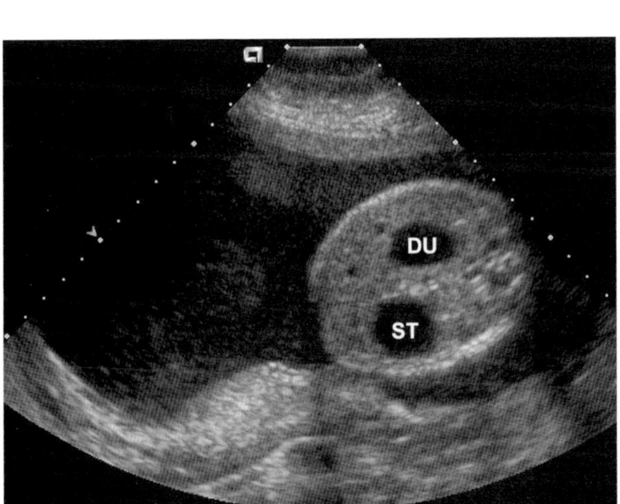

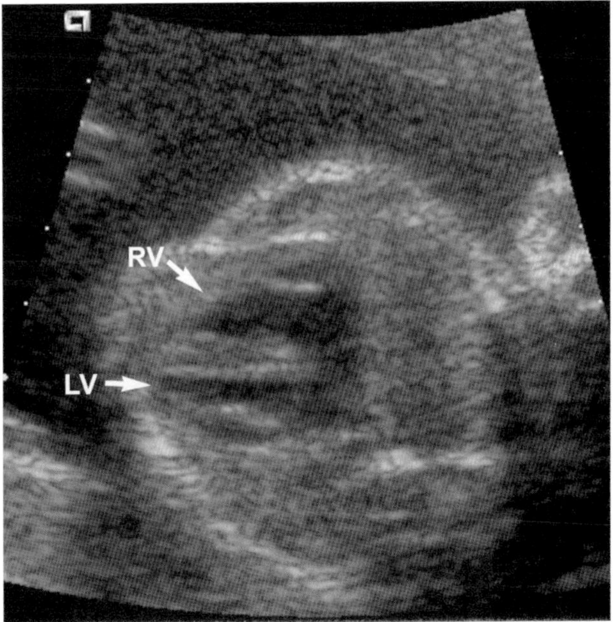

FIGURE 13.3-2. Duodenal atresia and hypoplastic left ventricle in a fetus with trisomy 21. A: Transverse view of the fetal abdomen reveals two fluid-filled structures ("double bubble"), representing a distended stomach (ST) and duodenum (DU). There is also polyhydramnios. **B:** Four-chamber view of the fetal heart reveals a hypoplastic left ventricle *(LV arrow)*, with a normal right ventricle *(RV arrow)*.

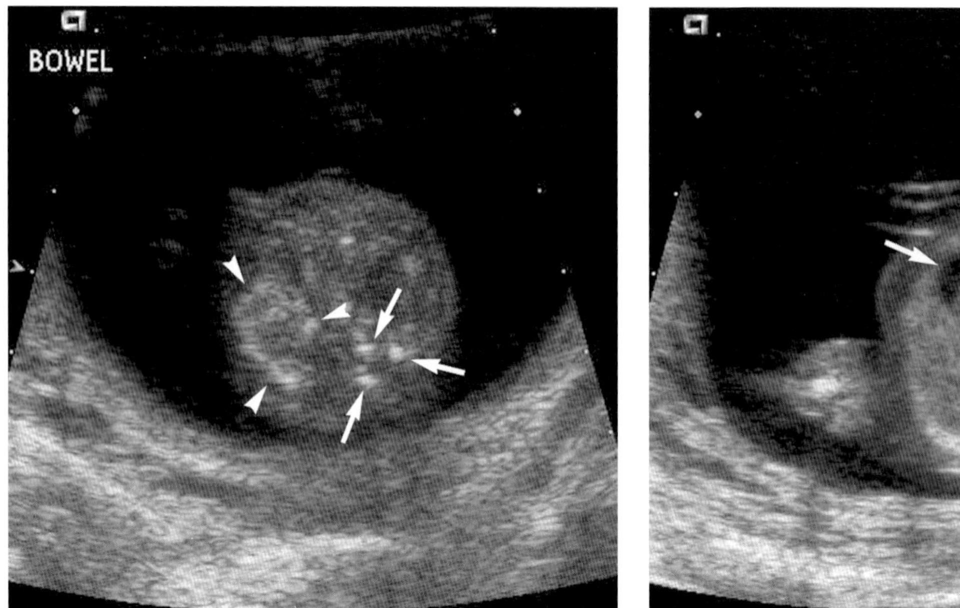

FIGURE 13.3-3. Echogenic bowel and pericardial effusion in a fetus with trisomy 21. A: Transverse view of the fetal abdomen reveals a region of bowel *(arrowheads)* that is equal in echogenicity to the vertebral ossification centers *(arrows)*. **B:** Transverse view of the fetal thorax demonstrates pericardial effusion *(arrows)*.

13.4. MONOSOMY X (TURNER SYNDROME, 45X)

Description and Clinical Features

Monosomy X, commonly known as Turner syndrome, is a chromosomal anomaly in which the fetus has an X chromosome as its only sex chromosome instead of the usual two sex chromosomes (XX in females and XY in males). Fetuses with Turner syndrome often have nuchal cystic hygromas and may have other abnormal fluid accumulations, including diffuse subcutaneous edema (lymphangiectasia), pleural effusions, and ascites. They also have an increased incidence of aortic coarctation and horseshoe kidneys.

Fetuses with Turner syndrome who have severe lymphangiectasia often die in the first or early second trimester. Newborns with this syndrome are phenotypically female. They typically have webbed necks (likely a result of regression of a prior cystic hygroma) and grow to a short stature. Most have ovarian dysgenesis, resulting in infertility in adult life.

Sonography

Turner syndrome is often detectable sonographically during the mid to late first trimester (Figure 13.4-1). The findings at this stage range from thickening of the nuchal translucency to a frank cystic hygroma (thickening with identifiable cystic spaces) to generalized subcutaneous edema (lymphangiectasia). Fetuses surviving into the second trimester will often be hydropic (Figure 13.4-2), with findings that include pleural effusions, pericardial effusion, ascites, and subcutaneous edema. When these findings are detected, the parents should be advised about the likelihood of Turner syndrome and offered karyotype testing via amniocentesis or chorionic villus sampling.

The cardiac and renal anomalies associated with Turner syndrome can sometimes be diagnosed by prenatal sonography. The finding of discrepant size of the cardiac ventricles, with the right ventricle being larger than the left ventricle, is suggestive of coarctation of the aorta. Most cases of coarctation, however, are not identified until after birth. A horseshoe kidney is more commonly diagnosed prenatally.

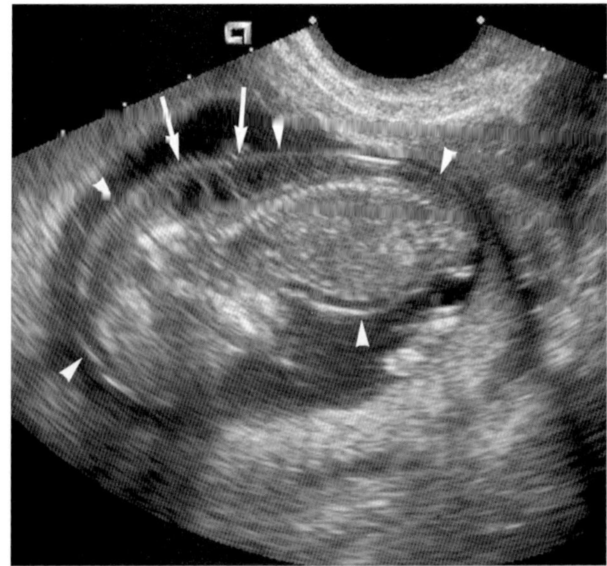
A

FIGURE 13.4-1. First-trimester fetus with Turner syndrome. A: Sagittal view through the fetus demonstrates skin thickening *(arrowheads)* around the entire fetus, including a septated fluid collection *(arrows)* in the posterior neck. **B:** Transverse view through the fetal neck demonstrates the septated fluid collection *(arrows)* posteriorly. **C:** Transverse view through the fetal abdomen demonstrates circumferential skin thickening *(arrowheads)*.

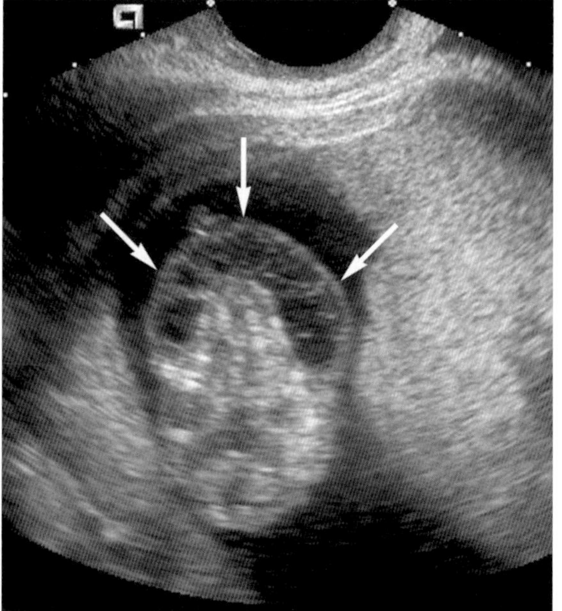
B

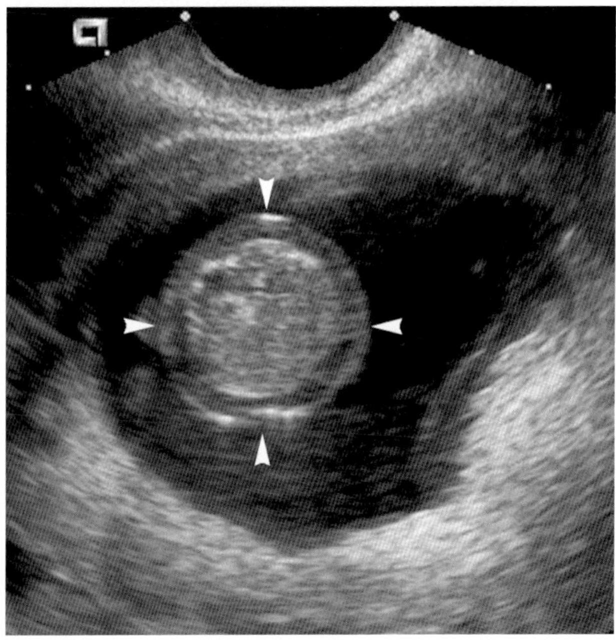
C

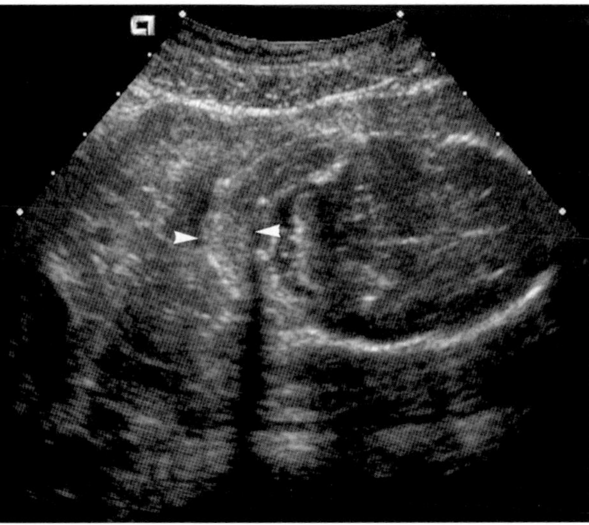
A

FIGURE 13.4-2. Second-trimester fetus with Turner syndrome. A: Axial view through the fetal head demonstrates nuchal edema with a thickened nuchal fold *(arrowheads)*. *(continued)*

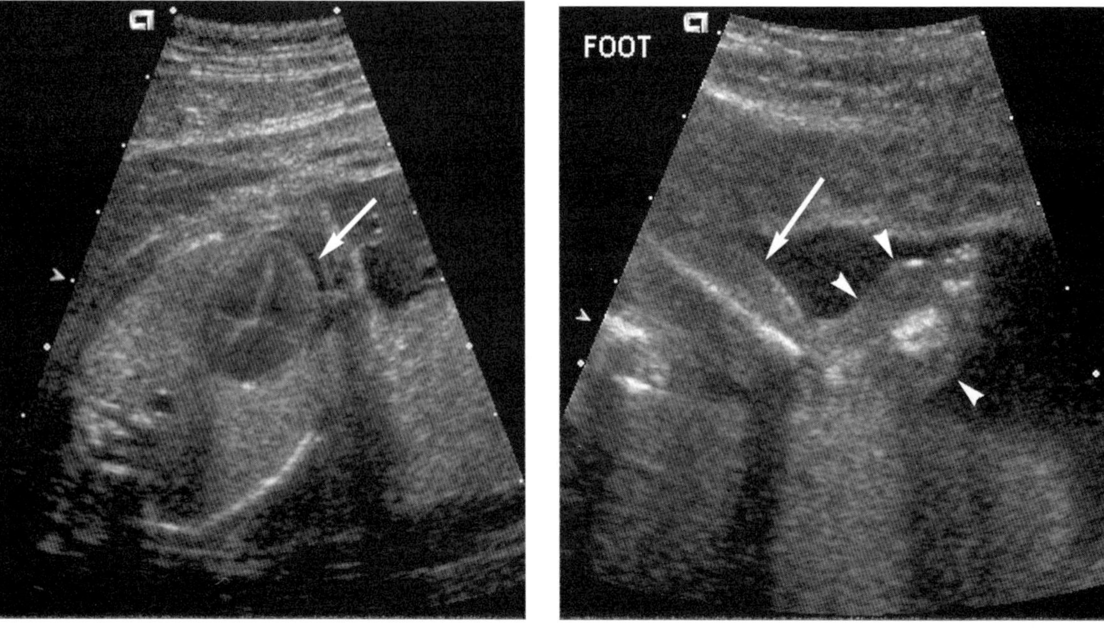

FIGURE 13.4-2. ***(continued)*** **Second-trimester fetus with Turner syndrome. B:** Transverse view of the chest demonstrates pericardial effusion *(arrow)*. **C:** A calf *(arrow)* and foot *(arrowheads)* are edematous.

13.5. TRIPLOIDY

Description and Clinical Features

Triploidy is a chromosomal anomaly in which the fetus has three (instead of the normal two) complete sets of chromosomes. That is, there are 69 chromosomes instead of the normal 46. In most cases, the extra set of chromosomes is paternal, resulting either from two sperm fertilizing a single ovum or a diploid sperm fertilizing an ovum. In a minority of cases, the extra set of chromosomes is maternal, occurring as a result of fertilization of a diploid ovum.

Triploid fetuses typically have severe growth restriction that begins early in pregnancy. They also have major structural anomalies involving multiple organ systems. Most die in the first or early second trimester. The rare cases of fetuses that survive into the third trimester either die *in utero* or shortly after birth.

When triploidy is due to two sets of paternal chromosomes, the placenta is usually enlarged and has multiple cysts. The combination of an enlarged cystic placenta and a triploid fetus is termed a partial mole. When triploidy results from two sets of maternal chromosomes, the placenta is usually small.

In some cases of triploidy, theca lutein cysts develop in the maternal ovaries. These are caused by high levels of human chorionic gonadotropin.

Sonography

The most common sonographic presentations of triploidy are:

- Dead embryo or fetus with an enlarged placenta containing multiple cysts
- Severe, early-onset growth restriction with a disproportionately small fetal abdomen (Figure 13.5-1); the placenta may or may not be enlarged and cystic.

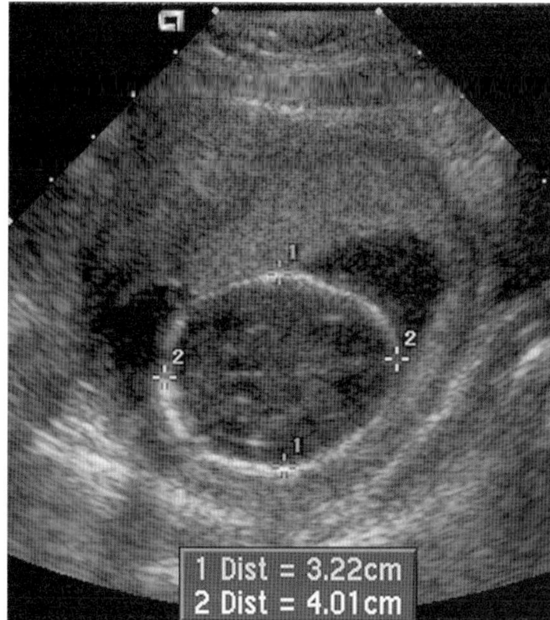

A

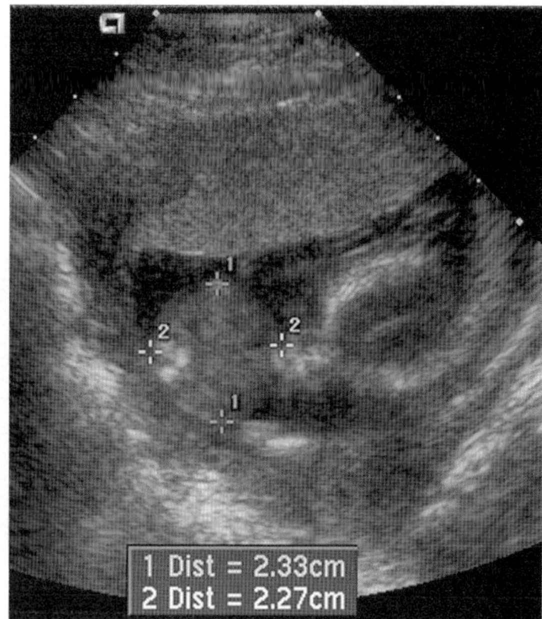

B

FIGURE 13.5-1. Growth-restricted triploid fetus at 18 weeks gestation. A: Measurements of the fetal head *(calipers)* reveal it to be small for 18 weeks gestation (biparietal diameter is 3.22 cm versus the expected biparietal diameter of 4.1 cm at this gestational age). **B:** Measurements of the fetal abdomen *(calipers)* reveal it to be small for 18 weeks gestation (mean abdominal diameter is 2.3 cm versus the expected abdominal diameter of 4.1 cm at this gestational age).

In addition to the intrauterine findings, the maternal ovaries may be enlarged and have multiple cysts (Figure 13.5-2). When triploidy is suspected, the diagnosis can be confirmed by amniocentesis or chorionic villus sampling if the fetus is alive or by examining the products of conception otherwise.

If a triploid fetus survives until 15–16 weeks or beyond, structural anomalies can be detected by ultrasound (Figures 13.5-2 and 13.5-3). These include:

- Central nervous system
  - Holoprosencephaly
  - Dandy-Walker malformation
  - Agenesis of the corpus callosum
- Face
  - Micrognathia
  - Microphthalmia
- Extremities
  - Syndactyly of the third and forth fingers
  - Clubfeet
- Omphalocele
- Cardiac anomalies
- Renal anomalies

If such anomalies are seen in a growth-restricted second- or third-trimester fetus, triploidy should be included in the differential diagnosis.

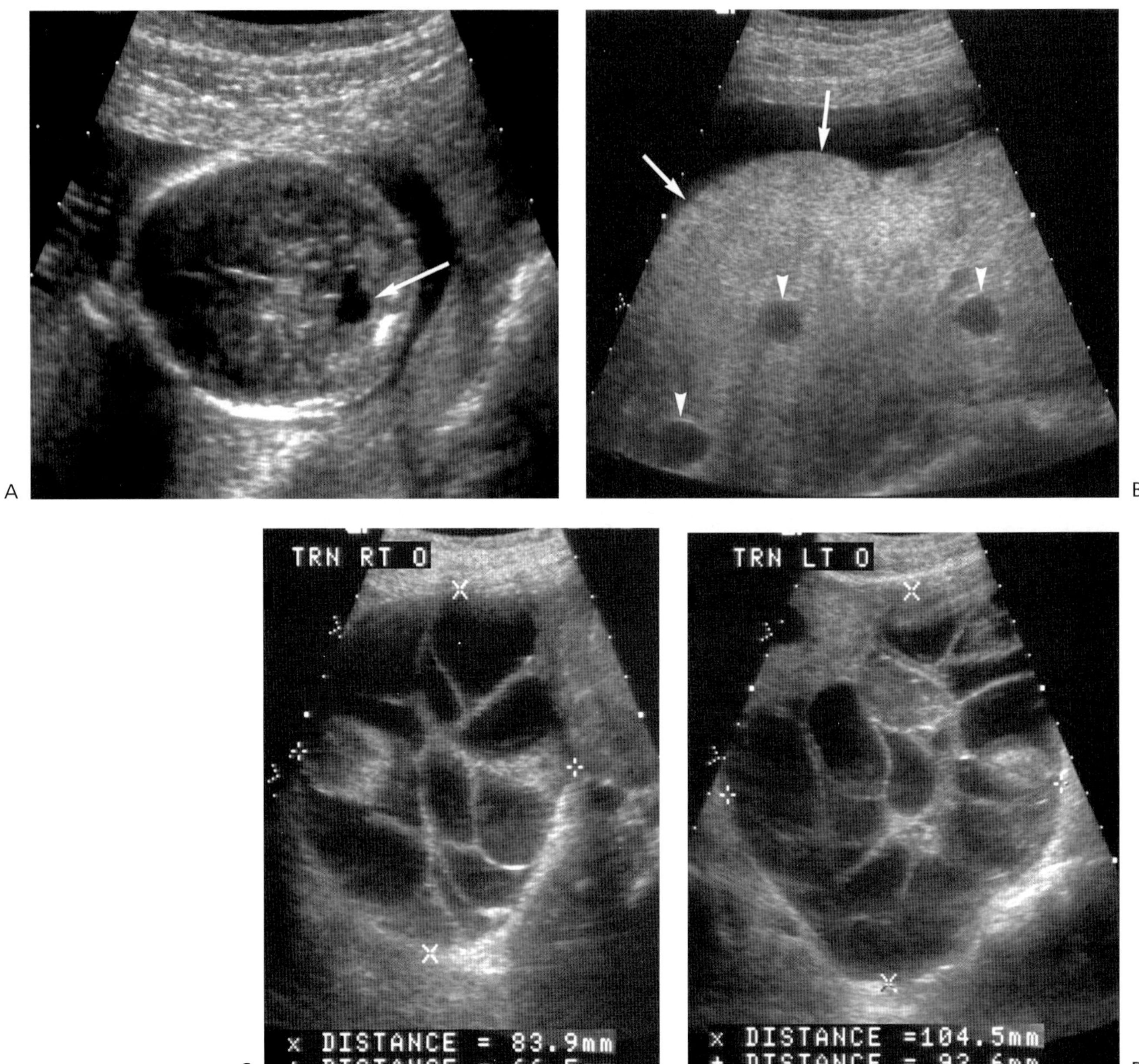

FIGURE 13.5-2. Fetal intracranial abnormality, thick cystic placenta, and enlarged cystic maternal ovaries in a case of triploidy. A: Axial view of the fetal head demonstrates a posterior fossa cyst *(arrow)*. **B:** The placenta *(arrows)* is thick and has multiple cysts *(arrowheads)*. **C and D:** The maternal ovaries (*calipers*; TRN RT O, transverse right ovary; TRN LT O, transverse left ovary) are enlarged with multiple cysts.

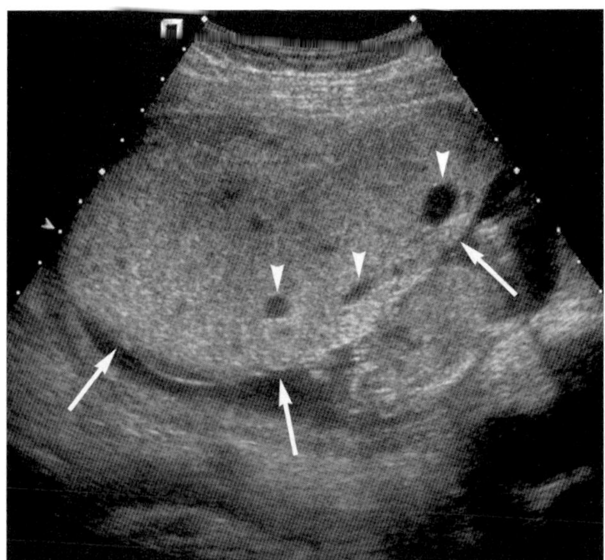
A

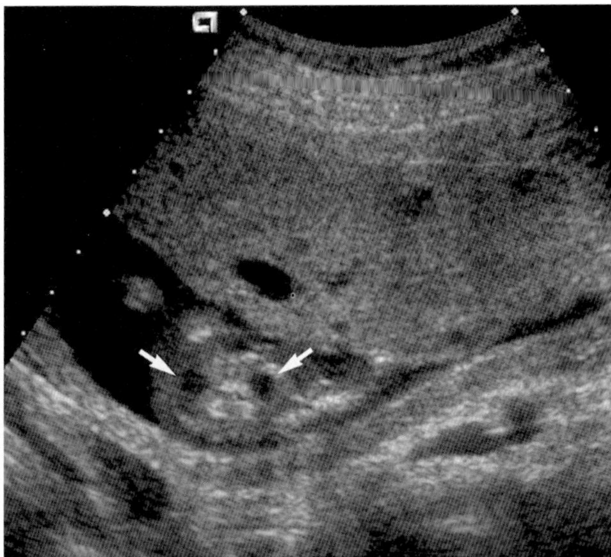
B

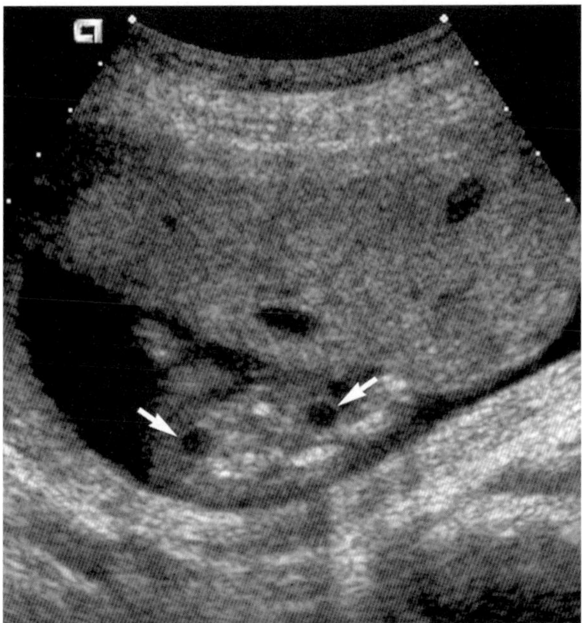
C

FIGURE 13.5-3. Fetal cystic hygromas and a thick cystic placenta in a case of triploidy. A: The placenta *(arrows)* is thick and has multiple cysts *(arrowheads)*. **B:** Transverse view of the fetal neck demonstrates cystic hygromas *(arrows)* on both lateral aspects of the neck. **C:** Transverse view through the upper thorax demonstrates cystic hygromas *(arrows)* in both axillae.

SUGGESTED READINGS

1. Benacerraf BR, Harlow B, Frigoletto FD Jr. Are choroid plexus cysts an indication for second-trimester amniocentesis? *Am J Obstet Gynecol* 1990;162:1001–1006.
2. Benacerraf BR, Neuberg D, Bromley B, et al. Sonographic scoring index for prenatal detection of chromosomal abnormalities. *J Ultrasound Med* 1992;11:449–458.
3. Benacerraf BR, Nadel A, Bromley B. Identification of second-trimester fetuses with autosomal trisomy by use of a sonographic scoring index. *Radiology* 1994;193:135–140.
4. Benacerraf BR. Ultrasound evaluation of chromosomal abnormalities. In: Callen PW, ed. *Ultrasonography in obstetrics and gynecology*, 4th ed. Philadelphia: WB Saunders, 2000:38–67.
5. Benacerraf BR. Should sonographic screening for fetal Down syndrome be applied to low risk women? *Ultrasound Obstet Gynecol* 2000;15:451–455.
6. Bromley B, Shipp T, Benacerraf BR. Genetic sonogram scoring index: accuracy and clinical utility. *J Ultrasound Med* 1999;18:523–528.
7. Chudleigh PM, Chitty LS, Pembrey M, et al. The association of aneuploidy and mild fetal pyelectasis in an unselected population: the results of a multicenter study. *Ultrasound Obstet Gynecol* 2001; 17:197–202.

8. DeVore GR. Trisomy 21: 91% detection rate using second-trimester ultrasound markers. *Ultrasound Obstet Gynecol* 2000;16:133–141.
9. DeVore G. Second trimester ultrasonography may identify 77 to 97% of fetuses with trisomy 18. *J Ultrasound Med* 2000;19:565–576.
10. Huggon IC, Cook AC, Simpson JM, et al. Isolated echogenic foci in the fetal heart as marker of chromosomal abnormality. *Ultrasound Obstet Gynecol* 2001;17:11–16.
11. Jauniaux E, Brown R, Rodeck C, et al. Prenatal diagnosis of triploidy during the second trimester of pregnancy. *Obstet Gynecol* 1996;88:983–989.
12. Jeanty P, Clavelli WA, Romaris SS. Ultrasound detection of chromosomal anomalies. In: Fleischer AC, Manning FA, Jeanty P, et al., eds. *Sonography in obstetrics & gynecology: principles and practice*, 6th ed. New York: McGraw-Hill, 2001:583–613.
13. Johnson JM, Nyberg DA. Chromosome abnormalities. In: Rumack CM, Wilson SR, Charboneau JW, eds. *Diagnostic ultrasound*, 2nd ed. St. Louis: Mosby, 1998:1177–1200.
14. Nadel AS, Bromley B, Frigoletto F, et al. Can the presumed risk of autosomal trisomy be decreased in fetuses of older women following a normal sonogram? *J Ultrasound Med* 1995;14:297–302.
15. Nyberg DA, Luthy A, Resta RG, et al. Age-adjusted ultrasound risk assessment for fetal Down's syndrome during the second trimester: description of the method and analysis of 142 cases. *Ultrasound Obstet Gynecol* 1998;12:8–14.
16. Sherer DM, Manning FA. First-trimester nuchal translucency screening for fetal aneuploidy. In: Fleischer AC, Manning FA, Jeanty P, et al., eds. *Sonography in obstetrics & gynecology: principles and practice*, 6th ed. New York: McGraw-Hill, 2001:89–112.
17. Twining P. Chromosomal markers. In: Dewbury K, Meire H, Cosgrove D, et al., eds. *Ultrasound in obstetrics and gynaecology*, 2nd ed. London: Churchill-Livingstone, 2001:475–496.
18. Winter TC, Uhrich SB, Souter VL, et al. The "genetic sonogram": comparison of the index scoring system with the age-adjusted ultrasound risk assessment. *Radiology* 2000;215:775–782.

14

FIRST TRIMESTER PREGNANCY COMPLICATIONS

14.1. FAILED PREGNANCY

Description and Clinical Features

There is a high rate of pregnancy loss in the first trimester, especially before 8 weeks gestation. The terms "failed pregnancy" and "early pregnancy failure" are preferred by many to describe early pregnancy loss. Various other terms have been used to describe early pregnancy loss, including "blighted ovum" or "anembryonic pregnancy", when no embryo is visible in the gestational sac of a failed pregnancy, "spontaneous abortion," and "missed abortion."

Early pregnancy failure may present clinically with pain, cramping, and bleeding (a symptom complex termed "threatened abortion"). Some early pregnancy losses are due to chromosomal anomalies, and other cases are thought to result from abnormalities of the corpus luteum or subclinical intrauterine infection. Most pregnancy failures, however, have no identifiable cause.

Sonography

Early pregnancy failure can be diagnosed with certainty when no embryonic heartbeat is seen on transvaginal sonography and either (1) the sonogram demonstrates an embryo of more than 5 mm in length (Figure 14.1-1) or (2) the gestational age is known with cer-

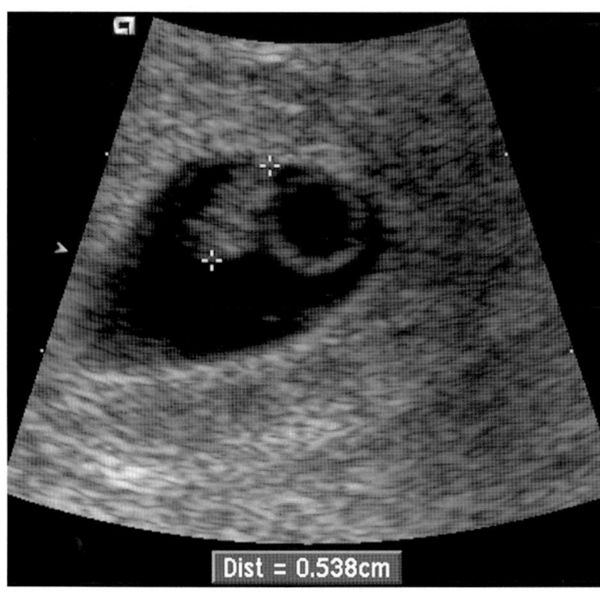

FIGURE 14.1-1. Definite pregnancy failure. There is an intrauterine gestational sac with an embryo *(calipers)* whose crown-rump length measures 5.38 mm. No cardiac activity was seen on real-time sonography.

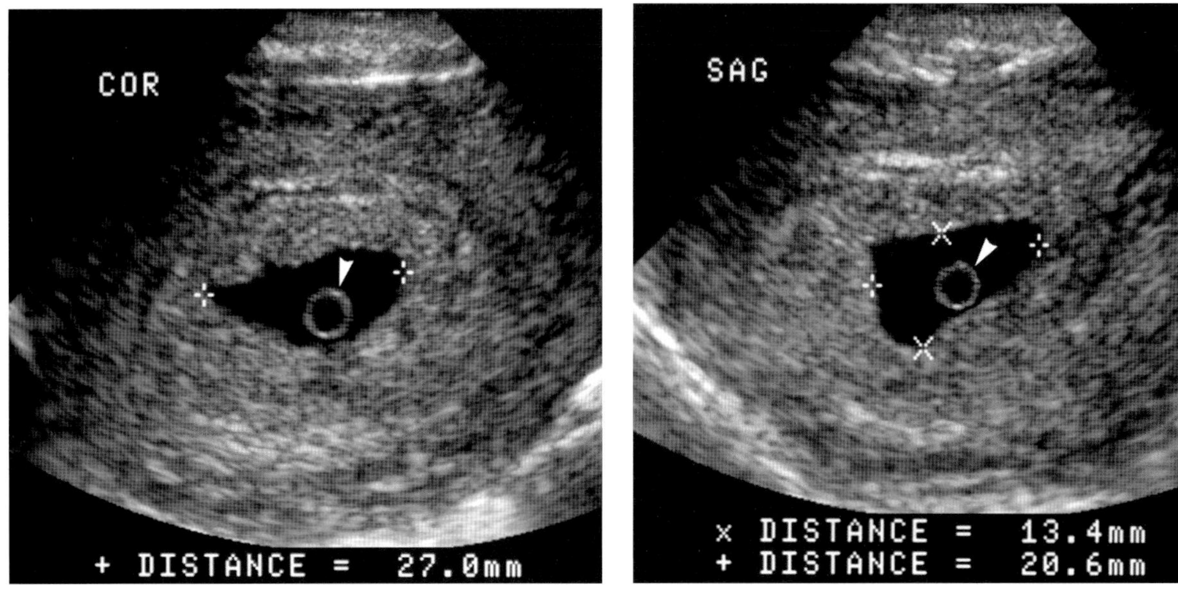

FIGURE 14.1-2. Probable pregnancy failure. Coronal *(COR)* **(A)** and sagittal *(SAG)* **(B)** views through the uterus demonstrate an intrauterine gestational sac *(calipers)* with a yolk sac *(arrowheads)*. The mean sac diameter is 20.3 mm (average of 27.0, 20.6, and 13.4 mm). Because no embryo is seen and the mean sac diameter is more than 16 mm, the likelihood of pregnancy failure is high.

tainty to be at least 6.5 weeks (e.g., age is known based on a previous sonogram or on *in vitro* fertilization with embryo transfer). Sonographic findings that are suspicious for, but not absolutely diagnostic of, early pregnancy failure include the following:

Mean sac diameter of more than 8 mm and no visible yolk sac.
Mean sac diameter of more than 16 mm and no visible embryo (Figure 14.1-2).
β-HCG above 1,000 mIU/ml (first or third International Preparation) and no gestational sac seen.
β-HCG above 10,000 mIU/ml and no embryo identified.

If any of these findings are present, pregnancy failure should be suspected and a follow-up sonogram should be performed to confirm the diagnosis.

14.2. SUBCHORIONIC HEMATOMA

Description and Clinical Features

Many women experience vaginal bleeding during the first trimester of pregnancy. Sometimes, in addition to blood passing per vagina, blood collects between the chorion of the developing gestation and the uterine wall, forming a subchorionic hematoma. When a hematoma is present, the pregnancy prognosis is related to the size of the hematoma. The prognosis is excellent if the hematoma is small, whereas large hematomas are associated with a fairly high risk of pregnancy loss.

Sonography

On ultrasound, a subchorionic hematoma appears as a hypoechoic or anechoic area around part of the gestational sac (Figure 14.2-1). It is often crescentic in shape. The hypo- or anechoic area representing a subchorionic hematoma must be distinguished

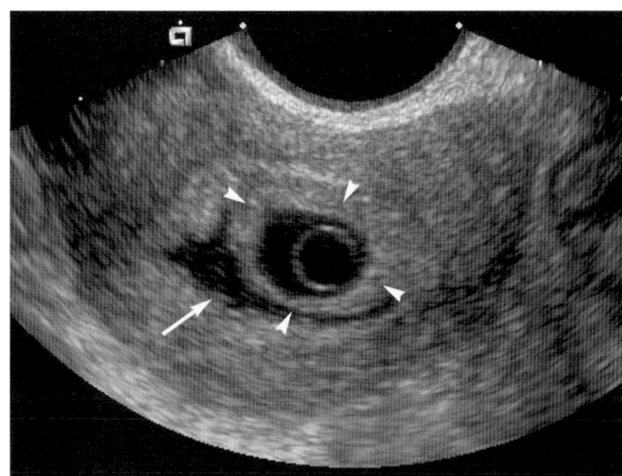

FIGURE 14.2-1. Subchorionic hematoma. Transverse view of the uterus demonstrates a crescentic fluid collection *(arrow)* surrounding approximately half of the gestational sac *(arrowheads).*

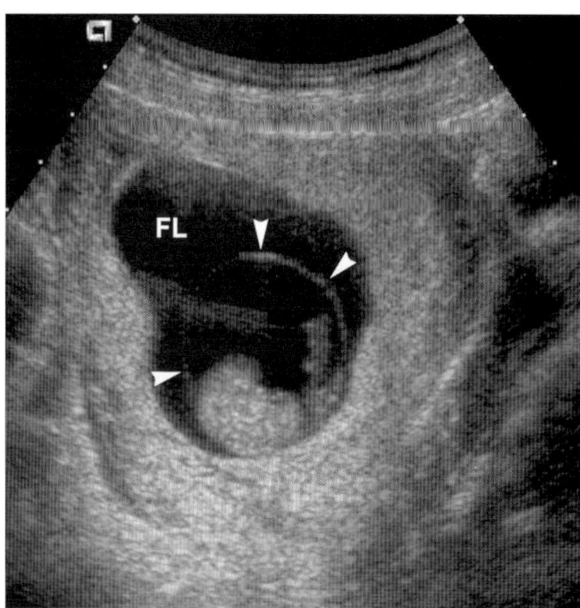

FIGURE 14.2-2. Normal separation of the chorion and amnion before fusion. Transverse view of the uterus at 9 weeks gestation demonstrates a thin membrane *(arrowheads),* the amnion, separated by a fluid collection *(FL)* from the outer (chorionic) margin of the gestational sac.

from fluid between the chorion and amnion, a normal finding in the first trimester (Figure 14.2-2). Distinguishing features include the following:

A subchorionic hematoma is bounded by a relatively thick and somewhat irregular membrane (the chorion) (Figure 14.2-1), whereas fluid between the chorion and amnion is bounded internally by a thin, smooth membrane (the amnion) (Figure 14.2-2).

A subchorionic hematoma may have some echoes within it, whereas fluid between the amnion and chorion is anechoic.

A subchorionic hematoma may track beneath the placenta (Figure 14.2-3), whereas fluid between the amnion and chorion never does.

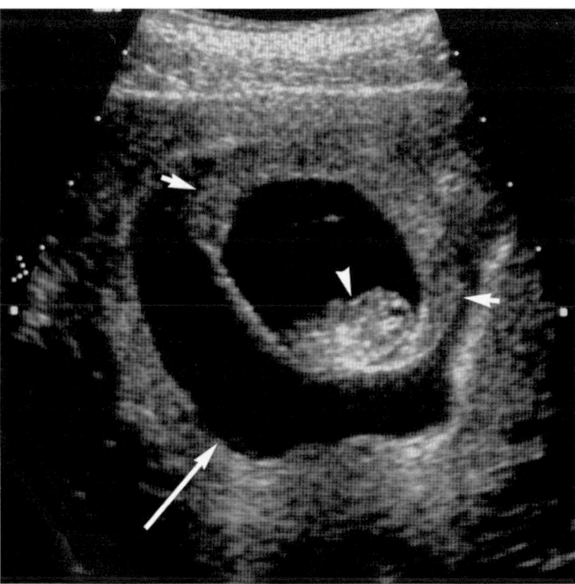

FIGURE 14.2-3. Subchorionic hematoma lifting the placental edge. A large crescentic fluid collection *(long arrow)* surrounds more than half of the gestational sac and lifts part of the placenta *(short arrows).* The fetus *(arrowhead)* lies within the gestational sac.

14.3. SLOW EMBRYONIC HEART RATE

Description and Clinical Features

Slow embryonic heart rates at 6.0–7.0 weeks gestation are associated with an increased risk of demise by the end of the first trimester, usually within 1–2 weeks after the slow heart rate is detected. In particular, at a gestational age less than 6.3 weeks (corresponding to a crown-rump length less than 5 mm), a heart rate less than 80 beats per minutes (bpm) is associated with a very high likelihood of subsequent demise, a rate of 80–89 bpm carries a moderately elevated risk of demise, and a rate of 90–99 bpm a slightly elevated risk of demise, compared with a rate of 100 bpm or higher. At 6.3–7.0 weeks (crown-rump length 5–9 mm), a heart rate less than 100 bpm is ominous, a rate of 100–109 bpm carries moderate risk of demise, and a rate of 110–119 bpm carries slight risk, compared with a rate of 120 bpm or more.

Sonography

Embryonic heart rate is easily measured by M-mode sonography, which is available on most modern ultrasound scanners. If the heart rate is less than 90 bpm at less than 6.3 weeks gestation (Figures 14.3-1 and 14.3-2) or less than 110 bpm at 6.3–7.0 weeks, a follow-up sonogram should be performed in 1–2 weeks. If cardiac activity is still present on this scan, periodic follow-up sonograms should be performed until the end of the first trimester, because demise occasionally occurs several weeks after the initial slow heart rate is detected (Figure 14.3-2). Follow-up sonography should also be considered for rates of 90–99 bpm at less than 6.3 weeks or 110–119 bpm at 6.3–7.0 weeks. Although the follow-up scan does not affect outcome, it can yield a more timely diagnosis of demise, thus minimizing the time that a dead embryo remains *in utero*.

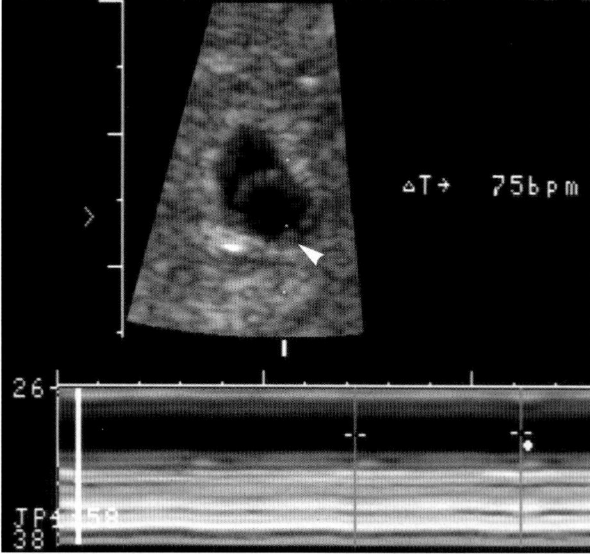

FIGURE 14.3-1. Markedly slow heart rate at 6 weeks gestation. *Dotted line* indicates the region of the image through which an M-mode tracing is obtained. There is cardiac activity at a site *(arrowhead)* on the edge of the yolk sac, measured *(lines with calipers)* on the M-mode tracing to be beating at a rate of 75 beats per minute. There was no cardiac activity on a follow-up scan 11 days later.

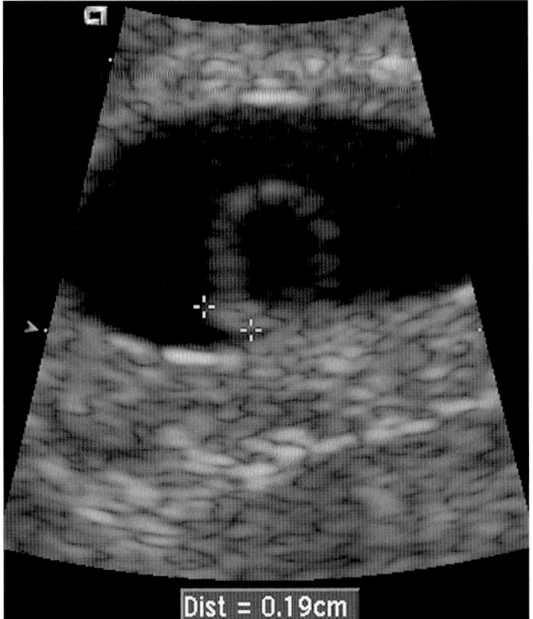

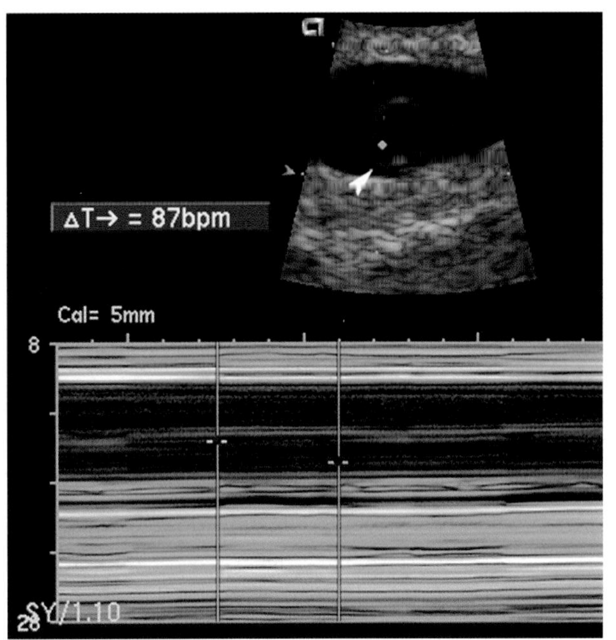

FIGURE 14.3-2. Slow heart rate at 6 weeks gestation. A: There is an embryo *(calipers)* adjacent to the yolk sac. The crown-rump length is 1.9 mm. **B:** M-mode through the embryo *(arrowhead)* demonstrates the heart rate to be 87 beats per minute *(calipers)*. There was still cardiac activity on a follow-up scan 11 days later, but a later follow-up scan at 10 weeks gestation showed no cardiac activity.

SUGGESTED READINGS

1. Benson CB, Doubilet PM. Slow embryonic heart rate in early first trimester: indicator of poor pregnancy outcome. *Radiology* 1994;192:343–344.
2. Brown DL, Emerson DS, Felker RE, et al. Diagnosis of early embryonic demise by endovaginal sonography. *J Ultrasound Med* 1990;9:631–636.
3. Doubilet PM, Benson CB. Embryonic heart rate in the early first trimester: what rate is normal? *J Ultrasound Med* 1995;14:431–434.
4. Doubilet PM, Benson CB. Emergency obstetrical ultrasound. *Semin Roentgenol* 1998;33:339–450.
5. Doubilet PM, Benson CB, Chow JS. Long-term prognosis of pregnancies complicated by slow embryonic heart rates in the early first trimester. *J Ultrasound Med* 1999;18:537–541.
6. Falco P, Milano V, Pilu G, et al. Sonography of pregnancies with first-trimester bleeding and a viable embryo: a study of prognostic indicators by logistic regression analysis. *Ultrasound Obstet Gynecol* 1996;7:165–169.
7. Frates MC, Benson CB, Doubilet PM. Pregnancy outcome after a first trimester sonogram demonstrating fetal cardiac activity. *J Ultrasound Med* 1993;12:383–386.
8. Goldstein SR. Embryonic death in early pregnancy: a new look at the first trimester. *Obstet Gynecol* 1994;84:294–297.
9. Laboda LA, Estroff JA, Benacerraf BR. First trimester bradycardia: a sign of impending fetal loss. *J Ultrasound Med* 1989;8:561–563.
10. Laing FC, Frates MC. Ultrasound evaluation during the first trimester of pregnancy. In: Callen PW, ed. *Ultrasonography in obstetrics and gynecology*, 4th ed. Philadelphia: WB Saunders, 2000:105–145.
11. Levi CS, Lyons EA, Lindsay DJ. Early diagnosis of nonviable pregnancy with endovaginal US. *Radiology* 1988;167:383–385.
12. Pedersen JF, Mantoni M. Prevalence and significance of subchorionic hemorrhage in threatened abortion: a sonographic study. *AJR Am J Roentgenol* 1990;154:535–537.

15

PLACENTA

15.1. PLACENTA PREVIA

Description and Clinical Features

Placenta previa refers to a placenta extending to or covering the internal cervical os. A *complete previa* covers the internal os entirely. A *marginal previa* extends to the edge of, but does not cover, the internal os. A *partial previa* partially covers the internal os.

A marginal or partial placenta previa in the second or early third trimester frequently resolves (i.e., no longer covers any part of the cervix) by the mid to late third trimester. When there is a placenta previa at the time of delivery, a vaginal delivery would put the mother and fetus at risk of life-threatening bleeding, and hence cesarean delivery is necessary.

Sonography

Placenta previa can be diagnosed by transabdominal, translabial, or transvaginal sonography. With any of these scanning techniques, a complete previa should be diagnosed when the placenta completely covers the cervix (Figure 15.1-1), and a marginal previa should be diagnosed if the placenta covers a portion of the cervix, ending in the vicinity of the internal os but not extending over the entire cervix (Figure 15.1-2). The term partial pre-

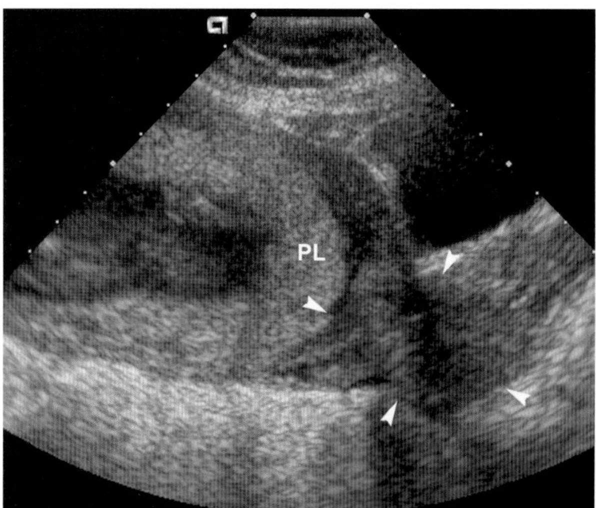

FIGURE 15.1-1. Complete placenta previa. Sagittal midline view of the lower uterus performed transabdominally demonstrates the placenta *(PL)* completely covering the cervix *(arrowheads)*.

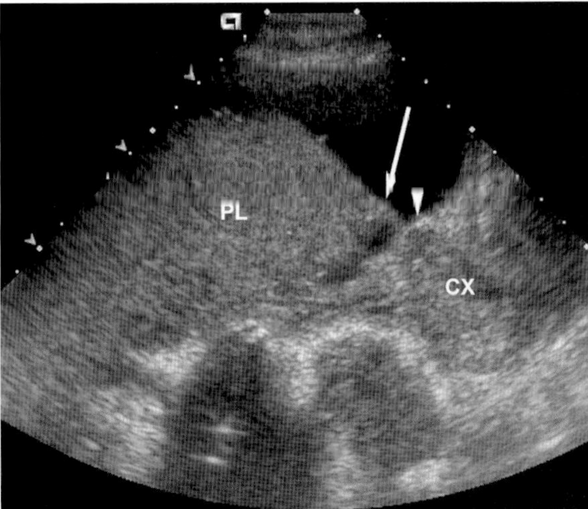

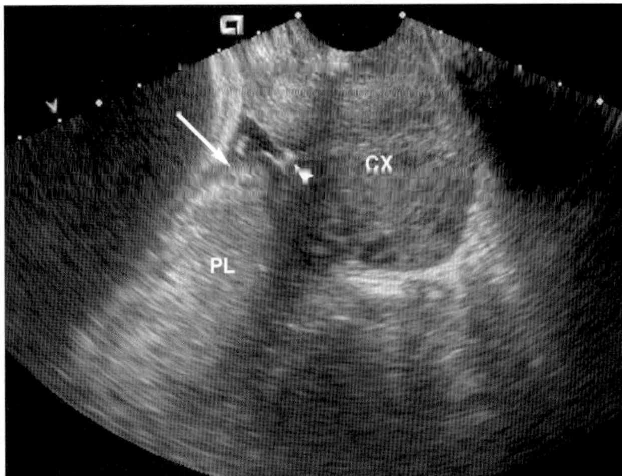

A B

FIGURE 15.1-2. Marginal placenta previa. Sagittal views of the cervix and lower uterine segment done transabdominally **(A)** and transvaginally **(B)** demonstrate the placenta *(PL)* with its edge *(arrow)* extending over part of the cervix (CX), ending close to the internal cervical os *(arrowhead)*.

via does not generally apply in the ultrasound setting because the internal os is usually closed at the time of sonography and, as such, cannot be partially covered. However, the term partial previa is sometimes used synonymously with marginal previa in ultrasound parlance.

Transabdominal sonography is the primary approach to diagnosing placenta previa and should be done with the bladder partially full. An empty bladder can make visualization of the relevant area difficult, and an overly full bladder can simulate a previa (pseudo-previa) by apposing the anterior and posterior walls of the lower uterine segment (Figure 15.1-3). If the lower segment is obscured by the presenting fetal part, manual ele-

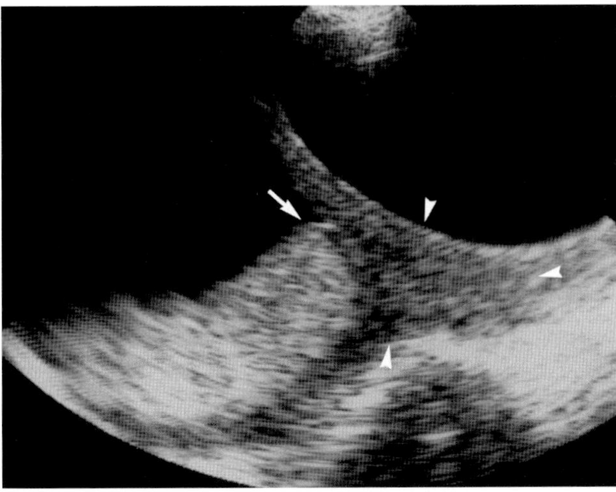

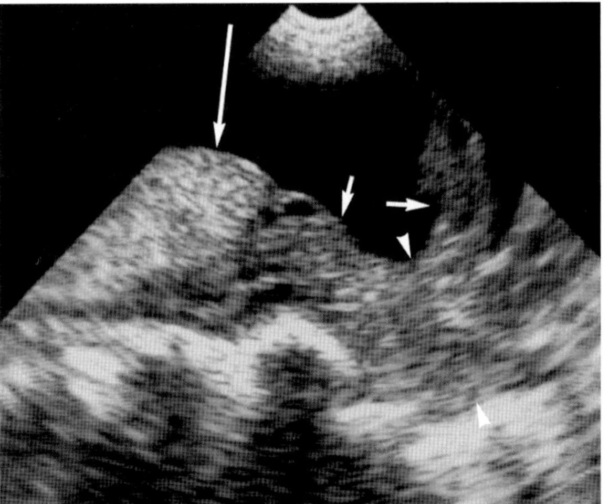

A B

FIGURE 15.1-3. Pseudo-previa caused by an overly full bladder. A: Sagittal view of the uterus through a very distended maternal bladder demonstrates the edge of the placenta *(short arrow)* extending over what might be mistaken to be the cervix *(arrowheads)*. **B:** The woman partially emptied her bladder, after which a sagittal view of the lower segment demonstrates that the placenta *(long arrow)* does not extend down to the cervix *(arrowheads)*. What had previously appeared to be the cervix were the anterior and posterior walls of the lower uterine segment *(short arrows)* pressed in apposition to one another by the overly full maternal bladder.

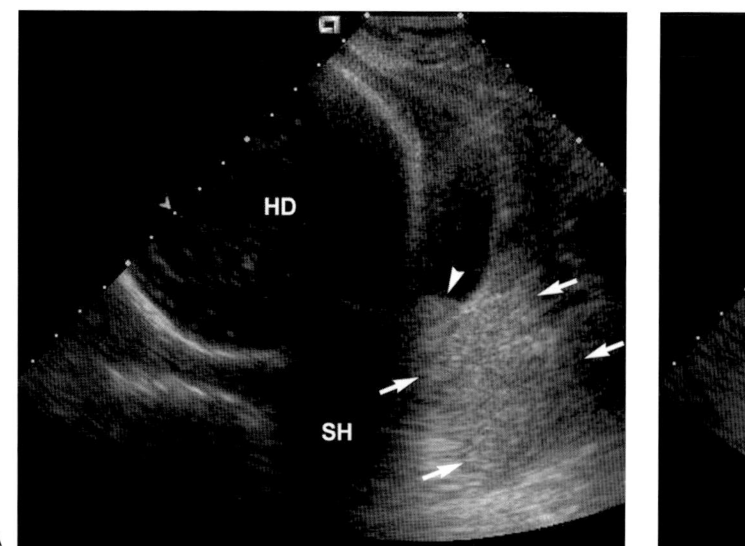

A

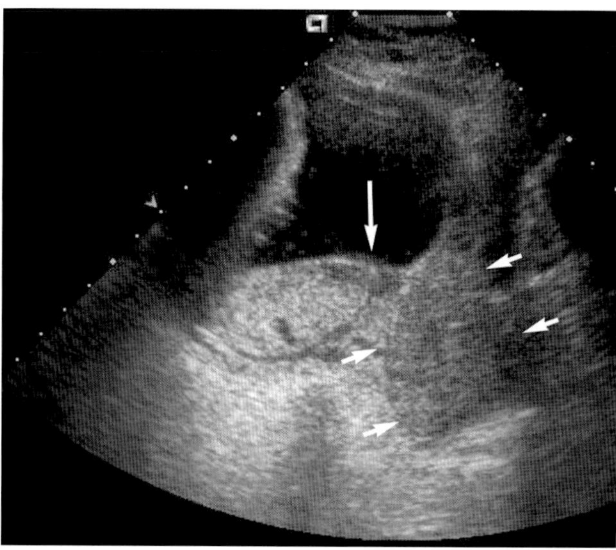
B

FIGURE 15.1-4. **Placenta previa demonstrated by manually lifting the fetal head. A:** On this sagittal view of the lower uterine segment, the fetal head *(HD)* casts an acoustic shadow *(SH)* that obscures the posterior lower uterine segment and a part of the cervix *(arrows)*. A small echogenic structure *(arrowhead)* that extends caudal to the shadow is suspicious, but not definitive, for a marginal placenta previa. **B:** Sagittal view of the lower uterine segment after manually lifting the fetal head definitively demonstrates a marginal placenta previa, with the placental edge *(long arrow)* partially covering the cervix *(short arrows)*.

vation of the fetus by abdominal palpation is often helpful (Figure 15.1-4). If the presenting part cannot be elevated, transvaginal (Figure 15.1-2) or translabial scanning can then be used to diagnose or exclude previa.

15.2. PLACENTAL ABRUPTION

Description and Clinical Features

Placental abruption refers to premature detachment of part or all of the placenta from the uterine wall before delivery of the fetus. The mother often presents clinically with pain and bleeding, but may be asymptomatic. Abruption can lead to fetal damage or death from hypoxia or exsanguination, and hence rapid and accurate diagnosis of abruption can be critical to pregnancy management.

Sonography

Ultrasound does not detect the placental separation itself but can identify a retroplacental hematoma (Figure 15.2-1) or a hematoma under the chorionic membrane (Figure 15.2-2) that is sometimes present with abruption. Hematomas vary in appearance, in that they may appear solid or complex and the solid component may be hypo- or hyperechoic relative to the placenta. If the hematoma is isoechoic to the placenta, color Doppler may aid in its detection.

It is important to note that ultrasound may be normal in a patient with an abruption when there is separation without a hematoma. Thus, identification of a retroplacental or submembranous hematoma is diagnostic of abruption, but a normal sonogram does not rule out abruption.

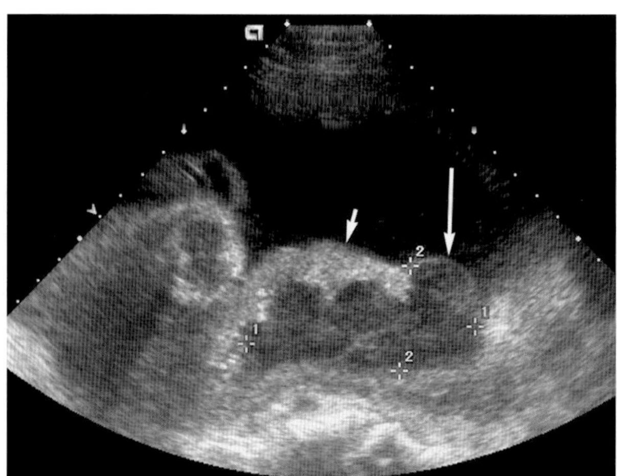

FIGURE 15.2-1. Placental abruption with retroplacental hematoma. There is a hypoechoic hematoma *(long arrow and calipers)* lifting the edge of the placenta *(short arrow).*

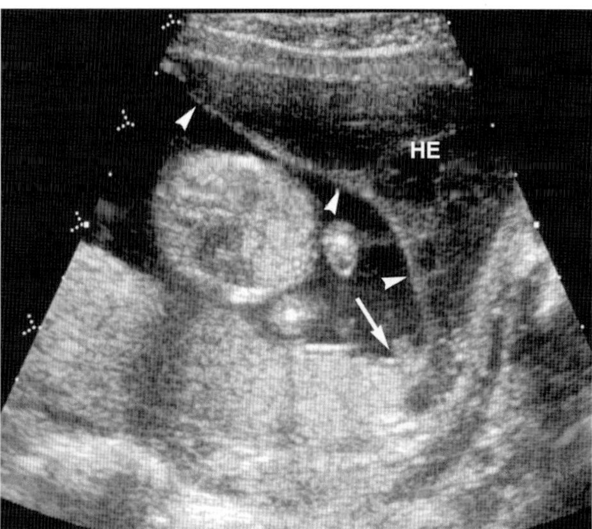

FIGURE 15.2-2. Placental abruption with a hematoma that is mainly under the chorionic membrane. There is a hypoechoic hematoma *(HE)* lifting the edge of the placenta *(arrow)* and the membranes *(arrowheads).*

15.3. PLACENTA ACCRETA, INCRETA, AND PERCRETA

Description and Clinical Features

The placenta does not normally come into contact with the myometrium because these two structures are separated by the decidualized endometrium. If the placenta implants on an area of scarred endometrium, however, the placenta can attach directly to, or even invade, the myometrium. This abnormal relationship between the placenta and myometrium, which results in difficulty separating the placenta from the uterus at delivery, has been divided into three types:

Accreta: attachment of the placenta directly to the myometrium, without invasion of chorionic villi into the myometrium
Increta: invasion of chorionic villi into the myometrium
Percreta: penetration of villi through the myometrium, to or through the serosa of the uterus

Placenta accreta, increta, and percreta occur most frequently at the site of a previous cesarean section, because this surgical procedure leads to endometrial scarring. A woman who has had one or more cesarean deliveries and whose current pregnancy has a placenta that overlies the cesarean section scar (i.e., a placenta previa or low-lying anterior placenta) is at high risk of accreta: there is an approximately 25% chance of accreta if she has had one cesarean section and an approximately 50% chance of accreta if she has had two or more cesarean sections.

Placenta accreta, increta, or percreta can lead to a number of serious complications including difficulty removing the placenta and heavy bleeding at delivery, which may necessitate hysterectomy, uterine rupture (if placenta increta or percreta), and hemorrhage into the bladder or other sites (if placenta percreta).

Sonography

The myometrium overlying the placenta normally appears as a hypoechoic band of tissue. The primary sonographic finding of placenta accreta, increta, or percreta is thinning of

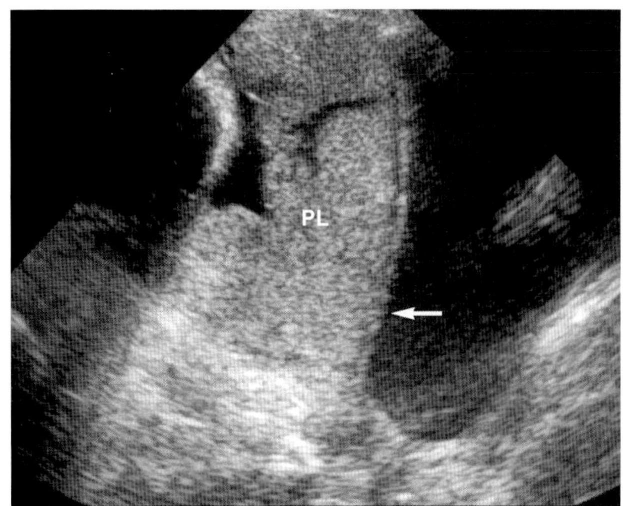

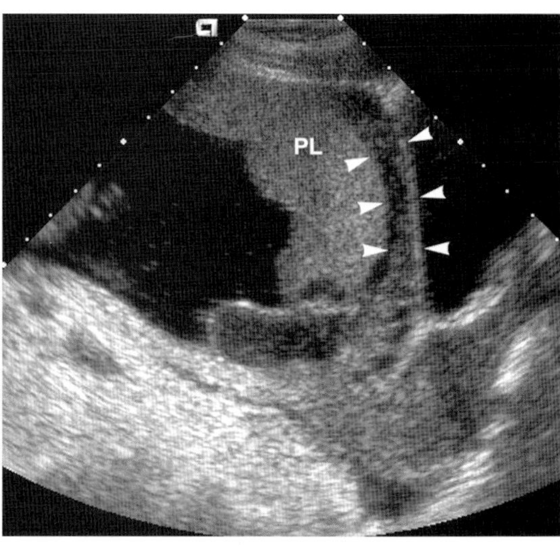

FIGURE 15.3-1. Placenta accreta or increta. A: Sagittal view of the lower uterus demonstrates that the myometrium is markedly thinned *(arrow)* beneath the placenta *(PL)*. **B:** A normal sagittal scan of the lower uterus for comparison, with the myometrium *(arrowheads)* appearing as a hypoechoic band under the placenta *(PL)*.

this hypoechoic band to a thickness of 1–2 mm or less (Figure 15.3-1) or complete absence of this band (Figure 15.3-2). A secondary finding with accreta, increta, or percreta is the presence of large irregular vascular spaces in the placenta (Figure 15.3-3).

The possibility of accreta or increta should be raised in one of two settings: (1) an anterior previa is seen on ultrasound in a woman who has had one or more cesarean sections; or (2) ultrasound demonstrates the absence or thinning of the myometrium overlying the placenta. The diagnosis can be made with confidence when both (1) and (2) apply. Percreta is diagnosed sonographically when the placenta extends through the serosal surface of the uterus. This is seen most clearly when the placenta protrudes into the bladder (Figure 15.3-3).

Placenta accreta, increta, or percreta is most often diagnosed sonographically when it is located in the anterior lower uterine segment. The diagnosis, however, can also be suggested in other locations within the uterus when there is thinning or absence of the myometrium overlying the placenta (Figure 15.3-4).

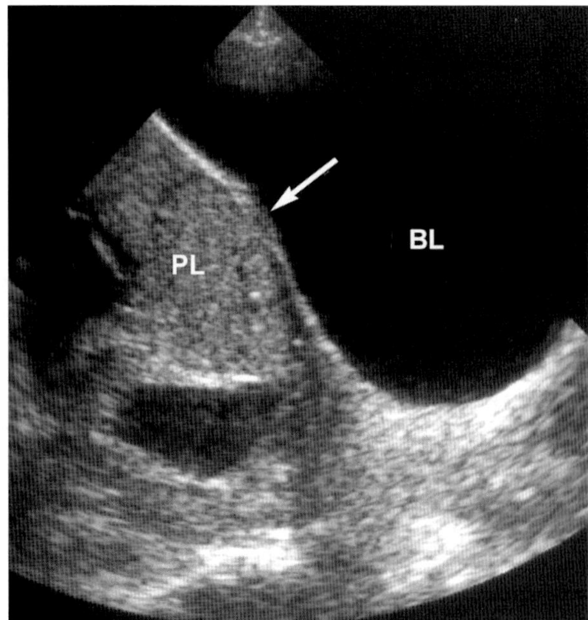

FIGURE 15.3-2. Placenta increta or percreta. Sagittal view through the lower uterus demonstrates an area *(arrow)* of complete absence of myometrium beneath the placenta *(PL)*. At this location, the placenta extends very close to, or possibly into, the maternal bladder *(BL)*.

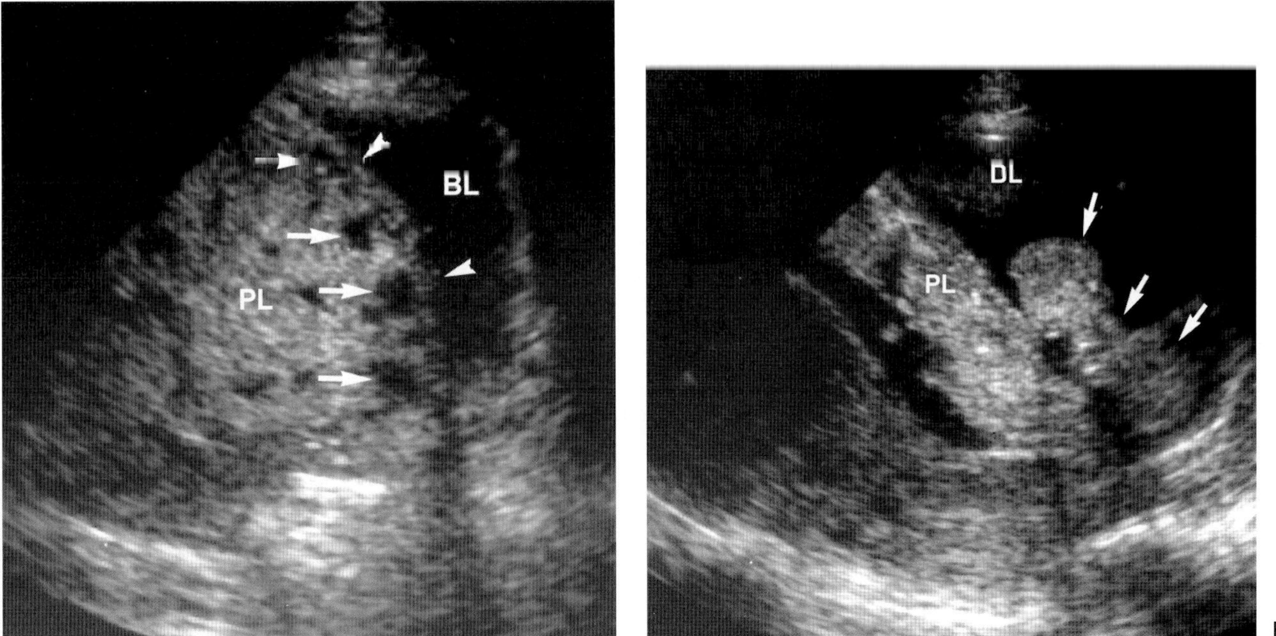

FIGURE 15.3-3. Placenta percreta. A: Sagittal view of the lower uterus reveals complete absence of myometrium *(arrowheads)* between the placenta *(PL)* and the maternal bladder *(BL)*. There are multiple prominent vascular spaces in the placenta *(arrows)*. **B:** Sagittal view of the lower uterus to the right of midline reveals the placenta *(PL)* lying primarily in the lower uterine segment, with portions of the placenta *(arrows)* extending into the maternal bladder *(BL)*.

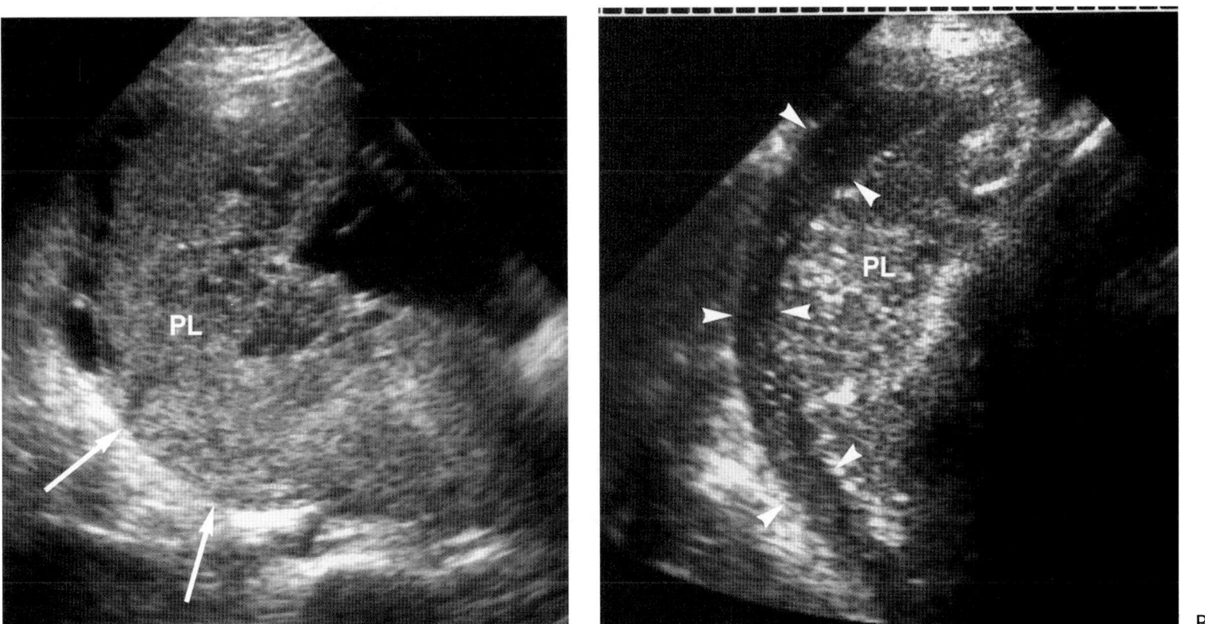

FIGURE 15.3-4. Placenta accreta or increta in the uterine fundus. A: Sagittal view of the uterine fundus reveals an area *(arrows)* of complete absence of the myometrium beneath the placenta *(PL)*. **B:** Normal scan for comparison, in which the myometrium *(arrowheads)* appears as a hypoechoic band beneath the placenta *(PL)*.

15.4. CHORIOANGIOMA

Description and Clinical Features

Chorioangiomas are benign tumors of the placenta. They arise from chorionic tissue and are generally highly vascular.

Large chorioangiomas can cause a number of problems, including fetal growth restriction and hydrops. The latter probably occurs as a result of high-output heart failure from vascular shunting through the tumor. Most chorioangiomas, however, cause no pregnancy complications and are incidental findings on sonography or at birth.

Sonography

On ultrasound, a chorioangioma appears as a solid mass within, or projecting from, the placenta (Figure 15.4-1). It may be difficult to diagnose in the latter part of pregnancy, when the placenta may develop infarcts or otherwise become fairly heterogeneous in appearance. A focal placental lesion can be diagnosed as a probable chorioangioma if it is well circumscribed and shows a high degree of vascularity on color Doppler (Figure 15.4-2).

When a chorioangioma is diagnosed, the fetus should be scanned to look for evidence of high-output heart failure. An early finding of this is distention of the umbilical vein (Figure 15.4-3) or right atrium. More advanced findings include fetal hydrops, with abnormal fluid collections (pleural, pericardial, intraperitoneal, or subcutaneous).

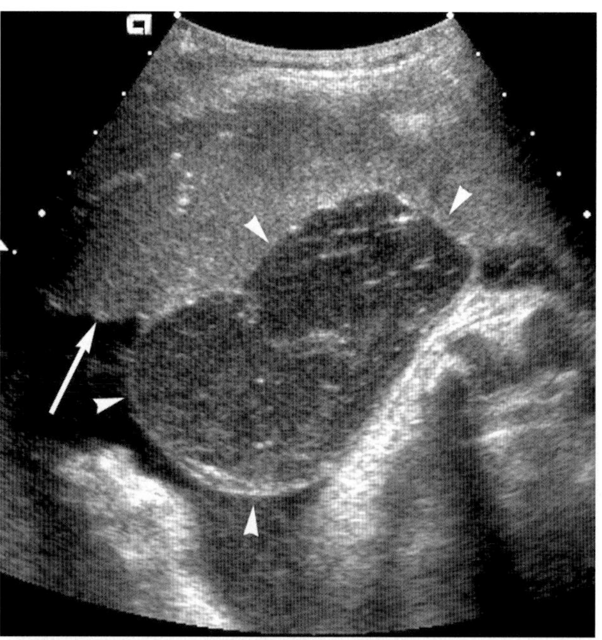

FIGURE 15.4-1. Placental chorioangioma. A large solid mass *(arrowheads)* extends from the surface of the placenta *(arrow)*.

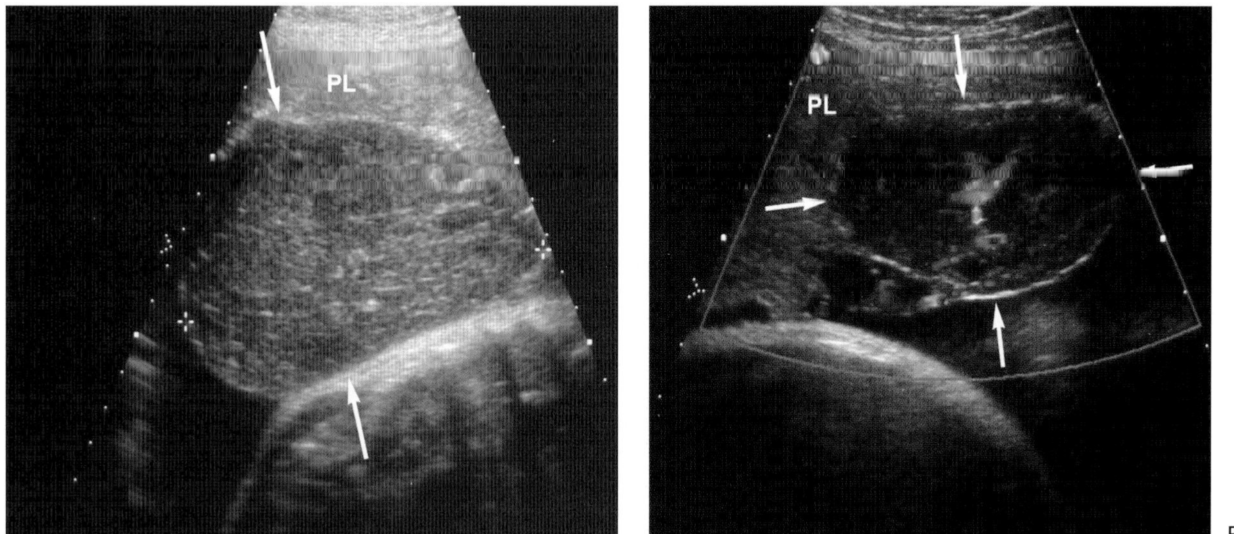

FIGURE 15.4-2. Placental chorioangioma on color Doppler. A: A large solid mass *(arrows and calipers)* arises from the surface of the placenta *(PL)*. **B:** Color Doppler demonstrates considerable blood flow in the placental *(PL)* mass *(arrows)*.

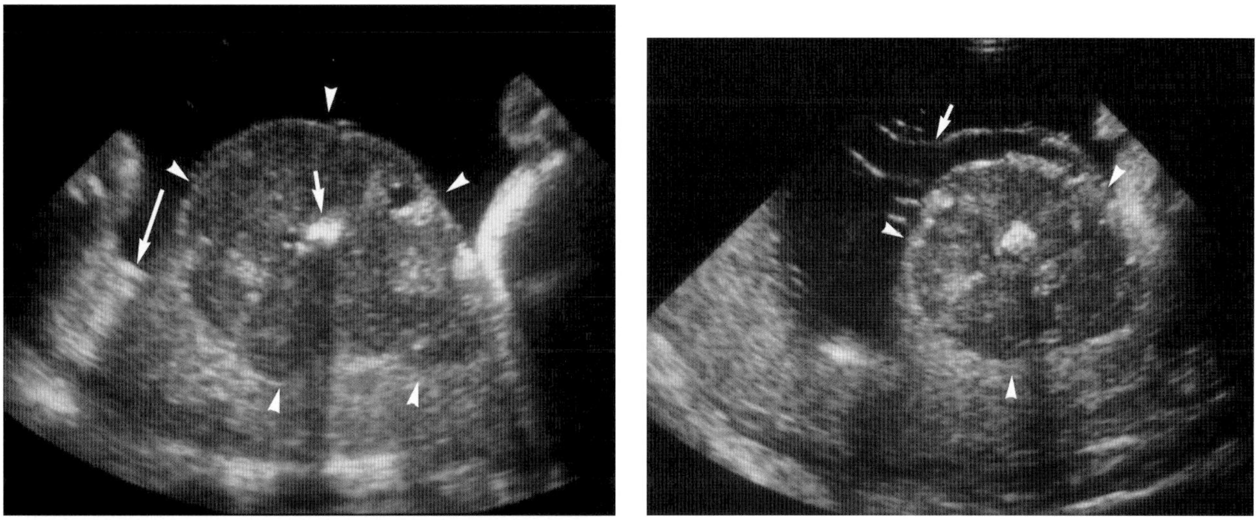

FIGURE 15.4-3. Placental chorioangioma with a distended umbilical vein. A: There is a large solid mass *(arrowheads)* with an internal calcification *(short arrow)* projecting from the surface of the placenta *(long arrow)*. **B:** The umbilical vein *(arrow)* implants close to the chorioangioma *(arrowheads)* and is dilated. **C:** The intrahepatic umbilical vein *(calipers)* is also dilated.

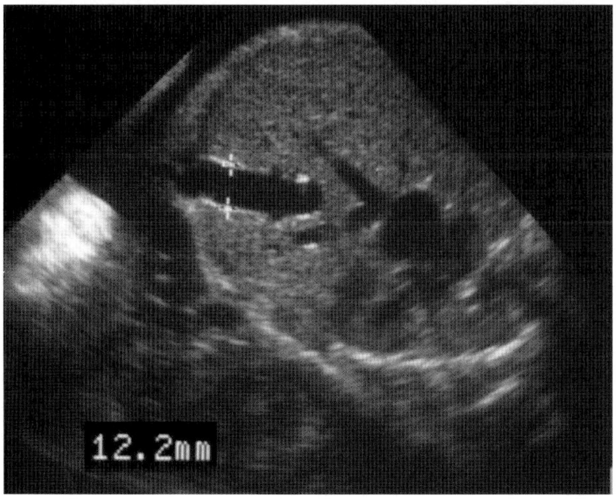

SUGGESTED READINGS

1. Clark SL, Koonings PP, Phelan JP. Placenta previa/accreta and prior cesarean section. *Obstet Gynecol* 1985;66:89–92.
2. Doubilet PM, Benson CB. Emergency obstetrical ultrasound. *Semin Roentgenol* 1998;33:339–450.
3. Finberg HJ, Williams JW. Placenta accreta: prospective sonographic diagnosis in patients with placenta previa and prior cesarean section. *J Ultrasound Med* 1992;11:333–343.
4. Hertzberg BS, Bowie JD, Carroll BA, et al. Diagnosis of placenta previa during the third trimester: role of transperineal sonography. *AJR Am Roentgenol* 1992;159:83–87.
5. Jauniaux E. The placenta. In: Dewbury K, Meire H, Cosgrove D, et al., eds. *Ultrasound in obstetrics and gynaecology*, 2nd ed. London: Churchill-Livingstone, 2001:527–555.
6. Leerentveld RA, Gilberts ECAM, Arnold MJCWJ, et al. Accuracy and safety of transvaginal sonographic placental localization. *Obstet Gynecol* 1990;76:759–762.
7. Levine D, Hulka CA, Ludmir J, et al. Placenta accreta: evaluation with color Doppler US, power Doppler US, and MR imaging. *Radiology* 1997;205:773–776.
8. Litwin MS, Loughlin KR, Benson CB, et al. Placenta percreta invading the urinary bladder. Report of three cases and review of the literature. *Br J Urol* 1989;64:283–286.
9. Nyberg DA, Cyr DR, Mack LA, et al. Sonographic spectrum of placental abruption. *AJR Am Roentgenol* 1987;148:161–164.
10. Pasto ME, Kurtz AB, Rifkin MD, et al. Ultrasonographic findings in placenta increta. *J Ultrasound Med* 1983;2:155–159.
11. Prapas N, Liang RI, Hunter D, et al. Color Doppler imaging of placental masses: differential diagnosis and fetal outcome. *Ultrasound Obstet Gynecol* 2000;16:559–563.
12. Spirt BA, Gordon LP. Sonography of the placenta. In: Fleischer AC, Manning FA, Jeanty P, et al., eds. *Sonography in obstetrics & gynecology: principles and practice*, 6th ed. New York: McGraw-Hill, 2001:195–224.

16

UTERUS AND CERVIX

16.1. CERVICAL INCOMPETENCE

Description and Clinical Features

"Incompetent cervix" refers to painless dilation of the cervix in the second or early third trimester of pregnancy. If left untreated, it leads to early delivery, which may result in a neonate that is too immature to survive or one that has major complications as a result of prematurity.

Before the availability of ultrasound, a woman was diagnosed as having an incompetent cervix if she had recurrent mid-trimester pregnancy losses. If she subsequently became pregnant, a suture (cerclage) could be placed tightly around the cervix to keep it closed. The cerclage would be removed late in pregnancy, permitting delivery. Since the advent of ultrasound, the condition can be diagnosed and treatment instituted before the mother experiences a pregnancy loss.

Sonography

The sonographic findings of an incompetent cervix are shortening (Figure 16.1-1) and "funneling" (Figure 16.1-2) of the cervix. Funneling refers to the typical configuration of

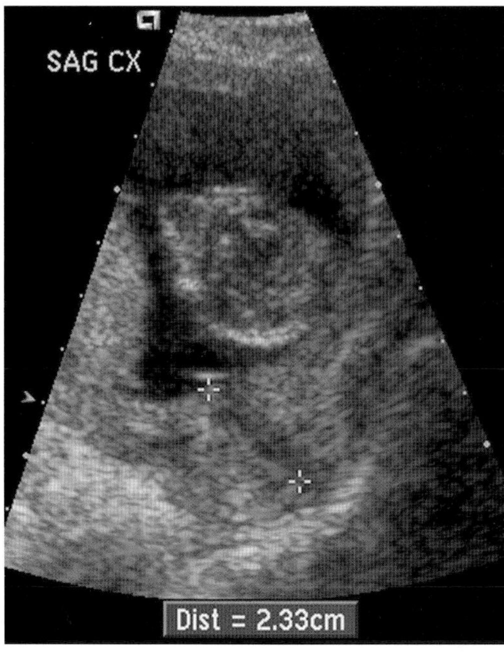

FIGURE 16.1-1. Short cervix. Sagittal view of the cervix *(SAG CX)* and lower uterus demonstrates a shortened cervix *(calipers)* measuring 23 mm.

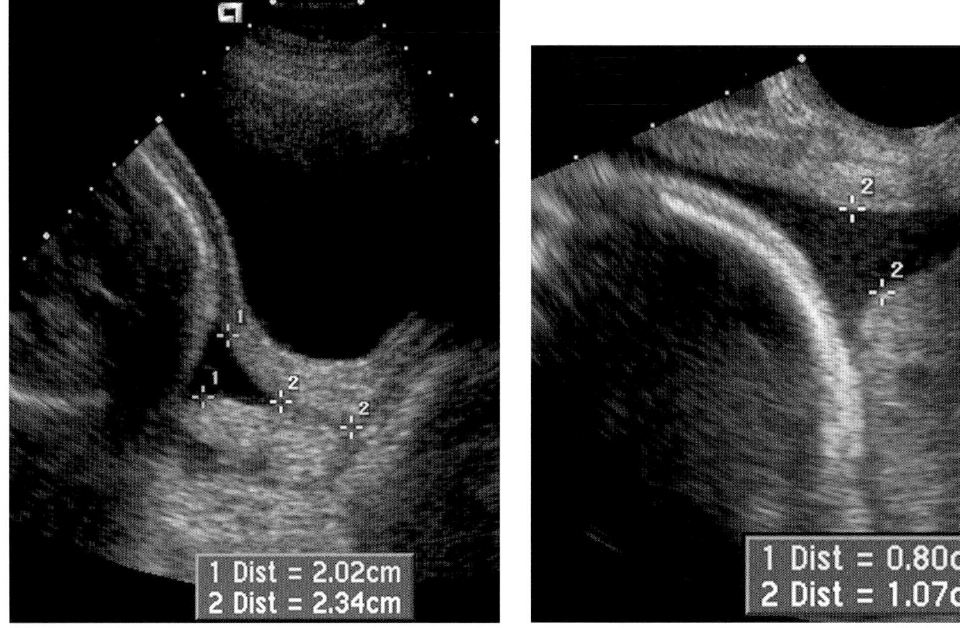

FIGURE 16.1-2. Short funneled cervix. A: Transabdominal view of the cervix demonstrates that the cervix is 20.2 mm dilated *(+1 calipers)* at the internal os. The length of the residual closed cervix is 23.4 mm *(+2 calipers)*. **B:** Transvaginal view of the cervix (in another case) demonstrates that the cervix is 10.7 mm dilated (*+2 calipers*) at the internal os. The length of the residual closed cervix is 8.0 mm (*+1 calipers)*.

a partially dilated cervical canal, in which the dilation is maximal at the internal os and tapers to a point of closure in the midportion of the canal. Cervical length is measured as the length of the closed portion of the cervix. That is, it is measured from the internal to external os in the absence of funneling, and from the tip of the funnel to the external os if the cervix is funneled (Figure 16.1-2).

Before the use of ultrasound, cervical competence was described as a dichotomous entity, a cervix is either competent or incompetent. Since ultrasound has come into common use in obstetrics, studies have shown that cervical incompetence is a continuous entity, in that the shorter the cervical length is, the greater the likelihood is of a preterm delivery. A cervical length more than 3 cm is normal, 2.5–3 cm is borderline, and one less than 2.5 cm is short. The most extreme finding is dilation of the full length of the cervical canal, with no remaining length of closed cervix (Figure 16.1-3).

When scanning transvaginally, care must be taken not to put too much pressure on the cervix with the transducer. An open cervix may be compressed and closed by excessive transducer pressure, thus leading to failure to diagnose an incompetent cervix (Figure 16.1-4).

The length and shape of the cervix may change during the course of the sonogram. This can occur spontaneously (Figure 16.1-5) or may be elicited by manual pressure on the uterine fundus. In either case, the likelihood of preterm delivery correlates with the shortest length of the cervix during the sonogram.

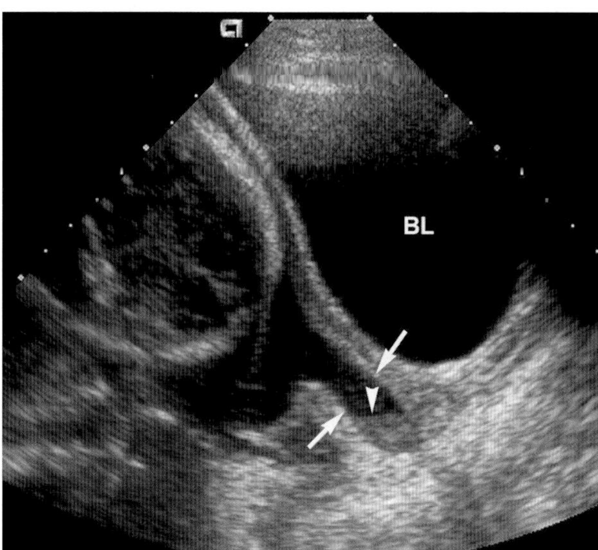

FIGURE 16.1-3. Dilation of the entire cervical canal. Transabdominal sagittal view of the lower uterus through a distended bladder *(BL)* reveals dilation of the entire length of the cervical canal *(arrows)*. The dilated cervical canal is filled with amniotic fluid as well as dependent debris *(arrowhead)*. No residual closed cervix is present.

A

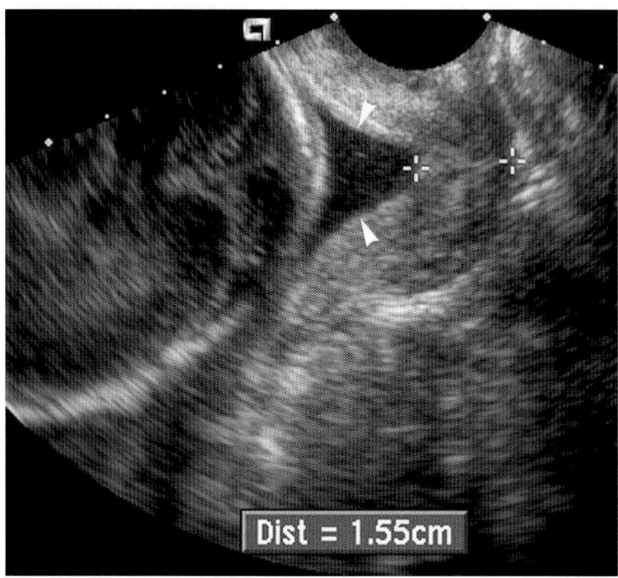

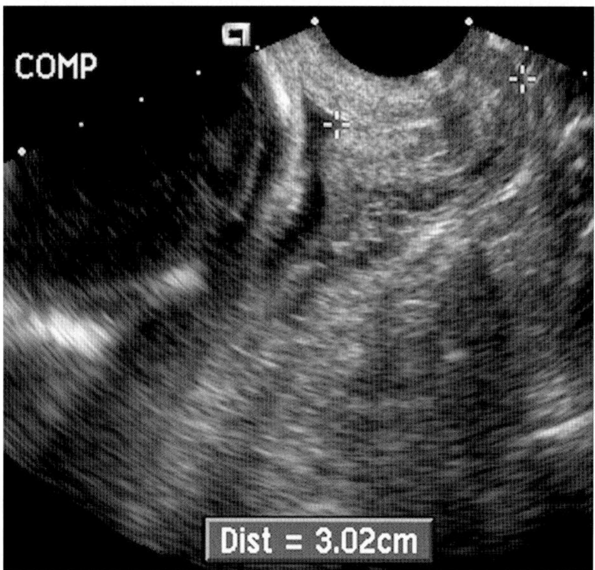

B

FIGURE 16.1-4. Transvaginal transducer pressure closing an open cervix. A: Transvaginal sonogram demonstrates cervical funneling *(arrowheads)*, with the length *(calipers)* of the residual closed cervix measuring 15.5 mm. **B:** When the cervix is compressed *(COMP)* by the transvaginal transducer, funneling disappears and the length *(calipers)* of the apparently closed cervix increases to 30.2 mm.

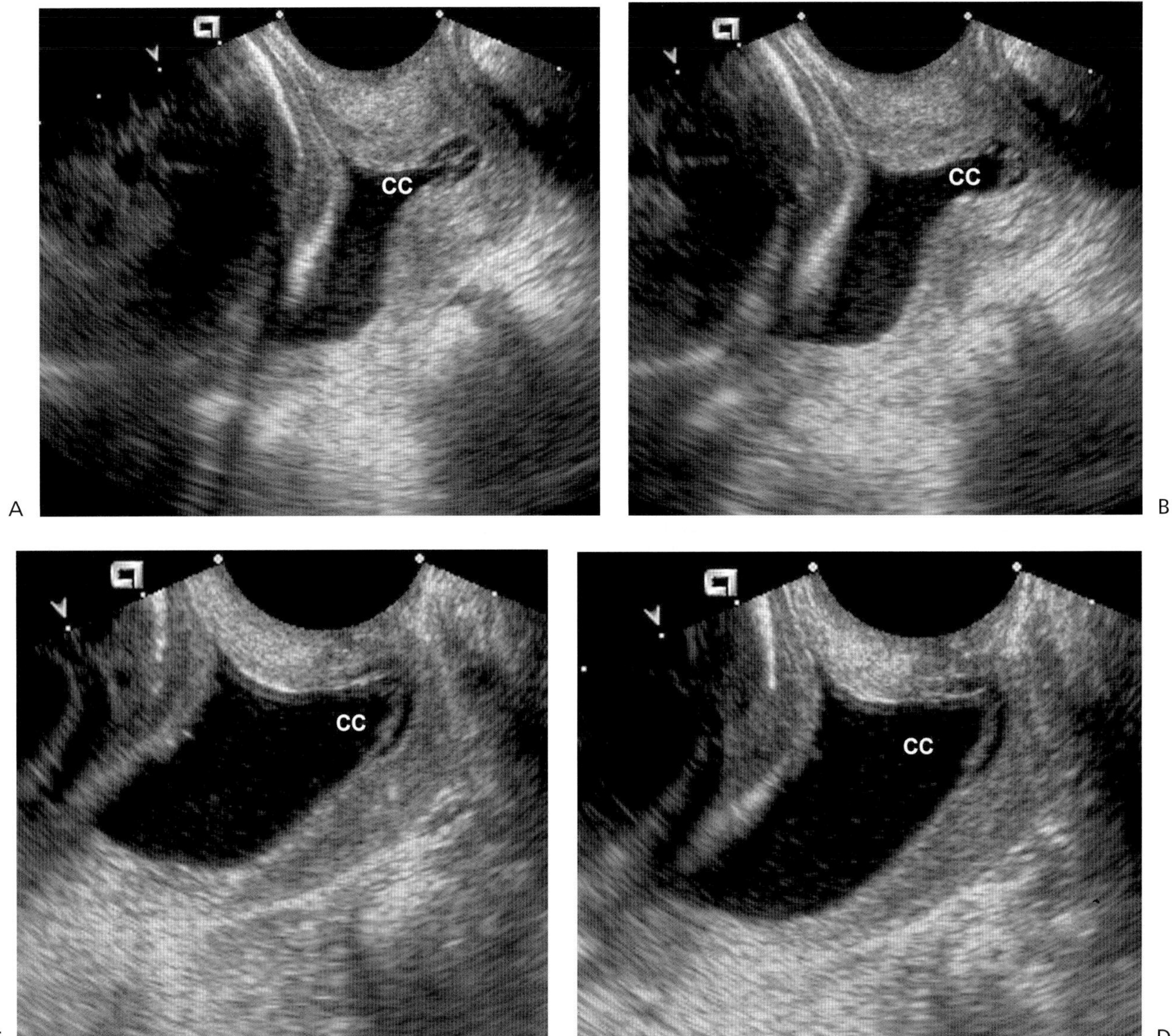

FIGURE 16.1-5. Spontaneously changing cervix. A–D: Sagittal scans through the lower uterine segment and cervix at 10- to 15-second intervals demonstrate progressive dilation of the cervical canal *(CC)*.

16.2. FIBROIDS IN PREGNANCY

Description and Clinical Features

Fibroids are common benign myometrial tumors. They are often asymptomatic during pregnancy. In some cases, however, they can lead to pregnancy complications, including the following:

Pregnancy loss: There is an elevated risk of pregnancy failure in the presence of fibroids.

Pain: Fibroids will, at times, cause considerable pain during pregnancy. This may be due to the tendency of fibroids to grow during pregnancy, because fibroid growth is often estrogen dependent. The pain is especially severe when a growing fibroid outstrips its blood supply and necroses centrally.

Obstruction of vaginal delivery: A large lower segment or cervical fibroid may obstruct vaginal delivery.

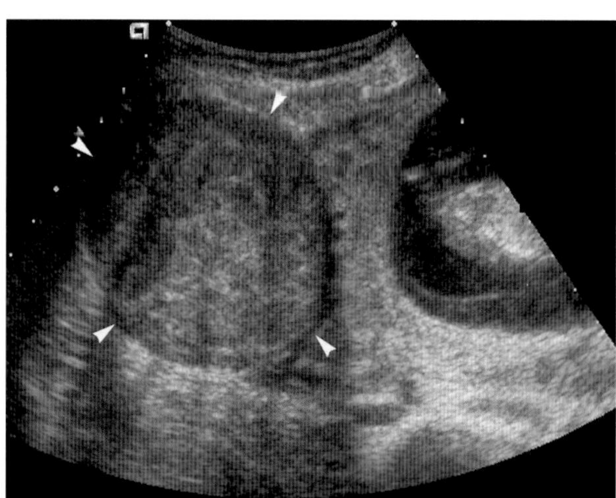

FIGURE 16.2-1. Uterine fibroid distorting the external contour of the gravid uterus. A large fibroid *(arrowheads)* extends out laterally from the right side of the uterus. The fibroid does not indent the gestational sac.

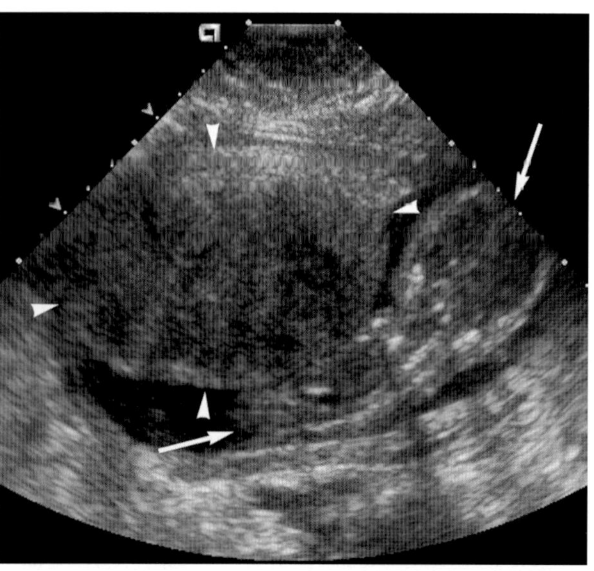

FIGURE 16.2-2. Uterine fibroid indenting the gestational sac. A large anterior fibroid *(arrowheads)* indents the gestational sac and presses against the fetus *(arrows)*.

Placental problems: When the placenta implants on a fibroid, there is increased risk of abruption or intrauterine growth restriction.

Sonography

A fibroid typically appears as a focal uterine mass that, if large, may bulge the outer uterine contour (Figure 16.2-1). It may indent the gestational sac (Figure 16.2-2) or be situated in the lower uterine segment (Figure 16.2-3), which can lead to complications as the fetus grows. The presence of anechoic areas within a fibroid suggests that it has undergone degeneration (Figure 16.2-4).

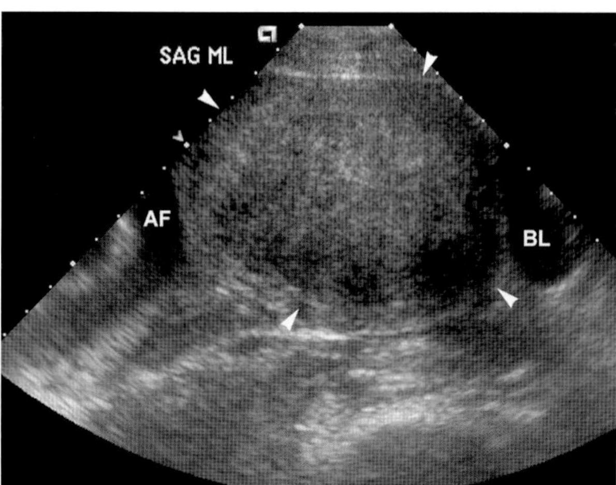

FIGURE 16.2-3. Uterine fibroid in the lower uterine segment. Sagittal midline *(SAG ML)* view of the lower uterine segment demonstrates a large fibroid *(arrowheads)* between the amniotic fluid *(AF)* in the gestational sac and the maternal bladder *(BL)*.

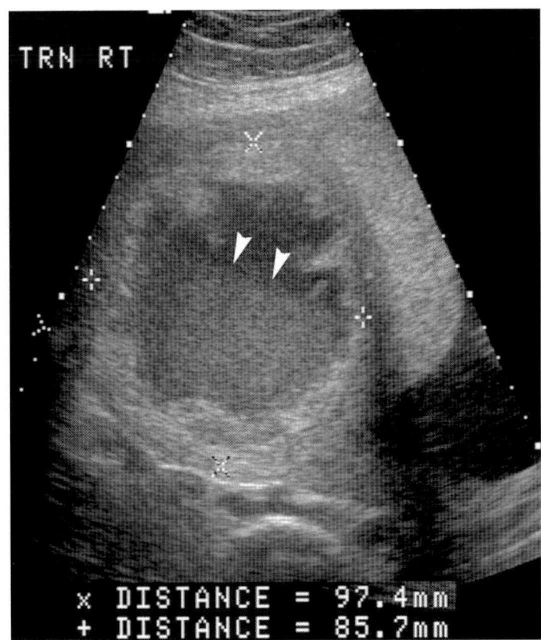

FIGURE 16.2-4. Necrotic fibroid in pregnancy. Transverse *(TRN)* view of the right *(RT)* gravid maternal pelvis demonstrates a fibroid *(calipers)* that has an irregular central cavity with fluid-debris level *(arrowheads)*.

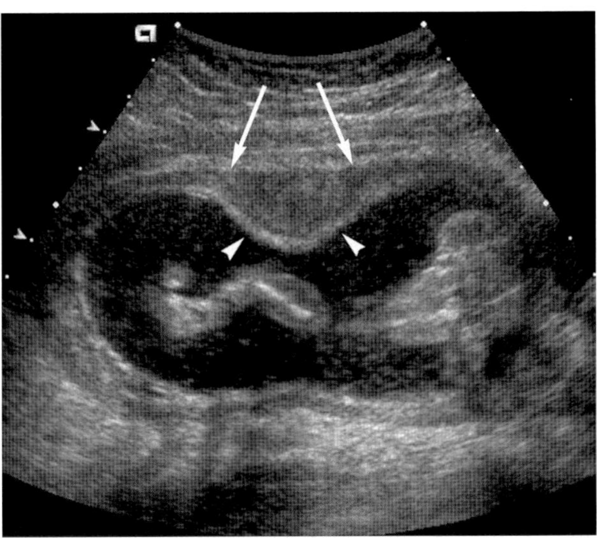

FIGURE 16.2-5. Uterine contraction. There is a focal bulge *(arrowheads)* in the myometrium that has no well-defined margin, but instead blends into the surrounding myometrium *(arrows)*.

In some cases, a uterine contraction can have a sonographic appearance similar to that of a fibroid. Differentiating features include the following:

A fibroid usually has distinct margins whereas a contraction appears as a focal area of myometrial thickening that blends into the adjacent myometrium (Figure 16.2-5).

A fibroid may bulge the outer contour of the uterus, whereas a contraction generally does not.

A fibroid has an unchanging appearance during the entire ultrasound examination, whereas a contraction generally resolves within 15–30 minutes.

16.3. UTERINE SYNECHIA AND AMNIOTIC SHEET

Description and Clinical Features

When a gestational sac develops in a uterus with an endometrial adhesion (synechia), the synechia pulls the amniotic and chorionic membranes toward the center of the gestational sac. This results in a sheet-like structure (amniotic sheet) extending into the amniotic cavity, composed of four layers: two layers of chorion internally and two layers of amnion externally. Unlike amniotic bands, the amniotic sheet created by a synechia is not attached to the fetus and does not cause fetal structural anomalies. Pregnancies with amniotic sheets, however, are more likely to require cesarean delivery due to fetal malposition than are pregnancies without sheets.

Sonography

When a synechia is present, ultrasound demonstrates the resulting amniotic sheet as a smooth, moderately thick projection of tissue into the gestational sac (Figures 16.3-1 and 16.3-2). The sheet is separate from the fetus and often has a slightly bulbous end. In some scan planes, the sheet may appear to divide the sac into two separate compartments, but it does not, in fact, do so (Figure 16.3-2). The placenta may partially implant on the sheet (Figure 16.3-3).

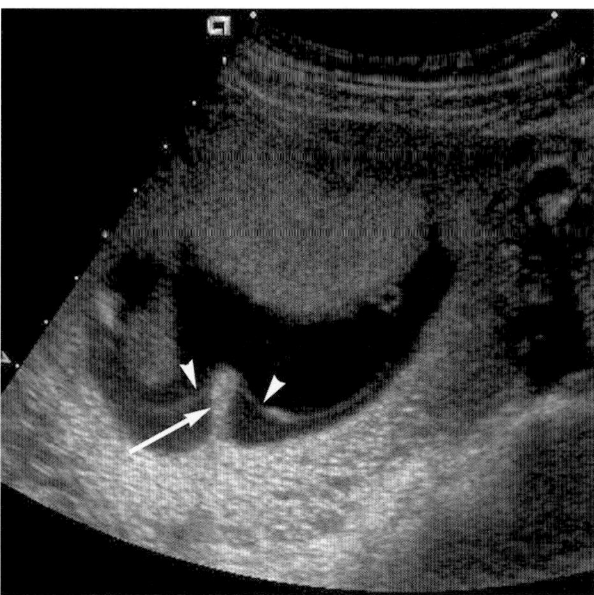

FIGURE 16.3-1. Amniotic sheet with amnion draped over it. There is a smooth, bulbous-ending projection into the gestational sac *(arrow)* that is completely separate from the fetus. The amnion *(arrowheads)* is seen draped over it.

It is important to distinguish an amniotic sheet from an amniotic band because the former is generally innocuous, whereas the latter can cause a variety of fetal structural abnormalities. The main differentiating features are as follows:

A band adheres to the fetus, whereas a sheet does not.

Fetal limb and body wall abnormalities are common with amniotic bands, whereas the fetus is generally normal when there is an amniotic sheet.

A sheet tends to be thicker than a band.

A sheet has a broad-based attachment to the uterine wall, whereas a sheet does not.

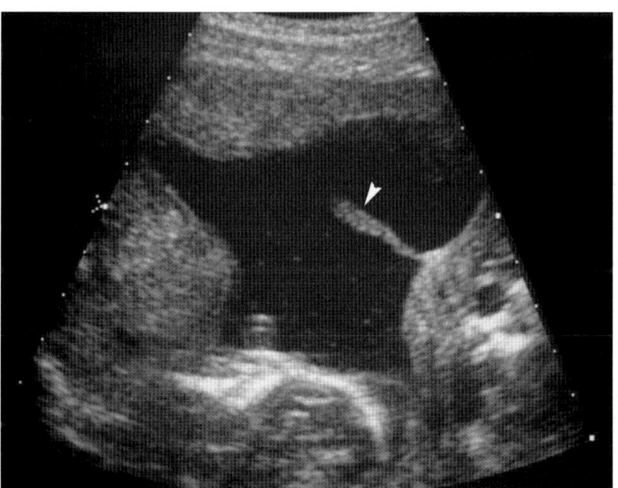

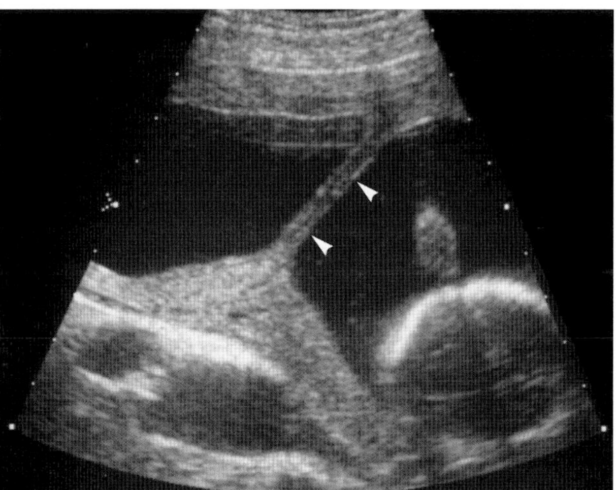

FIGURE 16.3-2. Amniotic sheet. A: An amniotic sheet *(arrowheads)* is seen as a thin, elongated projection of tissue into the gestational sac. The sheet is smooth and completely separate from the fetus. **B:** In another plane, the amniotic sheet appears to divide the gestational sac into two separate components, but the companion image **(A)** demonstrates that it does not do so in reality.

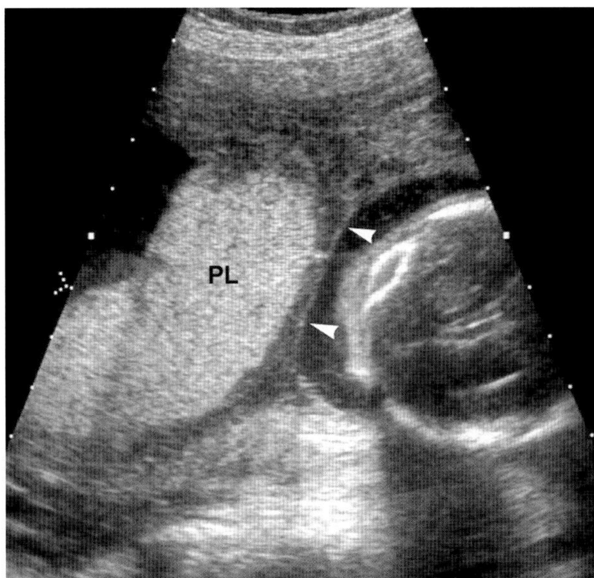

FIGURE 16.3-3. Placenta implanted on an amniotic sheet. A portion of the placenta *(PL)* implants on an amniotic sheet *(arrowheads)*.

SUGGESTED READINGS

1. Ball RH, Buchmeier SE, Longnecker M. Clinical significance of sonographically detected uterine synechiae in pregnant patients. *J Ultrasound Med* 1997;16:465–469.
2. Benson CB, Chow JS, Chang-Lee W, et al. Outcome of first trimester pregnancies in women with uterine leiomyomas identified by ultrasound. *J Clin Ultrasound* 2001;29:261–264.
3. Berghella V, Kuhlman K, Weiner S, et al. Cervical funneling: sonographic criteria predictive of preterm delivery. *Ultrasound Obstet Gynecol* 1997;10:161–166.
4. Cook CM, Ellwood DA. The cervix as a predictor of preterm delivery in "at-risk" women. *Ultrasound Obstet Gynecol* 2000;15:109–113.
5. Finberg HJ. Uterine synechiae in pregnancy: expanded criteria for recognition and clinical significance in 28 cases. *J Ultrasound Med* 1991;20:547–555.
6. Fong KW, Farine D. Cervical incompetence and preterm labor. In: Rumack CM, Wilson SR, Charboneau JW, eds. *Diagnostic ultrasound*, 2nd ed. St. Louis: Mosby, 1998:1323–1336.
7. Gomez R, Galasso M, Romero R, et al. Ultrasonographic examination of the uterine cervix is better than cervical digital exam as a predictor of the likelihood of premature delivery in patients with preterm labor and intact membranes. *Am J Obstet Gynecol* 1994;171:956–964.
8. Guzman ER, Rosenberg JC, Houlihan C, et al. A new method using vaginal ultrasound and transfundal pressure to evaluate the asymptomatic incompetent cervix. *Obstet Gynecol* 1994;83:248–252.
9. Guzman ER, Walters C, Ananth CV, et al. A comparison of sonographic cervical parameters in predicting spontaneous preterm birth in high-risk singleton gestations. *Ultrasound Obstet Gynecol* 2001;18:204–210.
10. Guzman ER, Ananth CV. Cervical length and spontaneous prematurity: laying the foundation for future interventional randomized trials for the short cervix. *Ultrasound Obstet Gynecol* 2001;18:195–199.
11. Hassan SS, Romero R, Berry SM, et al. Patients with an ultrasonographic cervical length <15 mm have nearly a 50% risk of early spontaneous preterm delivery. *Am J Obstet Gynecol* 2000;182:1458–1467.
12. Hertzberg BS, Kliewer MA, Farrell TA, et al. Spontaneously changing gravid cervix: clinical implications and prognostic features. *Radiology* 1995;196:721–724.
13. Iams JD, Goldenberg RL, Meis PJ, et al. The length of the cervix and the risk of spontaneous premature delivery. *N Engl J Med* 1996;334:567–572.
14. Iams JD. Cervical ultrasonography. *Ultrasound Obstet Gynecol* 1997;10:156–160.
15. Katz VL, Dotters DJ, Droegemueller W. Complications of uterine leiomyomas in pregnancy. *Obstet Gynecol* 1989;73:593–596.
16. Korbin CD, Benson CB, Doubilet PM. Pregnancy outcome with amniotic sheets/uterine synechiae: does placental implantation on the amniotic sheet matter? *Radiology* 1998;206:773–775.

17. Lev-Toaff AS, Coleman BG, Arger PH, et al. Leiomyomas in pregnancy: sonographic study. *Radiology* 1987;164:375–380.
18. Phelan JP. Myomas and pregnancy. *Obstet Gynecol Clin North Am* 1995;22:801–805.
19. Rosati P, Exacoustos C, Mancuso S. Longitudinal evaluation of uterine myoma growth during pregnancy: a sonographic study. *J Ultrasound Med* 1992;11:511–515.
20. Scheerer LJ, Bartolucci L. Ultrasound evaluation of the cervix. In: Callen PW, ed. *Ultrasonography in obstetrics and gynecology*, 4th ed. Philadelphia: WB Saunders, 2000:577–596.
21. Sonek J, Shellhaas C. Cervical sonography: a review. *Ultrasound Obstet Gynecol* 1998;11:71–78.
22. Stamm E, Waldstein G, Thickman D, et al. Amniotic sheets: natural history and histology. *J Ultrasound Med* 1991;10:501–504.
23. To MS, Skentou C, Liao AW, et al. Cervical length and funneling at 23 weeks of gestation in the prediction of spontaneous early preterm delivery. *Ultrasound Obstet Gynecol* 2001;18:200–203.

17

AMNIOTIC FLUID

17.1. OLIGOHYDRAMNIOS

Description and Clinical Features

Oligohydramnios refers to an abnormally low volume of amniotic fluid. Causes of oligohydramnios from the mid second trimester onward include the following:

- Ruptured membranes.
- Urinary tract abnormality with decreased fetal urine output: Oligohydramnios will result from any cause of decreased or absent urine output, including a bilateral renal parenchymal abnormality [e.g., bilateral renal agenesis, autosomal recessive (infantile) polycystic kidney disease] or obstruction of outflow from both kidneys (e.g., urethral obstruction).
- Placental insufficiency and intrauterine growth restriction: With placental insufficiency, blood is shunted away from the fetal kidneys, leading to decreased urine output.
- Postdates: Oligohydramnios may ensue after 40 weeks gestation and is especially likely if the pregnancy is permitted to continue past 42 weeks.

Oligohydramnios, if severe and prolonged, can lead to a number of fetal deformities from uterine pressure on the developing fetus, including pulmonary hypoplasia, abnormal facies, and clubfeet. These abnormalities are referred to as Potter syndrome if seen in

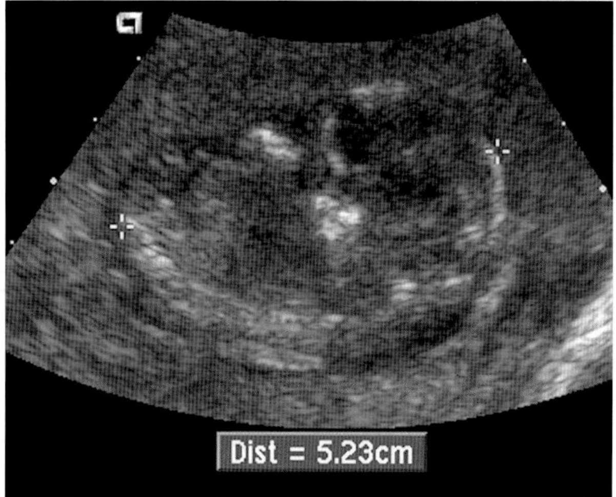

FIGURE 17.1-1. Oligohydramnios in the first trimester. This 12-week fetus *(calipers)* is surrounded by virtually no amniotic fluid. The fetus died within 1 week of this sonogram.

the setting of bilateral renal agenesis, and are sometimes termed "Potter sequence" when due to other causes of severe, prolonged oligohydramnios.

Sonography

The sonographic diagnosis of oligohydramnios can be established by subjective assessment of the amniotic fluid volume, deepest pocket measurement, or amniotic fluid index (AFI). A deepest pocket measurement less than 1–2 cm or an AFI less than 5 cm is generally considered diagnostic of oligohydramnios.

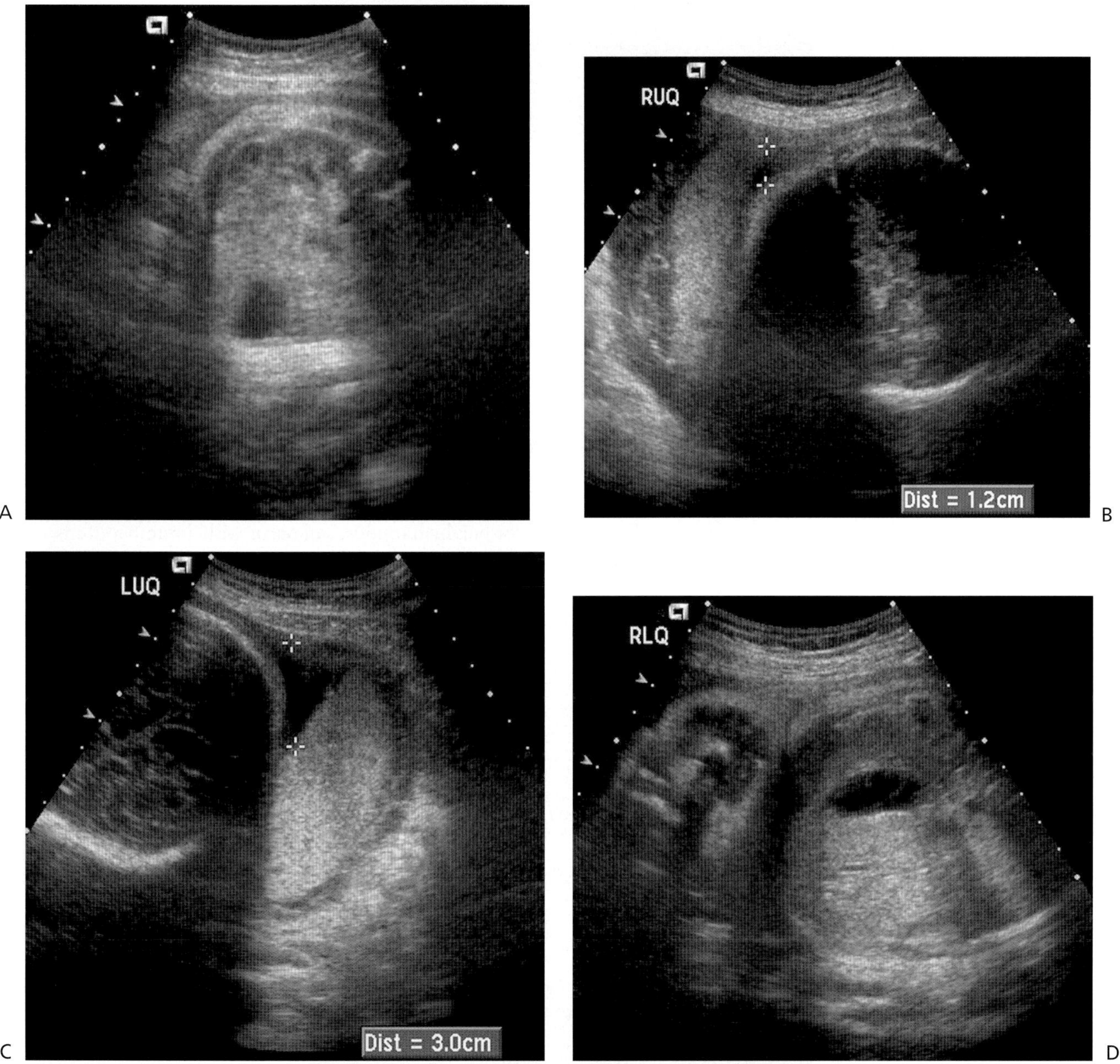

FIGURE 17.1-2. Oligohydramnios in the latter half of pregnancy. A: The amniotic fluid volume appears subjectively low in this 32-week gestation. Deepest pocket measurements in the right upper quadrant *(RUQ)* **(B)**, left upper quadrant *(LUQ)* **(C)**, right lower quadrant *(RLQ)* **(D)**, and left lower quadrant *(LLQ)* **(E)** yield an amniotic fluid index of 4.2 (1.2 + 3.0 + 0 + 0). *(continued)*

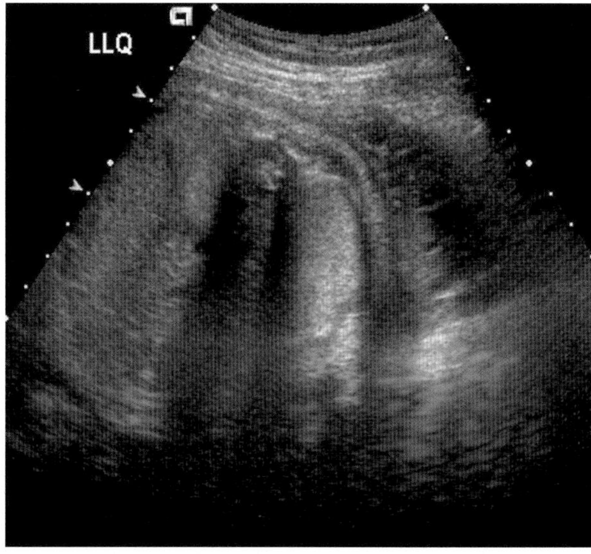

E

FIGURE 17.1-2E. ***(continued)***

Oligohydramnios is occasionally detected by ultrasound in the first trimester of pregnancy (Figure 17.1-1). It is more frequently seen from the mid-second trimester onward (Figure 17.1-2). When oligohydramnios is diagnosed, an effort should be made to ascertain its cause. The fetal urinary tract should be assessed, and fetal measurements should be obtained to evaluate for intrauterine growth restriction. If the oligohydramnios is severe and prolonged, measurement of the fetal thoracic diameter may be useful to assess for pulmonary hypoplasia.

17.2. POLYHYDRAMNIOS

Description and Clinical Features

Excessive amniotic fluid volume, or polyhydramnios, can occur with a number of maternal and fetal abnormalities. Diabetic mothers have a higher frequency of polyhydramnios

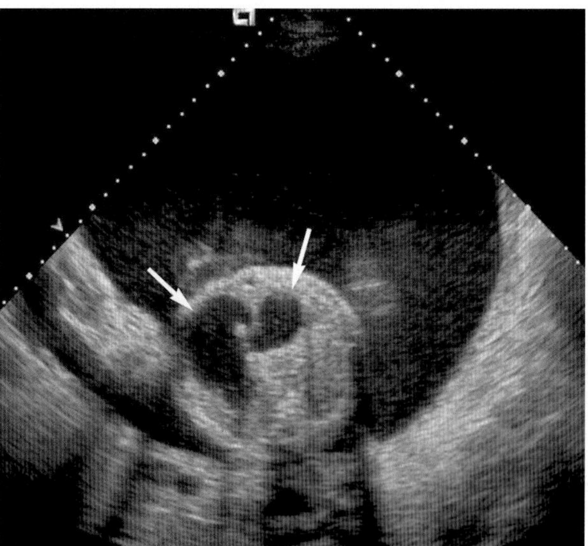

FIGURE 17.2-1. Severe polyhydramnios: subjective assessment. The volume of amniotic fluid appears markedly increased. Two dilated loops of bowel *(arrows)* are seen in the fetal abdomen. After birth, the neonate was found to have jejunal atresia.

than do nondiabetic mothers. Fetal anomalies that impair swallowing or decrease gastrointestinal tract absorption of amniotic fluid also lead to polyhydramnios. These anomalies include esophageal, duodenal, and proximal small bowel obstruction; [illegible] brain anomalies such as anencephaly; facial clefts and tumors; and intrathoracic masses. Hydropic fetuses are often surrounded by excessive amniotic fluid. Polyhydramnios may also be idiopathic in that no maternal or fetal cause is identified.

Polyhydramnios, regardless of its cause, may lead to a variety of maternal symptoms. The mother may experience pain or premature uterine contractions as a result of excessive stretching of the uterus. Pressure by the enlarged uterus on adjacent structures can cause maternal hydronephrosis, lower extremity edema, and respiratory problems.

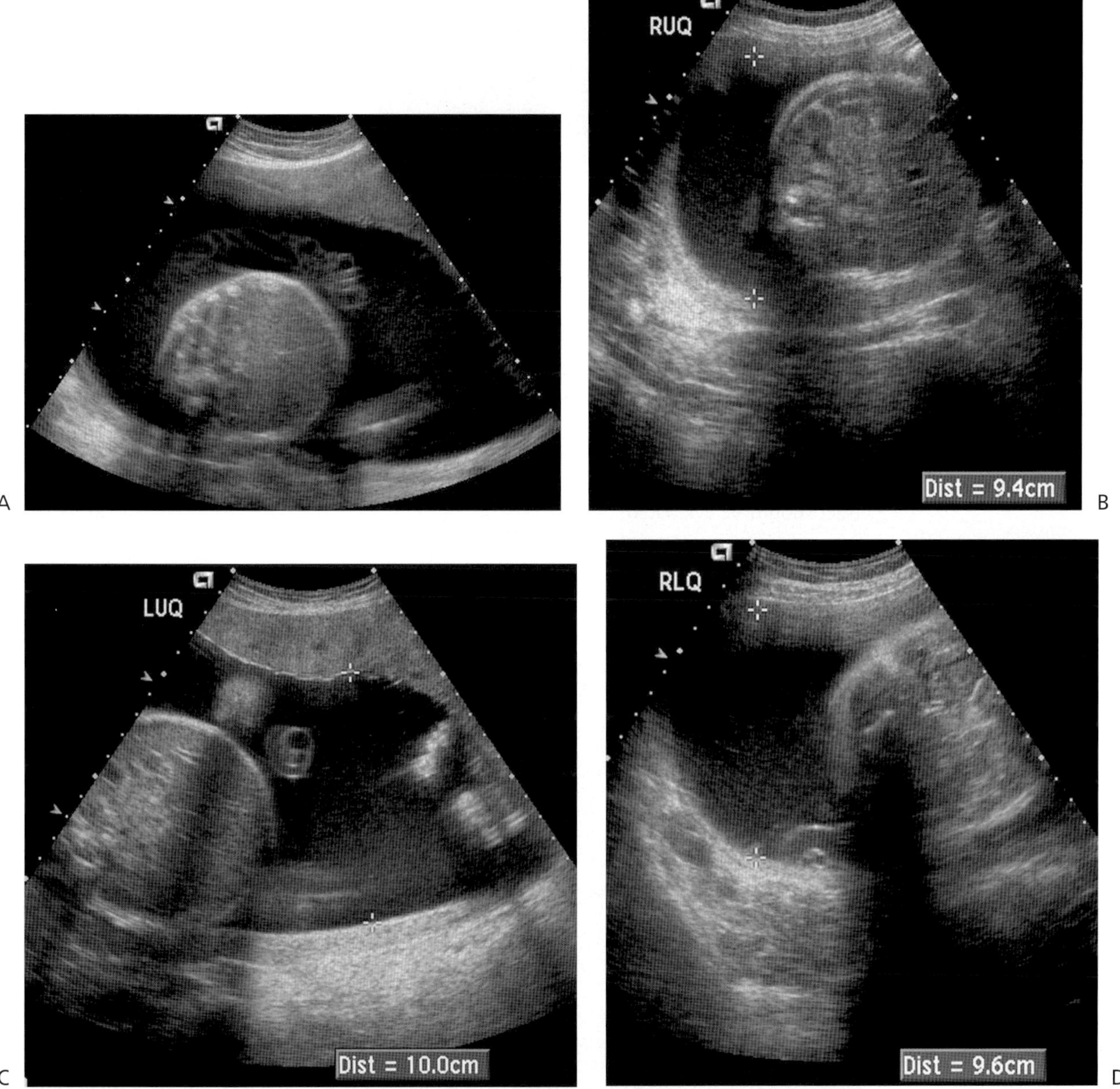

FIGURE 17.2-2. Moderate polyhydramnios: subjective assessment and amniotic fluid index. A: The amniotic fluid volume appears subjectively elevated in this 31-week gestation, in which the fetus had a neck mass that obstructed swallowing. Deepest pocket measurements in the right upper quadrant *(RUQ)* **(B)**, left upper quadrant *(LUQ)* **(C)**, right lower quadrant *(RLQ)* **(D)**, and left lower quadrant *(LLQ)* **(E)** yield an amniotic fluid index of 37.5 (9.4 + 10.0 + 9.6 + 8.5). *(continued)*

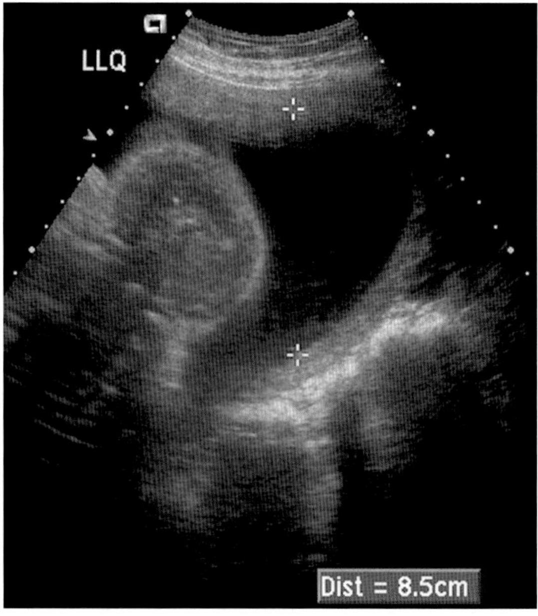

E

FIGURE 17.2-2E. ***(continued)***

Sonography

The sonographic diagnosis of polyhydramnios can be established by subjective assessment of amniotic fluid volume, deepest pocket measurement, or AFI (Figures 17.2-1 and 17.2-2). A deepest pocket measurement more than 8–10 cm or an AFI more than 18–20 cm is generally considered diagnostic of polyhydramnios.

When polyhydramnios is diagnosed, a careful fetal anatomic survey should be undertaken to search for a cause. In particular, the fetal head, face, thorax, and gastrointestinal tract should be evaluated.

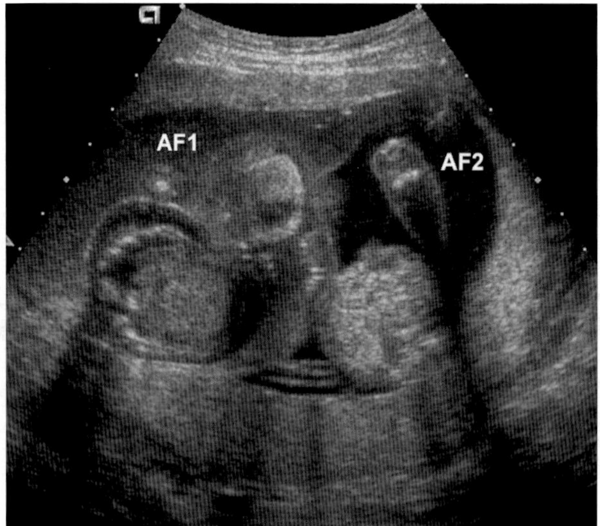

FIGURE 17.3-1. Intra-amniotic hemorrhage in one sac of a twin gestation. Sonogram performed 1 day after selective termination of a fetus with trisomy 21 demonstrates that the amniotic fluid *(AF1)* in this twin's sac has markedly increased echogenicity, representing intra-amniotic hemorrhage caused by the procedure. The amniotic fluid *(AF2)* in the other twin's sac is, appropriately, largely anechoic.

17.3. INTRA-AMNIOTIC HEMORRHAGE

Description and Clinical Features

Blood in the amniotic fluid can occur spontaneously, often in combination with a subchorionic hematoma or an abruption. It can also be iatrogenic, after an amniocentesis (especially when the needle traverses the placenta) or in patients taking anticoagulation medications. In most cases, the blood is resorbed, and there are no clinically significant sequelae.

Sonography

When there is an intra-amniotic hemorrhage, the amniotic fluid appears echogenic, causing the blood vessels in the umbilical cord to stand out in contrast to the surrounding fluid more distinctly than usual. On real-time sonography, swirling echogenic particles are seen within the amniotic fluid.

The sonographic diagnosis of blood in the amniotic fluid, however, is complicated by the fact that vernix or meconium in the fluid gives rise to the same sonographic appearance. As a result, the interpretation of echogenic fluid depends on the stage of pregnancy at which it is seen. Echogenic fluid in the first or second trimester most likely indicates blood in the fluid (Figure 17.3-1), whereas the same finding in the third trimester (especially the mid to late third trimester) likely represents vernix.

SUGGESTED READINGS

1. Barkin SZ, Pretorius DH, Beckett MK, et al. Severe polyhydramnios: incidence of anomalies. *AJR Am J Roentgenol* 1987;148:155–159.
2. Brace RA, Wolf EJ. Normal amniotic fluid volume changes throughout pregnancy. *Am J Obstet Gynecol* 1989;161:382–388.
3. Brown DL, Polger M, Clark PK, et al. Very echogenic amniotic fluid: ultrasound-amniocentesis correlation. *J Ultrasound Med* 1994;13:95–97.
4. Callen PW. Amniotic fluid: its role in fetal health and disease. In: Callen PW, ed. *Ultrasonography in obstetrics and gynecology*, 4th ed. Philadelphia: WB Saunders, 2000:638–659.
5. Hill LM, Breckle R, Thomas ML, et al. Polyhydramnios: ultrasonically detected prevalence and neonatal outcome. *Obstet Gynecol* 1987;69:21–25.
6. Magann EF, Chauhan SP, Whitworth NS, et al. Subjective versus objective evaluation of amniotic fluid volume of pregnancies of less than 24 weeks' gestation. *J Ultrasound Med* 2001;20:191–195.
7. Saltzman DH, Benson CB, Lavery MJ, et al. Echogenic amniotic fluid secondary to heparin therapy. *J Diagn Med Sonogr* 1985;1:155–156.
8. Sivit CJ, Hill MC, Larsen JW, et al. Second-trimester polyhydramnios: evaluation with US. *Radiology* 1987;165:467–469.
9. Sherer DM, Langer O. Oligohydramnios: use and misuse in clinical management. *Ultrasound Obstet Gynecol* 2001;18:411–419.

18

UMBILICAL CORD

18.1. SINGLE UMBILICAL ARTERY

Description and Clinical Features

The normal umbilical cord has three vessels: two umbilical arteries and one umbilical vein. When there is a single umbilical artery, the umbilical cord has two vessels: one artery and one vein. This abnormality is present in 0.2%–1% of pregnancies. It is more common in multiple gestations than singletons and more common in monozygotic twins than dizygotic twins.

Approximately 30% of fetuses with a single umbilical artery have structural anomalies; 4% have aneuploidy. Anomalies may involve any system but occur with highest frequency in the cardiovascular system, gastrointestinal tract, and central nervous system. The anomalies seen in association with a single umbilical artery can usually be identified by prenatal ultrasound.

Unusual variants of single umbilical artery are occasionally seen. For example, there may be two umbilical arteries in part of the umbilical cord and a single umbilical artery in the rest of the cord. In other cases, both arteries are present, but one is much smaller in diameter than the other.

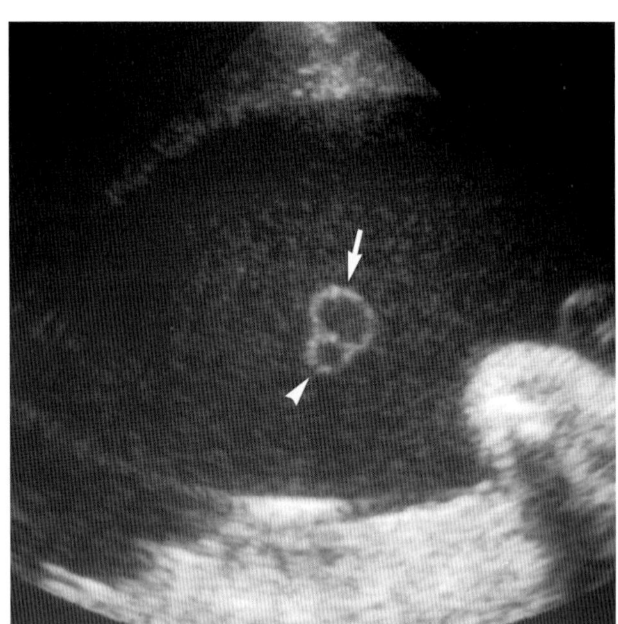

A

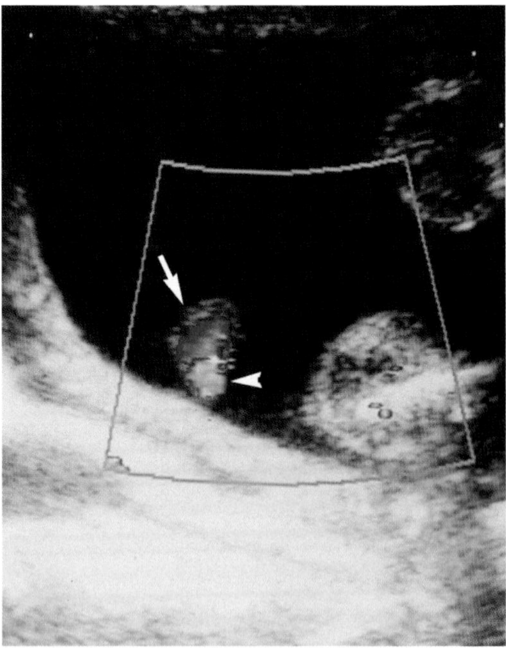

B

FIGURE 18.1-1. Cross-section of a two-vessel umbilical cord. A: Image of cord surrounded by polyhydramnios demonstrates two vessels, the larger one is the umbilical vein *(arrow)* and the smaller is the single umbilical artery *(arrowhead)*. **B:** Color Doppler demonstrates red in the umbilical vein *(arrow)* and blue in the umbilical artery *(arrowhead)*, proving that the flow is in opposite directions in the two vessels.

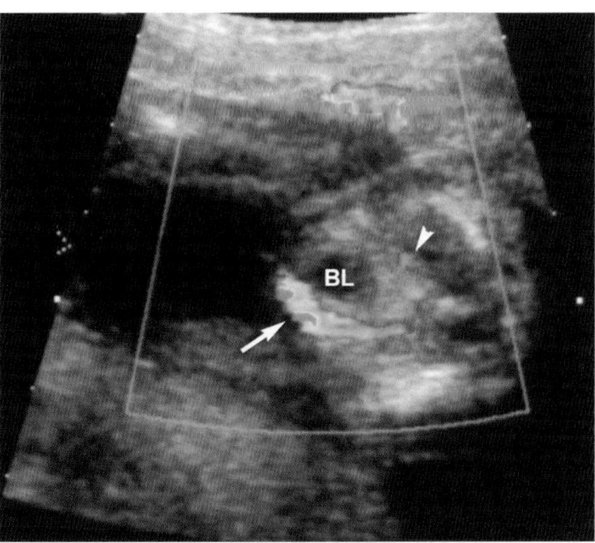

FIGURE 18.1-2. Single umbilical artery in the pelvis. Transverse image of a pelvis demonstrates a single umbilical artery *(arrow)* adjacent to one side of the bladder *(BL)*. On the contralateral side, no umbilical artery is seen arising from the iliac artery *(arrowhead)*.

Sonography

The diagnosis of a single umbilical artery can be made either on a transverse view of the umbilical cord surrounded by amniotic fluid or by identifying a single umbilical artery in the fetal pelvis. The transverse view of a two-vessel cord demonstrates two vessels: the larger umbilical vein and the smaller umbilical artery (Figure 18.1-1). Color Doppler will demonstrate opposite flow in the two vessels, toward the placenta in the umbilical artery and toward the fetus in the umbilical vein. A single umbilical artery can also be demonstrated with color Doppler of the fetal pelvis. The umbilical artery is seen adjacent to one side of the bladder, and no vessel is seen on the other side of the bladder (Figure 18.1-2).

18.2. ABNORMAL PLACENTAL CORD INSERTIONS

Description and Clinical Features

Marginal and velamentous insertions of the umbilical cord into the placenta are abnormal placental cord insertions associated with increased risks to the fetus. A marginal cord insertion is one that enters the placenta within 1 cm of the placental edge. A velamentous cord insertion is characterized by umbilical vessels traveling beneath the membranes before inserting into the edge of the placenta. Predisposing factors for these abnormal insertions include multiple gestations, a low-lying placenta, placenta previa, uterine anomalies, and uterine scarring. Risks include cord rupture and thrombosis.

Marginal cord insertions are thought to develop during the course of gestation as the placenta evolves. In particular, if the placental tissue on one side of the cord atrophies while the placental tissue on the other side of the cord grows, the position of the cord in the placental mass will be closer to one side of the placenta than the other. Marginal cord insertions implant directly into the placenta but close to the placental edge.

Velamentous cord insertions are thought to develop when there is atrophy of placental tissue on one side of the cord as well as placental tissue beneath the cord insertion site, leaving the umbilical vessels exposed beneath the membranes as they travel to the remaining placental mass. When the vessels of a velamentous umbilical cord travel across the cervix beneath the membranes, the configuration is termed vasa previa. Vasa previa car-

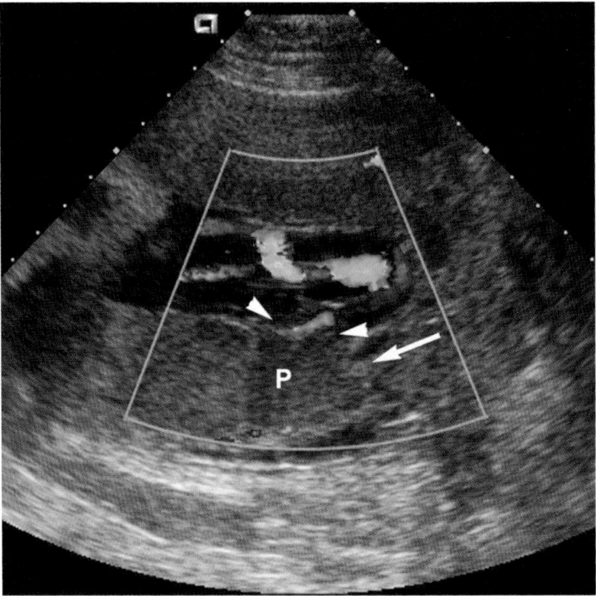

FIGURE 18.2-1. Marginal umbilical cord insertion. Color Doppler demonstrates placental cord insertion (arrowheads) located close to the edge *(arrow)* of the placenta (*P*).

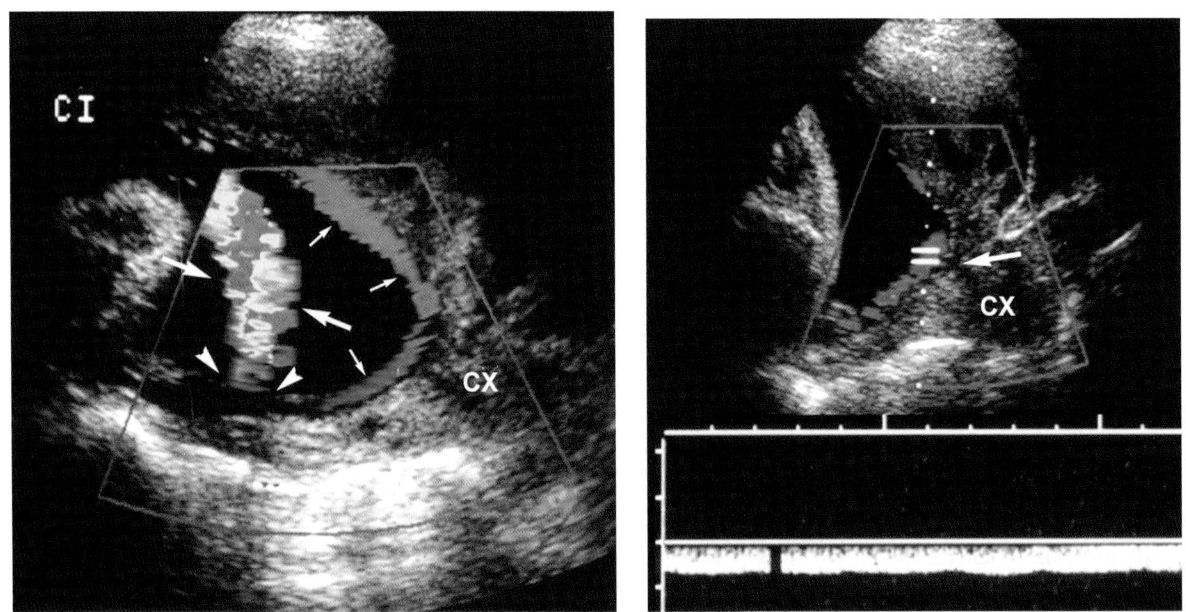

FIGURE 18.2-2. Velamentous cord insertion and vasa previa. A: Sagittal color Doppler image of the lower uterine segment and cord insertion *(CI, arrowheads)* demonstrates the umbilical cord *(large arrows)* inserting into membranes of the posterior wall away from the anterior placenta. Umbilical vessels *(small arrows)* travel beneath the membranes across the cervix *(CX)* to the anterior placenta. **B:** Sagittal color Doppler image of cervix *(CX)* demonstrates a Doppler gate on the umbilical vein that crosses directly over the internal cervical os *(arrow)*. Doppler waveform below demonstrates umbilical venous flow.

ries a high risk of perinatal mortality, because the fetal umbilical vessels coursing over the cervix are prone to bleeding.

Sonography

Color Doppler and gray-scale ultrasound are both useful for evaluating abnormal umbilical cord insertions. With a marginal cord insertion, the umbilical cord insertion into the placenta is seen near the edge of the placenta (Figure 18.2-1). With velamentous cord insertion, the intra-amniotic umbilical cord is seen terminating at the uterine wall away from the placenta, with the umbilical vessels traveling beneath the membranes to the placenta (Figure 18.2-2). The diagnosis of vasa previa is made when the vessels of a velamentous cord are seen crossing the cervix (Figure 18.2-2).

18.3. ALLANTOIC DUCT CYSTS

Description and Clinical Features

An allantoic duct cyst is a cyst of the umbilical cord. It may be an isolated finding or may be seen in association with fetal anomalies, especially omphaloceles, and aneuploidy. If a cyst is identified *in utero*, careful sonographic assessment of the fetus is warranted.

Sonography

The diagnosis of an allantoic duct cyst is made when a cyst is seen within the umbilical cord adjacent to the umbilical vessels (Figures 18.3-1 and 18.3-2). The cyst is anechoic with well-defined margins and a thin wall. Areas of excess Wharton's jelly within the cord should not be confused with allantoic duct cysts, because they are neither anechoic nor well-defined with thin walls.

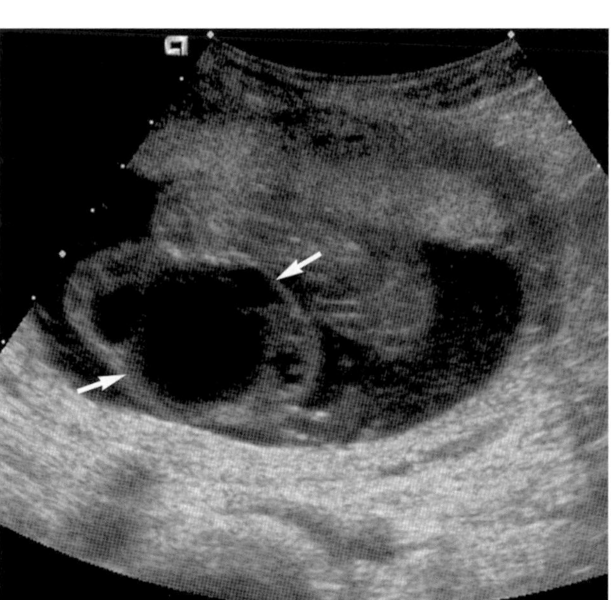

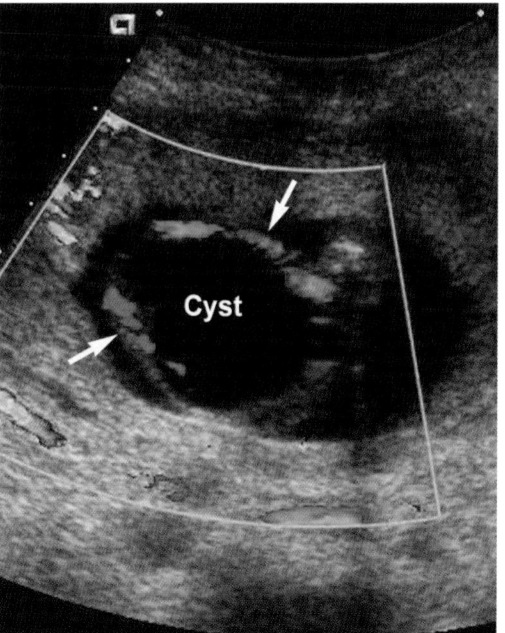

FIGURE 18.3-1. Allantoic duct cyst. A: Transverse image of the umbilical cord demonstrates a large cyst *(arrows)* within the cord. **B:** Color Doppler demonstrates umbilical vessels *(arrows)* draped around the cyst *(Cyst)*.

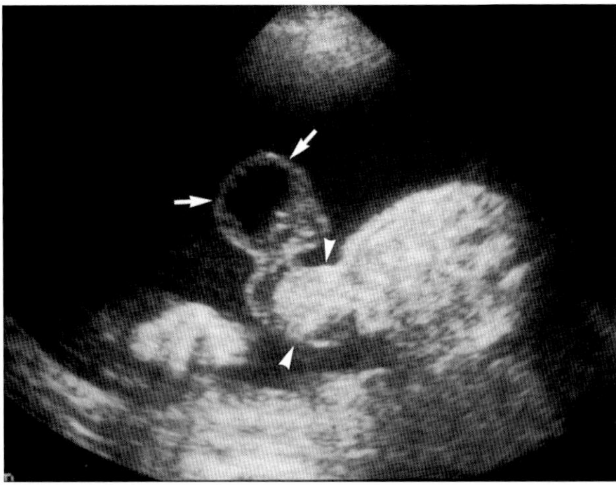

FIGURE 18.3-2. Allantoic duct cyst adjacent to an omphalocele. Allantoic duct cyst *(arrows)* in the umbilical cord adjacent to an omphalocele *(arrowheads)* protruding from the anterior abdominal wall.

18.4. UMBILICAL ARTERIAL DOPPLER

Description and Clinical Features

Doppler of the umbilical artery can be used to assess fetal well-being in the third trimester. Measuring the systolic/diastolic ratio (S/D ratio) on a spectral waveform of the umbilical artery provides information about vascular resistance in the placenta, which lies downstream from the umbilical artery. The normal S/D ratio decreases with increasing gestational age. Elevated S/D ratios indicate diminished diastolic flow, a sign of increased resistance in the placenta. The cutoff for an elevated S/D ratio depends on gestational age. At 26–30 weeks, the S/D ratio is elevated if it measures greater than 4.0, at 30–34 weeks if it measures greater than 3.5, and after 34 weeks if the S/D ratio is greater than 3.0. A fetus with an elevated S/D ratio, which indicates high placental resistance, is at increased risk of perinatal morbidity and mortality. Doppler measurements can be used to monitor the well-being of a high-risk fetus to determine optimal timing for delivery.

Absent or reversed end diastolic flow in the umbilical artery is associated with a poor prognosis. These findings are worse than an elevated S/D ratio because they indicate extremely elevated placental resistance, and have a higher association with perinatal morbidity and mortality.

Sonography

Umbilical arterial Doppler waveforms should be obtained from a free loop of cord in the amniotic fluid. When placental resistance is increased, the amount of diastolic flow is diminished and the S/D ratio is elevated (Figure 18.4-1). The waveform with absent diastolic flow demonstrates a sharp systolic peak that returns to the baseline during diastole, with no detectable blood flow in late diastole (Figure 18.4-2). When reversed diastolic flow is present, the sharp systolic peak is above the baseline, and the Doppler waveform is below the baseline in late diastole (Figure 18.4-3).

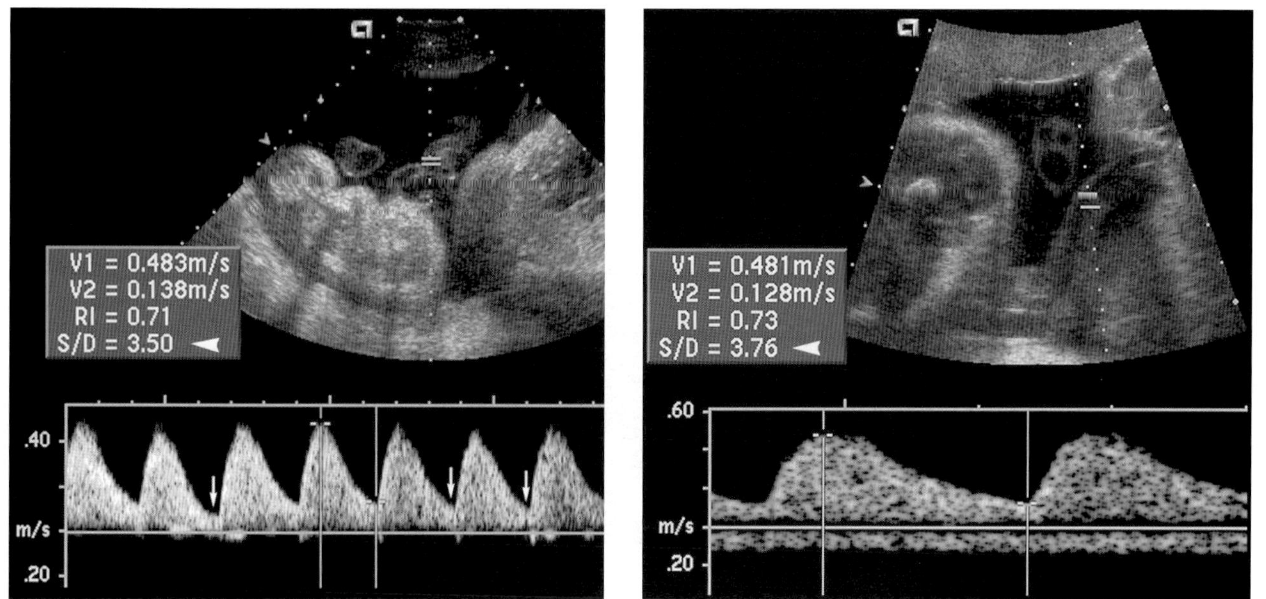

FIGURE 18.4-1. Diminished umbilical artery diastolic flow. A: Spectral Doppler of the umbilical artery in a 35 week fetus demonstrates diminished diastolic flow *(arrows)* with an elevated systolic/diastolic (S/D) ratio of 3.50 *(arrowhead, calipers)*. **B:** Umbilical artery Doppler of another 35 week fetus demonstrates elevated S/D ratio of 3.76 *(arrowhead, calipers)* due to diminished diastolic flow.

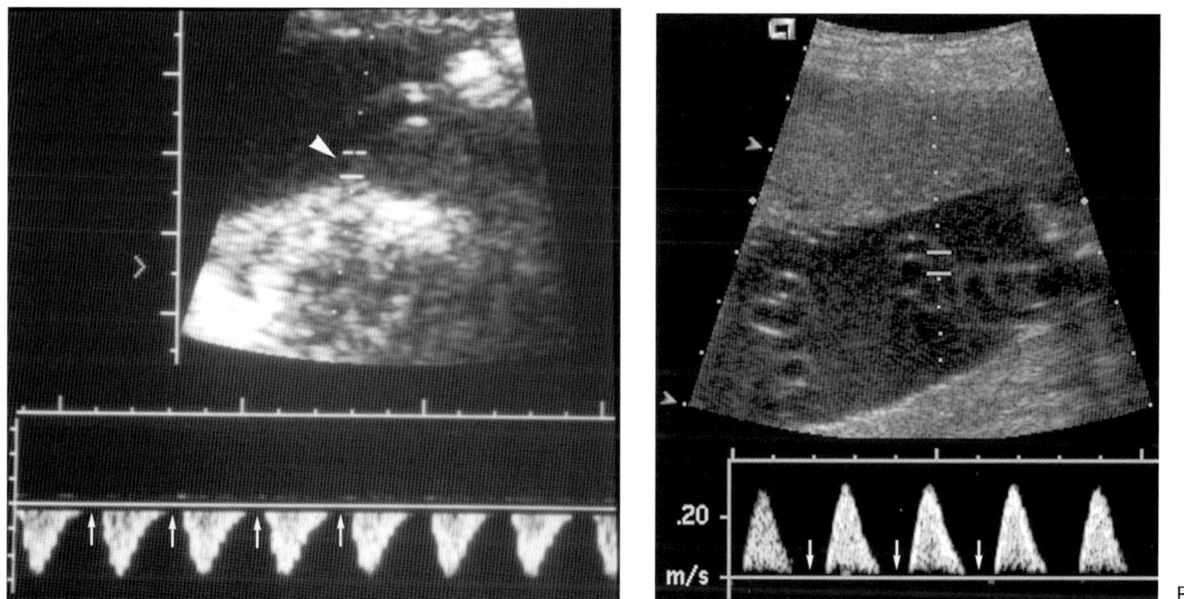

FIGURE 18.4-2. Absent diastolic flow in the umbilical artery. A: Doppler interrogation of the umbilical artery *(arrowhead)* demonstrates absence of diastolic flow *(arrows)* on the waveform below the image. **B:** Doppler of another fetus with absent diastolic flow *(arrows)* on the umbilical artery waveform.

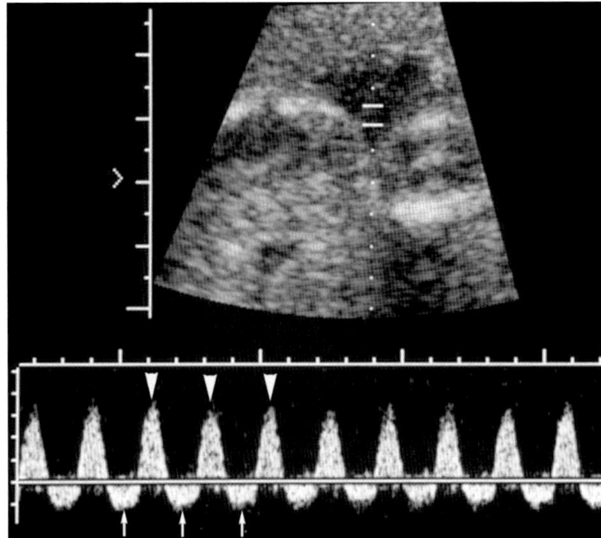

FIGURE 18.4-3. Reversed diastolic flow in the umbilical artery. Spectral Doppler of the umbilical artery demonstrates sharp systolic peaks *(arrowheads)* with reversed diastolic flow *(arrows)*, as the waveform extends below the baseline during diastole.

18.5. UMBILICAL VENOUS VARICES

Description and Clinical Features

Focal dilation of the umbilical vein is called an umbilical venous varix. It occurs most often in the intra-abdominal portion of the umbilical vein just beneath the umbilical cord insertion, between the anterior abdominal wall and the liver. An intra-abdominal umbilical venous varix may be an isolated sonographic finding or may be associated with fetal abnormalities, including fetal anomalies and fetal anemia. Focal dilation of the umbilical vein may be an early sign of hydrops.

Rarely, a varix of the umbilical vein will be present within the umbilical cord outside the fetus.

Sonography

An intra-abdominal umbilical venous varix is characterized by dilation of the umbilical vein. The dilation is usually saccular, producing focal, rounded expansion of the umbilical vein just deep to the umbilical cord insertion (Figure 18.5-1). Color Doppler can be used to confirm the vascular nature of this rounded cystic lesion and demonstrate its communication with the intrahepatic umbilical vein. Rarely, the varix will be more fusiform and extend into the intrahepatic portion of the umbilical vein (Figure 18.5-2).

A varix of the umbilical vein in the umbilical cord appears as a focal enlargement of the umbilical vein with flow on color Doppler (Figure 18.5-3).

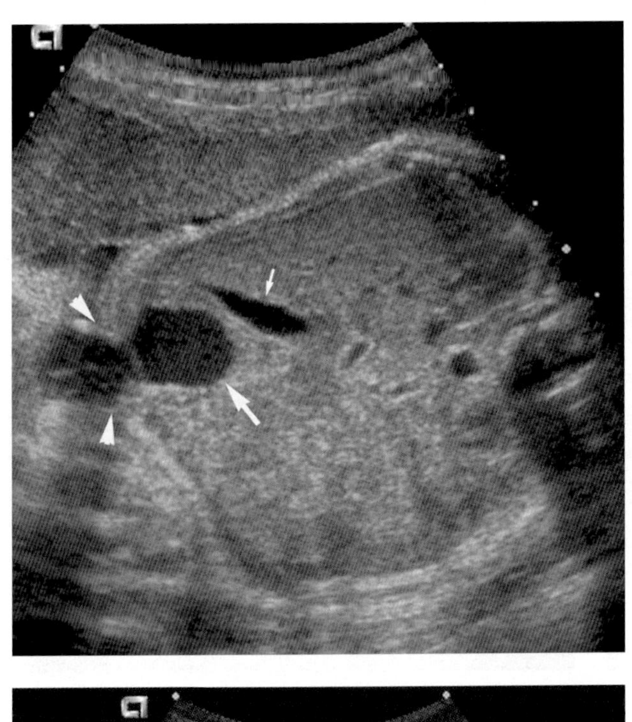

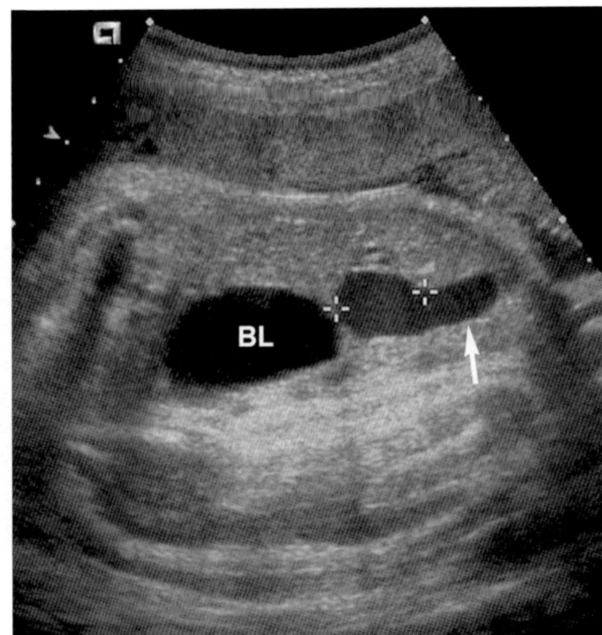

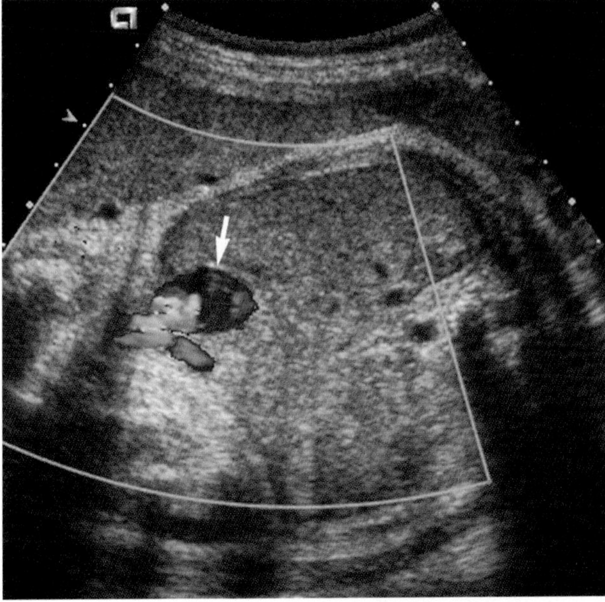

FIGURE 18.5-1. Umbilical venous varix. A: Transverse view of the abdomen demonstrates a cystic lesion *(large arrow)* just inside the abdomen at the umbilical cord insertion *(arrowheads)* adjacent to the gallbladder *(small arrow)*. **B:** Coronal image demonstrates focal dilation *(calipers)* of the umbilical vein *(arrow)* above the bladder *(BL)*. **C:** Color Doppler shows flow in the focally dilated portion of the umbilical vein *(arrow)* within the fetal abdomen.

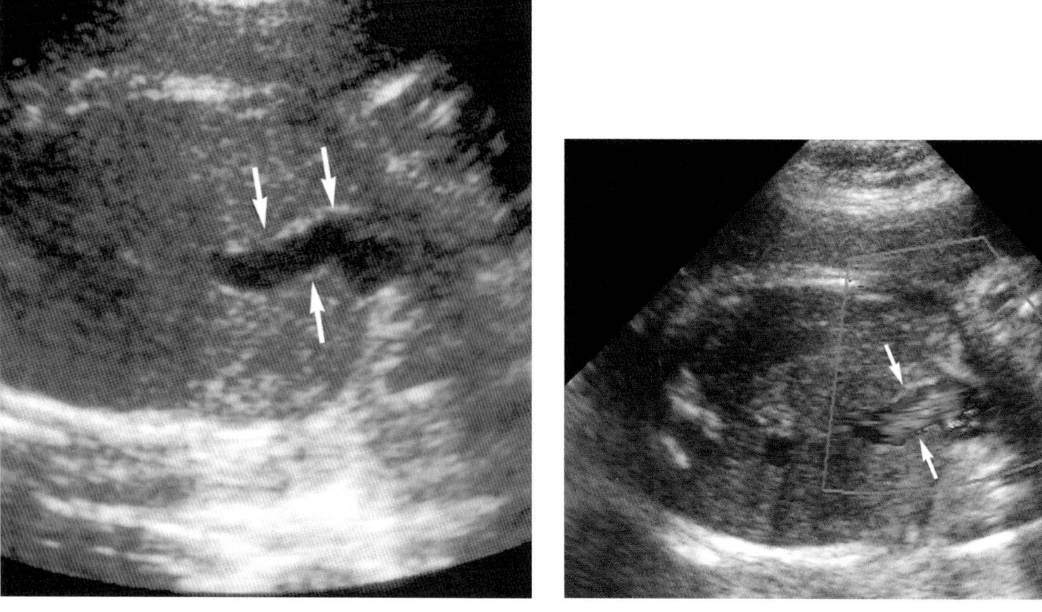

FIGURE 18.5-2. Fusiform umbilical venous varix. A: Transverse image of the abdomen demonstrates dilation of the entire intra-abdominal portion of the umbilical vein *(arrows)*. **B:** Color Doppler confirms umbilical blood flow in the diffusely dilated intra-abdominal portion of the umbilical vein *(arrows)*.

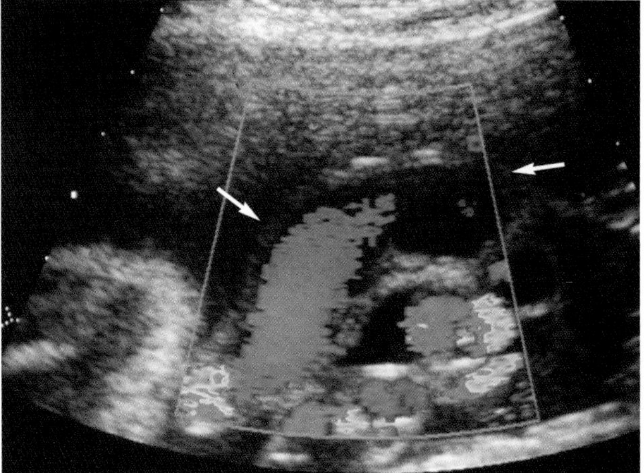

FIGURE 18.5-3. Varix of the umbilical vein in the umbilical cord. Color Doppler of the umbilical cord demonstrates marked dilation of a segment of the umbilical vein *(arrows)* within the umbilical cord. The fetus died *in utero* 2 days later.

SUGGESTED READINGS

1. Berkowitz GS, Mehalek JE, Chitkara U, et al. Doppler umbilical velocimetry in the prediction of adverse outcome in pregnancies at risk for intrauterine growth retardation. *Obstet Gynecol* 1988;71:742–746.
2. Catanzarite V, Maida C, Thomas W, et al. Prenatal sonographic diagnosis of vasa previa: ultrasound findings and obstetrics outcome in ten cases. *Ultrasound Obstet Gynecol* 2001;18:109–115.
3. Chow JS, Benson CB, Doubilet PM. The frequency and nature of structural anomalies in fetuses with single umbilical arteries. *J Ultrasound Med* 1998;17:765–768.
4. Di Salvo DN, Benson CB, Laing FC, et al. Sonographic evaluation of the placental cord insertion site. *AJR Am J Roentgenol* 1998;170:1295–1298.
5. Ferrazzi E, Vegni C, Bellotti M, et al. Role of umbilical Doppler velocimetry in the biophysical assessment of the growth-retarded fetus: answers from neonatal morbidity and mortality. *J Ultrasound Med* 1991;10:309–315.
6. Fleischer AC. Sonography of the umbilical cord and intrauterine membranes. In: Fleischer AC, Manning FA, Jeanty P, et al., eds. *Sonography in obstetrics & gynecology: principles and practice*, 6th ed. New York: McGraw-Hill, 2001:225–245.
7. Goncalves LF, Romero R, Gervasi MT, et al. Doppler velocimetry of the uteroplacental circulation. In: Fleischer AC, Manning FA, Jeanty P, et al., eds. *Sonography in obstetrics & gynecology: principles and practice*, 6th ed. New York: McGraw-Hill, 2001:285–313.
8. Harris RD, Alexander RD. Ultrasound of the placenta and umbilical cord. In: Callen PW, ed. *Ultrasonography in obstetrics and gynecology*, 4th ed. Philadelphia: WB Saunders, 2000:597–625.
9. Liu CC, Pretorius DH, Scioscia AL, et al. Sonographic prenatal diagnosis of marginal placental cord insertion, clinical importance. *J Ultrasound Med* 2002;21:627–632.
10. Nimrod CA, Nicholson SF. Doppler assessment of pregnancy. In: Rumack CM, Wilson SR, Charboneau JW, eds. *Diagnostic ultrasound*, 2nd ed. St. Louis: Mosby, 1998:1371–1389.
11. Nyberg DA, Mahony BS, Luthy D, et al. Single umbilical artery—prenatal detection of concurrent anomalies. *J Ultrasound Med* 1991;10:247–253.
12. Raga F, Ballester MJ, Osborne NG, et al. Role of color flow Doppler ultrasonography in diagnosing velamentous insertion of the umbilical cord and vasa previa: a report of two cases. *J Reprod Med* 1995;40:804–808.
13. Rahemtullah A, Lieberman E, Benson CB, et al. Outcome of pregnancy after prenatal diagnosis of umbilical venous varix. *J Ultrasound Med* 2001;20:135–139.
14. Reuter KL, Davidoff A, Hunter T. Vasa previa. *J Clin Ultrasound* 1988;16:346–348.
15. Sauerbrei EE, Davies GL. Diagnosis of vasa previa with endovaginal color Doppler and power Doppler sonography: report of two cases. *J Ultrasound Med* 1998;17:393–398.
16. Tekay A, Campbell S. Doppler ultrasonography in obstetrics. In: Callen PW, ed. *Ultrasonography in obstetrics and gynecology*, 4th ed. Philadelphia: WB Saunders, 2000:677–723.
17. Thompson RS, Trudinger BJ, Cook CM, et al. Umbilical artery velocity waveforms: normal reference values for A/B ratio and Pourcelot ratio. *Br J Obstet Gynaecol* 1988;95:589–591.
18. Trudinger BJ, Cook CM. Doppler umbilical and uterine flow waveforms in severe pregnancy hypertension. *Br J Obstet Gynaecol* 1990;97:142–148.

19

DIAGNOSIS AND CHARACTERIZATION OF MULTIPLE GESTATIONS

19.1. FETAL NUMBER

Description and Clinical Features

Twins can arise from a single fertilized ovum (zygote) that splits into two separate embryos within the first few days after conception or can occur from fertilization of two ova. The first of these mechanisms yields identical (monozygotic) twins, and the second results in fraternal (dizygotic) twins. Approximately two-thirds of naturally occurring twins are dizygotic and one-third are monozygotic. Higher order multiples can be of various types of zygosity. For example, triplets may arise from three zygotes (trizygotic triplets); two zygotes, one of which splits after conception, resulting in an identical pair together with a third nonidentical fetus; or, rarely, from one zygote that splits into three embryos.

Several factors influence the frequency of dizygotic twins. Specifically, dizygotic twinning occurs more frequently in:

- Pregnancies achieved after the use of follicle-stimulating drugs
- Mothers with a family history of dizygotic twins
- Mothers older than age 35
- Mothers of particular ethnic or racial backgrounds: Africans more often than Europeans, Europeans more often than Asians

The rate of monozygotic twinning, conversely, is fairly constant over all populations.

In pregnancies that begin as multiple gestations, one or more of the developing fetuses are often lost. Partial or complete pregnancy loss occurs most frequently in the early first trimester.

Sonography

Before 6 weeks, when the embryo and its heartbeat are not consistently identifiable, pregnancy number can be estimated by counting the number of gestational sacs (Figure 19.1-1) and yolk sacs (Figure 19.1-2). Each gestational sac will, in most cases, give rise to as many embryos as the number of yolk sacs contained within it. From 6 weeks gestational age onward, fetal number is determined by counting the number of embryos (or fetuses) with heartbeats (Figure 19.1-3).

Pregnancy number determined before 6 weeks, however, may prove to be an under- or overcount of the number found on a follow-up sonogram. The early sonogram may overcount the subsequent pregnancy number if one or more embryos fail to develop and, together with their gestational sacs, resorb completely ("vanishing twin") (Figure 19.1-4). The early sonogram can undercount the subsequent pregnancy number if the early gestational sacs are discrepant in size, with some visible and others not seen on ultrasound ("appearing twin") (Figure 19.1-5). Another situation in which undercounting occurs is when monochorionic twins are scanned at 5 weeks gestation (Figure 19.1-6). In such

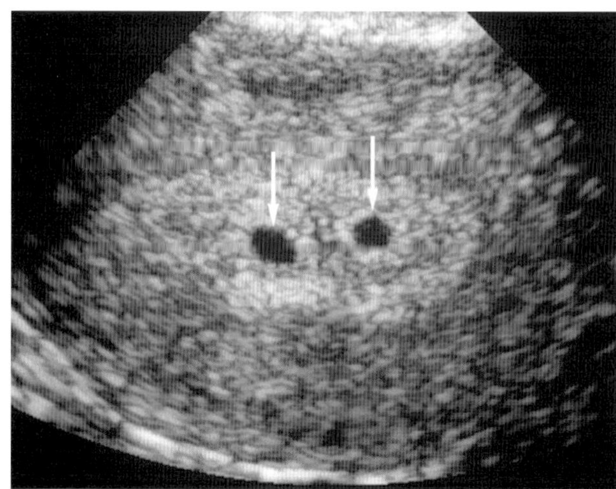

FIGURE 19.1-1. Twins at 5.0 weeks diagnosed by counting gestational sacs. Transverse view of the uterus demonstrates two gestational sacs *(arrows)*. No yolk sac or embryo is yet identifiable within either sac.

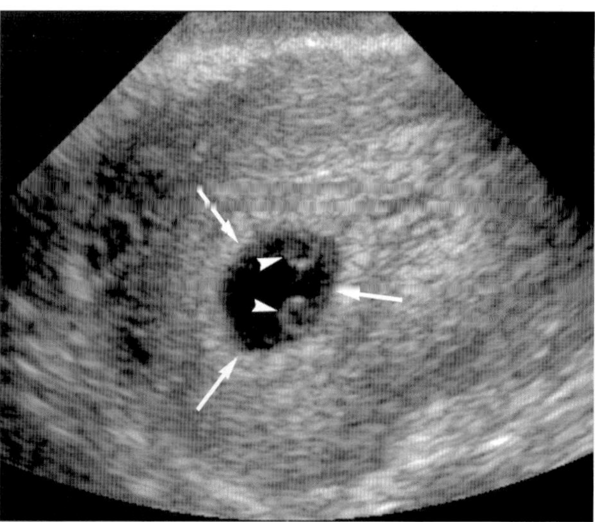

FIGURE 19.1-2. Twins at 5.5 weeks diagnosed by counting yolk sacs. There is a single gestational sac *(arrows)* with two yolk sacs *(arrowheads)*. Subsequent sonogram demonstrated a monochorionic diamniotic twin gestation.

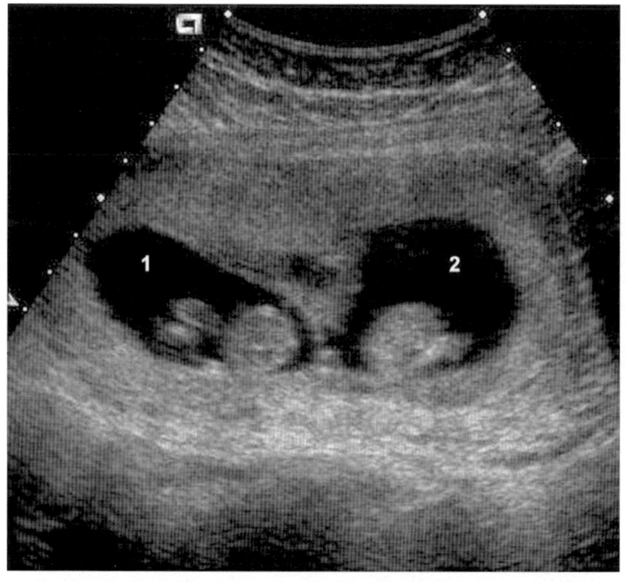

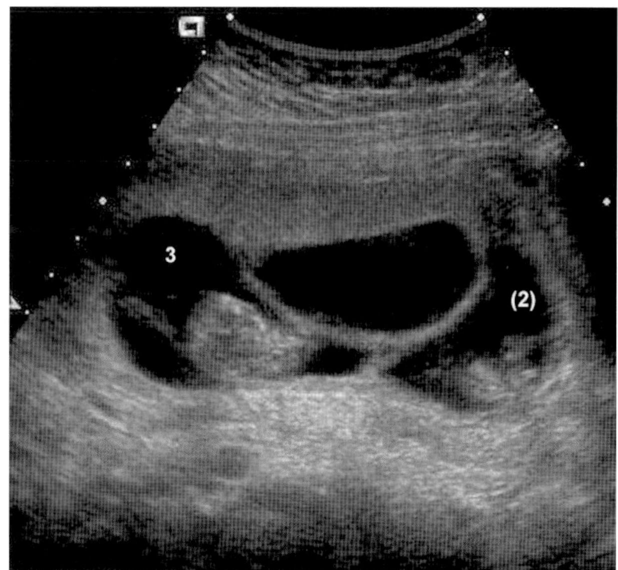

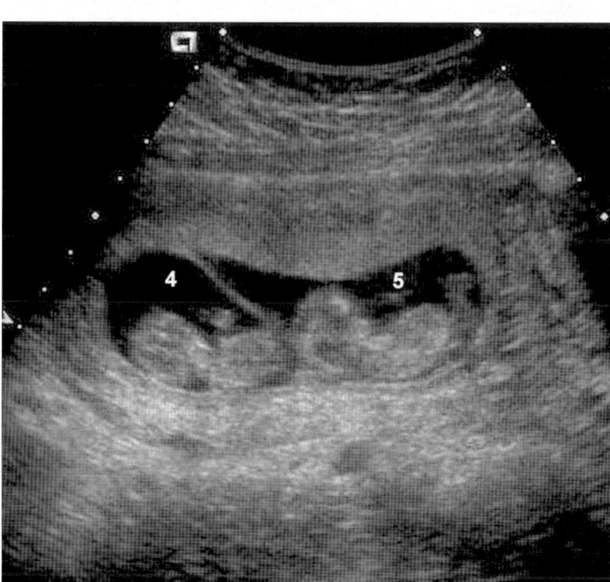

FIGURE 19.1-3. Quintuplets at 11 weeks diagnosed by counting fetuses with heartbeats. Transverse views of the lower **(A)**, mid **(B)**, and upper **(C)** portions of the gravid uterus demonstrate five fetuses *(labeled 1–5)*.

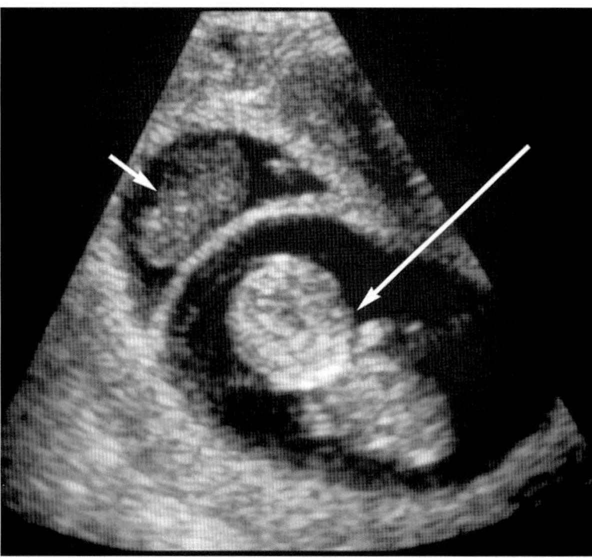

FIGURE 19.1-4. "Vanishing" twin. In this twin gestation, the fetuses *(arrows)* and gestational sacs are discrepant in size and only the larger fetus *(long arrow)* was alive at the time of the sonogram. One month later on a follow-up sonogram, the live fetus had grown normally and the second sac was no longer identifiable.

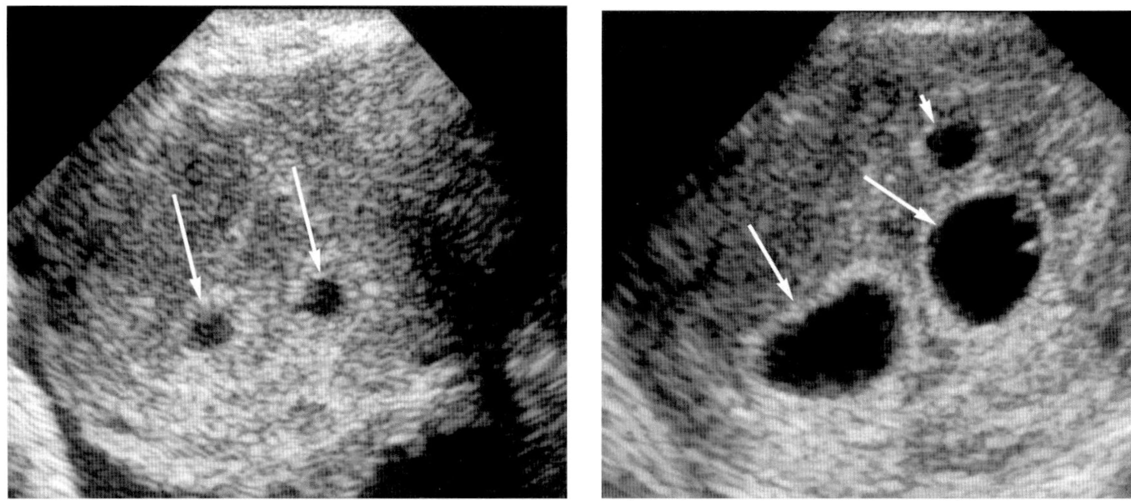

FIGURE 19.1-5. "Appearing" triplet. A: Sonogram at 5 weeks demonstrates two gestational sacs *(arrows)* within the uterus. No yolk sac or embryo was seen. **B:** Ten days later, the original two gestational sacs *(long arrows)* are again seen, but there is now a third smaller gestational sac *(shorter arrow)*. Embryos with heartbeats were visible in all three sacs. On subsequent sonograms, all three fetuses appeared normal and grew appropriately. Normal triplets were born.

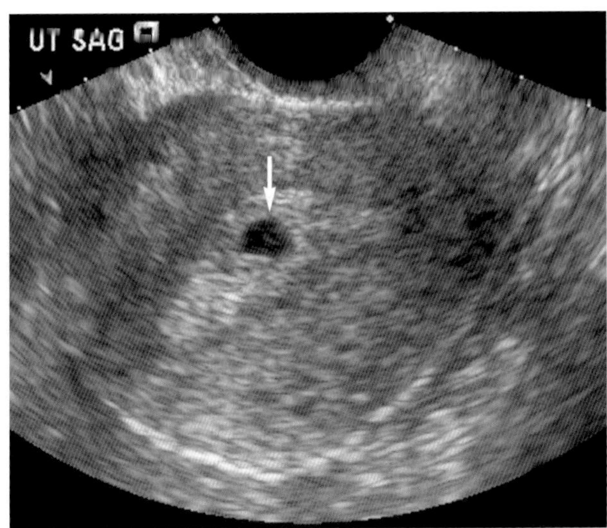

A

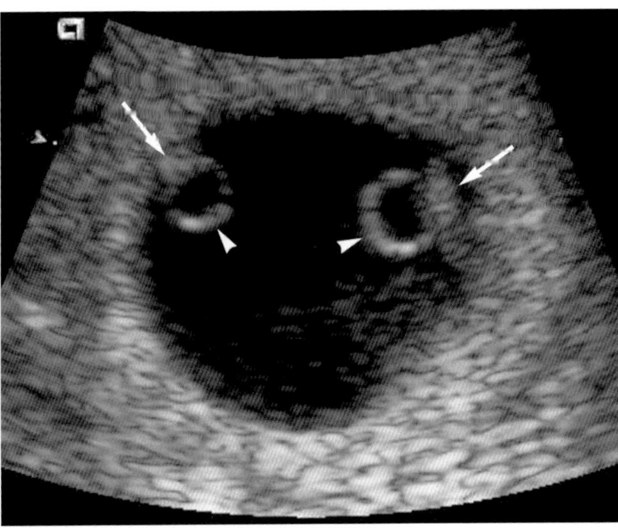

B

FIGURE 19.1-6. **"Appearing" twin. A:** Sonogram at 5 weeks demonstrates a single gestational sac *(arrow)* within the uterus. No yolk sac or embryo was seen. **B:** Eight days later, two yolk sacs *(arrowheads)* were seen within the gestational sac, and there were embryos *(arrows)* with heartbeats seen adjacent to the yolk sacs.

cases, the sonogram will demonstrate a single gestational sac without yolk sacs, thus providing no evidence of the existence of a multiple gestation.

19.2. PLACENTATION: CHORIONICITY AND AMNIONICITY

Description and Clinical Features

Twin gestations can be categorized according to their type of placentation (i.e., according to the number of chorions and amnions). A dichorionic diamniotic twin gestation is one in which each fetus is surrounded by its own chorion and amnion. With monochorionic diamniotic twins, each fetus lies within its own amniotic cavity, and a single chorion surrounds the two amniotic sacs. In a monochorionic monoamniotic twin gestation, both fetuses are surrounded by one chorion and one amnion.

Because the chorion forms the placenta, the number of placentas is directly related to chorionicity. That is, monochorionic twins share a single placenta, whereas each of dichorionic twins has its own placenta.

All dizygotic (fraternal) twins are dichorionic diamniotic because each twin forms separately and implants separately. The placentation type of a monozygotic (identical) twin gestation depends on the time of division of the fertilized ovum:

Dichorionic diamniotic if division occurs within 4 days of conception
Monochorionic diamniotic if division occurs between 4 and 8 days after conception
Monochorionic monoamniotic if it divides more than 8 days after conception

Approximately one-third of monozygotic twins are dichorionic diamniotic, two-thirds are monochorionic diamniotic, and 1%–3% are monochorionic monoamniotic.

Higher order multiples can have a variety of placentation types. For example, triplets might be triamniotic trichorionic, with each embryo having its own amnion and chorion, or they might be triamniotic dichorionic, with one embryo having its own amnion and chorion and the other two sharing a chorion but having separate amnions.

Sonography

In the first trimester, distinction between mono- and dichorionic twins is straightforward. Dichorionic twins are separated by a thick band of tissue or a thick membrane, whereas monochorionic twins have no membrane or a very thin membrane separating them (Figure 19.2-1).

Determination of amnionicity in the first trimester is straightforward if the twins are dichorionic, because all dichorionic twins are diamniotic. If the twins are monochorionic, the approach to distinguishing between mono- and diamniotic twins depends on gestational age.

In monochorionic twins before 7–8 weeks gestation, determination of amnionicity is based on the number of yolk sacs: if there is a single yolk sac, the twins are likely monoamniotic, whereas the presence of two yolk sacs indicates that the twins are likely diamniotic. At this stage of pregnancy, amnionicity is not determined by counting the number of amniotic sacs because the amnion is closely adherent to the embryo and thus not visible sonographically (Figure 19.2-2). As pregnancy progresses, the amniotic cavity fills with fluid and the amnion becomes visible at 7–8 weeks gestation, either as a separate membrane around each twin if diamniotic (Figure 19.2-3) or as a single membrane surrounding both twins if monoamniotic. In monochorionic diamniotic twins, by the end of the first trimester, the two amnions are apposed, appearing as a thin membrane across the gestational sac (Figure 19.2-2). If no dividing membrane is seen at this stage, the twins are likely, but not definitely, monoamniotic. Monoamnionicity can be diagnosed with certainty only if there is both nonvisualization of a dividing membrane and intermingling of the twin umbilical cords (Figure 19.2-4).

In the second and third trimesters, chorionicity may be more difficult to establish than in the first trimester because there is only a minor difference in thickness between a dichorionic and a monochorionic membrane (Figure 19.2-5). Twins are definitely dichorionic if they are of different sexes (because twins of different sexes must be dizygotic, and all dizygotic twins are dichorionic) (Figure 19.2-6) or if they have separate placentas (Figure 19.2-7). They are probably dichorionic if there is a triangle-shaped extension of placenta in the base of the membrane ("delta" or "twin peak" sign) (Figure 19.2-8). They are probably monochorionic

A 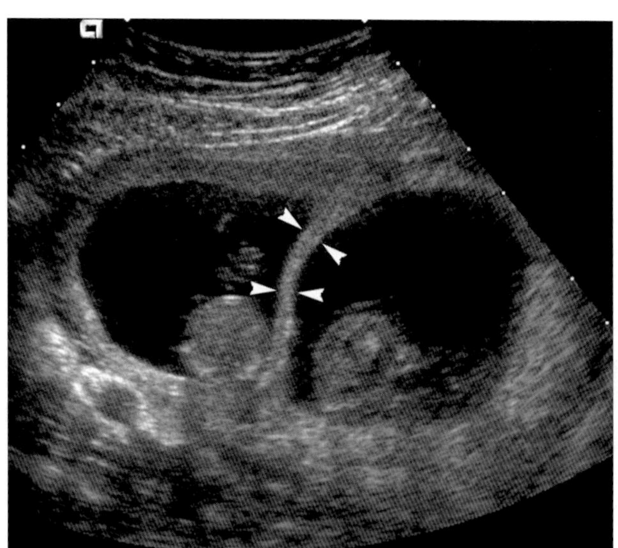

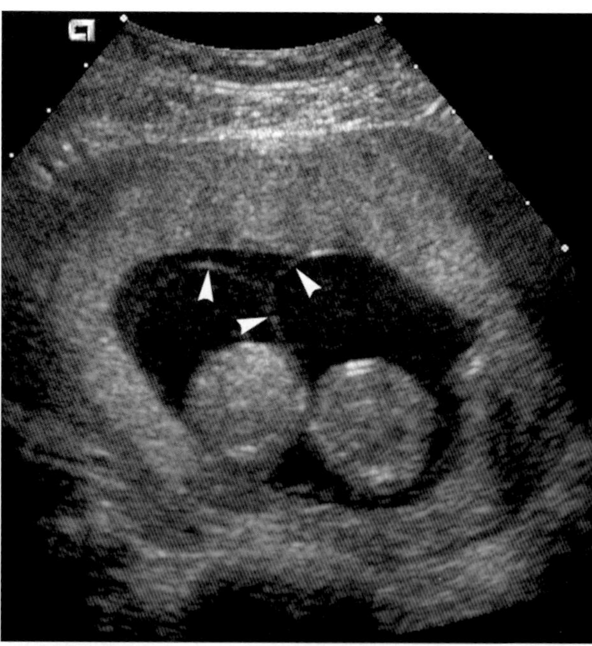 B

FIGURE 19.2-1. Determination of chorionicity in the first trimester. A: Dichorionicity: Sonogram demonstrates a twin gestation in which the two fetuses are separated by a thick membrane *(arrowheads)*, indicating that the twins are dichorionic. **B:** Monochorionicity: Sonogram demonstrates a twin gestation in which both fetuses lie within a single gestational sac, with no thick band of tissue or thick membrane between them, indicating that the twins are monochorionic. Each fetus is surrounded by a thin membrane, representing the amnion *(arrowheads)*.

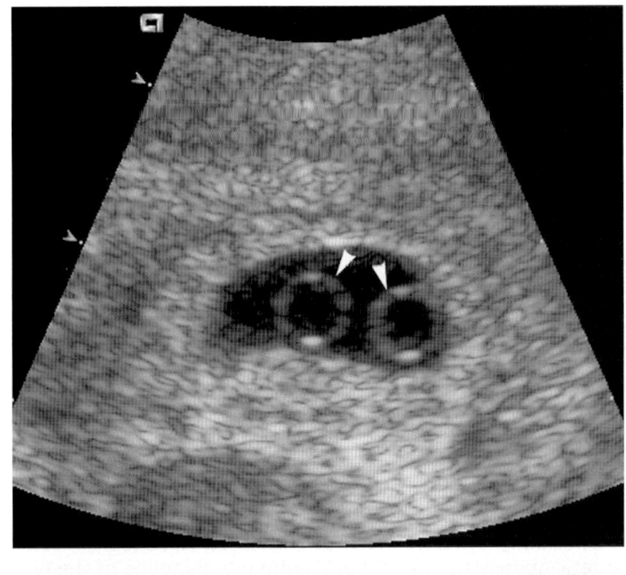

A

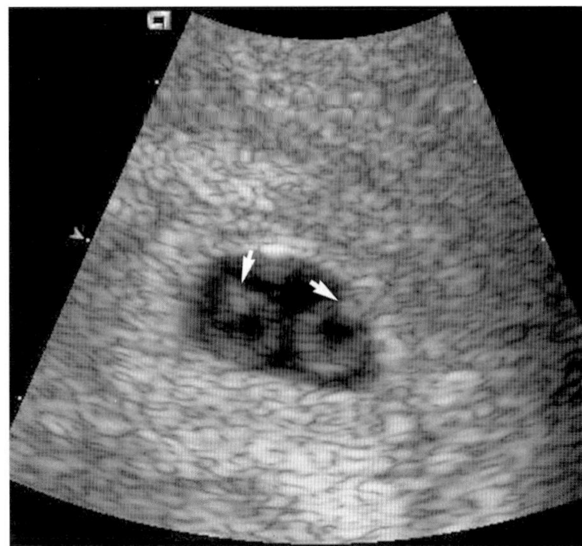

B

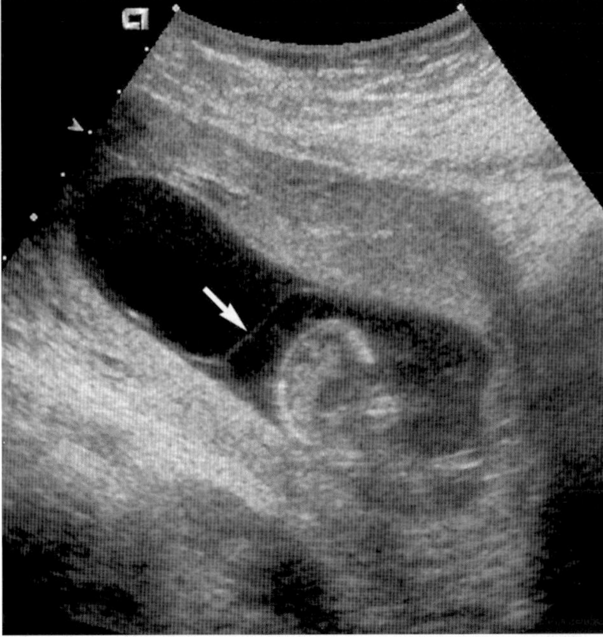

C

FIGURE 19.2-2. Diagnosis of diamniotic twins based on two yolk sacs at 6 weeks gestation. A: There is a single gestational sac with two yolk sacs *(arrowheads)*, a finding suggestive of monochorionic diamniotic twins. The amnionicity cannot be determined by direct visualization of the amnion at this gestational age because it is too early to identify the amnion sonographically. **B:** Beside each yolk sac, there is an embryo seen as an area of thickening *(arrows)* with cardiac activity on real-time sonography. **C:** Follow-up sonogram at 12 weeks demonstrates a thin intertwin membrane, indicative of a diamniotic gestation.

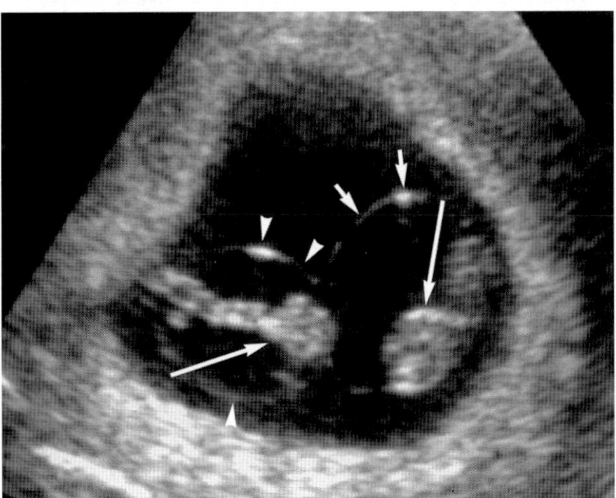

FIGURE 19.2-3. Diagnosis of diamniotic twins based on two amniotic sacs at 8 weeks gestation. There are two embryos *(long arrows)*, each surrounded by its own amnion (one amniotic membrane is designated by *arrowheads*, the other by *short arrows*).

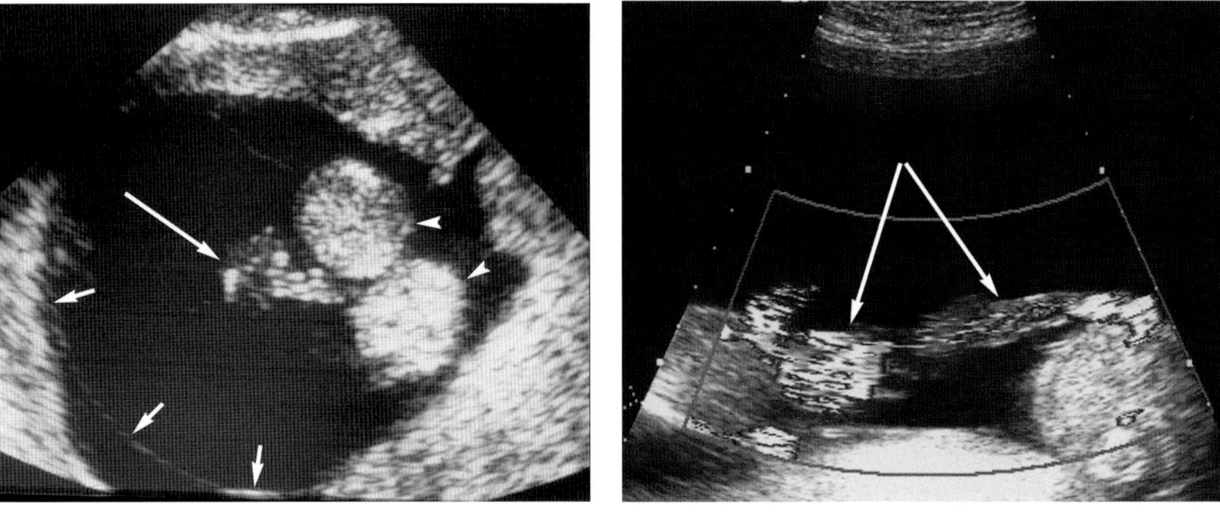

FIGURE 19.2-4. Monoamniotic twins diagnosed in the first trimester. A: Sonogram at 11 weeks gestation demonstrates two fetal abdomens *(arrowheads)*, with intermingling of the two umbilical cords *(long arrow)* and a single amniotic membrane *(short arrows)* surrounding both fetuses. **B:** On a subsequent sonogram at 22 weeks gestation, color Doppler better demonstrates intermingling of the twin umbilical cords *(arrows)*.

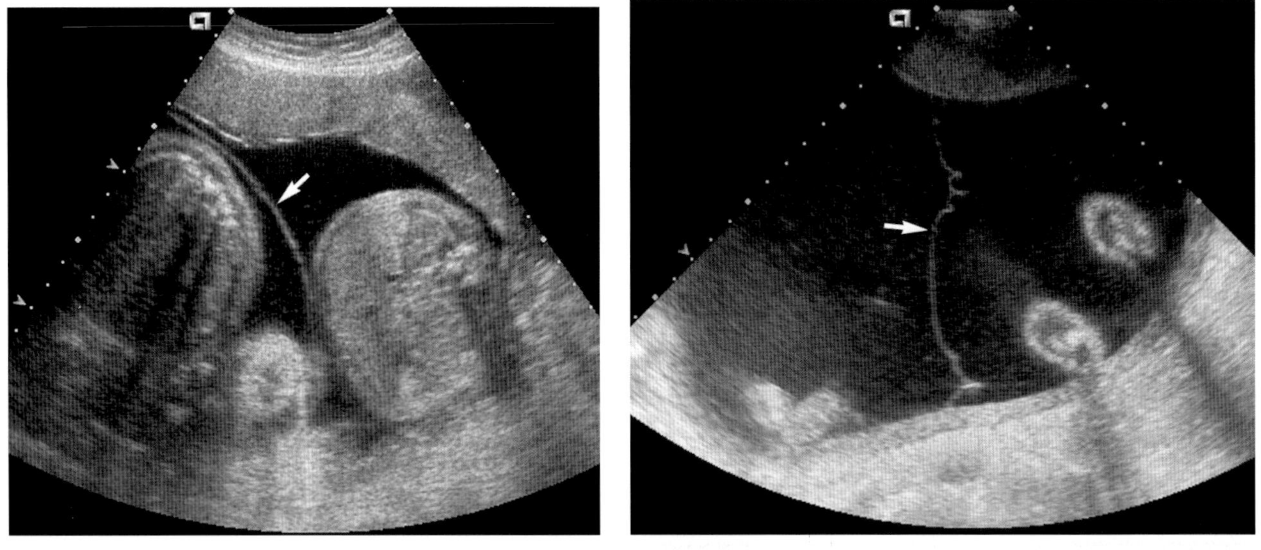

FIGURE 19.2-5. Determination of chorionicity via membrane thickness in second-trimester diamniotic twins. A: Dichorionicity: Sonogram demonstrates a twin gestation in which the two fetuses are separated by a relatively thick membrane *(arrow)*, suggesting that they are dichorionic. **B:** Monoamnionicity: In this case, the separating membrane *(arrow)* is very thin, suggesting that they are monochorionic.

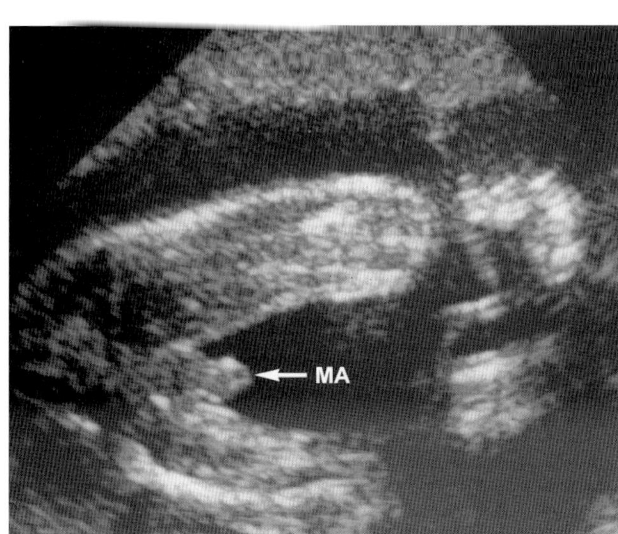

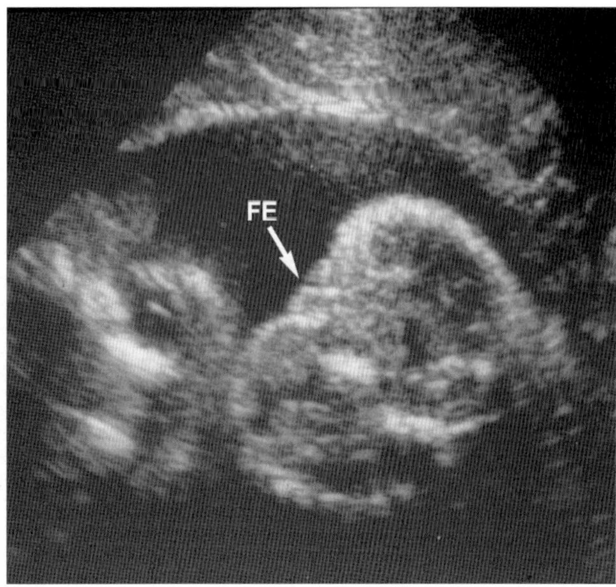

FIGURE 19.2-6. Diagnosis of dichorionicity based on different fetal sexes. Sonographic depiction of genitalia *(arrows)* demonstrates that one twin is male *(MA)* **(A)** and the other is female *(FE)* **(B)**. Because they are of different sexes, they must be dizygotic and hence dichorionic.

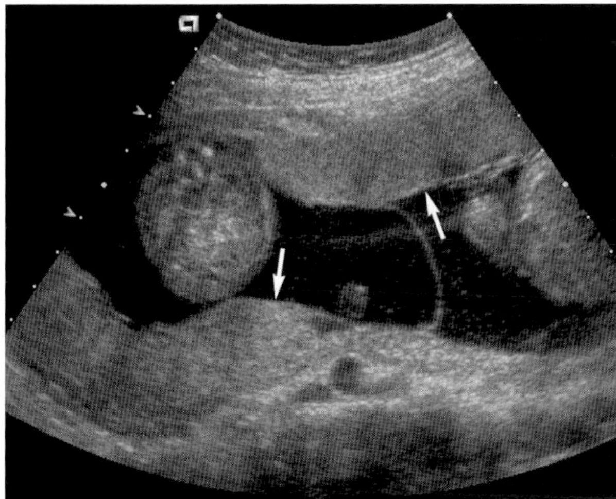

FIGURE 19.2-7. Diagnosis of dichorionicity based on separate placentas. Each twin has its own placenta *(arrows)*, indicating that the twins are dichorionic.

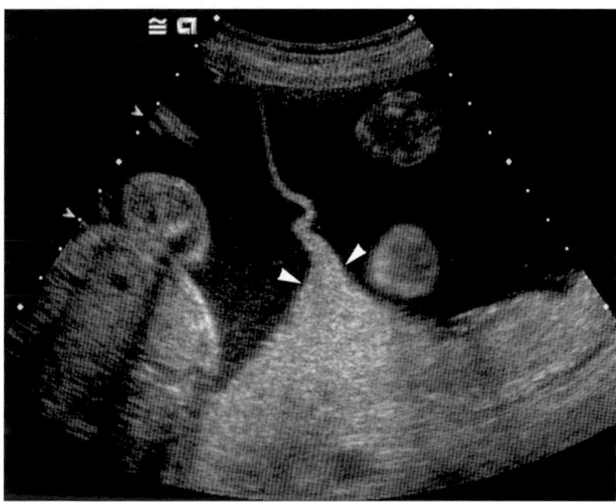

FIGURE 19.2-8. Diagnosis of dichorionicity based on the "delta" sign. There is a triangular wedge of placental tissue extending into the intertwin membrane *(arrowheads)*. This finding has been termed the "delta" (or "twin peak") sign and indicates a high likelihood of dichorionicity.

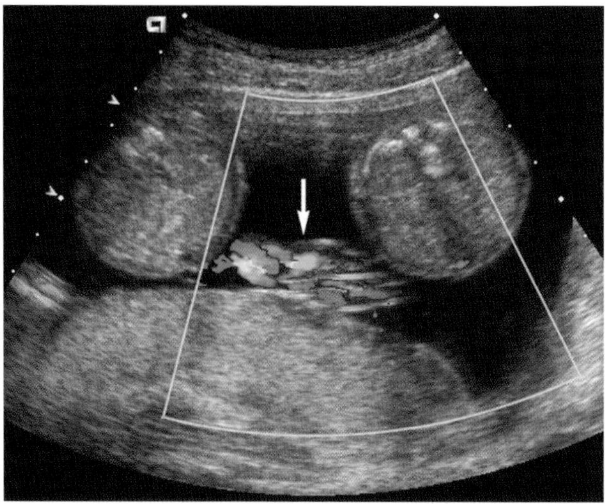

FIGURE 19.2-9. Monoamniotic twins in the second trimester. Twin gestation with intermingling of the twin umbilical cords *(arrow)* and no visible dividing membrane, indicative of a monoamniotic gestation.

if several findings are all present: a single placental mass is seen, the twins are of the same sex, and a very thin membrane is seen between them.

Second- and third-trimester twins are diamniotic if a membrane (thick or thin) can be identified between them, if they are of different sexes, or if they have separate placentas. Monoamnionicity can be diagnosed if none of these findings is present, and there is intermingling of the umbilical cords (Figure 19.2-9). If twins are of the same sex (or the sex of each cannot be determined), no membrane is visualized, there is a single placental mass, and the umbilical cords do not intermingle, it is indeterminate whether the twins are monoamniotic or diamniotic.

For triplets and higher order multiple gestations, the approach to determining placentation type by sonography is analogous to that for twins (Figures 19.2-10 and 19.2-11).

A

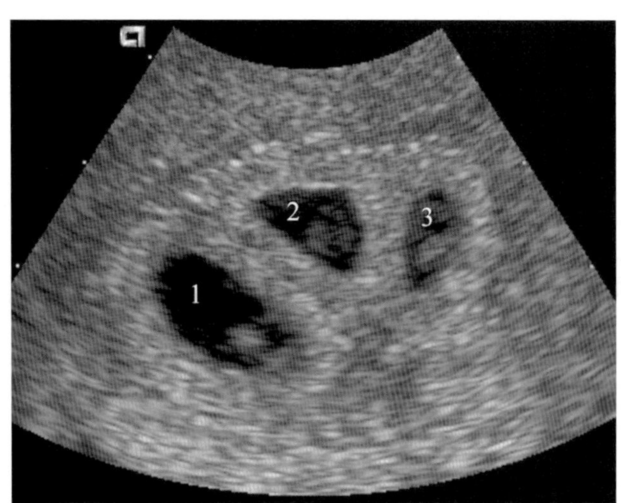

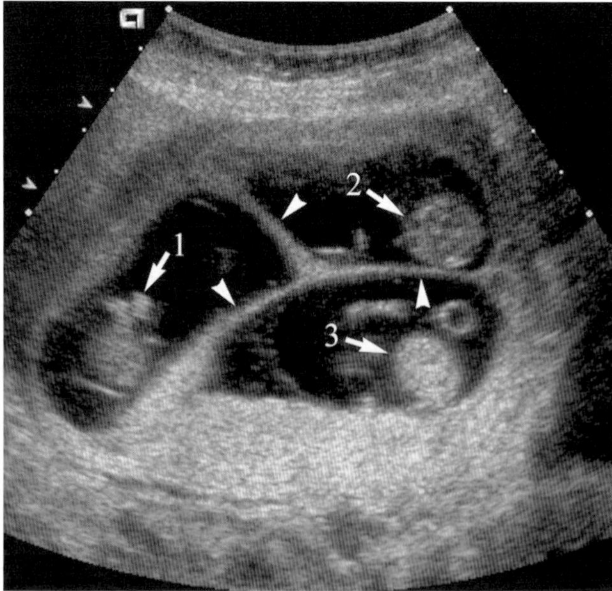

B

FIGURE 19.2-10. Trichorionic triamniotic triplets. A: Sonogram at 6 weeks gestation demonstrates three gestational sacs *(1, 2, and 3)* separated by thick bands of tissue. **B:** Sonogram at 12 weeks gestation in another pregnancy demonstrates three fetuses *(1, 2, and 3)* separated from one another by thick membranes *(arrowheads)*.

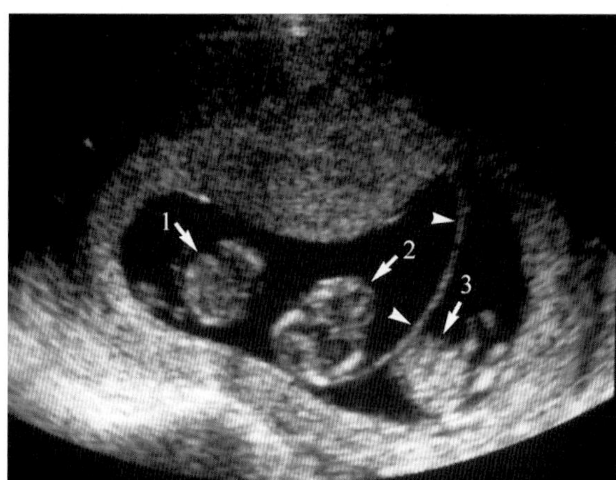

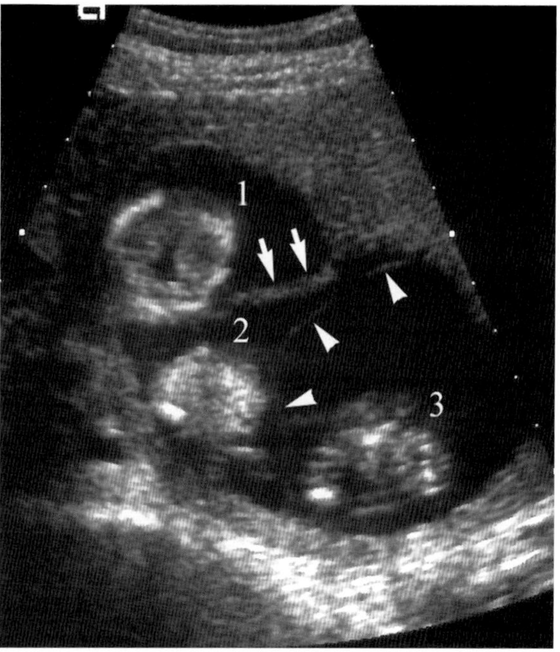

A B

FIGURE 19.2-11. Dichorionic triamniotic triplets. A: Sonogram at 13 weeks gestation demonstrates three fetuses *(1, 2, and 3)*. Fetuses 1 and 2 have no membrane visible between them on this image, but a thin membrane was identified on other images. There is a thick membrane *(arrowheads)* separating these two fetuses from fetus 3. **B:** Sonogram of another triplet gestation at 14 weeks demonstrates three fetuses *(1, 2, and 3)*. Fetuses 2 and 3 have a thin membrane *(arrowheads)* between them, and there is a thick membrane *(arrows)* separating these two fetuses from fetus 1.

SUGGESTED READINGS

1. Barth RA, Crowe HC. Ultrasound evaluation of multifetal gestations. In: Callen PW, ed. *Ultrasonography in obstetrics and gynecology*, 4th ed. Philadelphia: WB Saunders, 2000:171–205.
2. Benson CB, Doubilet PM, Laks MP. Outcome of twin gestations following a first trimester ultrasound demonstrating two heartbeats. *Ultrasound Obstet Gynecol* 1993;3:343–345.
3. Benson CB, Doubilet PM. Multiple gestations. *Ultrasound Q* 1998;14:234–246.
4. Benson CB, Doubilet PM. Twin pregnancy. In: McGahan JP, Goldberg BB, eds. *Diagnostic ultrasound: a logical approach*. Philadelphia: Lippincott–Raven, 1998:483–494.
5. Bromley BS, Benacerraf BR. Using the number of yolk sacs to determine amnionicity in early first trimester monochorionic twins. *J Ultrasound Med* 1995;14:415–419.
6. Doubilet PM, Benson CB. The "appearing twin": undercounting of multiple gestations on early first trimester sonograms. *J Ultrasound Med* 1998;17:199–203.
7. Filly RA, Goldstein RB, Callen PW. Monochorionic twinning: sonographic assessment. *AJR Am J Roentgenol* 1991;154:459–469.
8. Finberg HJ. The "twin peak" sign: reliable evidence of dichorionic twinning. *J Ultrasound Med* 1992;11:571–577.
9. Hertzberg BS, Kurtz AB, Choi HY, et al. Significance of membrane thickness in the sonographic evaluation of twin gestations. *AJR Am J Roentgenol* 1987;148:151–153.
10. Kurtz AB, Wapner RJ, Mata J, et al. Twin pregnancies: accuracy of first-trimester abdominal ultrasound in predicting chorionicity and amnionicity. *Radiology* 1992;185:759–762.
11. Nyberg DA, Filly RA, Golbus MS, et al. Entangled umbilical cords: a sign of monoamniotic twins. *J Ultrasound Med* 1984;3:29–32.
12. Sampson A, Ch. de Crespigny L. Vanishing twins: the frequency of spontaneous fetal reduction of a twin pregnancy. *Ultrasound Obstet Gynecol* 1992;2:107–109.
13. Townsend RR, Filly RA. Sonography of nonconjoined monoamniotic twin pregnancies. *J Ultrasound Med* 1988;7:665–670.
14. Townsend RR, Simpson GF, Filly RA. Membrane thickness in ultrasound prediction of chorionicity of twin gestations. *J Ultrasound Med* 1988;7:327–332.

20

COMPLICATIONS OF MULTIPLE GESTATIONS

20.1. TWIN-TWIN TRANSFUSION SYNDROME

Description and Clinical Features

Twin-twin transfusion syndrome is a complication of monochorionic twinning, resulting from unbalanced shunting of blood from one twin (the donor) to the other (the recipient) through arteriovenous anastomoses in their common placenta. The donor twin is anemic and growth restricted, whereas the recipient is polycythemic. In severe cases, the recipient may be hydropic.

Twin-twin transfusion syndrome occurs in approximately 10% of monochorionic twins. Complications may arise in the donor as a result of anemia and growth restriction and in the recipient due to high-output congestive heart failure. The mortality rate is high for both the donor and recipient twins, ranging from 40% to 87% in various studies. Treatment options include therapeutic amniocentesis from the sac of the recipient twin and endoscopically guided laser photocoagulation of communicating placental vessels. Use of the former treatment in mild to moderate cases of twin-twin transfusion syndrome and the latter in severe cases appears to increase the likelihood of the pregnancy resulting in at least one surviving fetus.

A
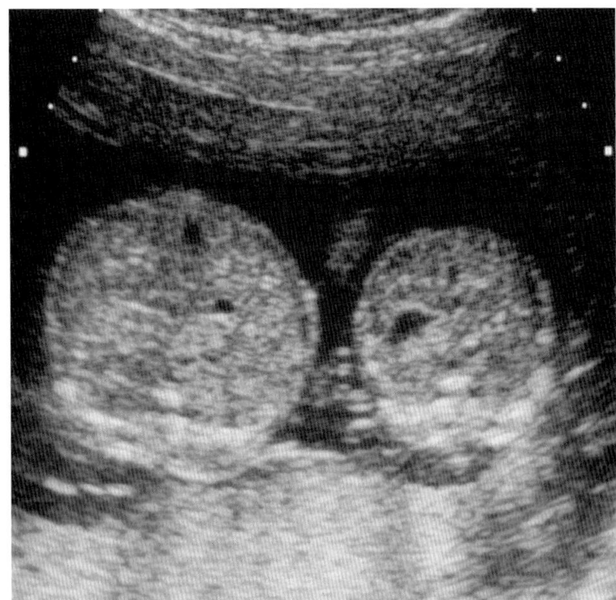
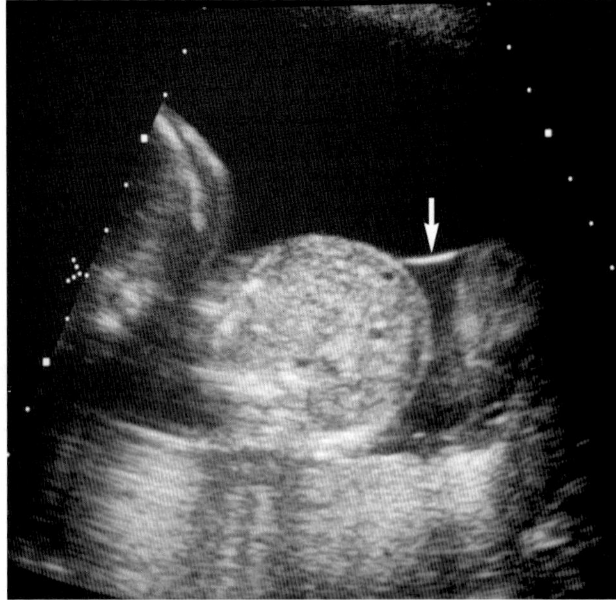
B

FIGURE 20.1-1. Twin-twin transfusion syndrome. A: Transverse view of the abdomens of monochorionic twins demonstrates a marked difference in size. **B:** There is oligohydramnios in the smaller twin's sac, with the intertwin membrane *(arrow)* closely applied to that fetus, and polyhydramnios in the larger twin's sac.

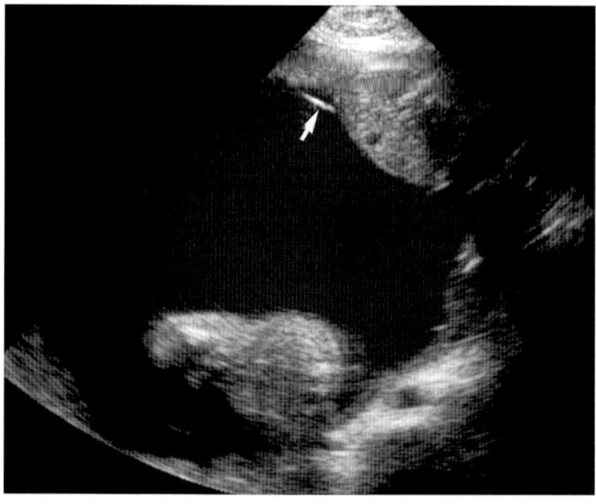

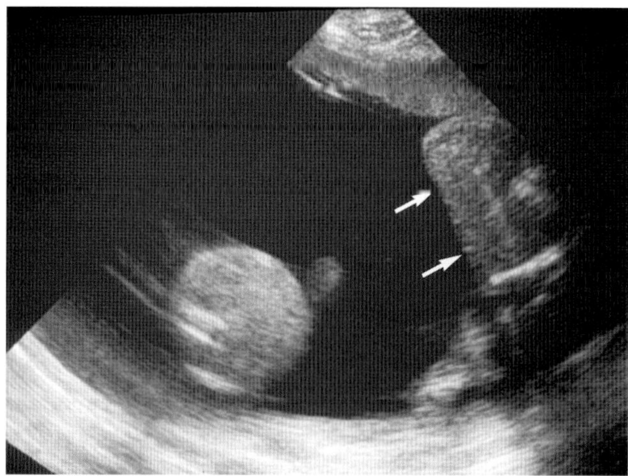

FIGURE 20.1-2. Twin-twin transfusion syndrome with a "stuck" twin. A: In this twin gestation, the intertwin membrane *(arrow)* is very closely applied to one twin's abdomen. This twin is termed a "stuck twin" because it is pressed against the uterine wall by the membrane and by the severe polyhydramnios in the co-twin's sac. **B:** The anterior abdominal wall of the stuck twin is flattened *(arrows)* by the membrane and polyhydramnios.

Sonography

The sonographic diagnosis of twin-twin transfusion syndrome is typically made when three findings are present (Figure 20.1-1):

Discrepant amniotic fluid volumes: Oligohydramnios in the smaller (donor) twin's sac, polyhydramnios in the larger (recipient) twin's sac. In severe cases, there is so little fluid around the donor twin that it is held fixed against the uterine wall by the intertwin membrane ("stuck twin") (Figure 20.1-2).

Discordant fetal size: Best defined as a difference in estimated weights of more than 25% of the larger twin's estimated weight (at or beyond 24 weeks gestation).

Monochorionic placentation (Note: If dichorionic twins are discordant in size, the leading diagnostic possibility is intrauterine growth restriction of the smaller twin).

In approximately 10% of cases of twin-twin transfusion syndrome, the recipient twin is hydropic (Figure 20.1-3).

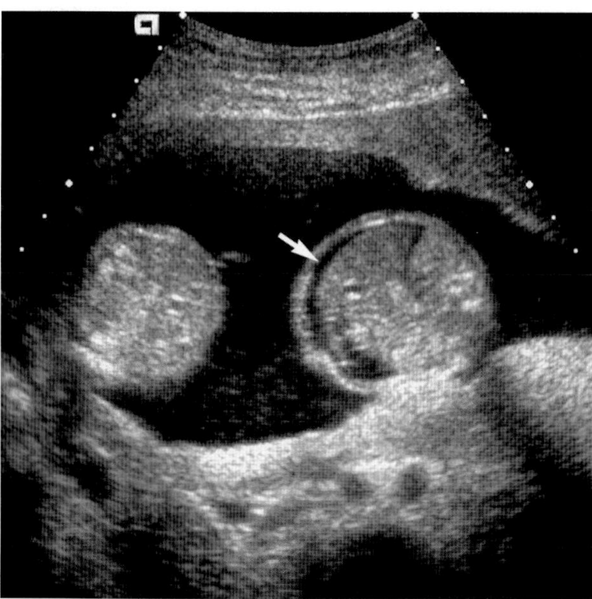

FIGURE 20.1-3. Twin-twin transfusion syndrome with a hydropic recipient twin. In this monochorionic twin gestation, the two fetal abdomens differ markedly in size, and there is ascites *(arrow)* in the abdomen of the larger twin.

20.2. ACARDIAC TWINNING

Description and Clinical Features

Acardiac twinning is a rare form of twinning in monochorionic gestations. It occurs as a result of large artery-to-artery and vein-to-vein anastomoses across the common placenta, which disrupt the hemodynamic balance between the twins, such that the cardiovascular system of one twin takes over the cardiovascular system of its co-twin. The twin whose cardiovascular system takes over is termed the pump twin, and the other twin, whose heart usually fails to develop, is termed the acardiac twin. The pump twin's heart propels blood through its umbilical arteries into the placenta and forces blood across the artery-to-artery anastomoses. This arterial blood then travels in a reverse direction, from the placenta through the acardiac twin's umbilical artery back to the acardiac twin. The acardiac twin receives its oxygen and nutrition from the incoming arterial blood that originated in the pump twin. Blood travels passively through the acardiac twin and returns through its umbilical vein to the placenta, where it crosses the vein-to-vein anastomoses back to the pump twin. The acardiac twin usually has a two-vessel cord, an abnormal or absent head, and only rudimentary upper extremities. The lower half of its body tends to be more normally formed, often with normal-appearing spine, kidneys, bladder, and lower extremities. The entire acardiac twin is typically surrounded by massive skin edema, particular in the upper portion of the body. The acardiac twin continues to grow during gestation.

The prognosis for the pump twin is related to whether this twin develops congestive heart failure *in utero* and to the size of the acardiac twin. Large acardiac twins may receive a large amount of blood, forcing the pump twin to increase cardiac output significantly. This can lead to hydrops or demise of the pump twin. Overall, the survival rate of pump twins is approximately 50%. The prognosis can be improved if the umbilical cord of the acardiac twin is ligated or occluded with laser before the pump twin has high-output heart failure.

The amnionicity of an acardiac twin gestation may be monoamniotic or diamniotic.

Sonography

Acardiac twinning is characterized by a monochorionic twin gestation in which one twin, the pump twin, is normally formed and the co-twin, the acardiac twin, is markedly abnor-

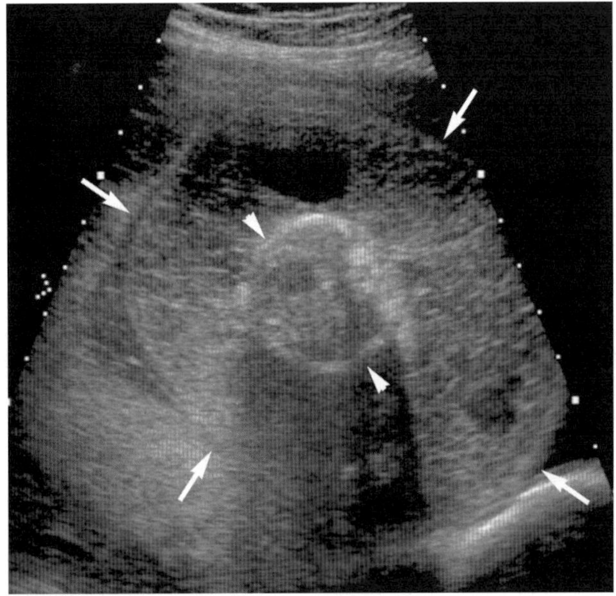

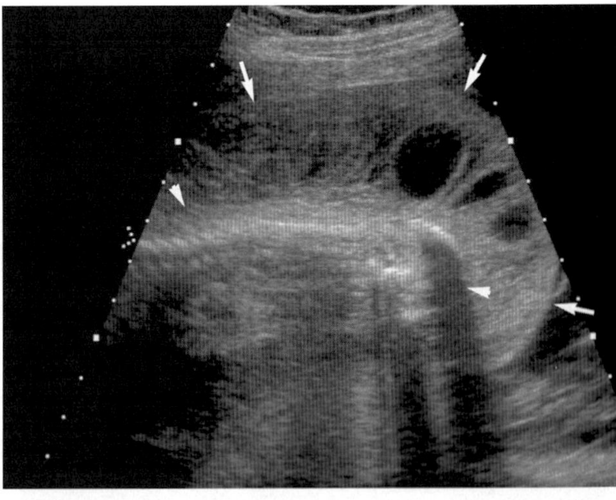

FIGURE 20.2-1. Acardiac twin. A: Transverse view of an acardiac twin demonstrates that the abdomen *(arrowheads)* is surrounded by massive skin edema *(arrows)*. **B:** Sagittal image shows marked skin thickening *(arrows)* around a small body *(arrowheads)*.

mal. The acardiac twin is incompletely formed, often missing the upper trunk, upper extremities, and head, and is encased by massive skin edema (Figure 20.2-1). Usually, no beating heart is found, although, in rare cases, a rudimentary heart is seen beating in the thorax (Figure 20.2-2). Its umbilical cord typically has only two vessels. The pathognomonic finding in these cases is reversed flow in the umbilical artery and vein of the acardiac twin. Umbilical arterial blood flows toward the acardiac twin and umbilical venous blood flows away from the anomalous twin toward the placenta (Figure 20.2-3).

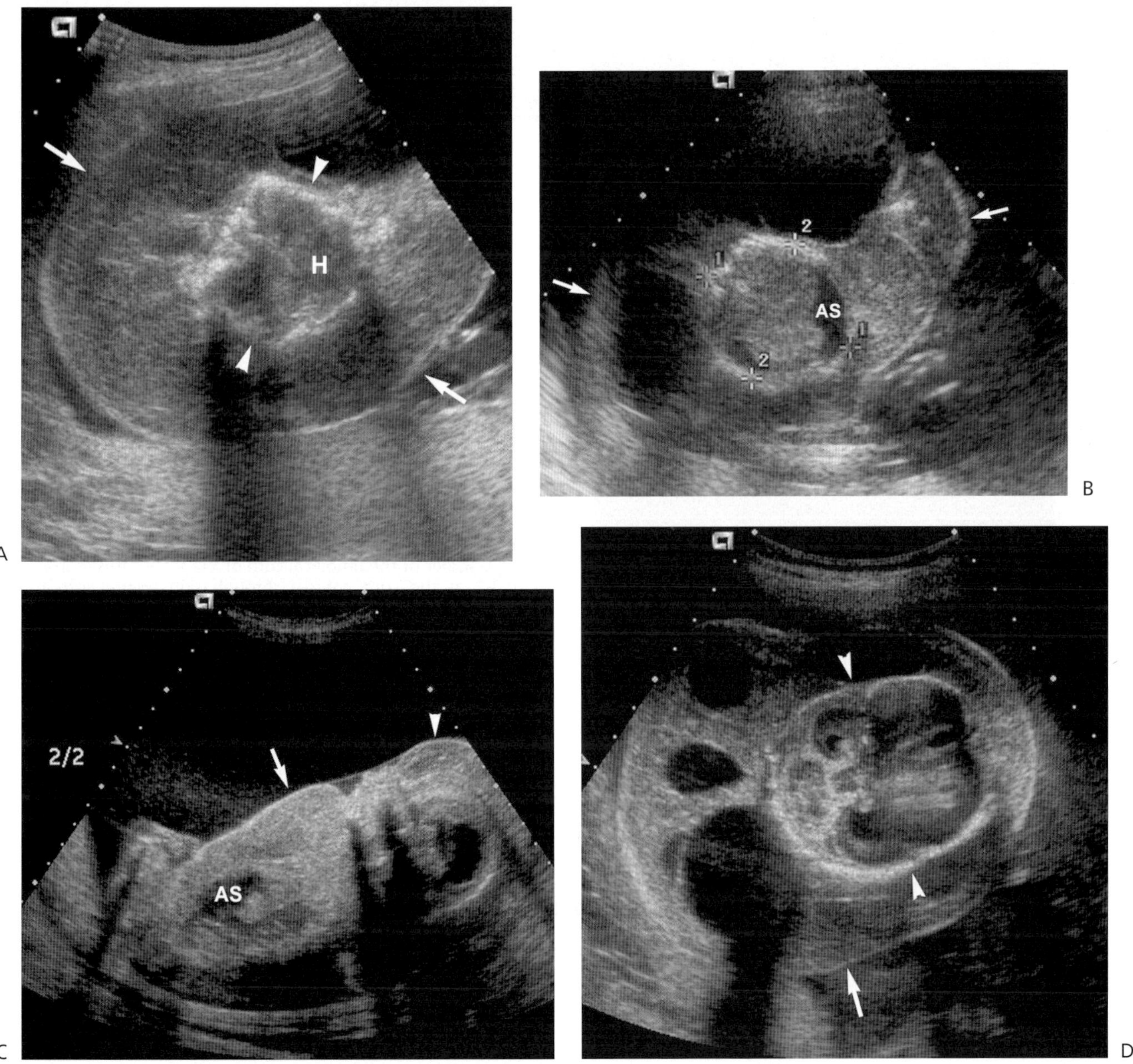

FIGURE 20.2-2. Acardiac twin with a rudimentary heart. A: Transverse image of the thorax *(arrowheads)* of an acardiac twin surrounded by massive skin thickening. A rudimentary heart *(H)* was seen beating. **B:** Transverse view of the fetal abdomen *(calipers)* shows massive skin edema *(arrows)* filled with fluid spaces. Ascites *(AS)* is also seen inside the abdomen. **C:** Sagittal image of the acardiac twin shows marked skin thickening over the thorax *(arrow)* and an abnormally formed head *(arrowhead)*. Ascites *(AS)* is again seen in the abdomen. **D:** Transverse image of the head *(arrowheads)* of the acardiac twin that contains an abnormally formed brain and is surrounded by marked skin thickening *(arrow)*.

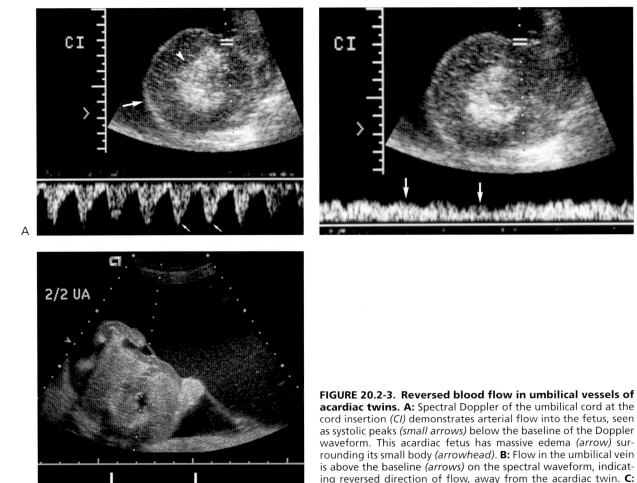

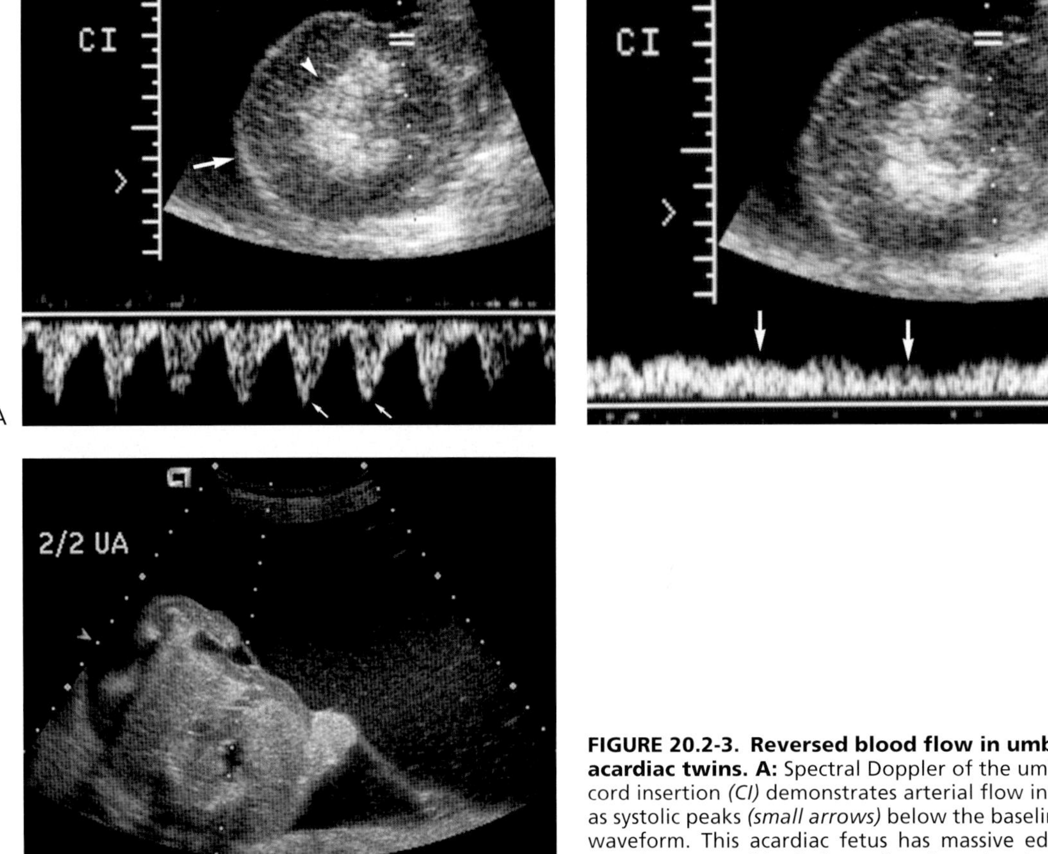

FIGURE 20.2-3. Reversed blood flow in umbilical vessels of acardiac twins. A: Spectral Doppler of the umbilical cord at the cord insertion *(CI)* demonstrates arterial flow into the fetus, seen as systolic peaks *(small arrows)* below the baseline of the Doppler waveform. This acardiac fetus has massive edema *(arrow)* surrounding its small body *(arrowhead)*. **B:** Flow in the umbilical vein is above the baseline *(arrows)* on the spectral waveform, indicating reversed direction of flow, away from the acardiac twin. **C:** Spectral Doppler of the umbilical cord of the same fetus as in Figure 20.2-2 as the cord courses through skin edema into the abdomen demonstrates reversed direction of flow in the umbilical vessels. The venous flow is away from the fetus, above the baseline on the Doppler waveform *(arrows)*, and arterial flow is toward the fetus, below the baseline on the waveform *(arrowheads)*.

The pump twin usually appears normal, unless it develops hydrops from high-output congestive heart failure.

20.3. CONJOINED TWINS

Description and Clinical Features

Conjoined twins result from the late splitting of a single fertilized egg, typically when the splitting occurs more than 12 days after conception. Various sites of union can occur, including:

Thoracopagus: joined at the thorax
Omphalopagus: joined at the anterior abdominal wall
Craniopagus: joined at the skull
Ischiopagus: joined at the pelvis

The prognosis of conjoined twins depends primarily on the nature and extent of organ sharing.

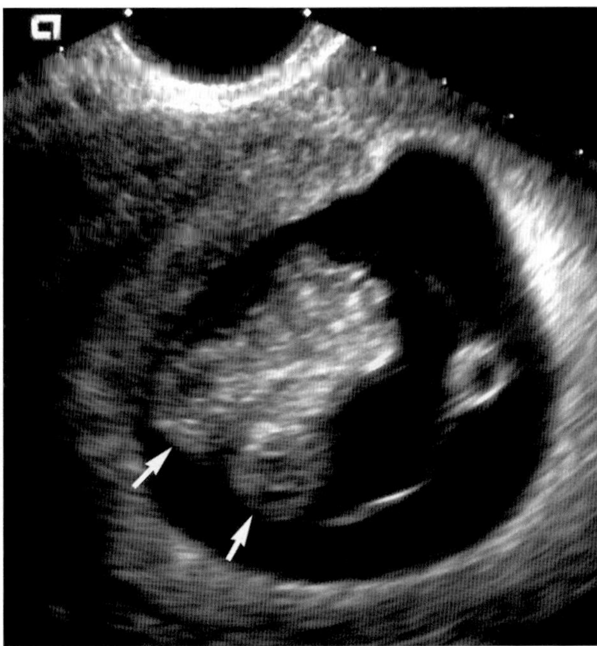

FIGURE 20.3-1. Conjoined twins at 11 weeks. Twins with separate heads *(arrows)* joined at their trunks.

Sonography

Conjoined twins are diagnosed by sonography by demonstrating continuity of the bodies of the twins. Careful evaluation may be needed to distinguish conjoined twins from monoamniotic twins whose bodies are contiguous but separate.

Sonography plays an important role in the diagnosis and evaluation of conjoined twins. The diagnosis of conjoined twins can be made in the first trimester (Figure 20.3-1), but the precise determination of organ sharing cannot usually be made until the second trimester (Figures 20.3-2 and 20.3-3). This information is useful for selecting the route of

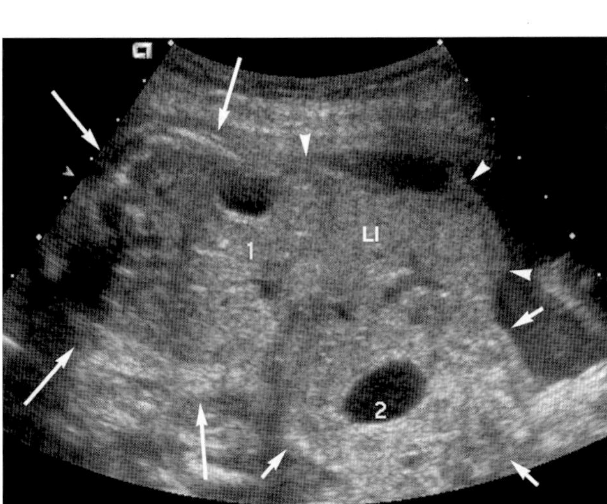

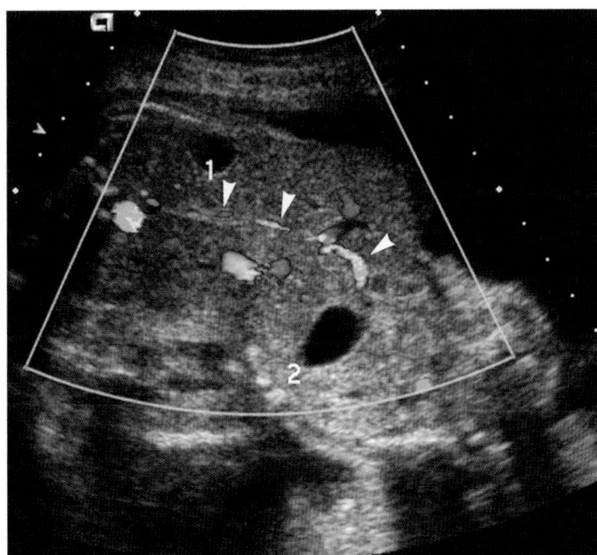

FIGURE 20.3-2. Conjoined twins with an omphalocele and a fused liver. A: Transverse view through the abdomens of twin 1 *(long arrows)* and twin 2 *(short arrows)* demonstrates that they are joined at their anterior abdominal walls and have a fused liver *(LI)*, with part of the liver herniated into an omphalocele sac *(arrowheads)*. **B:** A common blood vessel *(arrowheads)* communicates between the two fetuses through the fused liver. *(continued)*

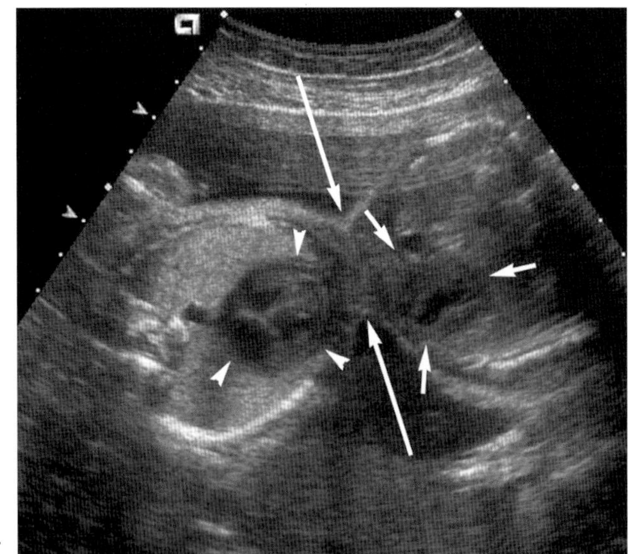
C

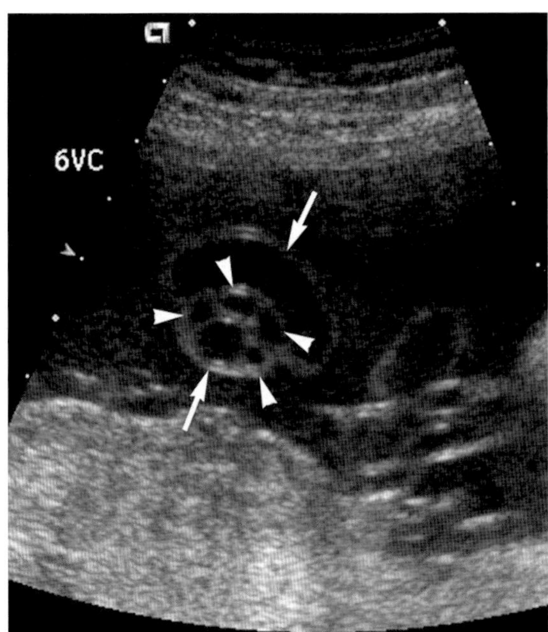

D

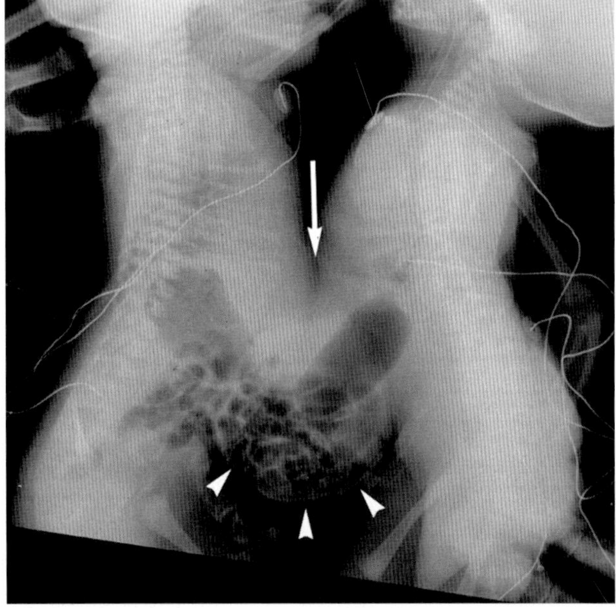
E

FIGURE 20.3-2. ***(continued)*** **C:** Transverse section through the twin lower thoraces demonstrates that the anterior subcutaneous tissues are joined *(long arrows)*, but their hearts *(arrowheads and short arrows)* are separate. **D:** The umbilical cord has six vessels *(6VC)*, including two veins *(arrows)* and four arteries *(arrowheads)*. **E:** Postnatal x-ray demonstrates joining from the lower thorax *(arrow)* to the omphalocele *(arrowheads)* in the mid abdomen.

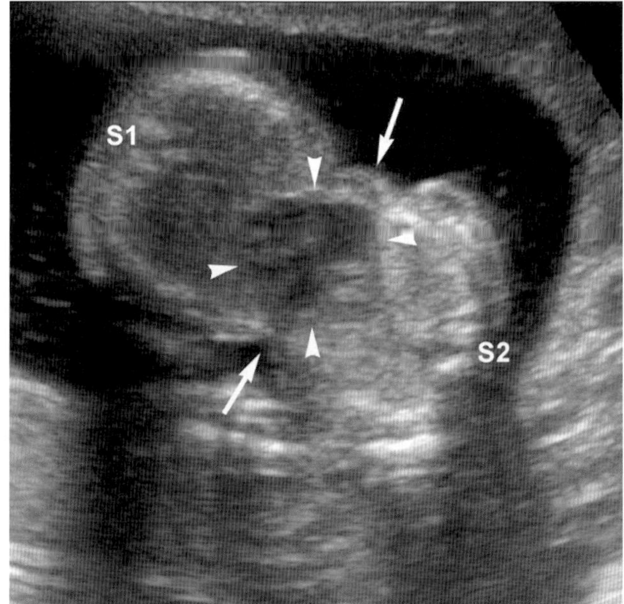

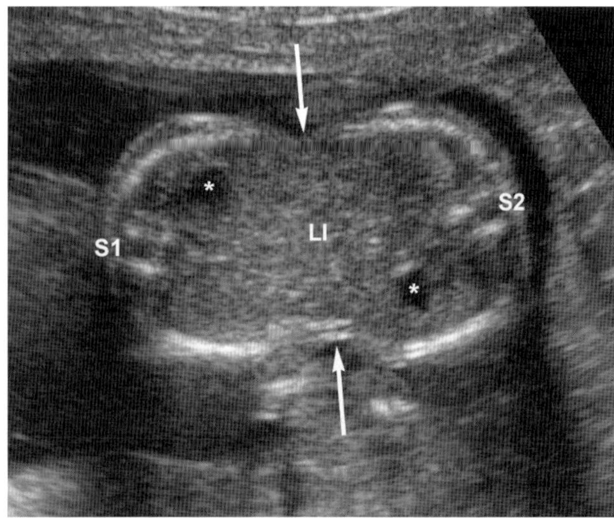

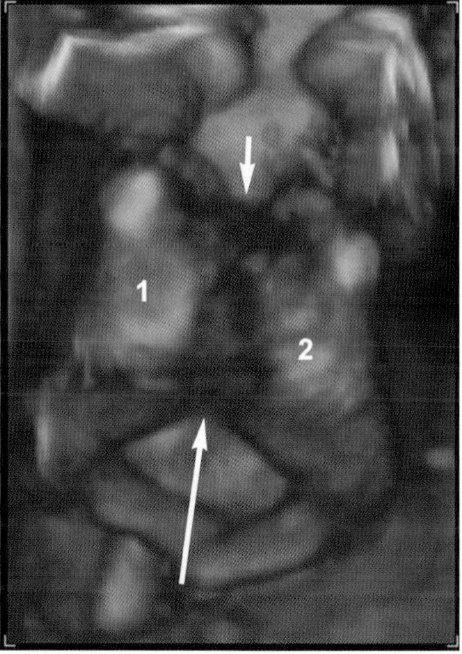

FIGURE 20.3-3. Conjoined twins sharing a heart and liver. A: Transverse view through twin thoraces *(S1, spine of twin 1; S2, spine of twin 2)* demonstrates that they are joined anteriorly *(arrows)* and share a heart *(arrowheads)*. **B:** Transverse view through the twin abdomens *(S1, spine of twin 1; S2, spine of twin 2; *, stomachs)* demonstrates that they are joined anteriorly *(arrows)* and share a liver (LI). **C:** Three-dimensional sonogram with surface rendering demonstrates fetuses 1 and 2 joined anteriorly from the thorax *(small arrow)* to the abdomen *(large arrow)*. (Courtesy of Dr. Beryl Benacerraf.)

delivery, determining prognosis, and getting an early start on surgical planning for separating the twins.

20.4. DEATH OF ONE TWIN *IN UTERO*

Description and Clinical Features

When one twin dies *in utero*, the prognosis for the surviving co-twin depends on the chorionicity of the twin gestation and the gestational age at which death occurs. When one twin of a dichorionic pair dies, there are usually no sequelae to the surviving co-twin. The dead twin will be completely resorbed ("vanishing twin") if death occurs by approximately 10 weeks gestation and partially resorbed if death occurs later.

The prognosis is worse when the twins are monochorionic, because such twins frequently have vascular anastomoses through their common placenta. Death of one of a monochorionic pair in the first trimester often leads to the subsequent death of the co-twin. Death of one of a monochorionic pair during the second trimester may lead to ischemic damage to the survivor's brain, gastrointestinal tract, or other organs, a complication termed twin embolization syndrome. This term may be a misnomer because the ischemic damage to the surviving twin may be due to hypotension at the time of death of its co-twin, as opposed to emboli from the dead co-twin.

Sonography

Ultrasound can diagnose the death of one twin and, when clinically appropriate, monitor the status of the surviving co-twin. When one of a dichorionic pair dies in the first trimester, the dead fetus will remain visible sonographically for a few weeks, but within 1–2 weeks will be smaller than its live co-twin and have less fluid around it (Figure 20.4-1). On subsequent scans, there may be little or no sonographic evidence of the dead fetus. When one of a dichorionic pair dies in the second trimester (Figure 20.4-2), the dead fetus will remain visible throughout gestation, becoming a small, thin remnant of its original body.

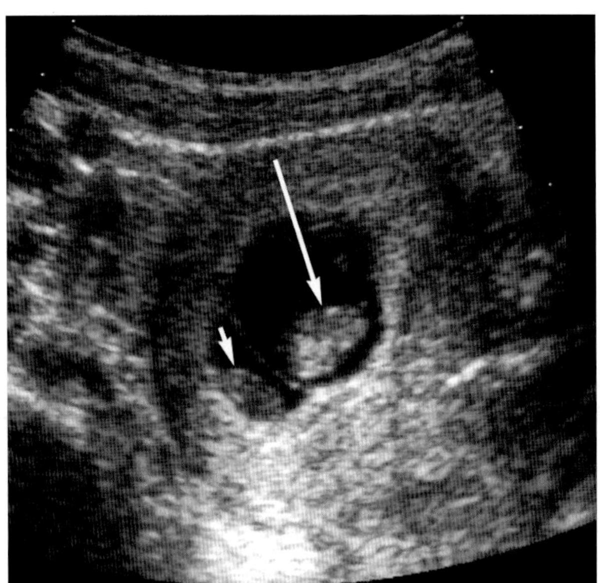

FIGURE 20.4-1. Death of one twin in the first trimester. Twin gestation with one live fetus *(long arrow)* and a smaller dead fetus *(short arrow)*. On follow-up sonograms, the live fetus developed normally, whereas the dead fetus was completely resorbed.

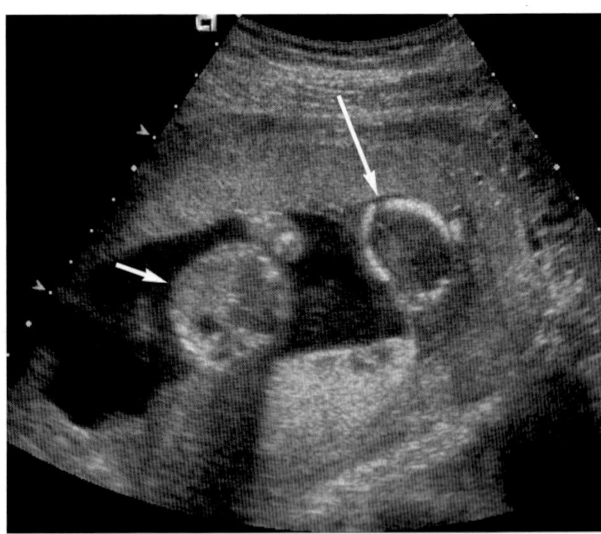

FIGURE 20.4-2. Death of one twin in the second trimester. Twin gestation with one live fetus *(short arrow)* and the skull of a dead fetus *(long arrow)*. There is oligohydramnios in the sac of the dead fetus, and its skull has overlapping bones.

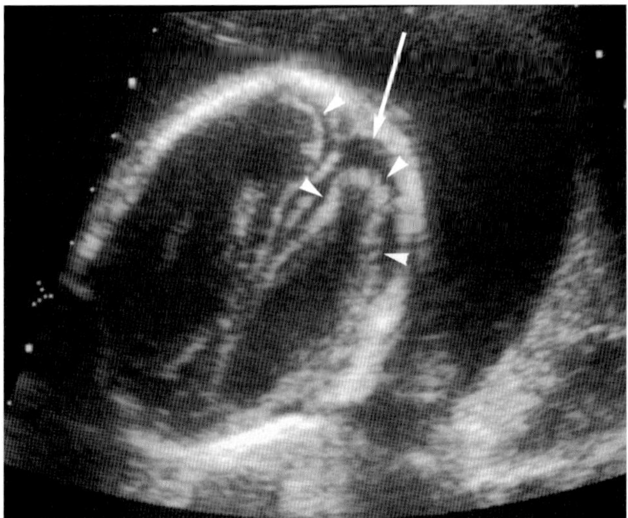
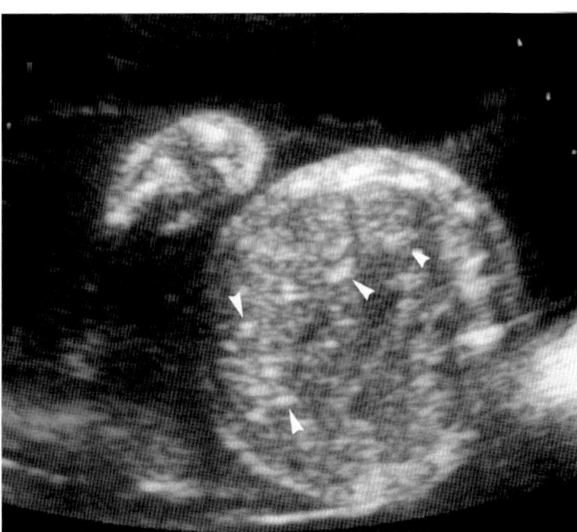

A B

FIGURE 20.4-3. Twin embolization syndrome. A: Axial image of the head of a 23 week twin whose monochorionic co-twin died a week earlier demonstrates an irregular cortical contour *(arrowheads)* and increased extra-axial space *(arrow)* due to cerebral atrophy. **B:** Transverse view of the fetal abdomen of the surviving twin demonstrates a mottled heterogeneous hepatic echotexture with focal areas of increased echogenicity *(arrowheads)*, indicating multiple infarcts. (From Benson CB, Doubilet PM. Sonograph of multile gestations. *Radiologist* 1994;1:147–154, with permission.)

When one of a monochorionic twin pair dies during the second trimester, the co-twin should be monitored sonographically for signs of ischemic damage. Sonographic findings of such damage include focal or diffuse lesions in the brain, gastrointestinal tract, liver, or other structures in the surviving co-twin. In particular, cerebral cortical thinning and ventricular dilation may be seen in the brain, and the liver may display focal areas of altered echogenicity or calcifications (Figure 20.4-3).

SUGGESTED READINGS

1. Anderson RL, Golbus MS, Curry CJR, et al. Central nervous system damage and other anomalies in surviving fetus following second trimester antenatal death of co-twin. *Prenat Diagn* 1990;10: 513–518.
2. Barth VA, Filly RA, Goldberg JD, et al. Conjoined twins: prenatal diagnosis and assessment of associated malformations. *Radiology* 1990;177:201–207.
3. Barth RA, Crowe HC. Ultrasound evaluation of multifetal gestations. In: Callen PW, ed. *Ultrasonography in obstetrics and gynecology*, 4th ed. Philadelphia: WB Saunders, 2000:171–205.
4. Benson CB, Bieber FR, Genest DR, et al. Doppler demonstration of reversed umbilical blood flow in an acardiac twin. *J Clin Ultrasound* 1989;17:291–295.
5. Benson CB, Doubilet PM. Multiple gestations. *Ultrasound Q* 1998;14:234–246.
6. Brown DL, Benson CB, Driscoll SG, et al. Twin-twin transfusion syndrome: sonographic findings. *Radiology* 1989;170:61–63.
7. Caballero P, Del Campo L, Ocon E. Cystic encephalomalacia in twin embolization syndrome. *Radiology* 1991;178:892–893.
8. Campbell S, De Lia J, Fisk N, et al. Twin-to-twin transfusion syndrome--debates on the etiology, natural history and management. *Ultrasound Obstet Gynecol* 2000;16:210–213.
9. Gibson JY, D'Cruz CA, Patel RB, et al. Acardiac anomaly: review of the subject with case report and emphasis on practical sonography. *J Clin Ultrasound* 1986;14:541–545.
10. Kalchbrenner M, Weiner S, Templeton J, et al. Prenatal ultrasound diagnosis of thoracopagus conjoined twins. *J Clin Ultrasound* 1987;15:59–63.
11. Machin GA, Feldstein VA, Van Gemert MJC, et al. Doppler sonographic demonstration of arterio-venous anastomosis in monochorionic twin gestation. *Ultrasound Obstet Gynecol* 2000;16:214–217.
12. Papa T, Dao A, Bruner JP. Pathognomonic sign of twin reversed arterial perfusion using color Doppler sonography. *J Ultrasound Med* 1997;16:501–503.

13. Patten RM, Mack LA, Nyberg DA, et al. Twin embolization syndrome: sonographic detection and significance. *Radiology* 1989;173:685–689.
14. Quintero RA, Comas C, Bornick PW, et al. Selective versus non-selective laser photocoagulation of placental vessels in twin-to-twin transfusion syndrome. *Ultrasound Obstet Gynecol* 2000;16: 230–236.
15. Reisner DP, Mahony BS, Petty CN, et al. Stuck twin syndrome: outcome in thirty-seven consecutive cases. *Am J Obstet Gynecol* 1993;169:991–995.
16. Taylor MJO, Farquharson D, Cox PM, et al. Identification of arterio-venous anastomoses in vivo in monochorionic twin pregnancies: preliminary report. *Ultrasound Obstet Gynecol* 2000;16:218–222.
17. Urig MA, Clewell WH, Elliott JP. Twin-twin transfusion syndrome. *Am J Obstet Gynecol* 1990;163: 1522–1526.

21

DIAGNOSTIC OBSTETRICAL PROCEDURES

21.1. AMNIOCENTESIS

Description and Clinical Features

Amniocentesis is aspiration of amniotic fluid through a percutaneously inserted needle. This procedure is most commonly performed in the early to mid second trimester to determine the fetal karyotype. The karyotype is assessed by culturing fetal cells that have been shed into the amniotic fluid. It can also be performed for a variety of other diagnostic purposes, such as testing for levels of α-fetoprotein or acetylcholinesterase to assess risk of open neural tube defect, testing for fetal lung maturity, and checking for fetal hemoglobin breakdown products in cases of suspected hemolysis due to maternal antibodies to fetal blood. Less frequently, amniocentesis is performed therapeutically to reduce the amniotic fluid volume (e.g., to relieve maternal symptoms in a pregnancy complicated by polyhydramnios or to treat twin-twin transfusion syndrome by taking fluid from the recipient twin's sac).

Risks of amniocentesis include amniotic fluid leak, chorioamnionitis, and unexplained postprocedure fetal demise. The pregnancy loss rate after second-trimester amniocentesis has been estimated to be approximately 0.4% above the "background" loss rate.

Sonography

Although amniocentesis can be performed without ultrasound guidance (and, in fact, was done that way before the availability of ultrasound), the use of ultrasound to select a site, guide the needle insertion, and monitor the procedure is advisable. Before the needle is inserted, ultrasound is used to select a site that permits safe access to the fluid, avoiding

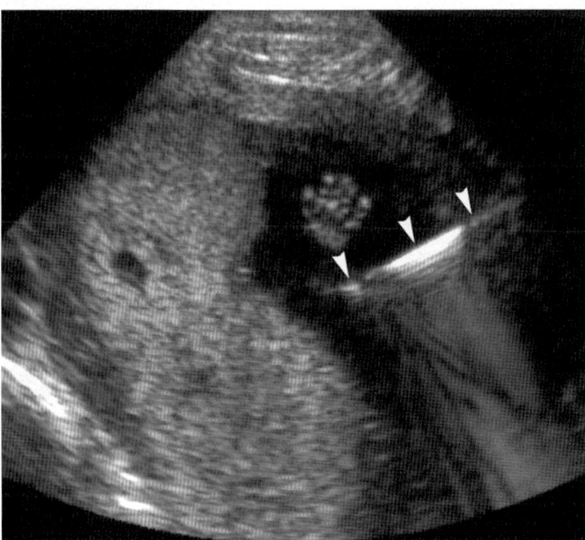

FIGURE 21.1-1. Ultrasound-guided amniocentesis. Ultrasound has been used to guide a needle *(arrowheads)* into the amniotic fluid.

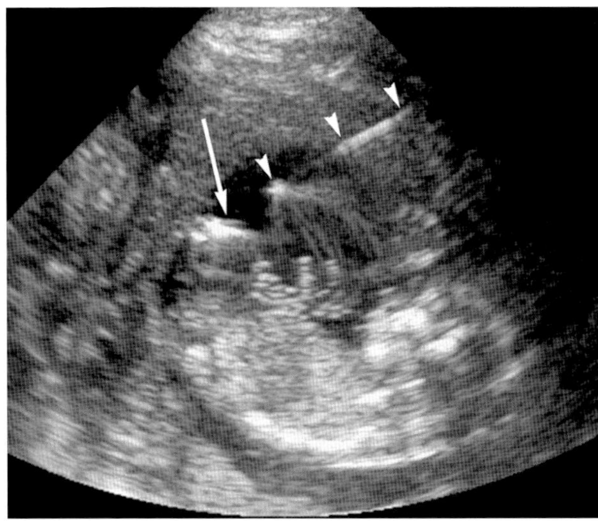

FIGURE 21.1-2. Continuous sonographic monitoring during amniocentesis. A fetal lower extremity *(arrow)* is in close proximity to the needle *(arrowheads)* during amniocentesis.

the fetus, umbilical cord, large uterine blood vessels, and, if possible, the placenta. Real-time guidance, with a sector, linear, or curvilinear transducer, is used to direct the needle into the site (Figure 21.1-1), and continuous real-time monitoring (Figure 21.1-2) is used throughout the procedure in case fetal movement or uterine contraction requires the needle position to be changed.

If the needle traverses the placenta, blood is often seen streaming from the placenta into the amniotic fluid as soon as the needle is removed (Figure 21.1-3). This placental bleeding usually stops within a short time and carries no sequelae, especially with amniocenteses performed before the third trimester.

A

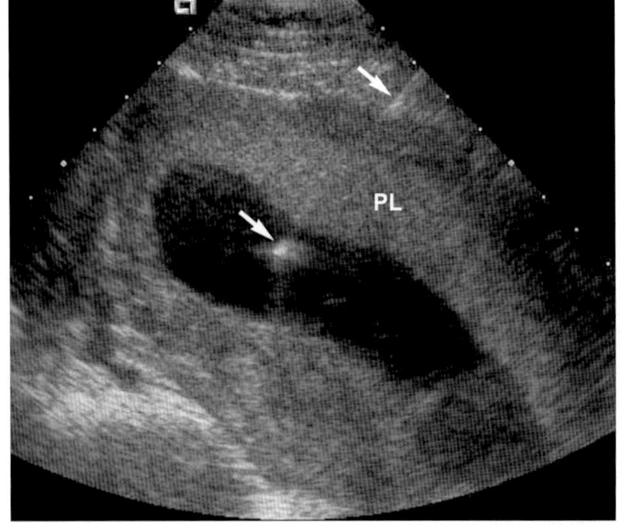

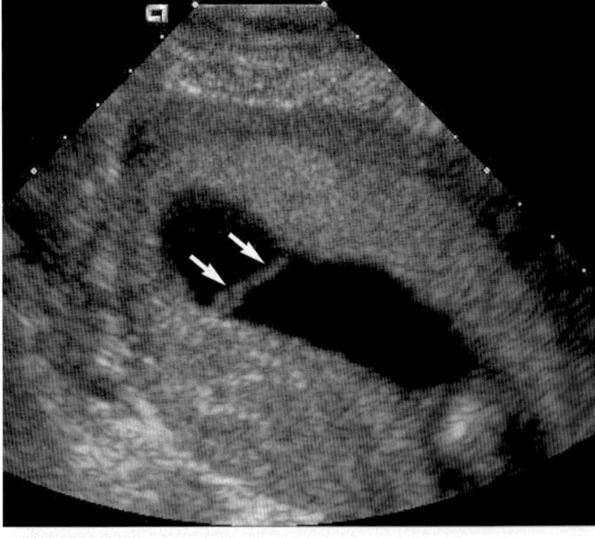

B

FIGURE 21.1-3. Ultrasound-guided amniocentesis through the anterior placenta. **A:** The amniocentesis needle *(arrows)* traverses the anterior placenta *(PL)*. **B:** After the needle was removed, streaming of blood *(arrows)* is seen into the amniotic cavity from the puncture site in the placenta. The bleeding stopped after approximately 30 seconds.

21.2. CHORIONIC VILLUS SAMPLING

Description and Clinical Features

In the mid first trimester, chorionic villi proliferate at the implantation site to form the chorion frondosum, which interdigitates with the maternal decidua basalis to form the placenta. Because the chorionic villi develop from the fertilized egg, these cells have the same genetic makeup as the fetus. Sampling and testing the villi, via direct examination of the mitotically active cytotrophoblasts and culture of the mesenchymal cells, provide chromosomal and biochemical information about the fetus.

Chorionic villus sampling (CVS) is usually performed at 10–12 weeks gestation, and karyotypic results are available within 1–7 days. CVS thus yields chromosomal information earlier in the pregnancy and more quickly than amniocentesis. Potential disadvantages of CVS include the following:

Pregnancy loss: Some studies suggest a slightly higher rate of pregnancy loss after CVS than amniocentesis, but the risks are difficult to compare because CVS is performed earlier in pregnancy when background loss rates are higher.

Inaccurate karyotype: The placenta and fetus can occasionally have different karyotypes. When this happens, CVS provides incorrect information about the fetal karyotype. Contamination of the sample by maternal decidual cells is another potential source of error.

Fetal malformations: An increased incidence of limb reduction anomalies after CVS has been reported. This risk appears to be restricted to CVS performed before 10 weeks gestation.

Sonography

CVS is performed under continuous ultrasound guidance. The procedure can be performed via one of two approaches:

Transabdominal (Figure 21.2-1): The needle is inserted percutaneously through the maternal abdominal wall and directed into the placenta. Suction is applied as the sampling device is moved back and forth through the placenta.

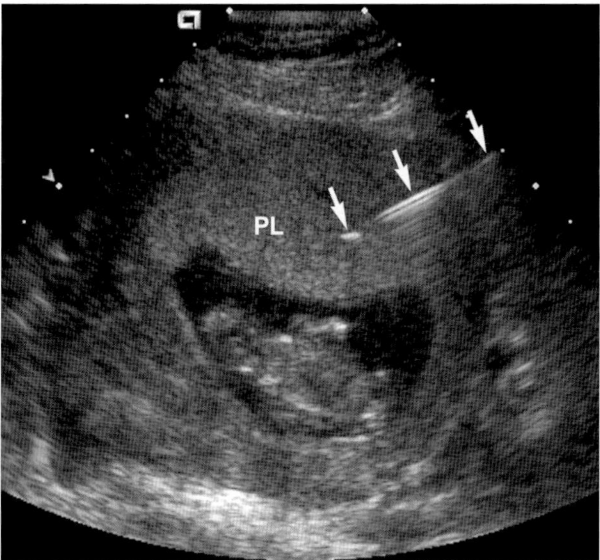

FIGURE 21.2-1. Transabdominal chorionic villus sampling. A catheter *(arrows)*, inserted percutaneously through the anterior abdominal wall of the mother, extends into the placenta (PL).

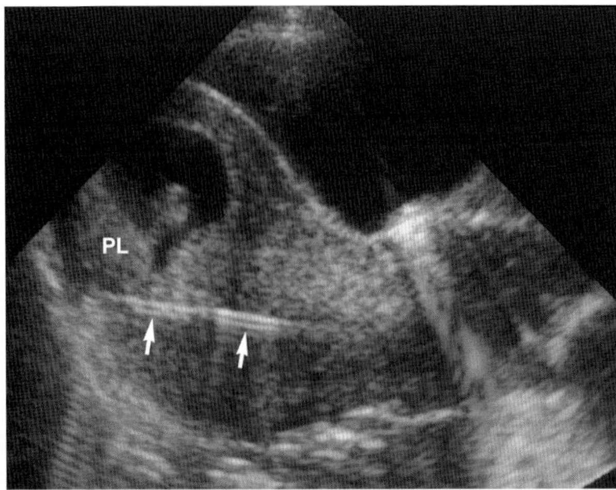

FIGURE 21.2-2. Transcervical chorionic villus sampling. A catheter *(arrows)*, introduced through the mother's cervix, courses beneath the placenta *(PL)*.

Transcervical (Figure 21.2-2): A catheter is inserted through the cervix and directed via transabdominal ultrasound guidance into the placenta. Suction is applied as the catheter is moved back and forth through the placenta.

21.3. PERCUTANEOUS UMBILICAL BLOOD SAMPLING

Description and Clinical Features

Percutaneous umbilical blood sampling, also termed cordocentesis, is an ultrasound-guided procedure in which a sample of fetal blood is withdrawn from the umbilical cord. The procedure is performed for a variety of diagnostic purposes, including determination of fetal hematocrit when fetal anemia is suspected and assessment of fetal karyotype when this information is needed more quickly than can be determined from amniocentesis.

Percutaneous umbilical blood sampling carries a somewhat higher risk than amniocentesis because its potential complications include all those of amniocentesis together with others specific to percutaneous umbilical blood sampling: bleeding from the puncture site in the cord and fetal bradycardia (likely due to umbilical arterial spasm). Bleeding or bradycardia is most often transient, but if either complication persists, it may be necessary to deliver the fetus emergently.

Sonography

Continuous real-time ultrasound guidance is essential for directing the needle into the umbilical cord and monitoring the procedure. Guidance can be provided using a sector, linear, or curvilinear transducer and can be done either freehand or using a needle guide.

If the placenta is anterior, the needle is inserted through the placenta and advanced into the umbilical vein at its insertion into the placenta (Figure 21.3-1). Because the needle does not puncture the free wall of the umbilical vein, there is no intra-amniotic bleeding when the needle is removed.

If the placenta is located laterally, fundally, or posteriorly, the needle is directed through the wall of the umbilical cord. If possible, the puncture should be 1–2 cm from the placental insertion site of the cord (Figure 21.3-2) because the cord is fairly immobile at this location. If the placental cord insertion site is blocked by the fetus, an attempt can be made to insert the needle into a free loop of cord (Figure 21.3-3).

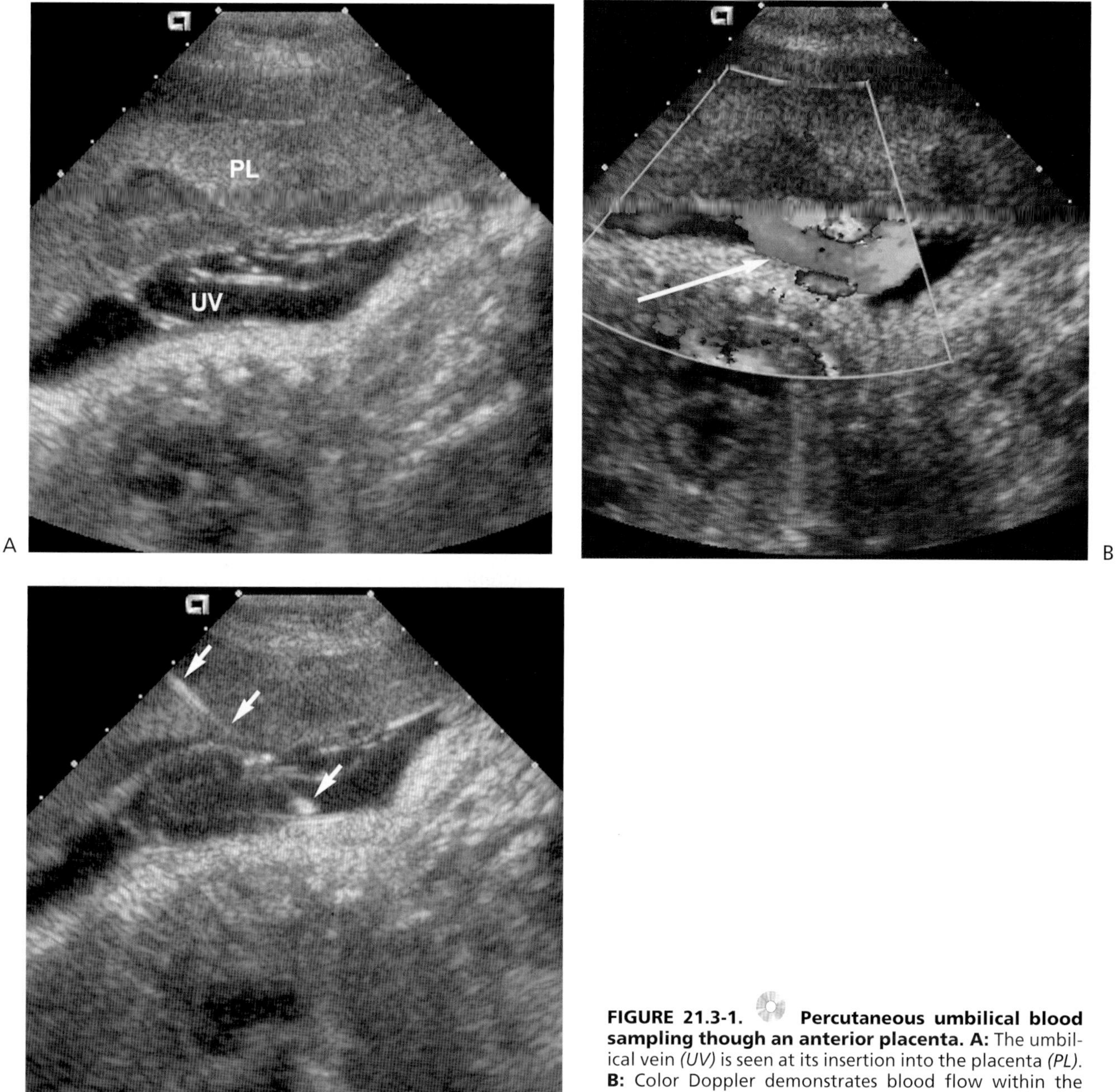

FIGURE 21.3-1. Percutaneous umbilical blood sampling though an anterior placenta. A: The umbilical vein *(UV)* is seen at its insertion into the placenta *(PL)*. **B:** Color Doppler demonstrates blood flow within the umbilical vein *(arrow)*. **C:** A needle *(arrows)* traverses the placenta, and its tip is situated in the umbilical vein.

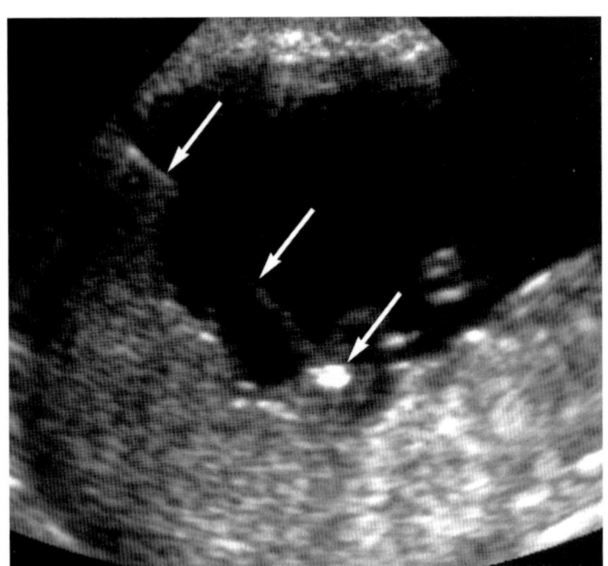

FIGURE 21.3-2. Percutaneous umbilical blood sampling with a posterior placenta. A needle *(arrows)* traverses the amniotic fluid and ends in the umbilical vein near the umbilical cord insertion site into the placenta.

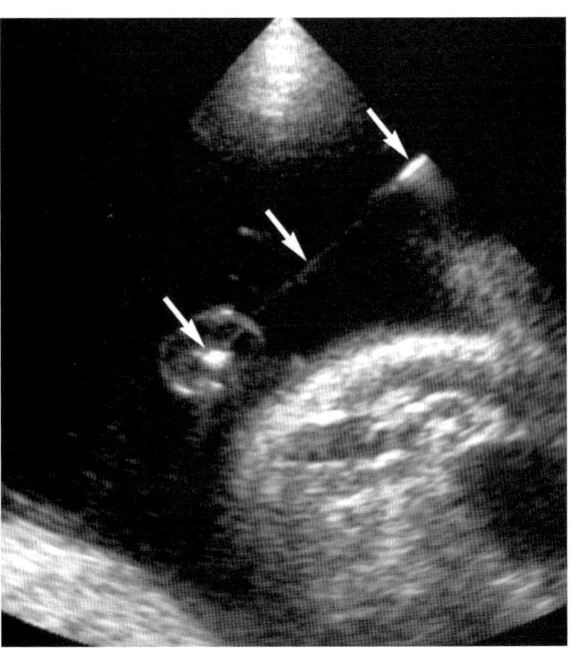

FIGURE 21.3-3. Percutaneous umbilical blood sampling from a free loop of the umbilical cord. A needle *(arrows)* traverses the amniotic fluid and ends in a free loop of the umbilical cord.

SUGGESTED READINGS

1. Benacerraf BR, Frigoletto FD. Amniocentesis under continuous ultrasound guidance: a series of 232 cases. *Obstet Gynecol* 1983;62:760–763.
2. Copel JA, Grannum PA, Hobbins JC. Interventional procedures in obstetrics. *Semin Roentgenol* 1991;26:87–94.
3. Daffos F, Capella-Pavlovsky M, Forestier F. Fetal blood sampling during pregnancy with use of a needle guided by ultrasound: a study 606 consecutive cases. *Am J Obstet Gynecol* 1985;82:6556–6560.
4. Ghezzi F, Romero R, Maymon E, et al. Fetal blood sampling. In: Fleischer AC, Manning FA, Jeanty P, et al., eds. *Sonography in obstetrics & gynecology: principles and practice*, 6th ed. New York: McGraw-Hill, 2001:775–804.
5. Maymon E, Romero R, Goncalves L, et al. Amniocentesis. In: Fleischer AC, Manning FA, Jeanty P, et al, eds. *Sonography in obstetrics & gynecology: principles and practice*, 6th ed. New York: McGraw-Hill, 2001:741–774.
6. Wapner RJ. Chorionic villus sampling. In: Fleischer AC, Manning FA, Jeanty P, et al., eds. *Sonography in obstetrics & gynecology: principles and practice*, 6th ed. New York: McGraw-Hill, 2001:721–740.

22

THERAPEUTIC OBSTETRICAL PROCEDURES

22.1. FETAL BLOOD TRANSFUSION

Description and Clinical Features

If a fetus is found to be anemic based on umbilical blood sampling, it can be treated with a blood transfusion. The most direct way to add blood to the fetal circulation is to transfuse it into the umbilical vein, either in the umbilical cord or intrahepatically. If the umbilical vein cannot be accessed, an alternative approach is to inject blood into the fetal peritoneal cavity, where the erythrocytes are absorbed into fetal circulation.

Sonography

Continuous real-time guidance is essential for fetal blood transfusion, whether the transfusion is into the umbilical vein in the umbilical cord (Figures 22.1-1 and 22.1-2), the intrahepatic umbilical vein (Figure 22.1-3), or intraperitoneally (Figure 22.1-4). When monitoring an intravascular transfusion, the observation of streaming echoes in the umbilical vein confirms that the transfusion is proceeding appropriately (Figures 22.1-1,

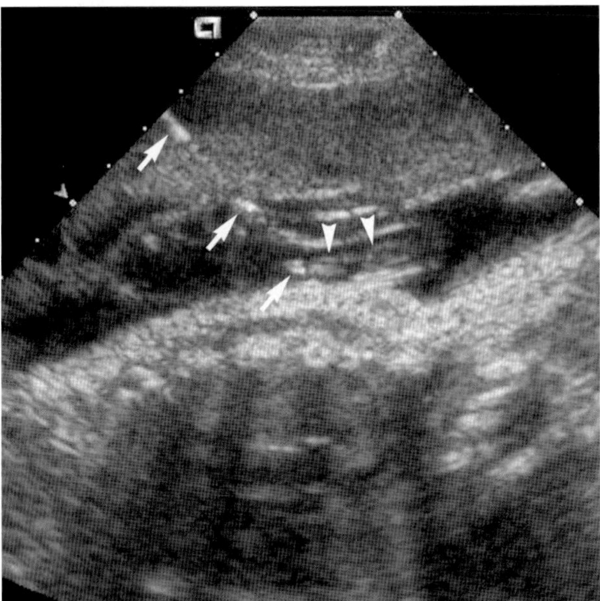

FIGURE 22.1-1. Intravascular blood transfusion into the umbilical vein at its placental insertion. There is a needle *(arrows)* with its tip in the umbilical vein. Blood is seen streaming *(arrowheads)* into the vein as it is injected through the needle.

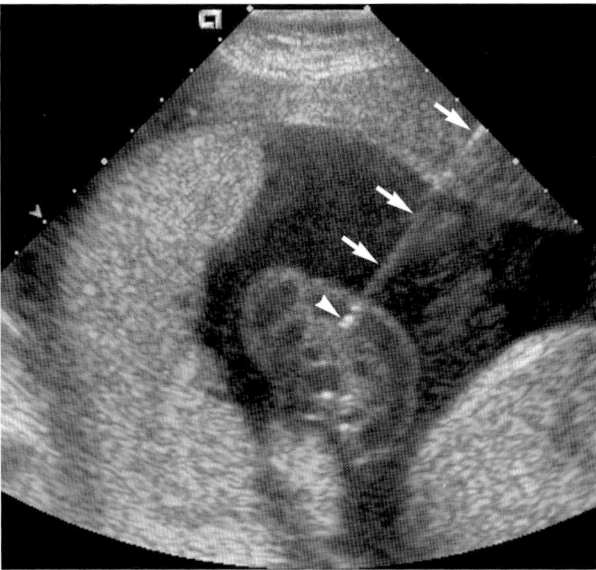

FIGURE 22.1-2. Intravascular blood transfusion into the umbilical vein in a free loop of cord. A needle *(arrows)* travels through the gestational sac, with its tip *(arrowhead)* ending in the umbilical vein in a free loop of cord. Blood was transfused through the needle.

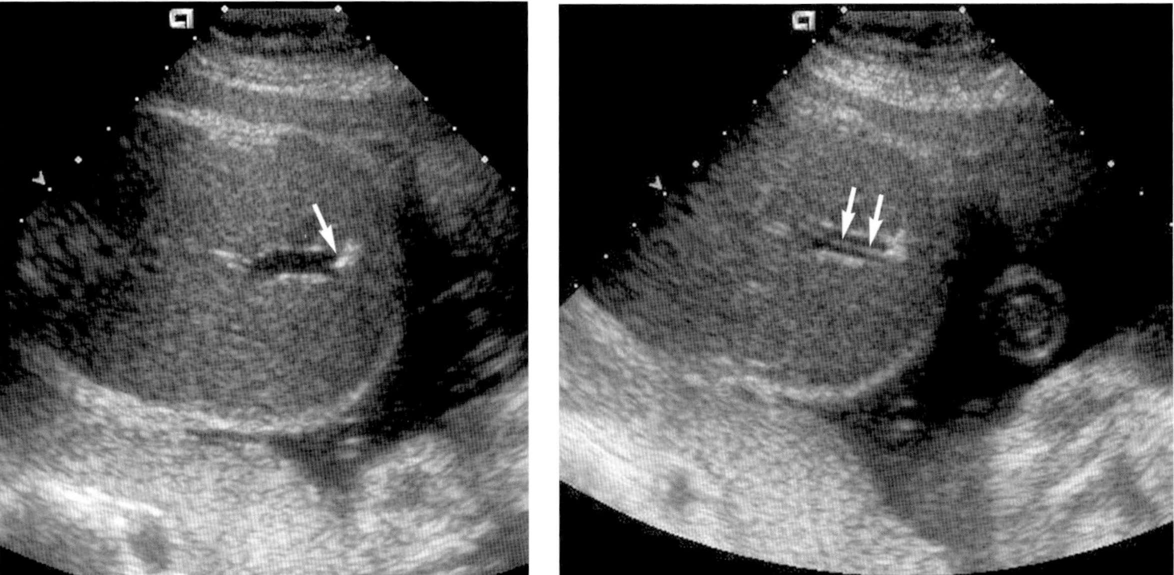

FIGURE 22.1-3. Intravascular blood transfusion into the intrahepatic umbilical vein. A: Transverse section through the fetal abdomen demonstrates the tip of a needle *(arrow)* within the intrahepatic umbilical vein. **B:** There is streaming of blood *(arrows)* as it is transfused into the umbilical vein.

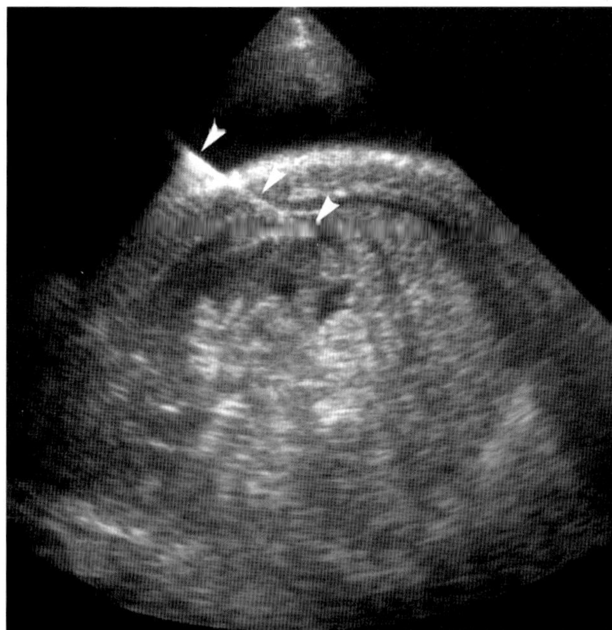

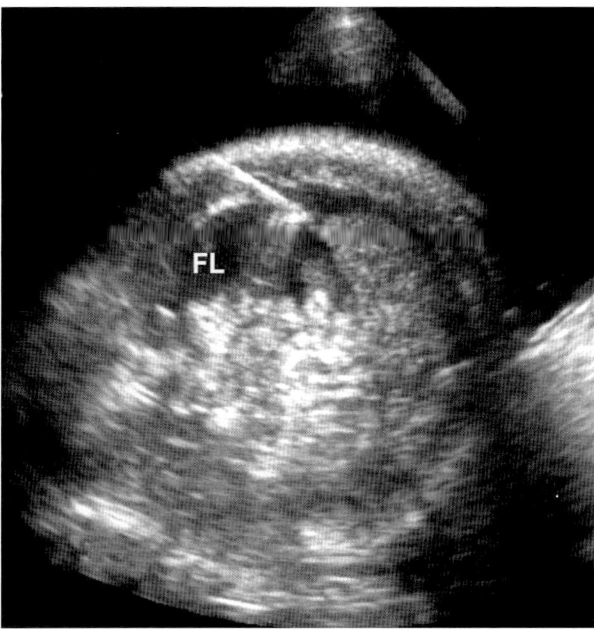

A B

FIGURE 22.1-4. **Intraperitoneal blood transfusion. A:** A needle *(arrowheads)* traverses the fetal abdominal wall and ends within the abdomen. **B:** After injection of blood into the peritoneal space, additional fluid *(FL)* is seen in the fetal abdomen.

22.1-2, and 22.1-3). When monitoring an intraperitoneal transfusion, free fluid should be seen collecting in the fetal abdomen as the blood is injected.

22.2. THORACENTESIS AND THORACOAMNIOTIC SHUNTING

Description and Clinical Features

Drainage of fetal pleural effusions may improve pregnancy outcome in a number of situations. Examples include the following:

Hydrops with a large unilateral pleural effusion: Drainage of the unilateral effusion may increase venous return to the fetal heart by correcting mediastinal shift, thereby improving or alleviating hydrops.

Large bilateral pleural effusions in a fetus immediately before delivery: Bilateral thoracenteses, followed immediately by delivery, will allow the neonatal lungs to expand and will obviate the need for emergency postnatal thoracenteses.

Fluid may be removed by thoracentesis, whereby a needle is inserted into the fetal thorax, fluid is aspirated, and the needle is removed. When continuous drainage is required, as in the first of the examples above, a thoracoamniotic shunt can be placed.

Sonography

Sonographic guidance for thoracentesis is provided in the same manner as for amniocentesis, using real-time sonographic monitoring to guide the needle into the fetal thorax (Figure 22.2-1). Placement of a thoracoamniotic shunt involves several steps, all directed by ultrasound (Figure 22.2-2). First, a large-bore needle is directed into the fetal thorax. The trocar is removed and a double-pigtail catheter is threaded through the needle until one end of the catheter coils in the fetal thorax. The needle is then pulled back until its tip is in the amniotic fluid, and the remaining part of the catheter is

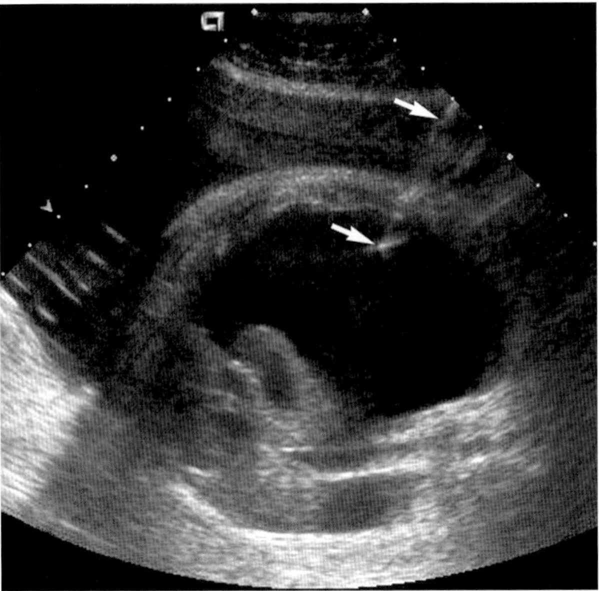

FIGURE 22.2-1. **Fetal thoracentesis.** A needle *(arrows)*, inserted percutaneously through the maternal anterior abdominal wall, ends in the thorax of a fetus with a large pleural effusion.

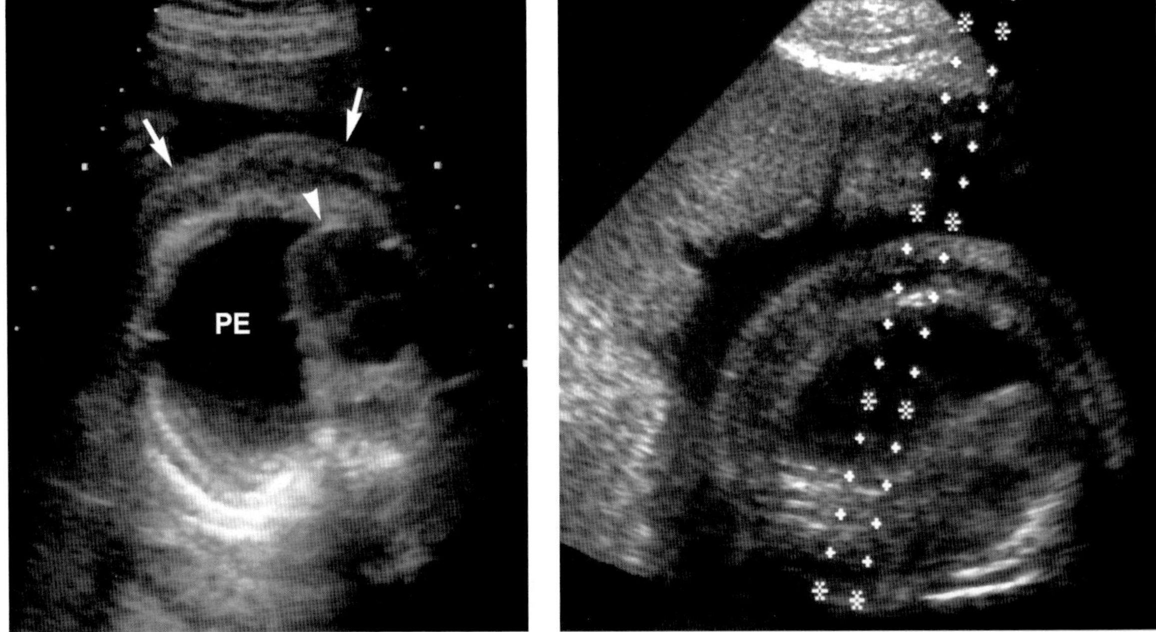

FIGURE 22.2-2. **Thoracoamniotic shunt placement. A:** Transverse section of the fetal thorax reveals a large, left-sided pleural effusion *(PE)* deviating the heart *(arrowhead)* to the right. Subcutaneous edema *(arrows)* is seen around the thorax. **B:** In preparation for thoracentesis, a needle guide was placed on the transducer and guide marks on the image indicate the path that a needle inserted through the guide will follow.

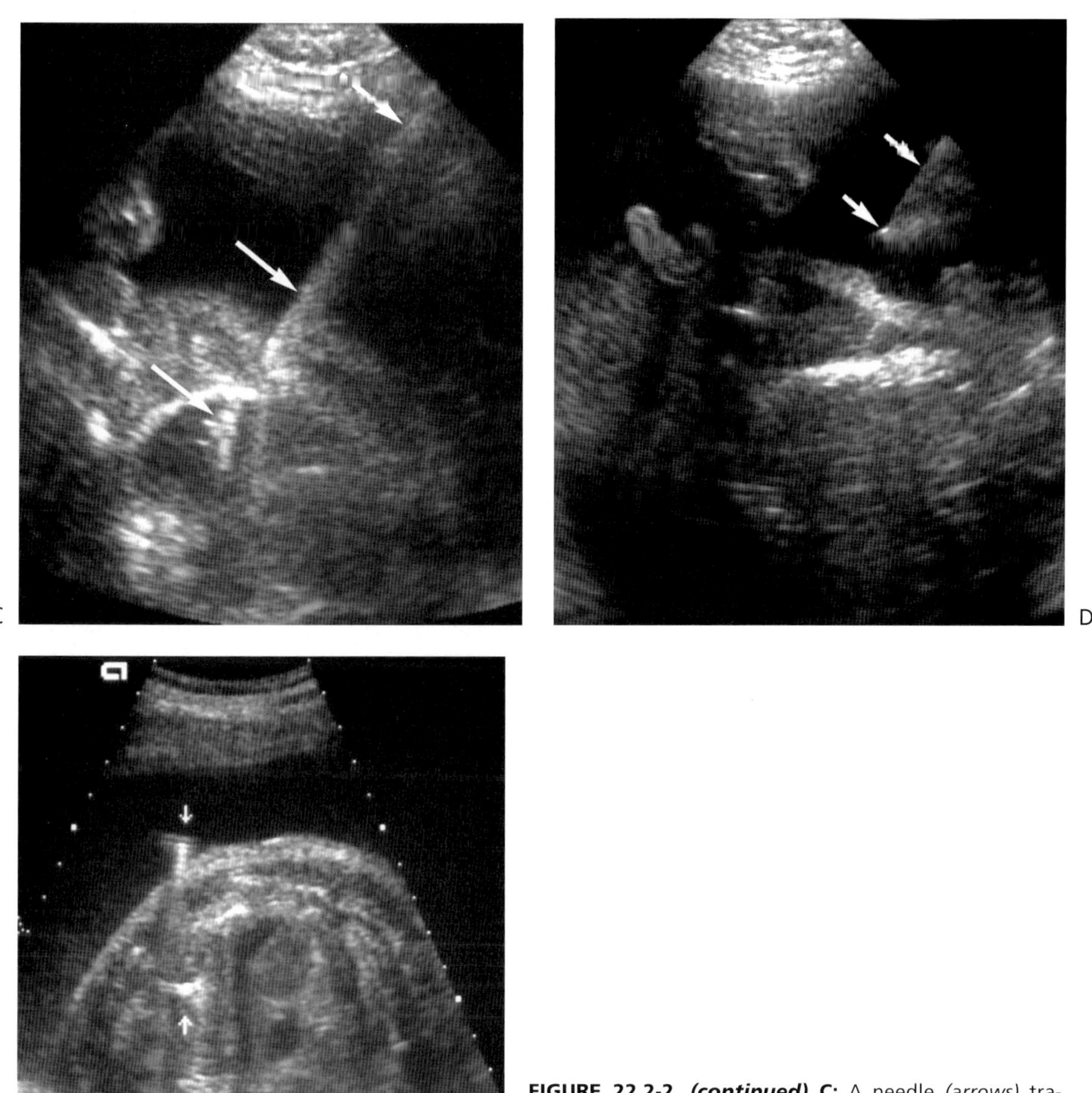

FIGURE 22.2-2. *(continued)* **C:** A needle *(arrows)* traverses the amniotic fluid and ends within the pleural effusion in the fetal thorax. **D:** After one end of a double-pigtail catheter is inserted into the fetal thorax, the needle is withdrawn into the amniotic fluid *(arrows)*. **E:** At the conclusion of the procedure, one end of the shunt catheter is seen in the amniotic fluid and the other within the fetal thorax *(arrows)*.

pushed out of the needle into the amniotic cavity. The needle is then withdrawn to complete the procedure.

22.3. BLADDER DRAINAGE AND VESICOAMNIOTIC SHUNTING

Description and Clinical Features

Urethral obstruction, which is most commonly due to posterior urethral valves, is likely to cause life-threatening pulmonary hypoplasia and renal dysplasia if left untreated *in utero*. The obstruction can be treated *in utero* either by open surgery or by ultrasound-guided percutaneous placement of a vesicoamniotic shunt. A fetus diagnosed with urethral obstruction must meet several criteria before a corrective procedure is considered:

Severe oligohydramnios: In the absence of severe oligohydramnios, the prognosis is good without surgery because bladder outlet obstruction is incomplete.
Gestational age incompatible with viability outside the uterus.
No other major structural anomaly.
Normal karyotype.
Renal parenchyma appears normal on ultrasound.
Normal fetal renal function: If the above criteria are met, fetal renal function is evaluated by performing an ultrasound-guided fetal bladder drainage. The presence of normal fetal urinary electrolyte levels and reaccumulation of urine in the fetal bladder over the next 24 hours indicate adequate renal function.

If all these criteria are met, in utero treatment of the urethral obstruction should be contemplated.

Sonography

Ultrasound plays a central role in all aspects of the diagnosis and treatment of urethral obstruction, including diagnosing the condition, assessing whether the fetus is a candidate for *in utero* intervention, and guiding the drainage procedure and placement of the vesicoamniotic shunt. After the diagnosis is established by ultrasound, ultrasound is used to assess the amniotic fluid volume, evaluate the fetal renal parenchyma for evidence of dysplasia (parenchymal cysts or thin echogenic cortex), conduct a comprehensive fetal anatomic survey to assess for coexisting anomalies, assign gestational age, and guide amniocentesis or umbilical blood sampling to determine fetal karyotype. If these demonstrate no contraindication to proceeding, ultrasound is then used to guide a needle into the fetal urinary bladder (Figure 22.3-1) to assess renal function.

If the decision is made to proceed with vesicoamniotic shunting, shunt placement is performed under ultrasound guidance (Figure 22.3-2). The procedure generally begins with an amnioinfusion (reverse amniocentesis): instillation of saline into the amniotic space to create a pocket of fluid in which to place the amniotic end of the vesicoamniotic shunt. A large-bore needle is then inserted into the fetal bladder and a double-pigtail catheter is inserted through the needle. One end of the catheter is advanced into the fetal bladder. The needle is then withdrawn into the amniotic space, and the rest of the catheter is pushed out of the needle, so that the second coil of the catheter is in the amniotic cavity. The needle is then removed.

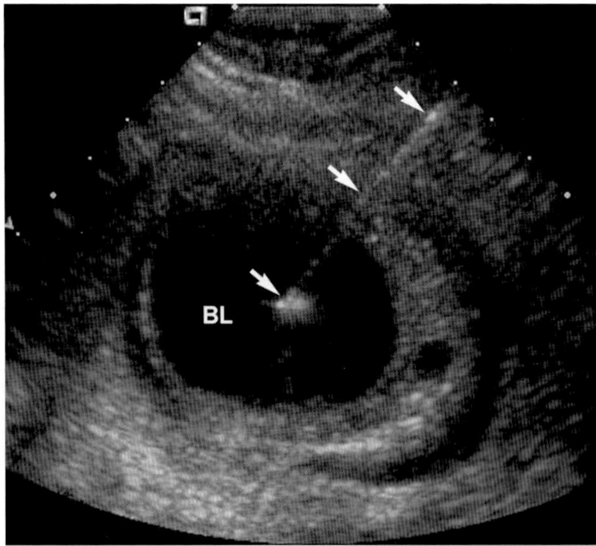

FIGURE 22.3-1. Fetal bladder drainage. A needle *(arrows)* has been guided by ultrasound into a distended fetal bladder (BL).

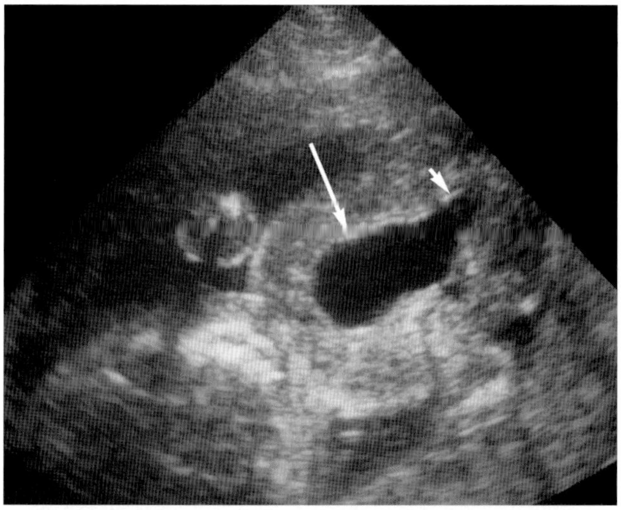

A

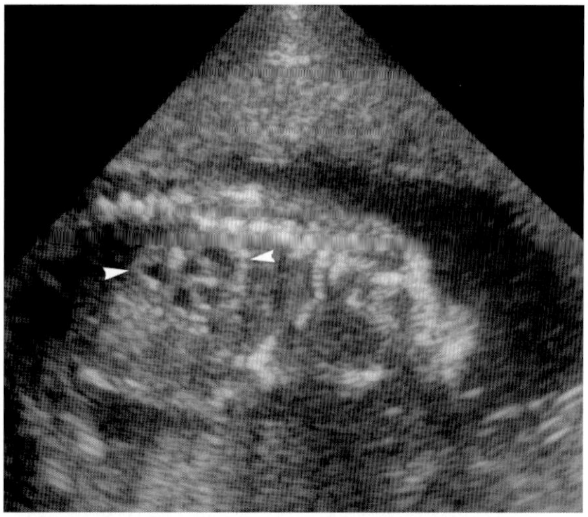

B

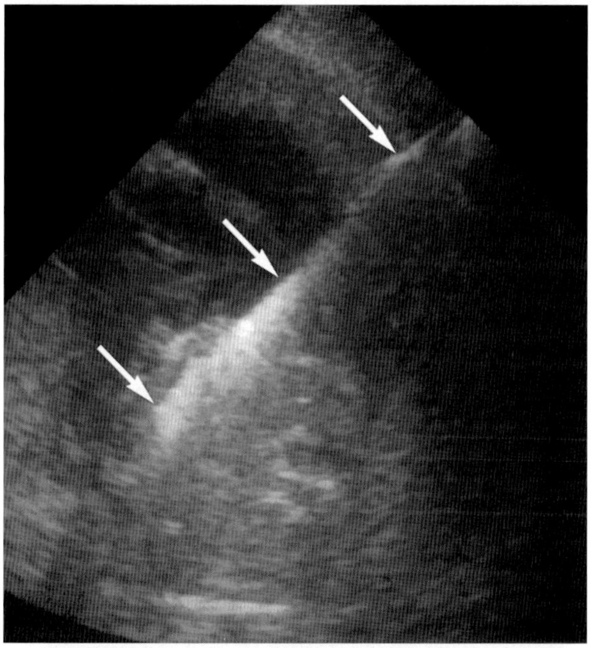

C

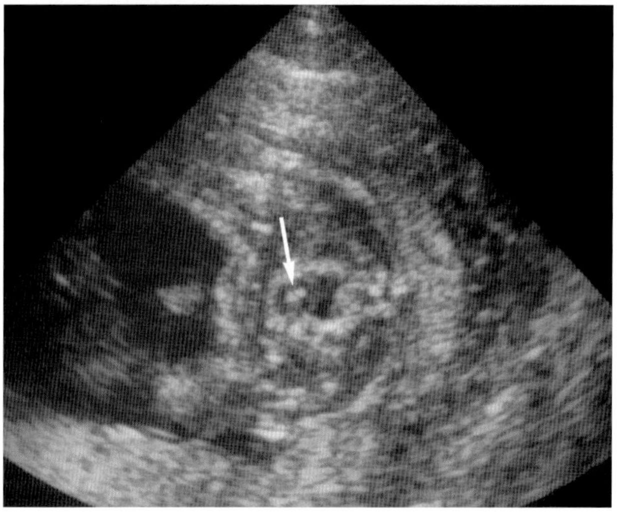

D

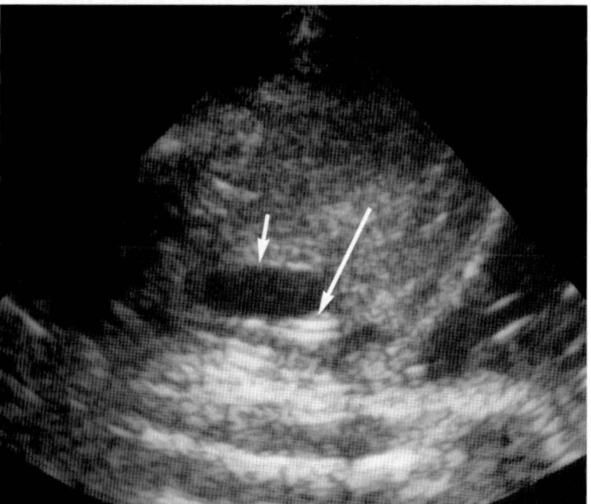

E

FIGURE 22.3-2. Vesicoamniotic shunt placement. The diagnosis of posterior urethral valves was made based on a dilated fetal bladder *(long arrow)* and posterior urethra *(short arrow)* **(A)** and hydronephrosis *(arrowheads)* **(B)**. At the time of diagnosis, there was severe oligohydramnios. The fluid surrounding this fetus **(A,B)** was not amniotic fluid, but saline infused into the amniotic space in preparation for placement of a vesicoamniotic shunt. **C:** A large-bore needle *(arrows)* was inserted in the fetal bladder. This needle was used for placement of a double-pigtail catheter, with one end in the fetal bladder and the other in the amniotic cavity. **D:** After the procedure, the fetal bladder was decompressed and contained one end of the shunt catheter *(arrow)*. The other end of the catheter, not visualized on this image, was in the amniotic fluid space. **E:** Eight weeks later, the bladder *(short arrow)* was once again distended because the catheter *(long arrow)* became clogged with debris. The fetus was delivered shortly after this sonogram, and the neonate underwent transurethral resection of posterior urethral valves. (From Benson CB, Doubilet PM. Fetal genitourinary system. In: Fleischer AC, Manning FA, Jeanty P, Romero R (eds). *Sonography in obstetrics and gynecology, principles and practice*. 6th ed. New York: McGraw-Hill, 2000, pp. 431–444, with permission.)

Once a shunt has been placed, the fetus should be monitored closely by ultrasound. If the shunt is working properly, the fetal bladder will remain decompressed. Redistention of the bladder (Figure 22.3-2) indicates shunt malfunction, due either to debris clogging the shunt or dislodgment of the shunt, which necessitates either delivery of the fetus or insertion of a new shunt.

22.4. PARACENTESIS

Description and Clinical Features

Fetal ascites is often seen as a component of hydrops. It can also occur in other settings, such as urine ascites in a fetus with calyceal rupture due to urinary tract obstruction. In most cases of fetal ascites, there is no benefit to performing prenatal paracentesis. Occasionally, however, removing the fluid can improve the outcome (e.g., decreasing abdominal girth at term to permit vaginal delivery or relieving upward pressure on the diaphragm to facilitate lung growth).

Sonography

Fetal paracentesis is performed under continuous ultrasound guidance (Figures 22.4-1 and 22.4-2). The needle is advanced through the maternal abdominal and uterine walls and directed toward a site on the fetal abdominal wall overlying a pocket of ascites. When the needle is in an appropriate location adjacent to the fetal abdomen and there is no fetal motion, the needle is quickly advanced through the abdominal wall into the ascites.

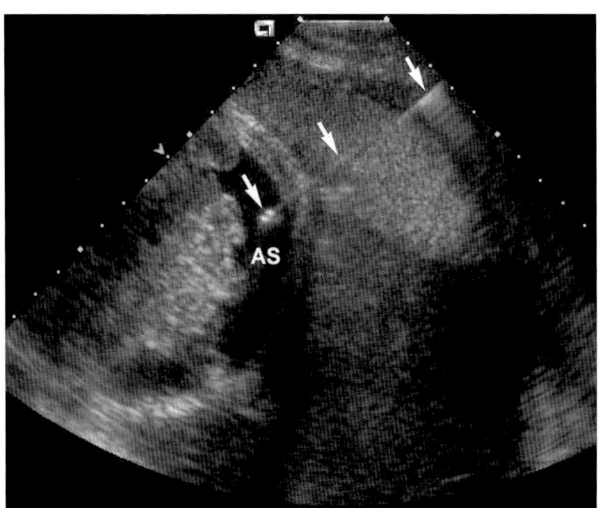

FIGURE 22.4-1. Fetal paracentesis with a small-to-moderate amount of ascites. A needle *(arrows)*, inserted percutaneously through the maternal anterior abdominal wall, ends in the abdomen of this fetus with ascites *(AS)*.

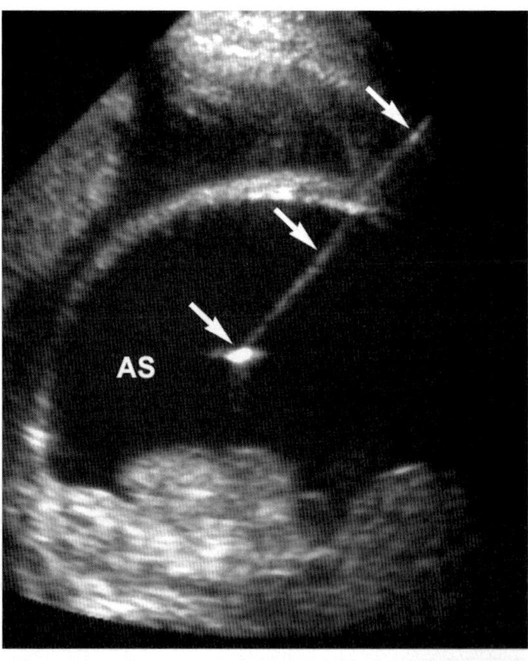

FIGURE 22.4-2. Fetal paracentesis with a large amount of ascites. Transverse view of the fetal abdomen demonstrates a needle *(arrows)* within a large amount of ascites *(AS)*. The procedure was performed to diminish fetal abdominal girth so that the baby could be delivered vaginally, and to decrease upward pressure on the diaphragm so that the lungs could expand after birth.

22.5. TRACHEAL OCCLUSION FOR DIAPHRAGMATIC HERNIA

Description and Clinical Features

Neonates born with a congenital diaphragmatic hernia are at risk of pulmonary hypoplasia and pulmonary hypertension, both of which occur as a result of herniated abdominal organs occupying space in the rigid thorax. These complications are most frequent and severe when the volume of herniated material is large, especially if a portion of the liver is herniated into the thorax.

Early attempts at *in utero* therapy of diaphragmatic hernias that included a herniated liver employed an open surgical procedure: hysterotomy, exposing the fetal diaphragm, returning the herniated tissue to the abdomen, and repairing the diaphragmatic defect. Results were disappointing, in part because there was a high incidence of complications arising from kinking of the umbilical vein and the resultant obstruction of umbilical venous blood flow after the herniated portion of the liver was abruptly moved from above to below the diaphragm.

An alternative approach, occluding the fetal trachea via a metallic clip or balloon using combined laparoscopic and sonographic guidance, has been performed at a number of centers. The rationale for tracheal occlusion is that secretions trapped in the lungs force expansion and growth of alveoli, thus diminishing the pulmonary complications in the neonate with a congenital diaphragmatic hernia.

A fetus diagnosed with a diaphragmatic hernia must satisfy a number of criteria before tracheal occlusion may be considered. These include:

- Left-sided hernia
- Diagnosis before 24 weeks
- No other major structural or chromosomal anomaly
- Features suggestive of a poor prognosis if left untreated, including presence of liver in the thorax and small size of the contralateral lung

When these criteria have been satisfied, tracheal clipping under endoscopic and sonographic guidance has been performed in some cases. The procedure is best performed at 24–26 weeks gestation. Because the neonate will not be able to breathe until the clip is removed, delivery must be done via cesarean section using the *ex utero* intrapartum treatment procedure. The fetal head and shoulders are delivered while the abdomen and umbilical cord remain in the maternal uterus, allowing the tracheal clip to be removed and the neonate to be intubated while umbilical blood flow continues. Once the airway is established, delivery is completed.

The tracheal clipping procedure has largely fallen out of favor because its success rate has been disappointing. Furthermore, experience has shown that similar results can be obtained without *in utero* treatment using the following approach: perform the *ex utero* intrapartum treatment procedure at the time of delivery, carry out a trial of intubation while umbilical blood flow continues, and proceed to extracorporeal membrane oxygenation if respiration via intubation is unsuccessful.

Sonography

Ultrasound plays an important role when the tracheal clipping procedure is considered for prenatal treatment of a left diaphragmatic hernia. After the diagnosis of a left diaphragmatic hernia is established by ultrasound, the nature and size of the herniated contents and the size of the right lung should be assessed sonographically. In particular, intervention should only be considered if liver has herniated into the thorax and the lung/head ratio (the product of the anteroposterior and transverse diameters of the lung divided by the head circumference, all measured in millimeters) is less than 1.4, because fetuses without these findings are likely to have a good prognosis without *in utero* treatment.

If a decision is made to proceed with tracheal clipping, the procedure is performed under combined sonographic and endoscopic guidance (Figure 22.5-1). Ultrasound is

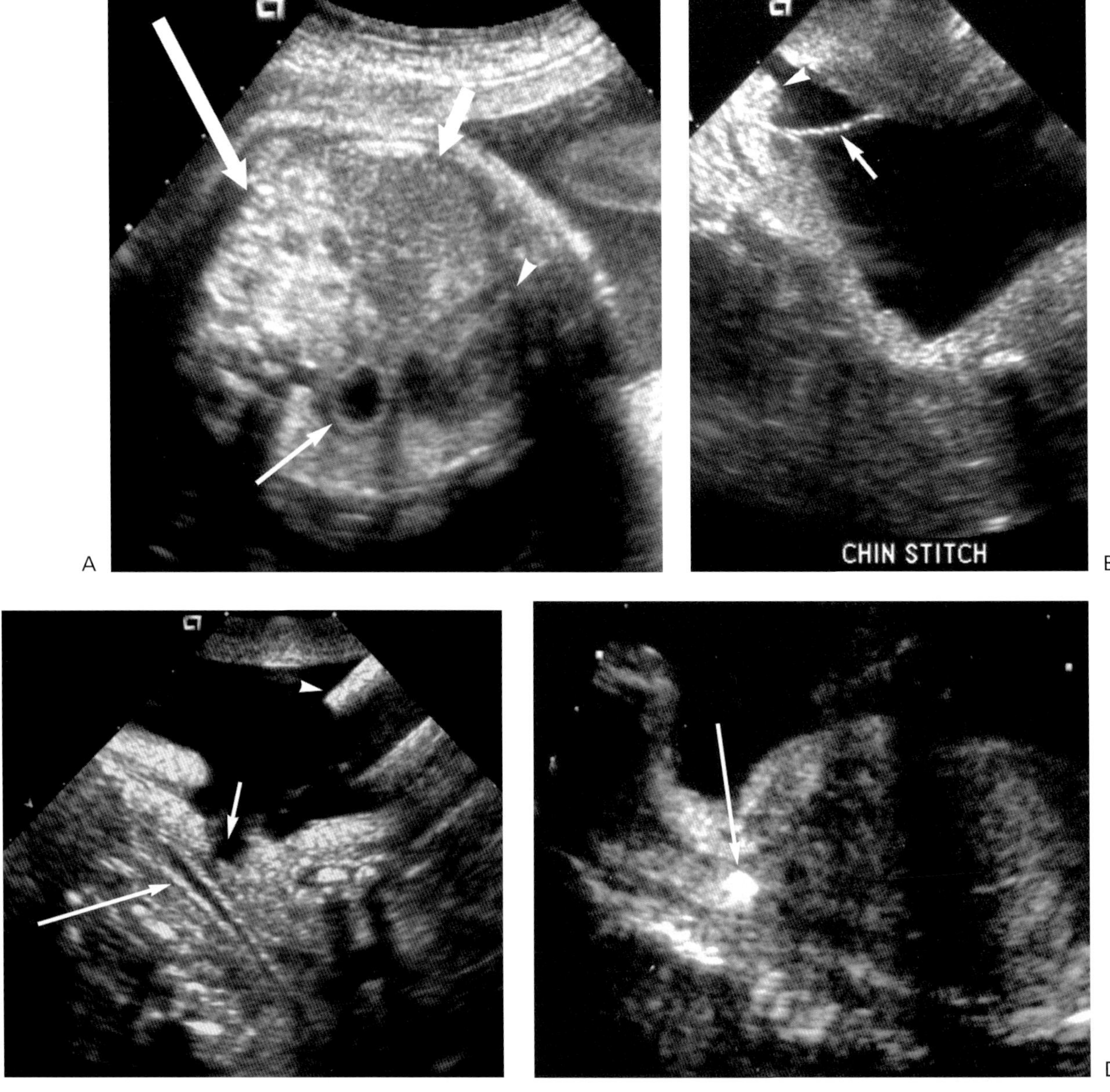

FIGURE 22.5-1. Tracheal clipping for treatment of a diaphragmatic hernia. A: Transverse section of the fetal thorax reveals intra-abdominal contents within the thorax, including stomach *(thin arrow)*, liver *(short thick arrow)*, and bowel *(long thick arrow)*. The heart *(arrowhead)* is deviated to the right side of the thorax. **B:** After the fetus was paralyzed by an intramuscular injection of pancuronium bromide (Pavulon), the fetal chin *(arrowhead)* was stitched *(arrow)* to the anterior uterine wall. **C:** Using sonographic and laparoscopic *(arrowhead)* guidance, the soft tissues of the anterior fetal neck were dissected *(short arrow)* to expose the trachea *(long arrow)*. **D:** A metallic clip *(arrow)* was placed to occlude the trachea.

used to determine where to insert the endoscope, selecting a site that is close to the fetal neck and avoids traversing the placenta. Once the endoscope has been inserted, ultrasound is used to direct it to the anterior neck and to monitor fetal heart rate.

22.6. MULTIFETAL PREGNANCY REDUCTION AND SELECTIVE TERMINATION

Description and Clinical Features

Multifetal pregnancy reduction is a procedure performed on a multiple gestation to decrease the number of living fetuses in the uterus. This procedure is usually performed on a gestation with three or more fetuses to reduce the pregnancy to fewer fetuses, usually twins. The resulting pregnancy carries a significantly reduced risk of perinatal morbidity and mortality. The procedure is typically performed in the late first trimester. Before the procedure, chorionicity for each fetus must be determined. If two fetuses are a monochorionic pair, reduction of one will invariably cause death of the other within several days. When a reduced fetus has its own placenta, there is minimal risk to the remaining fetuses.

Selective termination is a procedure performed in a multiple gestation to eliminate an abnormal fetus, allowing the pregnancy to continue with the remaining normal fetus or fetuses. This procedure is typically performed during the early to mid second trimester because this is when structural or chromosomal anomalies are most often diagnosed. When the anomalous or aneuploid fetus is one of a monochorionic pair, this procedure is contraindicated because of the risk to the other fetus sharing that placenta.

Sonography

Multifetal pregnancy reduction is generally performed by passing a needle transabdominally under ultrasound guidance into the thorax or heart of the fetus to be reduced (Figure 22.6-1 and 22.6-2). Approximately 3 ml potassium chloride is then injected. After the procedure, it is important to confirm the absence of a heart beat in the reduced fetus and normal cardiac activity in the remaining fetus or fetuses.

Selective termination is performed by a similar technique. A needle is passed under ultrasound guidance through the maternal abdomen and uterine wall into the thorax or heart of the abnormal fetus (Figure 22.6-3 and 22.6-4); 3–5 ml potassium chloride is then injected.

A

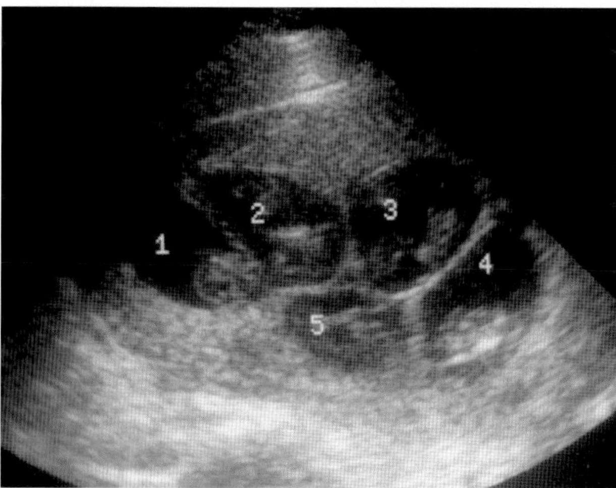

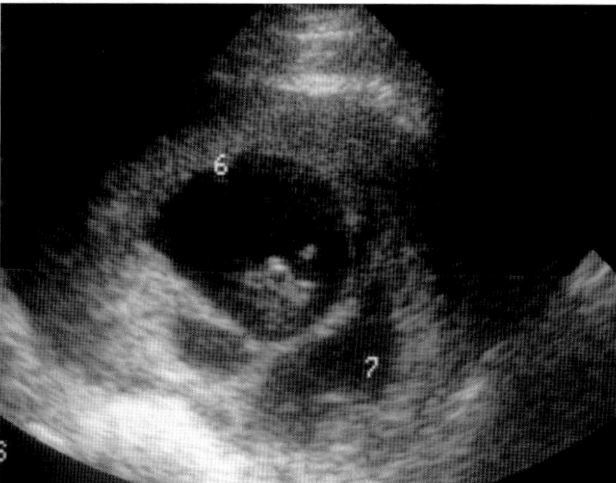

B

FIGURE 22.6-1. Multifetal pregnancy reduction of septuplets. Images of a uterus demonstrate five *(1, 2, 3, 4, and 5)* **(A)** and two more *(6 and 7)* **(B)** gestational sacs. *(continued)*

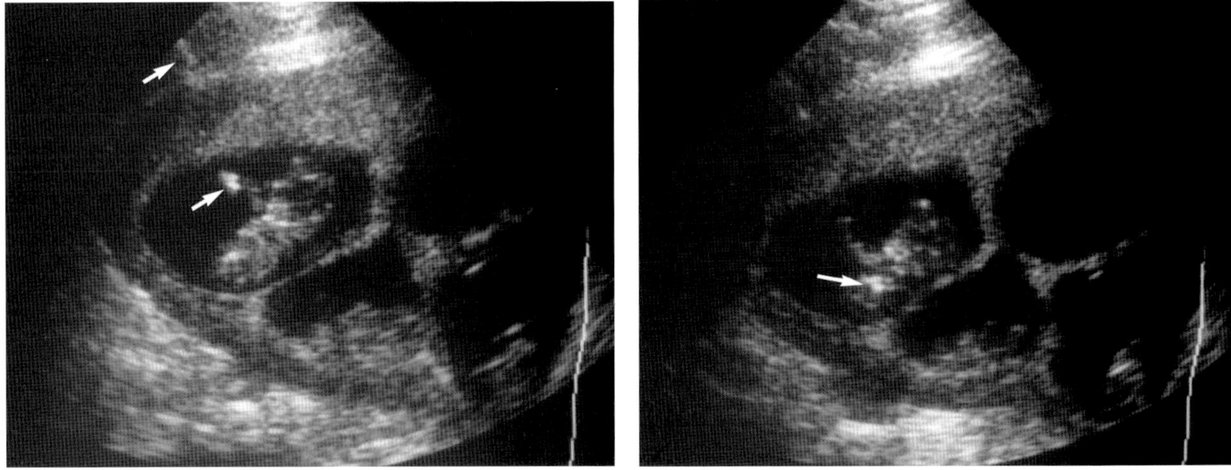

FIGURE 22.6-1. *(continued)* C: A needle *(arrows)* has been inserted in the sac of one of the fetuses to be reduced. **D:** The needle is inserted further, with the tip *(arrow)* in the thorax of the septuplet to be reduced.

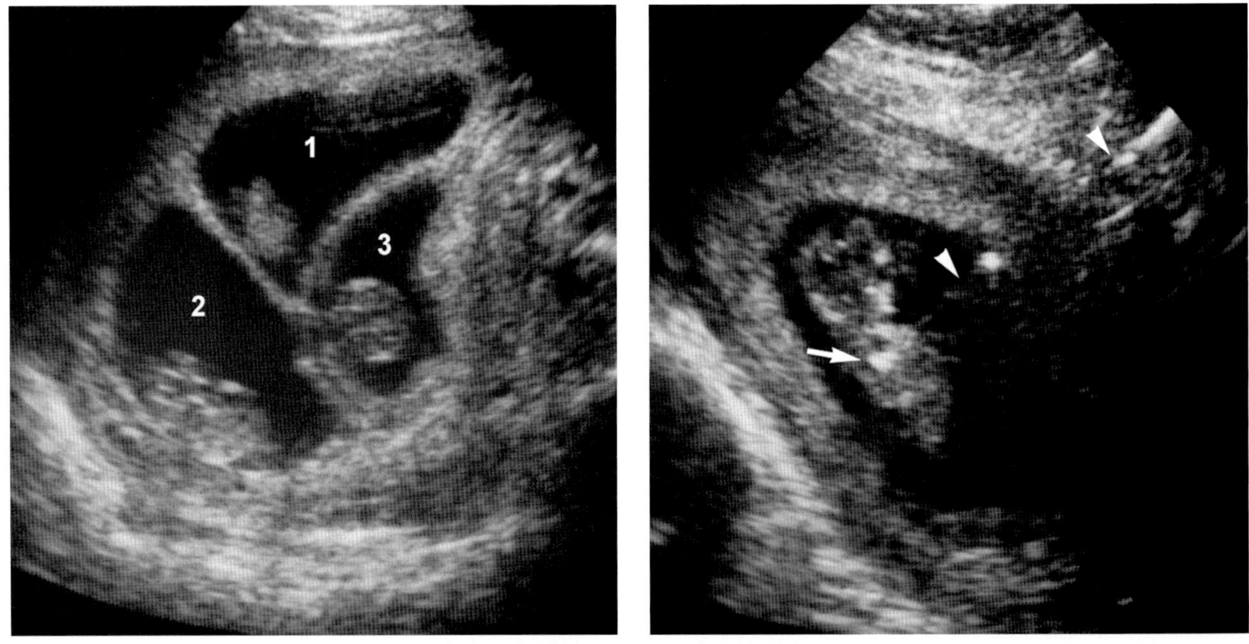

FIGURE 22.6-2. Multifetal pregnancy reduction of triplets to twins. A: Image of a uterus demonstrates three separate gestational sacs *(1, 2, and 3)*, each containing a fetus with a heartbeat. **B:** A needle *(arrowheads)* is inserted until its tip *(arrow)* is within the thorax or heart of the triplet to be reduced.

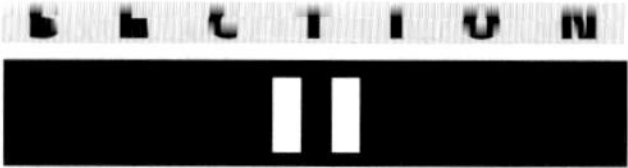

GYNECOLOGICAL ULTRASOUND

23

UTERUS

23.1. MYOMETRIUM

Description and Clinical Features

The myometrium is the muscular portion of the uterus. It is bounded internally by the endometrium and externally by the serosa, a membrane derived from the peritoneum. The myometrium forms the bulk of the uterus from the cervix, the caudal portion of the uterus, through the body, to the fundus. It is thickest during a woman's menstrual years, and atrophies substantially after menopause.

Cysts within the cervix, termed nabothian cysts, occur frequently. They result from the retention of mucus within obstructed endocervical glands. These cysts are of little or no clinical significance unless large or infected.

The arterial blood supply to the myometrium comes from the uterine artery, which arises from the internal iliac artery. Numerous branches of the uterine artery penetrate the uterus, forming the arcuate arteries that course within the myometrium.

Sonography

The myometrium is moderately hypoechoic, especially in relation to the more echogenic endometrium. Although the normal myometrium is fairly homogeneous in echotexture, several features stand out, especially when scanning transvaginally. The inner myometrium is less echogenic than the outer myometrium, and the arcuate arteries and veins are often visible as serpiginous structures in the outer myometrium (Figure 23.1-1).

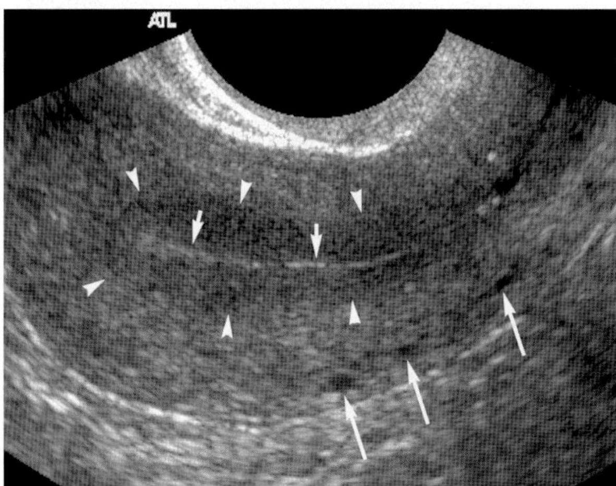

FIGURE 23.1-1. Normal premenopausal uterus. Sagittal transvaginal view of the uterus demonstrates the hypoechoic inner myometrium *(arrowheads)* and the more hyperechoic outer myometrium. The thin echogenic line *(short arrows)* represents the endometrium and marks the location of the uterine cavity. Arcuate vessels are seen as anechoic serpiginous structures *(long arrows)* in the peripheral aspect of the myometrium.

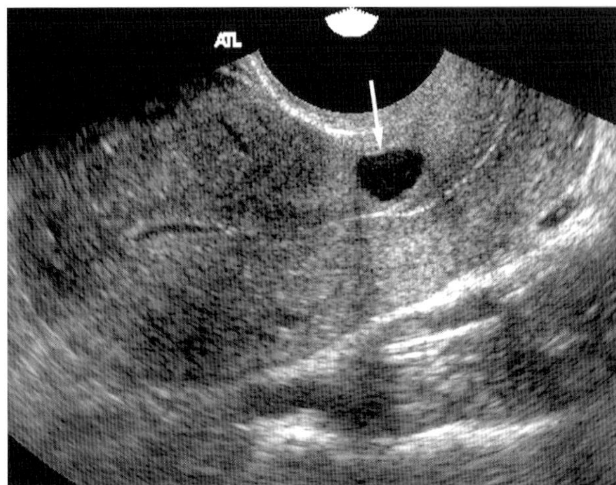

FIGURE 23.1-2. Nabothian cyst. Sagittal transvaginal view of the uterus reveals a nabothian cyst *(arrow)* in the cervix.

The cervix is identifiable at the caudal end of the uterus. The cervical myometrium is generally homogeneous, except where nabothian cysts are present (Figure 23.1-2).

The myometrium atrophies after menopause. In the elderly woman, 20–30 years post-menopause, the uterus tends to be smaller and thinner than in the premenopausal woman (Figure 23.1-3).

Color Doppler can demonstrate the uterine and arcuate arteries and veins. The uterine vessels can be seen coursing along the lateral margins of the uterus, beginning at the junction between the cervix and body, and extending to the fundus. The arcuate vessels are seen most prominently within the peripheral myometrium (Figure 23.1-4).

A

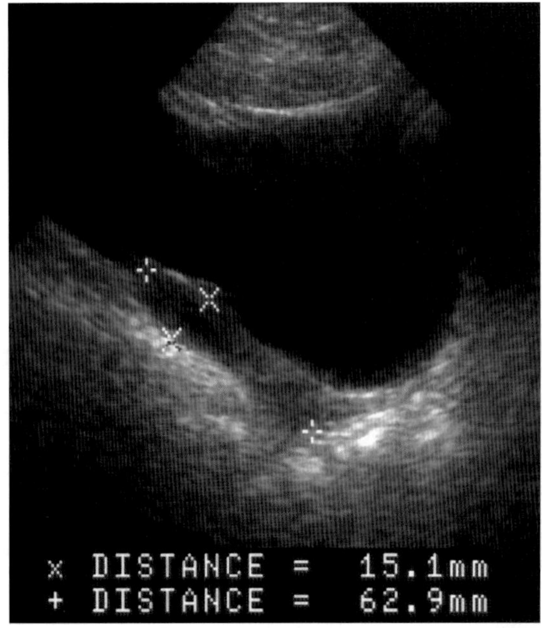

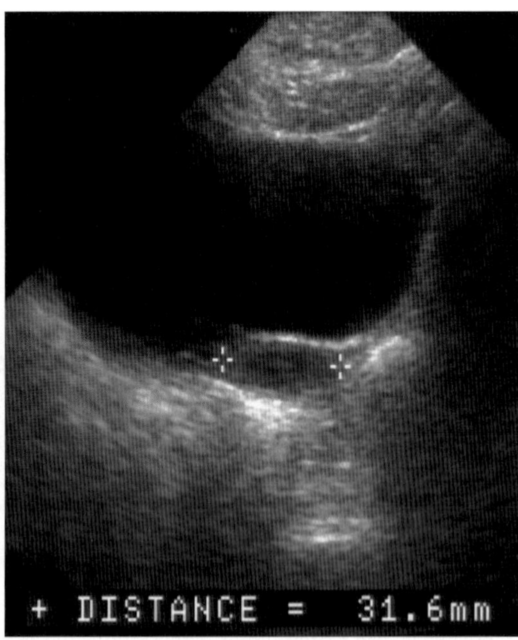

B

FIGURE 23.1-3. Postmenopausal uterus. Sagittal **(A)** and transverse **(B)** views demonstrate an atrophic postmenopausal uterus *(calipers)*.

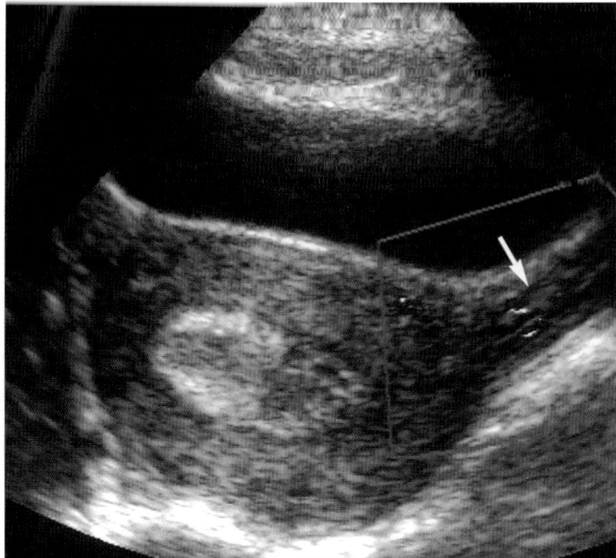
A

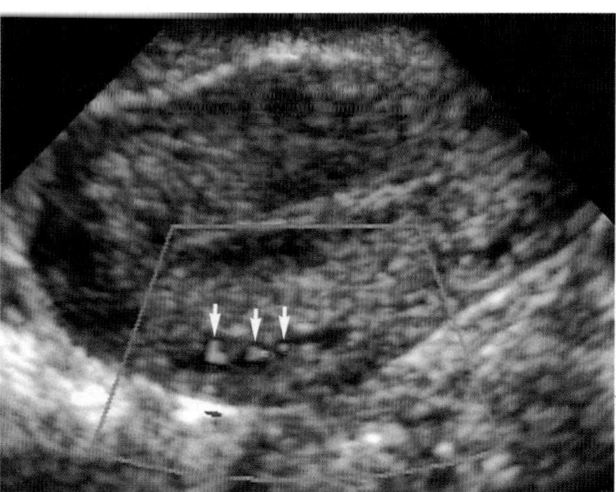
B

FIGURE 23.1-4. Color Doppler of uterine and arcuate vessels. A: Transverse view of the uterus with color Doppler demonstrates the left uterine artery *(arrow)* just lateral to the uterus. **B:** Sagittal view of the uterus with color Doppler demonstrates the arcuate arteries and veins *(arrows)* in the peripheral aspect of the myometrium.

23.2. ENDOMETRIUM

Description and Clinical Features

The endometrium is the innermost layer of the uterus that lines the uterine cavity. It is adherent to the inner myometrium and is continuous with the fallopian tubes.

The endometrium has a basal layer adjacent to the myometrium and a functional layer containing glandular tissue. In women of menstrual age, the functional layer changes markedly during the menstrual cycle. The functional layer is shed during menstruation, leaving the thin basal layer as the only remnant of the endometrium. There is often blood and shed tissue in the uterine cavity during this part of the cycle. After menstruation, the endometrium enters its proliferative phase, during which the functional layer regenerates in response to stimulation by estrogen produced by ovarian follicles, mainly by a single dominant ovarian follicle. This phase continues until ovulation, around midcycle, when the dominant ovarian follicle ruptures. The resulting corpus luteum produces progesterone. Under the influence of progesterone, the endometrium enters its secretory phase, during which its glands begin to secrete. The secretory phase continues until menstruation begins anew.

After menopause, the endometrium atrophies. This can lead to vaginal bleeding because the atrophic endometrium is prone to ulceration and bleeding.

Sonography

In a woman of menstrual age, the sonographic appearance of the endometrium varies during the menstrual cycle corresponding to the anatomic changes described above (Figure 23.2-1). During menses, blood or debris is often detectable in the uterine cavity. In the early proliferative phase, the endometrium appears as a thin echogenic line, corresponding to the apposed thin basal layers. In the late proliferative phase, the functional layer is thicker and hypoechoic, so that the endometrium has a multilayered appearance: a thin echogenic line anteriorly (anterior basal layer), then a thick hypoechoic zone (anterior functional layer), followed by a thin echogenic line in the middle (junction between the

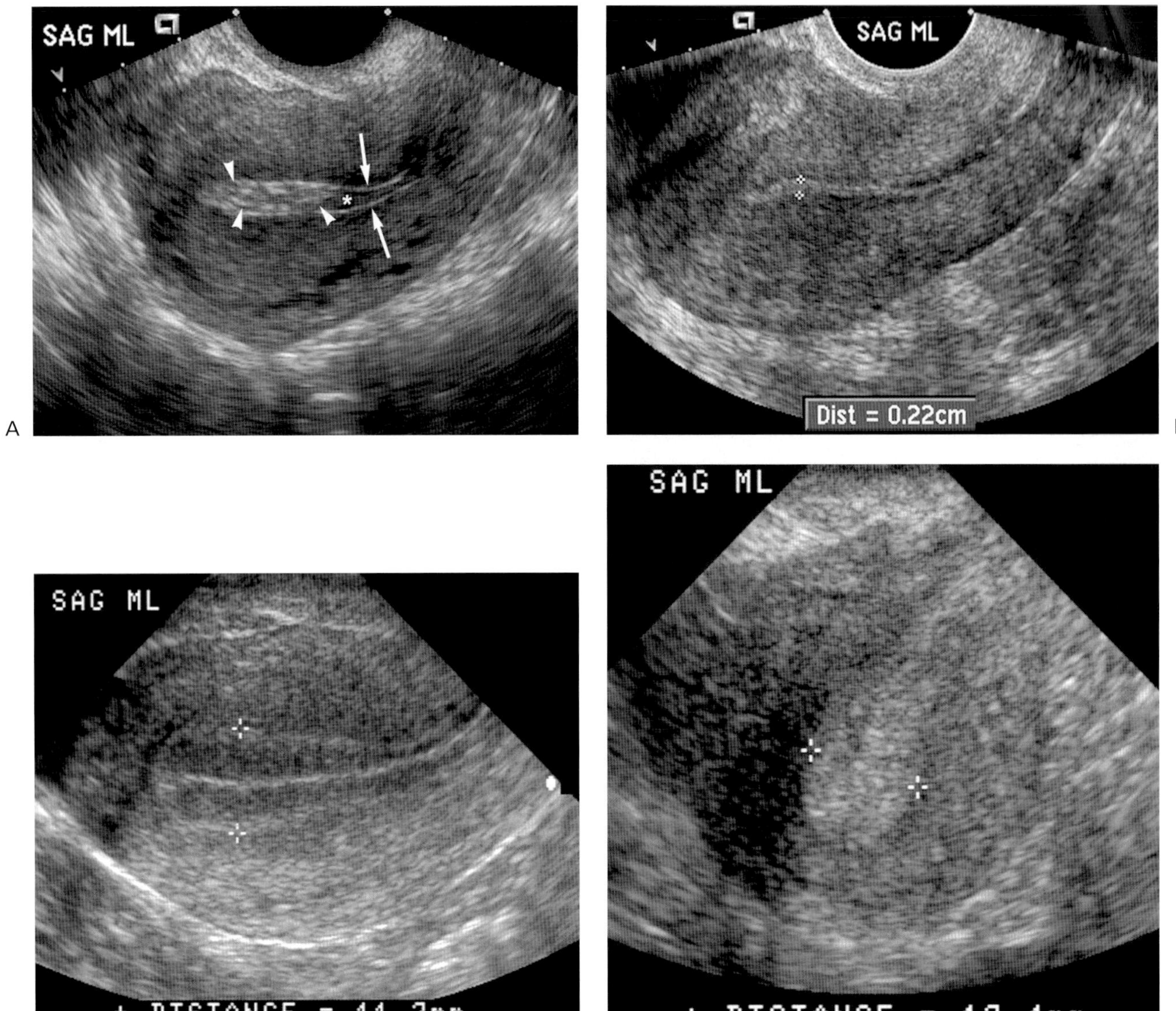

FIGURE 23.2-1. Normal endometrial appearance during the menstrual cycle. Sagittal midline *(SAG ML)* views of the uterus in women at different stages of the menstrual cycle depict the variations in endometrial appearance. **A:** Sonogram during menses demonstrates a clot *(arrowheads)* and fluid *(*)* within the uterine cavity; the endometrium *(arrows)*, outlined by fluid in the cavity, is very thin. **B:** The endometrium *(calipers)* appears as a thin echogenic line during the early proliferative phase, shortly after menses. **C:** During the late proliferative phase, the endometrium *(calipers)* has a multilayered appearance: echogenic around its periphery and in the midline and hypoechoic in between. **D:** During the secretory phase, the endometrium *(calipers)* is thick and echogenic.

two functional layers), then a thick hypoechoic zone (posterior functional layer), and finally a thin echogenic line posteriorly (posterior basal layer). During the secretory phase, the functional layer becomes more echogenic until it merges with the equally echogenic basal layers to appear as a single thick echogenic band.

In the postmenopausal woman, the normal endometrium appears on ultrasound as a thin homogeneously echogenic structure (Figure 23.2-2). Using the generally accepted approach for measuring endometrial thickness (from the anterior to posterior endometrial-myometrial junction on a sagittal transvaginal sonogram of the uterus), the thickness is generally 4–5 mm or less after menopause.

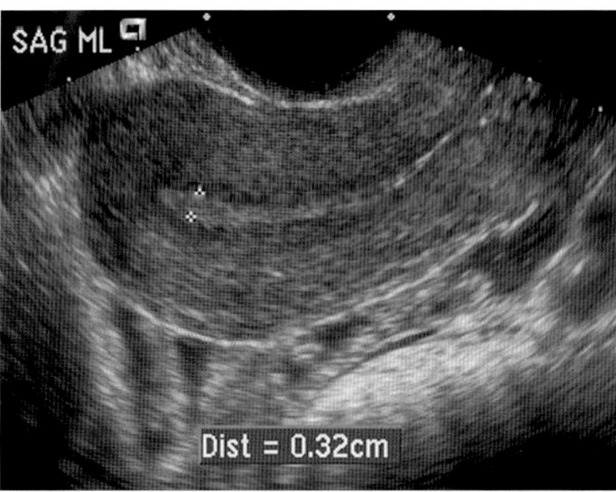

FIGURE 23.2-2. Normal postmenopausal endometrium. The endometrium *(calipers)* appears as a thin echogenic line on a sagittal midline *(SAG ML)* view of the uterus in this postmenopausal woman.

SUGGESTED READINGS

1. Forrest TS, Elyaderani MK, Muilenberg MI, et al. Cyclic endometrial changes: US assessment with histologic correlation. *Radiology* 1988;167:233–237.
2. Levi CS, Holt SC, Lyons EA, et al. Normal anatomy of the female pelvis. In: Callen PW, ed. *Ultrasonography in obstetrics and gynecology*, 4th ed. Philadelphia: WB Saunders, 2000:781–813.
3. Lyons EA, Gratton D, Harrington C. Transvaginal sonography of normal pelvic anatomy. *Radiol Clin North Am* 1992;30:663–675.
4. Merz E, Miric-Tesanic D, Bahlmann F, et al. Sonographic size of uterus and ovaries in pre- and postmenopausal women. *Ultrasound Obstet Gynecol* 1996;7:38.
5. Platt JF, Bree RL, Davidson D. Ultrasound of the normal nongravid uterus. *J Clin Ultrasound* 1990;18:15–19.
6. Richenberg J, Cooperberg P. Ultrasound of the uterus. In: Callen PW, ed. *Ultrasonography in obstetrics and gynecology*, 4th ed. Philadelphia: WB Saunders, 2000:814–846.

24

ADNEXA

24.1. OVARIES

Description and Clinical Features

The ovaries are paired ovoid pelvic organs located on each side of the uterus. They are mobile intraperitoneal structures. They lie anterior to the retroperitoneal structures, such as the ureter and internal iliac vessels. The ovary receives its blood supply both from the ovarian artery, which arises from the aorta, and from branches of the uterine artery.

In women of menstrual age, two types of functional cysts may be found in the ovaries: follicular cysts and corpus luteal cysts. During the first half of the menstrual cycle, multiple follicles develop until one (or occasionally more) becomes dominant. The dominant follicle ruptures midcycle at ovulation and involutes to become a corpus luteum. The corpus luteum regresses at the end of the menstrual cycle. Functional cysts are generally less than 2 cm in diameter but may become larger if they fail to involute or regress and fill up with fluid or blood.

After menopause, the ovaries decrease in size, both because ovarian tissue atrophies and ovarian cysts occur infrequently. When cysts occur in the postmenopausal ovary, they require follow-up or removal only if they are large or complex.

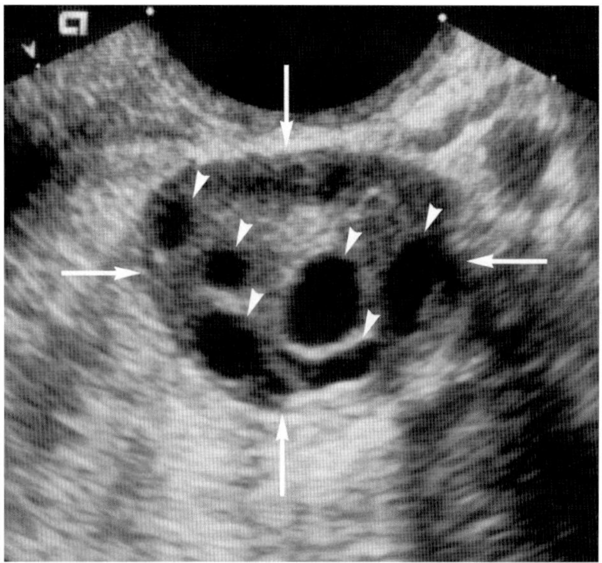

FIGURE 24.1-1. Normal ovary in a woman of menstrual age. The ovary *(arrows)* appears as a structure of moderate echogenicity, containing several small functional cysts *(arrowheads)*.

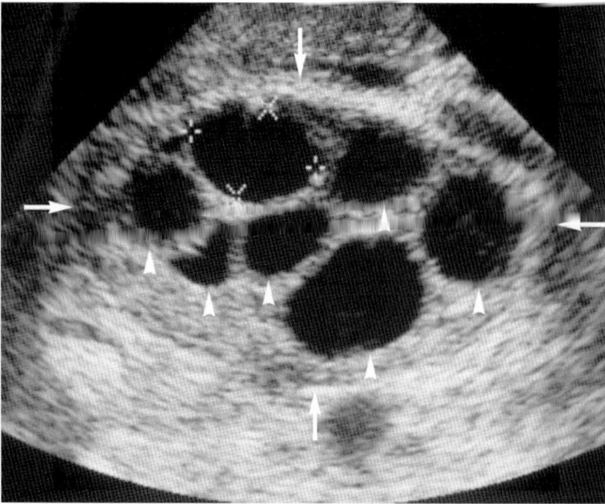

FIGURE 24.1-2. Ovary in a woman undergoing treatment for infertility. In this woman taking medication to stimulate development of ovarian follicles, ultrasound demonstrates multiple cysts *(calipers, arrowheads)* throughout the ovary *(arrows)*. The cysts occupy a relatively larger portion of the ovary than they do in a normal, nonstimulated ovary.

Sonography

The ovaries are generally visualized better by transvaginal than transabdominal sonography. An exception is the ovary located high in the pelvis, which may only be seen transabdominally. The premenopausal ovary appears on ultrasound as a soft-tissue structure with multiple small cysts, corresponding to functional cysts (Figure 24.1-1). In a woman taking follicular-stimulating medication to treat infertility, the number and size of cysts are greater than in normal nonstimulated ovaries (Figure 24.1-2).

The postmenopausal ovary is smaller than the premenopausal ovary. Its echotexture is usually homogeneous (Figure 24.1-3). As such, postmenopausal ovaries are more frequently undetectable on ultrasound than are premenopausal ovaries.

A

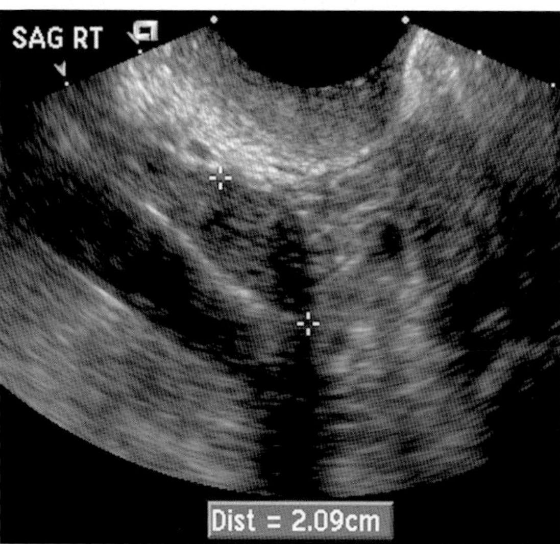

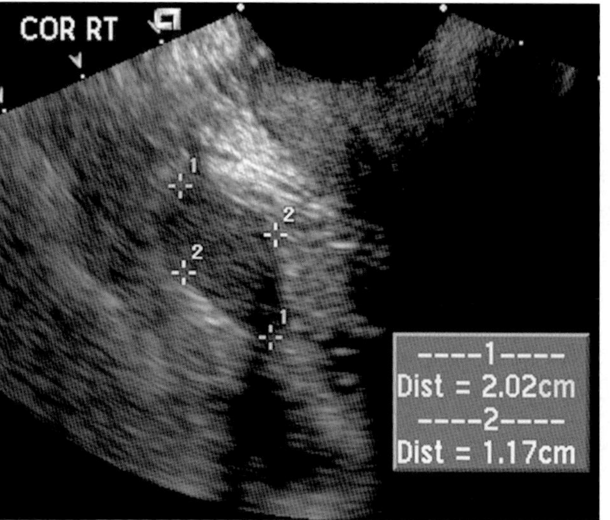

B

FIGURE 24.1-3. Normal ovary in a postmenopausal woman. Sagittal *(SAG RT)* **(A)** and coronal *(COR RT)* **(B)** transvaginal images demonstrate the right ovary *(calipers)* in a postmenopausal woman. The ovary is small and homogeneous, without the physiologic cysts seen in the typical premenopausal ovary.

24.2. EXTRAOVARIAN ADNEXAL STRUCTURES

Description and Clinical Features

The adnexa lie lateral to the uterus. The main components of the adnexa on each side are the ovary, fallopian tube, and broad ligament. The fallopian tube consists of several segments, the most medial of which is the intramural portion, which runs through the cornu of the uterus. This portion is continuous, in turn, with the isthmus, ampulla, and infundibulum of the tube. The isthmus is narrower than the ampulla. The infundibulum,

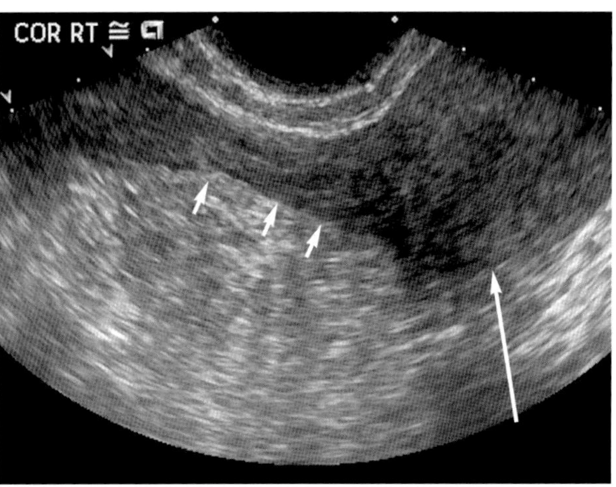

FIGURE 24.2-1. Broad ligament. Coronal transvaginal view of the uterus *(long arrow)* and right adnexa demonstrates the broad ligament *(short arrows)* extending laterally from the superior aspect of the uterus.

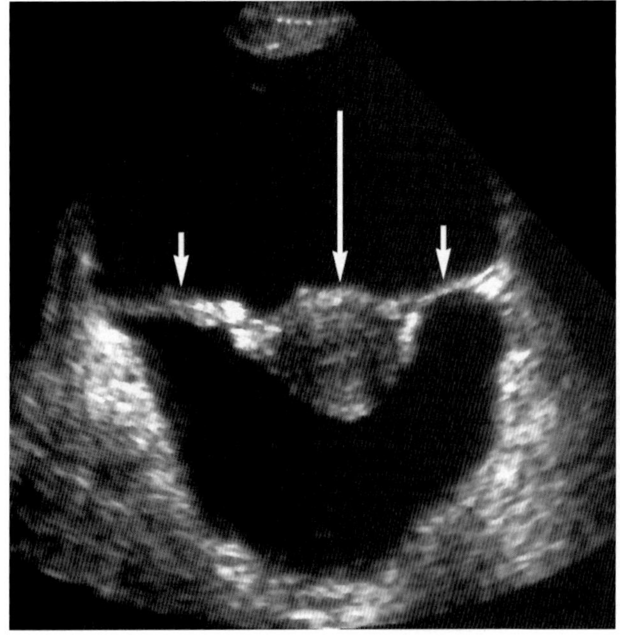
A

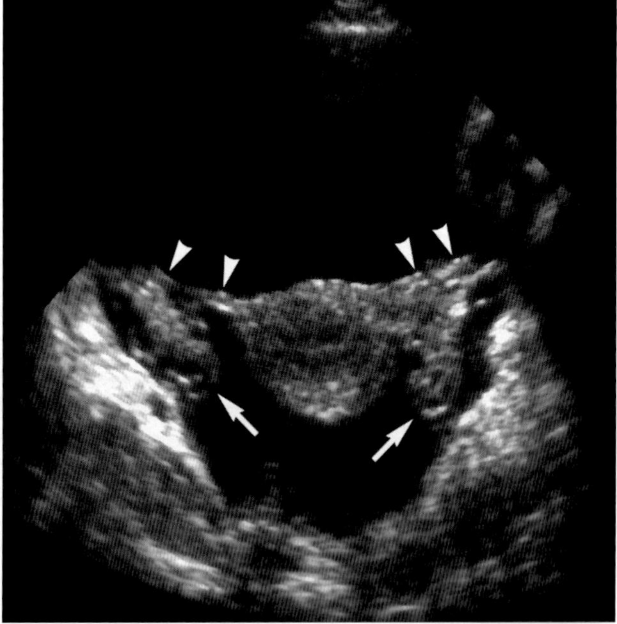
B

FIGURE 24.2-2. Broad ligament outlined by ascites. A: Transverse view of the pelvis in a woman with a large amount of ascites demonstrates the broad ligaments *(short arrows)* surrounded by fluid as they extend from the uterus *(long arrow)* to the pelvic sidewalls. **B:** The ovaries *(arrows)*, surrounded by ascites, are seen connected to the broad ligaments *(arrowheads)*.

which opens into the abdomen, has fimbriae at its end, one of which is attached to the ovary.

The broad ligament lies lateral to the uterus and is covered on both surfaces by the peritoneum. Lying within the broad ligament are the fallopian tube and uterine artery. The ovary is connected to the broad ligament by a mesenteric attachment.

Sonography

On ultrasound, the broad ligament can sometimes be seen extending laterally from the fundus of the uterus (Figure 24.2-1). Its visualization is enhanced if it is surrounded by ascites (Figure 24.2-2).

The normal fallopian tube is rarely identifiable by ultrasound. It becomes visible if it is distended with fluid due to a pathologic process (hydro- or pyosalpinx).

SUGGESTED READINGS

1. Cohen HL, Tice HM, Mandell FS. Ovarian volumes measured by ultrasound. *Radiology* 1990;177: 189–192.
2. Dill-Macky MJ, Atri M. Ovarian sonography. In: Callen PW, ed. *Ultrasonography in obstetrics and gynecology*, 4th ed. Philadelphia: WB Saunders, 2000:857–896.
3. Fleischer AC, McKee MS, Gordon AN, et al. Transvaginal sonography of postmenopausal ovaries with pathologic correlation. *J Ultrasound Med* 1990;9:637–644.
4. Levi CS, Holt SC, Lyons EA, et al. Normal anatomy of the female pelvis. In: Callen PW, ed. *Ultrasonography in obstetrics and gynecology*, 4th ed. Philadelphia: WB Saunders, 2000:781–813.
5. Lyons EA, Gratton D, Harrington C. Transvaginal sonography of normal pelvic anatomy. *Radiol Clin North Am* 1992;30:663–675.
6. Merz E, Mirio-Tesanic D, Bahlmann F, et al. Sonographic size of uterus and ovaries in pre- and postmenopausal women. *Ultrasound Obstet Gynecol* 1996;7:38–42.

25

MYOMETRIUM

25.1. FIBROIDS (LEIOMYOMAS) AND LEIOMYOSARCOMAS

Description and Clinical Features

Fibroids, or uterine leiomyomas, are commonly occurring benign myometrial tumors composed of smooth muscle and connective tissue. They are found in approximately 20% of women over the age of 35 and are more common in women of African than European origin. They often enlarge during pregnancy and may shrink after menopause. Most are located in the uterine body and fundus, but they can also occur in the cervix. Fibroids are classified as:

Intramural: confined to the myometrium
Submucosal: projecting into the endometrium
Subserosal: projecting from the serosal surface of the uterus

Fibroids can cause a variety of symptoms, including pain and abnormal vaginal bleeding. They can cause ureteral compression, leading to hydronephrosis. They can cause several complications during pregnancy, including miscarriage, pain, obstruction of vaginal delivery (if the fibroid is large and in the lower segment or cervix), and placental abruption (if the placenta implants on a fibroid).

Leiomyosarcomas are rare malignant tumors of the myometrium, occurring most often after menopause. Leiomyosarcomas enlarge over time, a finding that distinguishes them from fibroids in postmenopausal women.

Sonography

The appearance of fibroids on ultrasound is variable. In some cases, ultrasound demonstrates a single or multiple discrete, heterogeneous, highly attenuating masses in the myometrium. In others, the entire uterus is enlarged and heterogeneous, often with a nodular external contour.

A discrete fibroid may be submucosal, intramural, or subserosal and may be in the body, fundus, or (less commonly) cervix (Figure 25.1-1). Submucosal fibroids project into and distort the endometrium. The diagnosis of a submucosal fibroid can be aided by instilling fluid into the uterine cavity (saline infusion sonohysterogram) (Figure 25.1-2). Subserosal fibroids are diagnosed when a myometrial mass is seen extending from the outer surface of the uterus.

Calcification, either within the fibroid or around its rim, is fairly common (Figure 25.1-3). Cystic areas are occasionally seen within fibroids and may represent necrosis.

Fibroids are usually highly vascular. On color Doppler, multiple vessels can be identified throughout the mass (Figure 25.1-4).

Leiomyosarcomas have a sonographic appearance similar to that of fibroids. Because they are much less common than fibroids, they are not generally diagnosed preoperatively. If a mass that appears to be a fibroid enlarges in a postmenopausal woman, the possibility of leiomyosarcoma should be considered.

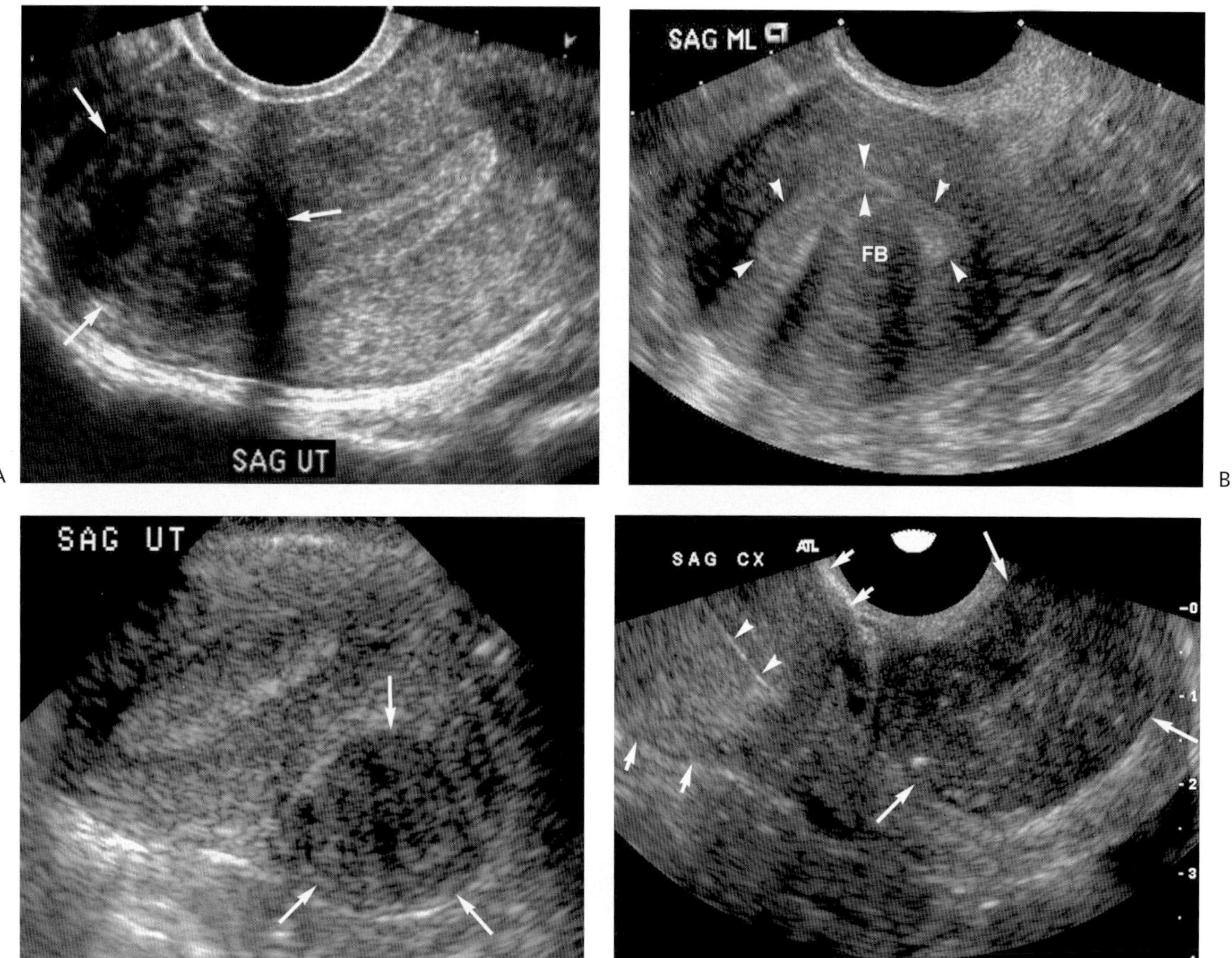

FIGURE 25.1-1. Fibroids in various locations. A: Sagittal view of the uterus *(SAG UT)* demonstrates an intramural fibroid *(arrows)* in the uterine fundus. **B:** Sagittal midline *(SAG ML)* view of the uterus demonstrates a submucosal fibroid *(FB)* indenting the endometrium *(arrowheads)*. **C:** Sagittal view of the uterus demonstrates a subserosal fibroid *(arrows)* projecting from the posterior aspect of the uterus. **D:** Sagittal view of the cervix *(SAG CX)* demonstrates a large cervical fibroid *(long arrows)* located caudal to the uterine body *(short arrows)*; the endometrium *(arrowheads)* is visible within the body.

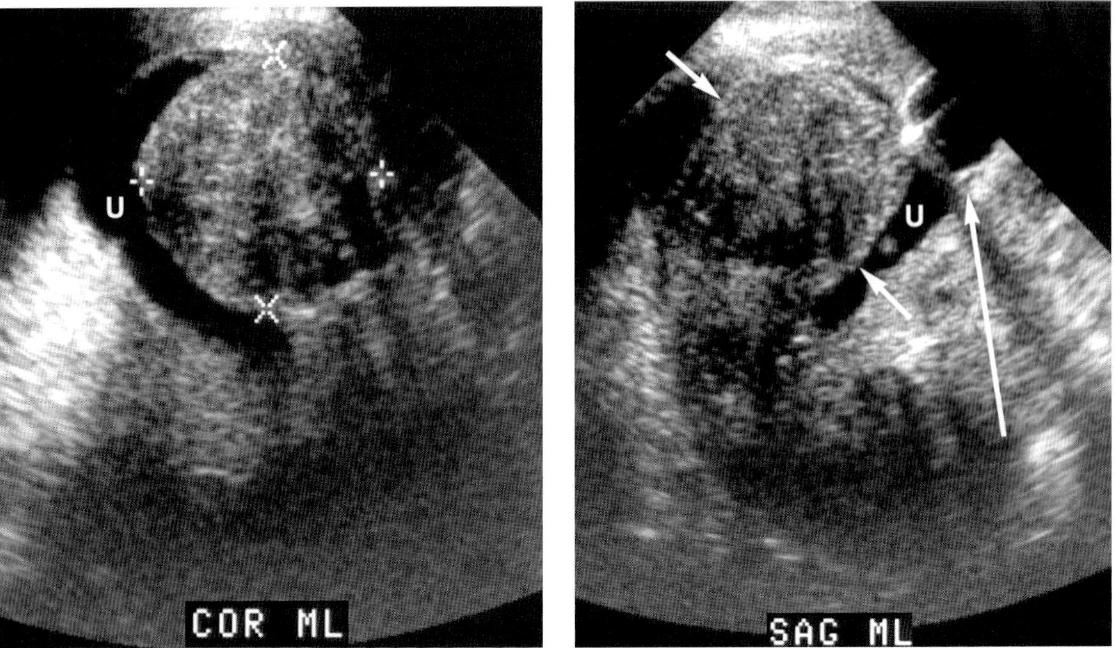

FIGURE 25.1-2. Submucosal fibroid demonstrated by saline infusion sonohysterography. A: Coronal view *(COR ML)* of the uterus after instillation of saline into the uterine cavity *(U)* demonstrates a submucosal fibroid *(calipers)* protruding into the saline-filled cavity. **B:** Sagittal view *(SAG ML)* demonstrates the submucosal fibroid *(short arrows)* adjacent to the balloon-tipped catheter *(long arrow)* in the saline-filled uterine cavity *(U)*.

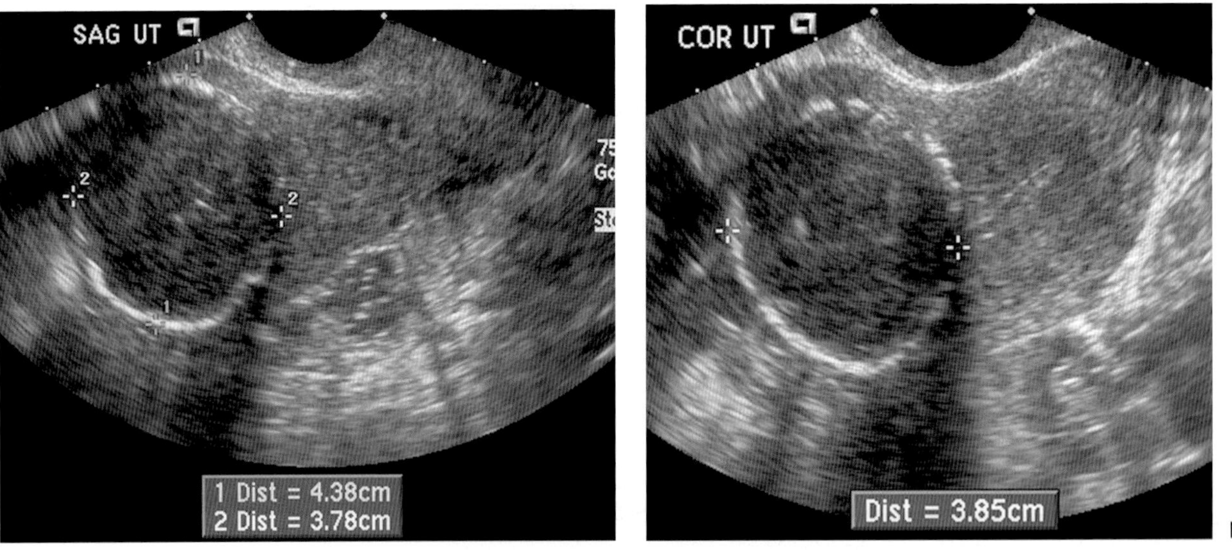

FIGURE 25.1-3. Calcified fibroid. Sagittal *(SAG UT)* **(A)** and coronal *(COR UT)* **(B)** transvaginal views of the uterus demonstrate a fibroid *(calipers)* with a calcified rim.

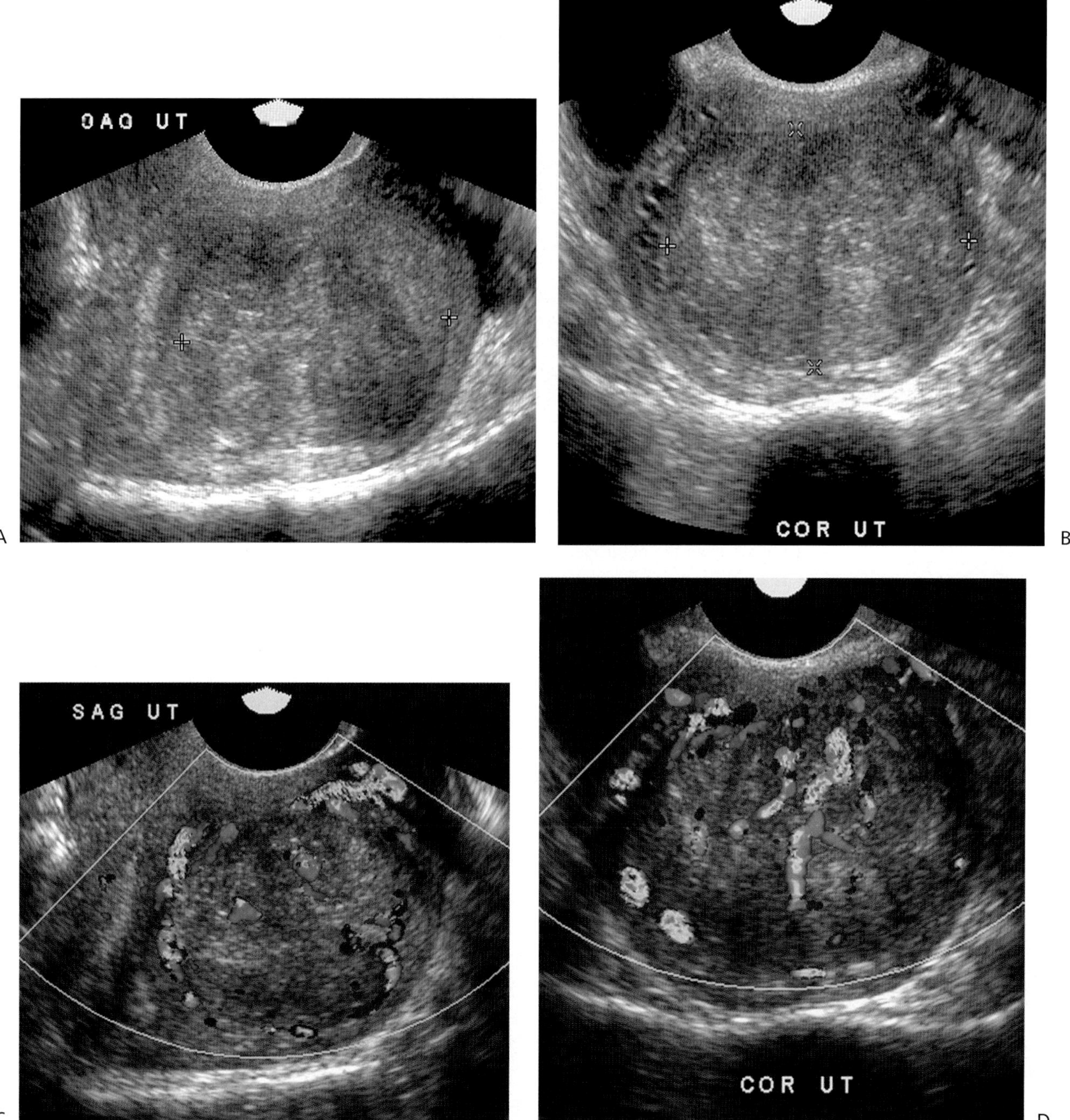

FIGURE 25.1-4. Color Doppler of a fibroid. Sagittal *(SAG UT)* **(A)** and coronal *(COR UT)* **(B)** transvaginal views of the uterus demonstrate a large fibroid *(calipers)*. Color Doppler images in sagittal **(C)** and coronal **(D)** planes demonstrate considerable blood flow around and within the fibroid, indicating that it is highly vascular.

25.2. ADENOMYOSIS

Description and Clinical Features

Adenomyosis is a form of endometriosis in which aberrant endometrial tissue is located within the myometrium. It may be diffuse or focal. Symptoms include abnormal vaginal bleeding, pain, and infertility.

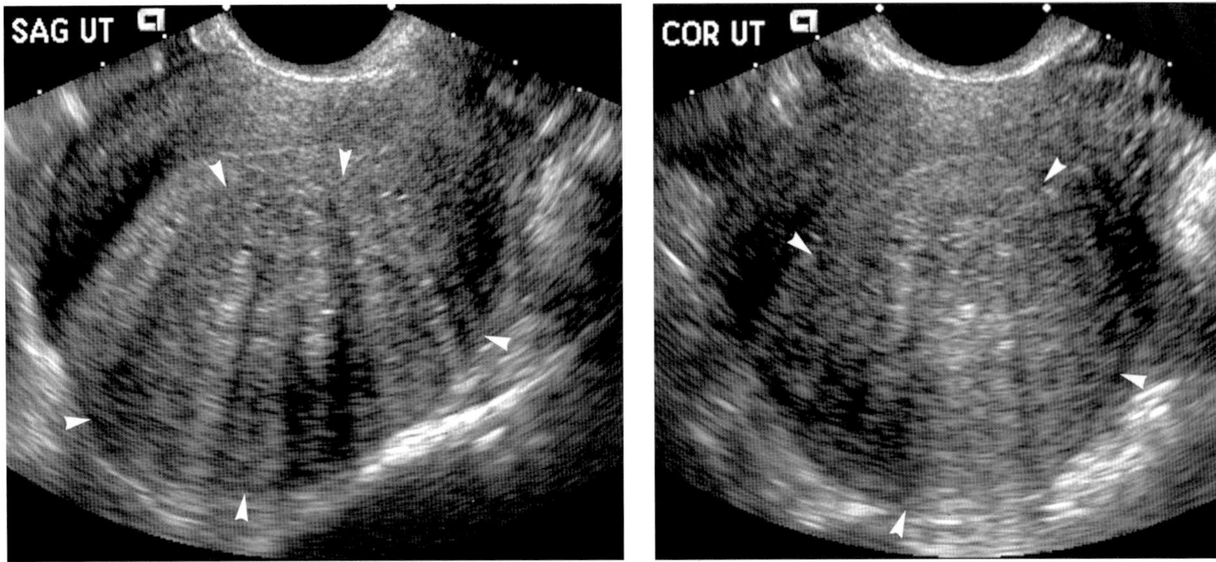

FIGURE 25.2-1. Adenomyosis involving the posterior myometrium. Sagittal *(SAG UT)* **(A)** and coronal *(COR UT)* **(B)** transvaginal views of the uterus demonstrate that the posterior aspect of the uterus is enlarged and heterogeneous *(arrowheads)*. Multiple areas of shadowing emanate from the heterogeneous posterior myometrium.

Sonography

Adenomyosis presents sonographically as a poorly defined, localized (Figure 25.2-1) or diffuse (Figure 25.2-2) area of uterine enlargement and abnormal echogenicity. In most cases, the echotexture is heterogeneous, sometimes with irregular shadowing and multiple small (2–3 mm) myometrial cysts intermixed with hyperechoic tissue. In other cases, the echotexture is homogeneously hyperechoic.

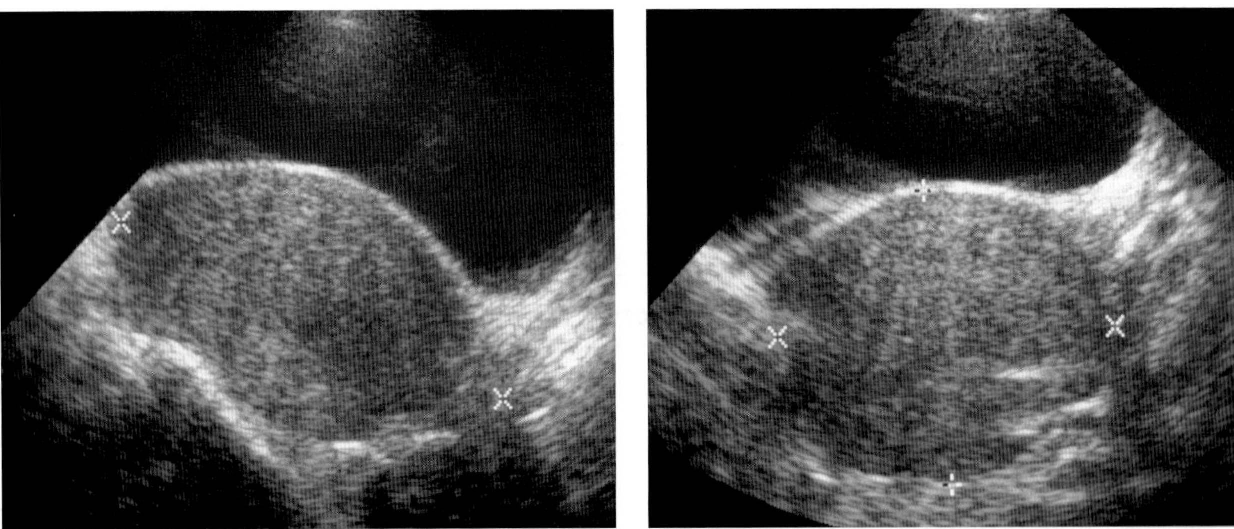

FIGURE 25.2-2. Diffuse adenomyosis. Sagittal **(A)** and transverse **(B)** transabdominal views demonstrate a large homogeneously hyperechoic uterus *(calipers)*. The woman, who was having symptoms of pain and excessive vaginal bleeding, underwent a hysterectomy, and diffuse adenomyosis was found.

Although there is considerable overlap in the sonographic appearances of adenomyosis and fibroids, a number of features can be used to make the correct diagnosis in many cases:

The presence of one or more well-defined myometrial masses with identifiable margins is highly suggestive of fibroids.
The presence of small cysts and/or hyperechoic areas within the myometrial lesion is suggestive of adenomyosis.
Variation of the lesion's appearance during the menstrual cycle is suggestive of adenomyosis.

25.3. UTERINE DUPLICATION ANOMALIES

Description and Clinical Features

The uterus and vagina arise embryologically from paired m¸llerian ducts that fuse in the midline. The medial walls of the ducts form a median septum that is subsequently resorbed. The normal embryologic sequence can go awry in a number of ways, leading to a variety of uterine anomalies:

Didelphic uterus: two separate uteri and cervices, with a normal or septate vagina, caused by complete failure of fusion of the müllerian ducts.
Bicornuate uterus: two separate uterine horns that join at a variable level above the cervix, caused by partial failure of fusion of the müllerian ducts.
Septate or subseptate uterus: normal outer uterine contour, with the presence of a septum completely (septate) or partially (subseptate) dividing the uterine cavity; caused by complete or partial failure of resorption of the median septum.

In addition to these duplication anomalies, failure of one or both of the müllerian ducts to develop leads to a unicornuate uterus or uterine aplasia.

The embryologic development of the uterus and kidneys are closely related. As a result, renal anomalies, especially unilateral renal agenesis or renal ectopia, are common in women with uterine anomalies.

Women with uterine anomalies are at increased risk of infertility and early pregnancy loss. The anomaly that appears to carry the greatest risk is a septate uterus.

Sonography

With any uterine duplication anomaly, a transverse view through an affected area of the uterus demonstrates separation of the endometrium into two parts. On coronal or transverse images, the endometrium appears as side-by-side, rounded echogenic areas separated by hypoechoic tissue (Figure 25.3-1). Depending on the extent of duplication or septation, this appearance may be seen through the entire length of the uterus or only near the fundus.

Differentiation between a septate or subseptate uterus and a bicornuate or didelphic uterus can be made by ultrasound in some cases. If a transverse view demonstrates two completely distinct uterine horns, separated by nonuterine tissue, the diagnosis of a bicornuate or didelphic uterus is established (Figure 25.3-2). An alternative approach is to obtain a coronal view of the uterus by means of planar reformatting from a three-dimensional sonogram (Figure 25.3-3). On this view, the fundal uterine contour is smooth with a septate or subseptate uterus and indented with a bicornuate or didelphic uterus.

Whenever a uterine anomaly is detected, the kidneys should be evaluated sonographically. In particular, the presence and location of both kidneys should be assessed (Figure 25.3-4).

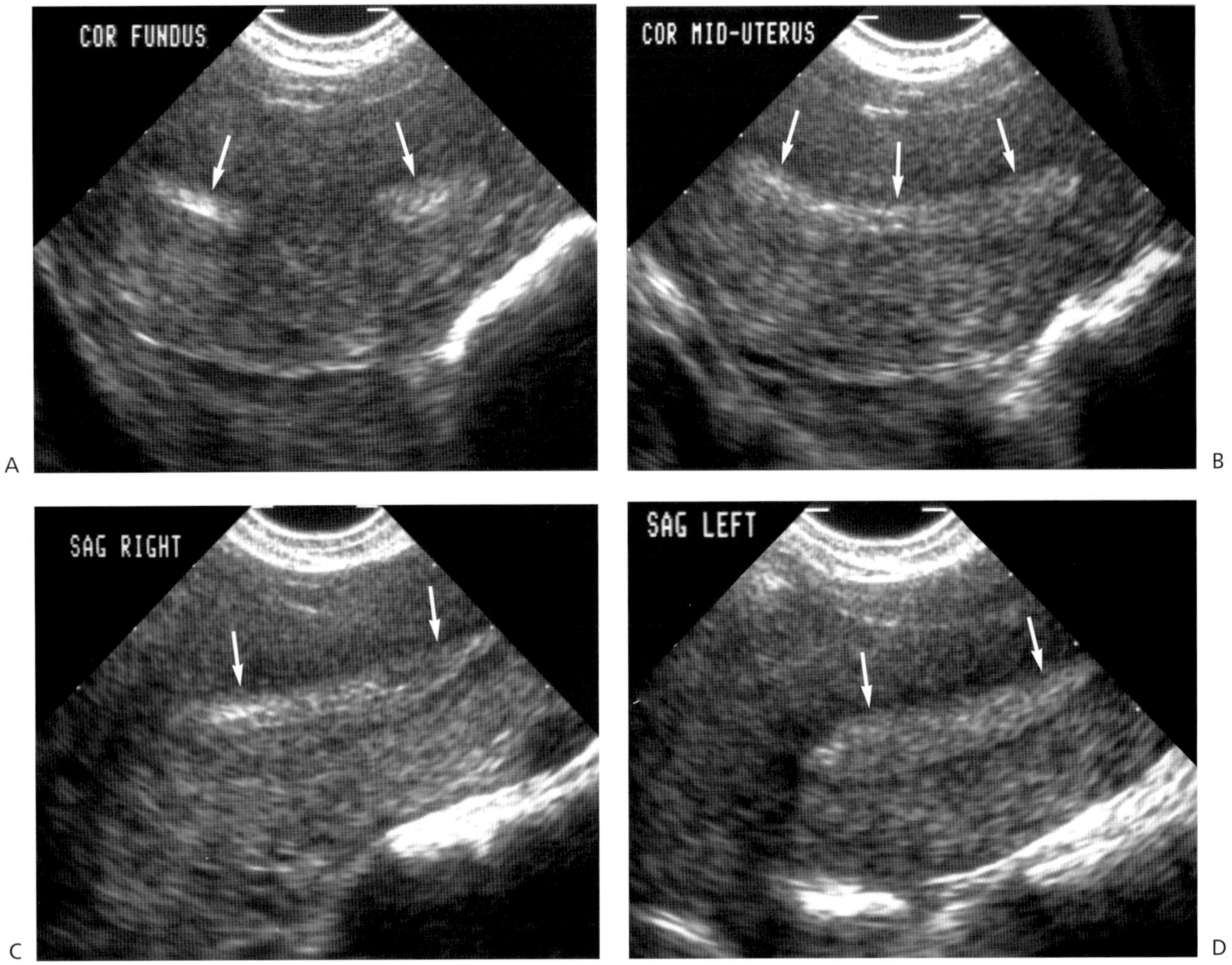

FIGURE 25.3-1. Uterine duplication anomaly. A: Coronal transvaginal view of the uterine fundus *(COR FUNDUS)* demonstrates separation of the endometrium into two parts *(arrows)*. **B:** Coronal view through the body of the uterus *(COR MID-UTERUS)* demonstrates that the endometrium is not separated at this level, because there is a single expanse of endometrium *(arrows)* extending across the uterus. Right *(SAG RIGHT)* **(C)** and left *(SAG LEFT)* **(D)** parasagittal views of the uterus reveal endometrial tissue *(arrows)* extending up each side of the uterus.

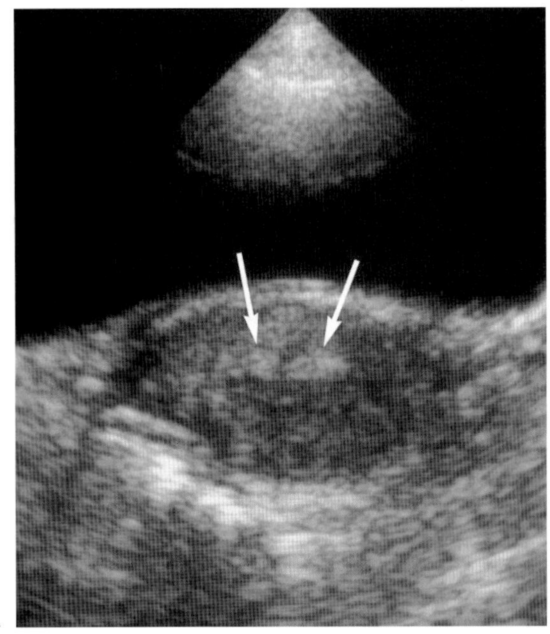

FIGURE 25.3-2. Didelphic uterus. A: Transverse transabdominal view of the cervix demonstrates two separate echogenic structures *(arrows)* representing two endocervical canals.

(continued)

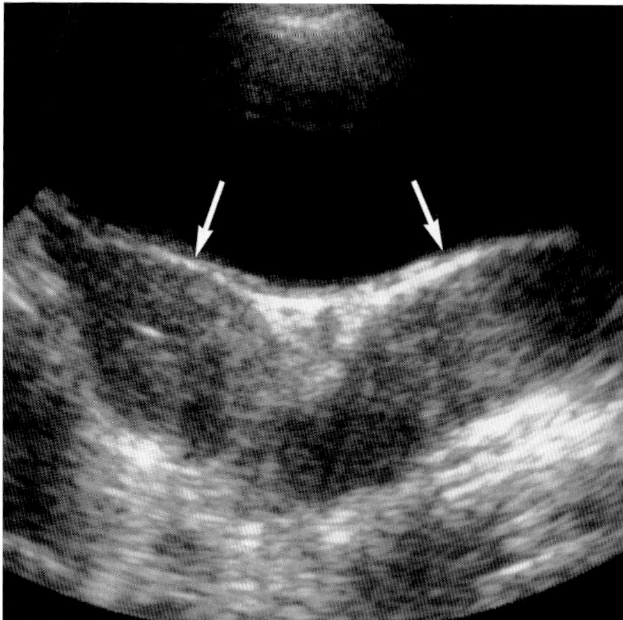
B

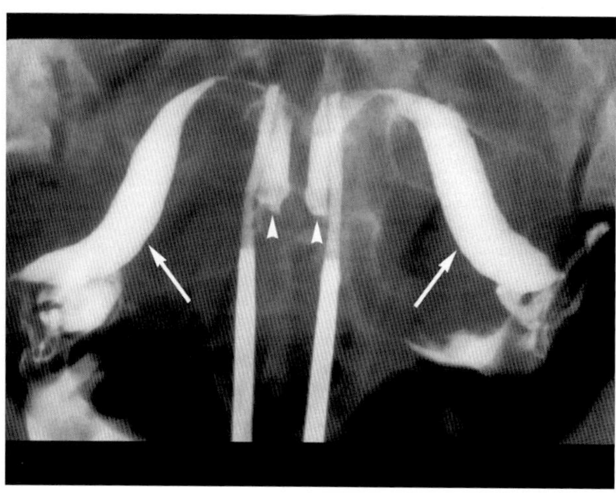
C

FIGURE 25.3-2. *(continued)* **B:** Transverse view through the mid to upper uterus demonstrates separate right and left uterine horns *(arrows)*. **C:** X-ray hysterosalpingogram confirms a didelphic uterus, with paired contrast-filled cervical canals *(arrowheads)* and uterine cavities *(arrows)*.

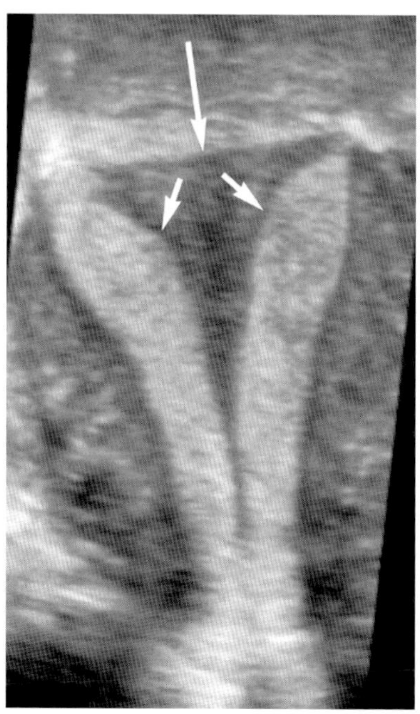

FIGURE 25.3-3. Septate uterus diagnosed via planar reformatting from a three-dimensional sonogram. Coronal view of the uterus obtained by three-dimensional reformatting demonstrates that the endometrium is separated into two components *(short arrows)* and the uterine fundus *(long arrow)* has a smooth external contour, establishing a diagnosis of septate uterus. (Courtesy of Dr. Beryl Benacerraf.)

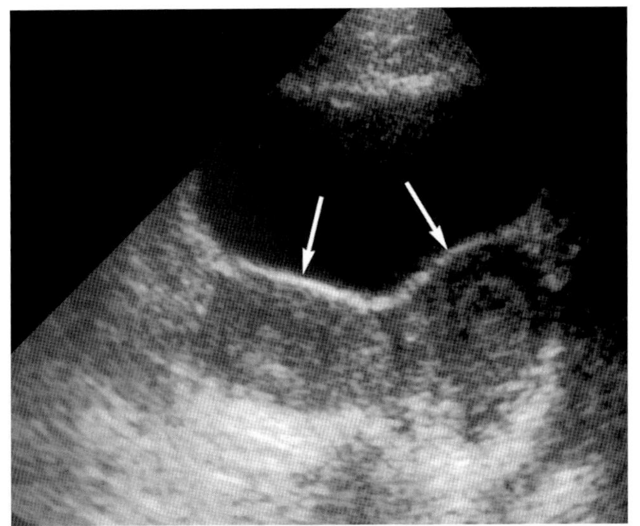
A

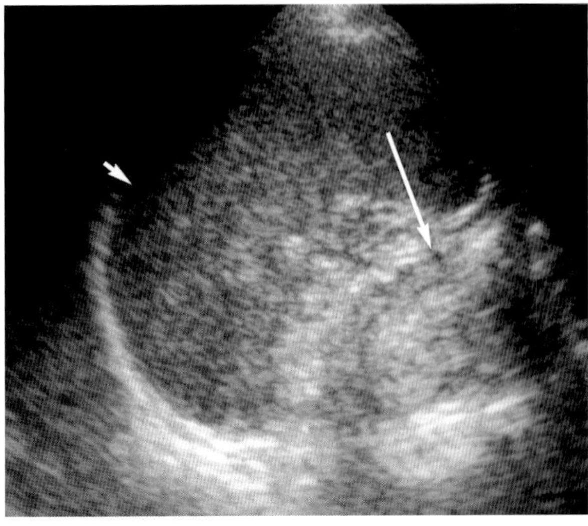
B

FIGURE 25.3-4. Uterine duplication anomaly with unilateral renal agenesis. A: Transverse transabdominal view reveals two separate uterine bodies *(arrows)*. **B:** On this longitudinal view of the left upper quadrant, no kidney is seen in the left renal fossa *(long arrow)* below the spleen *(short arrow)*.

SUGGESTED READINGS

1. Ascher SM, Arnold LL, Patt RH. Adenomyosis: prospective comparison of MR imaging and transvaginal sonography. *Radiology* 1994;190:803–806.
2. Fleischer AC, Entman SS. Sonographic evaluation of uterine disorders. In: Fleischer AC, Manning FA, Jeanty P, et al., eds. *Sonography in obstetrics & gynecology: principles and practice*, 6th ed. New York: McGraw-Hill, 2001:949–977.
3. Huang R, Chou C, Chang C. Differentiation between adenomyoma and leiomyoma with transvaginal sonography. *Ultrasound Obstet Gynecol* 1995;5:47–50.
4. Karasik S, Lev-Toaff AS, Lev-Toaff ME. Imaging of uterine leiomyomas. *AJR Am J Roentgenol* 1992; 158:799–805.
5. Mintz MC, Grumbach K. Imaging of congenital uterine anomalies. *Semin Ultrasound CT MR* 1988; 9:167–174.
6. Reinhold C, Atri M, Mehio A, et al. Diffuse uterine adenomyosis: morphologic criteria and diagnostic accuracy of endovaginal sonography. *Radiology* 1995;197:609–614.
7. Richenberg J, Cooperberg P. Ultrasound of the uterus. In: Callen PW, ed. *Ultrasonography in obstetrics and gynecology*, 4th ed. Philadelphia: WB Saunders, 2000:814–846.

26

ENDOMETRIUM

26.1. ENDOMETRIAL POLYPS

Description and Clinical Features

Endometrial polyps are fairly common lesions that can occur at any age. They can be pedunculated or broad-based, are generally benign, and, if benign, have little potential to become malignant. In a woman of menstrual age, polyps can cause intermenstrual bleeding, menorrhagia (heavy menstrual bleeding), or infertility. In the postmenopausal woman, the most common symptom of polyps is vaginal bleeding.

When a woman presents with abnormal vaginal bleeding, endometrial tissue sampling using either a suction catheter (office endometrial biopsy) or dilation and curettage is often performed. These sampling techniques, however, can miss polyps entirely because they blindly sample a portion of the endometrium. Ultrasound and saline-infusion sonohysterography (SIS) can be used to detect polyps, after which they can be sampled or resected under hysteroscopic guidance.

Sonography

On ultrasound, endometrial polyps are either homogeneously echogenic (Figure 26.1-1) or complex lesions with echogenic tissue and one or more small cysts (Figure 26.1-2). If fluid (blood or secretions) is present in the uterine cavity, the polyp is seen as a focal mass surrounded by fluid (Figure 26.1-3). Color Doppler typically reveals a single feeding vessel (Figures 26.1-1 and 26.1-3).

A polyp should be suspected when ultrasound demonstrates a focal area of endometrial thickening or a focal echogenic lesion within less echogenic endometrium, and should be included in the differential diagnosis when ultrasound demonstrates diffuse endometrial thickening. In any of these situations, the diagnosis can be confirmed using SIS, which depicts polyps as focal projections of endometrial tissue into the saline-filled uterine cavity (Figure 26.1-4).

When an endometrial polyp is present, ultrasound is most likely to detect it if the surrounding endometrium is thin or hypoechoic. Thus, polyps are most likely to produce an abnormal ultrasound in a postmenopausal woman or during the proliferative stage of the menstrual cycle in a premenopausal woman. They are most likely to be missed during the secretory phase of the menstrual cycle, when they may be indistinguishable from the normal thick echogenic endometrium.

Polyps may also occur in the cervix. They are most easily identifiable on sonography if outlined by fluid, such as secretions or blood, in the cervical canal (Figure 26.1-5).

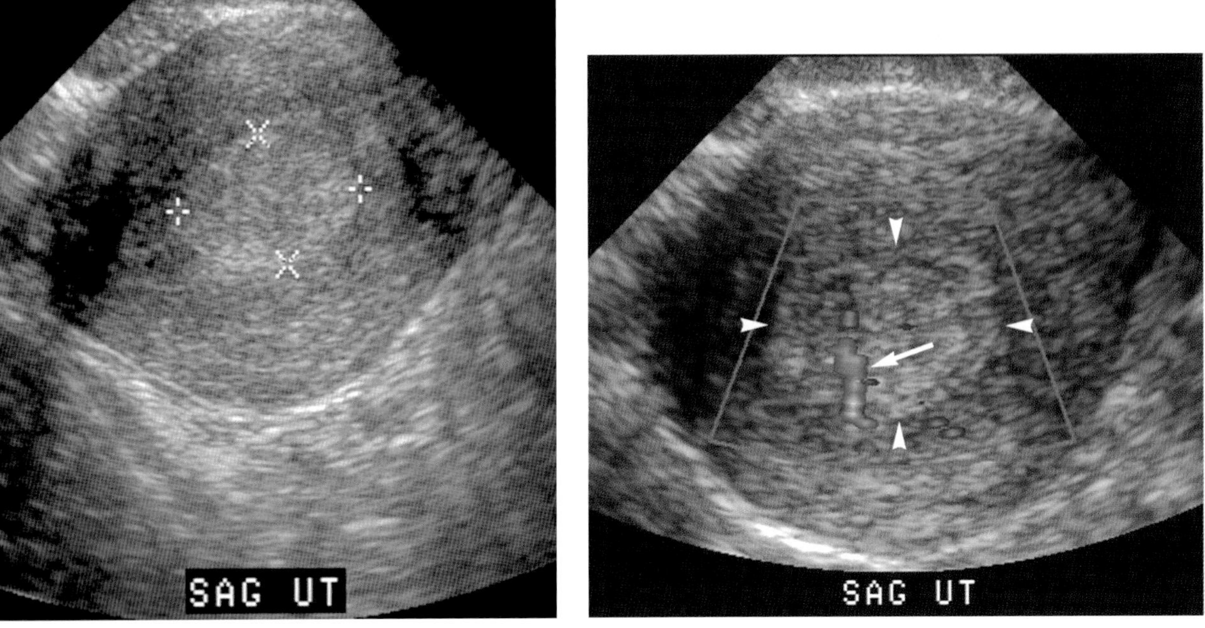

FIGURE 26.1-1. Endometrial polyp with a feeding vessel. A: Sagittal transvaginal view of the uterus *(SAG UT)* demonstrates a homogeneously echogenic mass *(calipers)* in the endometrium. **B:** Color Doppler demonstrates a single feeding vessel *(arrow)* into the endometrial mass *(arrowheads)*.

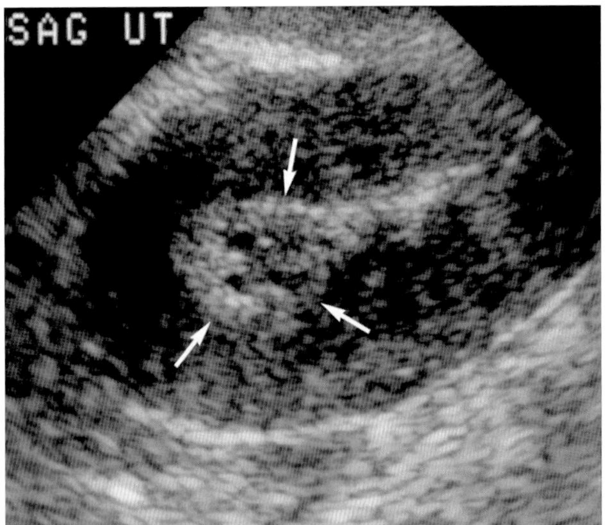

FIGURE 26.1-2. Endometrial polyp containing multiple small cysts. Sagittal transvaginal view of the uterus *(SAG UT)* demonstrates a complex endometrial lesion *(arrows)* consisting of echogenic tissue with multiple small cysts.

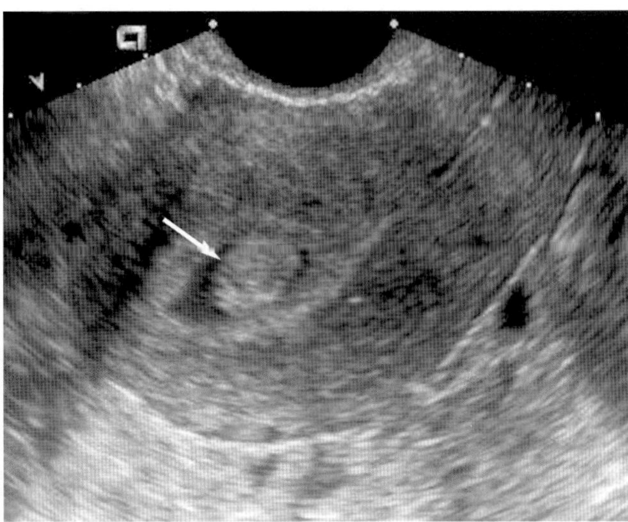

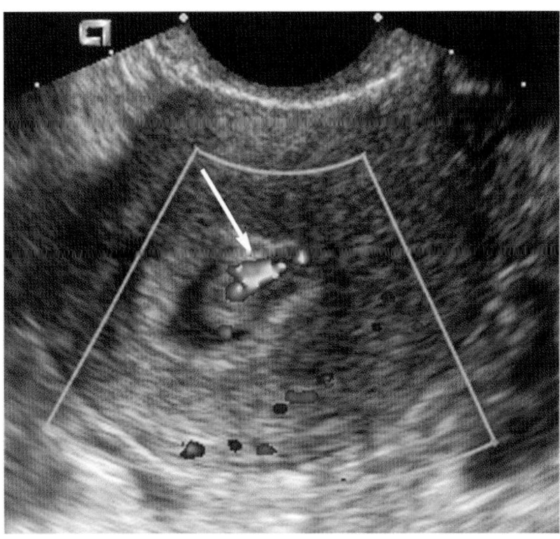

FIGURE 26.1-3. Endometrial polyp surrounded by fluid. A: Sagittal transvaginal view of the uterus demonstrates a polypoid projection of tissue *(arrow)* into the fluid-filled uterine cavity. The fluid likely represents blood or secretions. **B:** Color Doppler demonstrates a single feeding vessel *(arrow)* into the polyp.

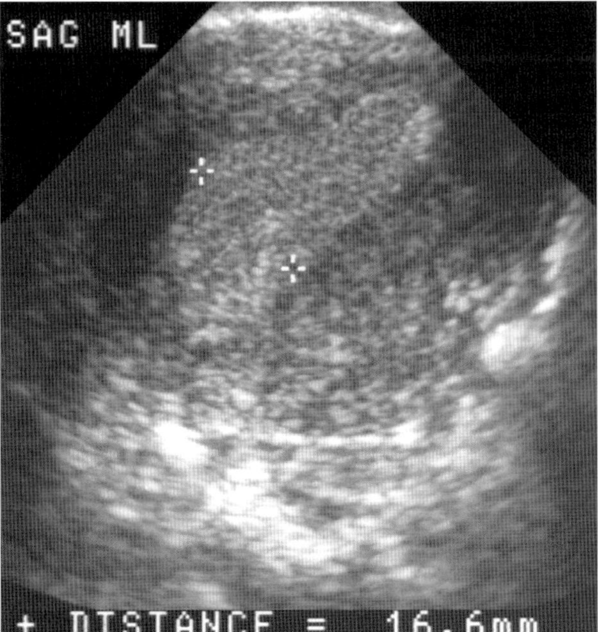

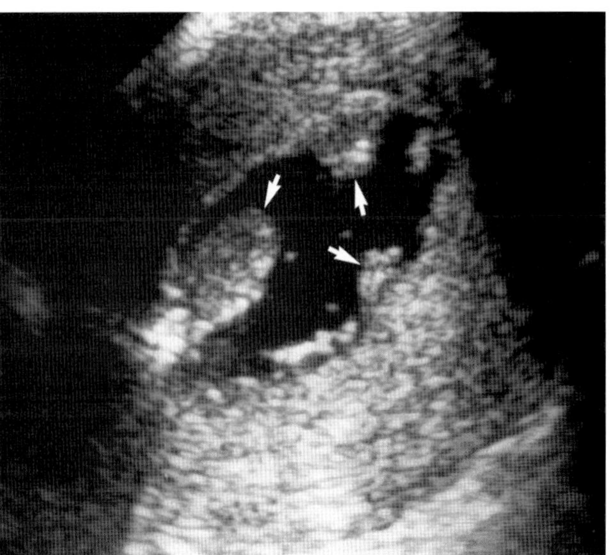

FIGURE 26.1-4. Endometrial polyps depicted by saline infusion sonohysterography. A: Sagittal midline *(SAG ML)* transvaginal view of the uterus demonstrates homogeneous thickening of the endometrium *(calipers)*, measuring 16.6 mm in thickness. **B:** After instillation of saline, multiple polyps *(arrows)* are seen projecting into the fluid-filled uterine cavity.

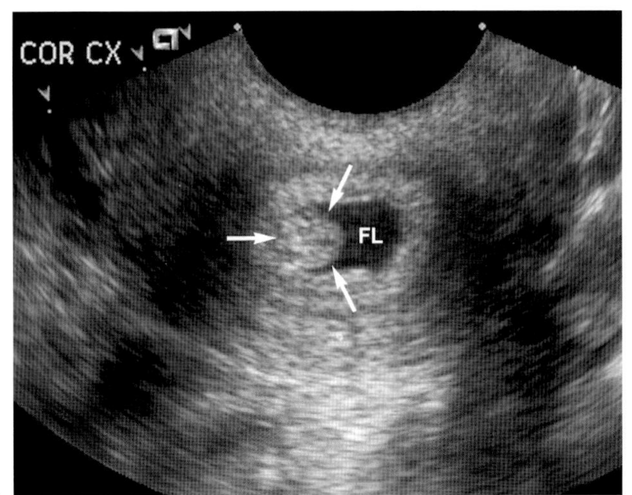

A

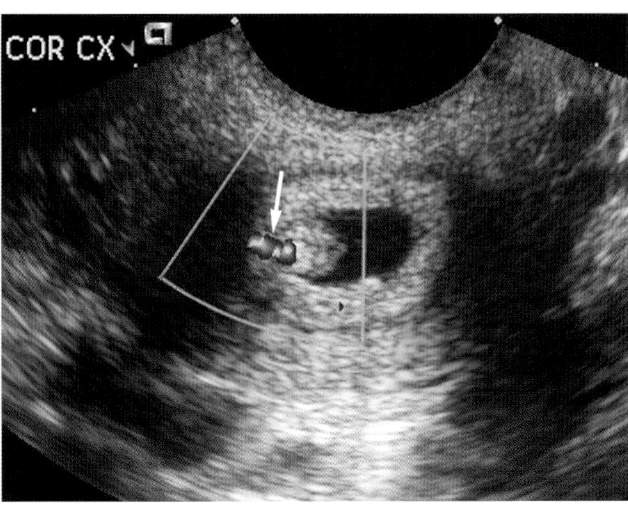

B

FIGURE 26.1-5. **Cervical polyp. A:** Coronal transvaginal view of the cervix *(COR CX)* demonstrates a polypoid soft-tissue mass *(arrows)* outlined by fluid *(FL)* in the cervical canal. **B:** Color Doppler demonstrates a single feeding vessel *(arrow)* into the polyp.

26.2. ENDOMETRIAL HYPERPLASIA

Description and Clinical Features

Endometrial hyperplasia refers to abnormal proliferation of the endometrial glands. It is caused by unopposed estrogen stimulation, which can result from estrogen given as hormone replacement therapy, hormonal disorders (e.g., polycystic ovary syndrome), or estrogen-producing tumors.

Hyperplasia is usually a diffuse endometrial process. It can occur with or without cellular atypia. If cellular atypia is present, there is a substantial risk of progression to endometrial carcinoma. The risk is far lower in the absence of atypia.

Endometrial hyperplasia can occur in women of any age. It generally presents with abnormal vaginal bleeding and is among the most common causes of such bleeding.

Sonography

In most cases of endometrial hyperplasia, the endometrium appears diffusely thick and homogeneously echogenic on ultrasound. On SIS, the saline-filled uterine cavity is surrounded in its entirety by thick endometrial tissue (Figure 26.2-1).

Endometrial hyperplasia is diagnosed based on abnormal thickening of the endometrium, and is best detected by ultrasound when the normal endometrium is thin. In a postmenopausal woman not on hormone replacement therapy, the sonogram can be performed at any time. In a postmenopausal woman on sequential hormone replacement therapy, the sonogram should be performed shortly after progesterone withdrawal bleeding, when the endometrium is expected to be at its thinnest. In a premenopausal woman, sonography should be done during the early proliferative phase of the menstrual cycle. During the secretory phase of the cycle, the presence of endometrial hyperplasia is likely to be missed sonographically because hyperplastic endometrium and normal secretory endometrium have similar sonographic appearances.

When ultrasound demonstrates diffuse thickening of the endometrium, endometrial hyperplasia should be included in the differential diagnosis, along with endometrial polyps and carcinoma. SIS can exclude polyps, but a definitive diagnosis of hyperplasia can only be made by tissue sampling (office biopsy or dilation and curettage).

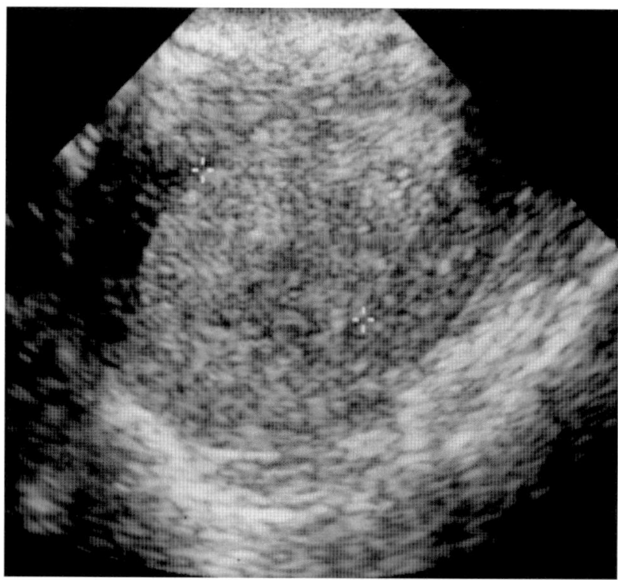

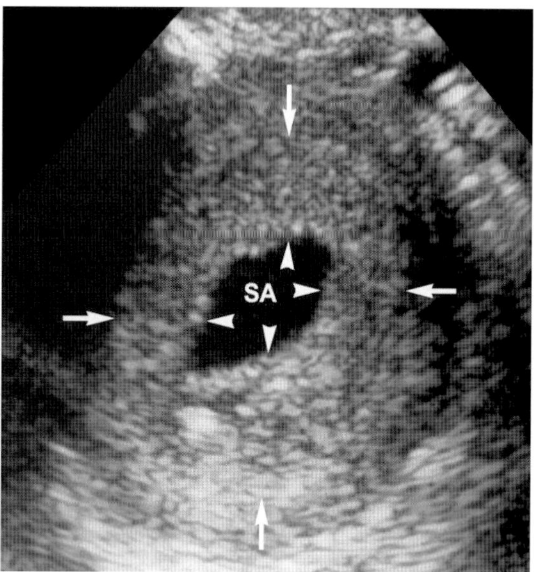

A B

FIGURE 26.2-1. Endometrial hyperplasia. A: Sagittal transvaginal view of the uterus demonstrates marked thickening of the endometrium *(calipers)*, which is fairly homogeneous in appearance. **B:** After instillation of saline *(SA)* into the uterine cavity, the endometrium *(between arrows and arrowheads)* is seen to be diffusely thick, suggesting endometrial hyperplasia. The diagnosis of hyperplasia was confirmed by endometrial biopsy. (From Doubilet PM. Vaginal bleeding—Postmenopausal. In: Bluth EI, Arger PH, Benson CB, Ralls PW, Siegel MJ, eds. *Ultrasound: a practical approach to clinical problems.* New York: Thieme Medical and Scientific Publishers, 2000, pp. 237–244, with permission.)

26.3. ENDOMETRIAL CARCINOMA

Description and Clinical Features

Endometrial cancer is the fourth most common malignancy in women in the United States, and the most common pelvic gynecologic malignancy. Most cases occur in women older than the age of 50, and thus it is mainly a disease of postmenopausal women. The typical presenting symptom is abnormal vaginal bleeding, which, after menopause, refers to any bleeding other than that occurring at the expected time in the cycle of a woman on sequential hormone replacement therapy.

Approximately 10% of postmenopausal women with abnormal vaginal bleeding have endometrial carcinoma. The cause in the remaining 90% is either another form of endometrial pathology (polyps or hyperplasia) or endometrial atrophy. The definitive diagnosis of endometrial carcinoma can only be made from a tissue sample, which may be obtained by either an office biopsy or dilation and curettage. These techniques, however, may fail to detect a focal area of endometrial carcinoma because they blindly sample a portion of the endometrium. Ultrasound and SIS can be helpful in cases of endometrial carcinoma, both by detecting endometrial pathology and by determining whether the abnormality is diffuse, in which case a blind biopsy can be performed, or focal, in which case a hysteroscopically guided biopsy should be done.

Sonography

The sonographic appearance most suggestive of endometrial carcinoma in a postmenopausal woman is marked endometrial thickening (>8–10 mm) with an ill-defined endometrium-myometrium interface (Figures 26.3-1 and 26.3-2). (Note: As indicated in the section on the normal endometrium (p. 278), endometrial thickness should be measured from the anterior to posterior endometrium-myometrium junction on a sagittal

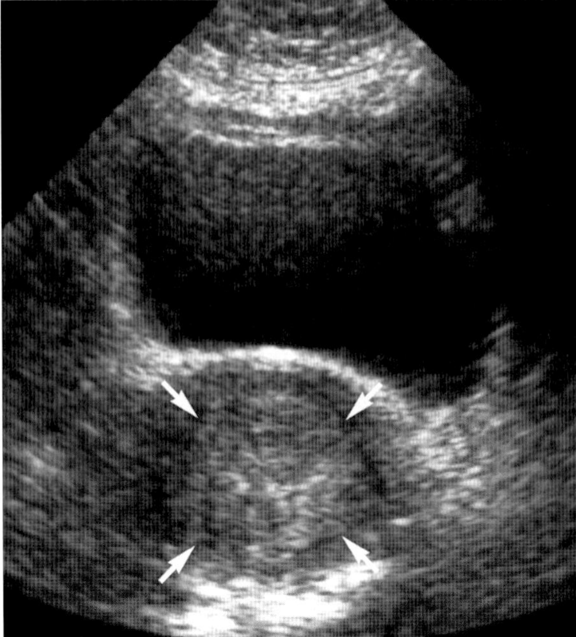

FIGURE 26.3-1. Endometrial carcinoma. Transverse transabdominal view of the uterus in a postmenopausal woman demonstrates a heterogeneous thickened endometrium with ill-defined margins *(arrows)*. This appearance is highly suggestive of endometrial carcinoma, which was confirmed via biopsy.

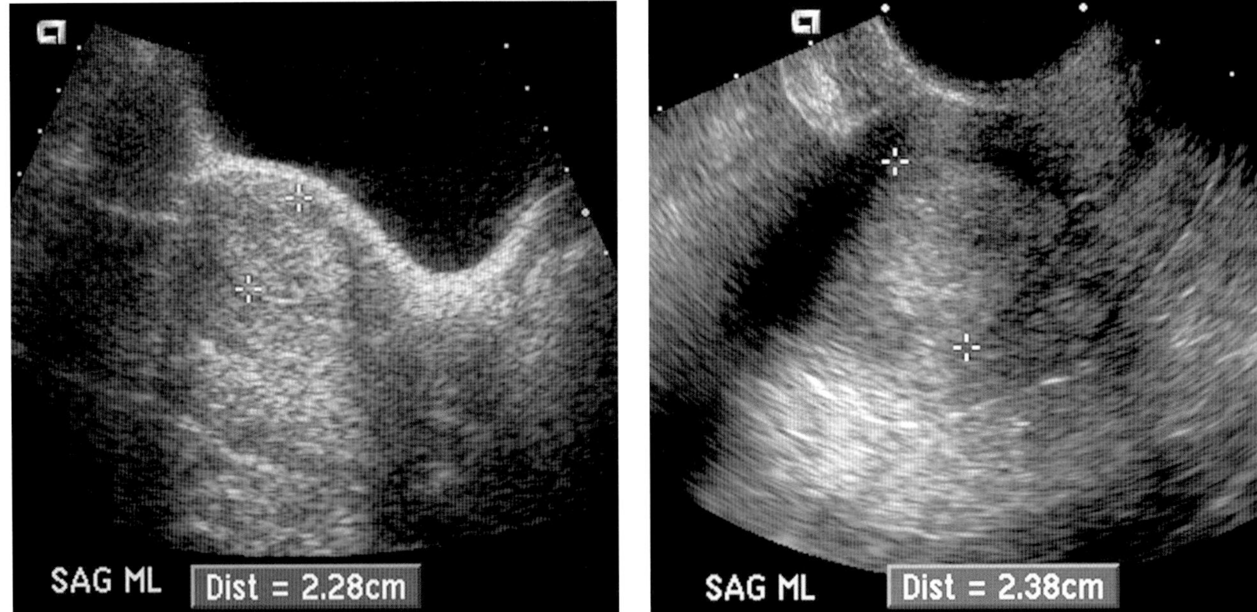

FIGURE 26.3-2. Endometrial carcinoma. Transabdominal **(A)** and transvaginal **(B)** sagittal midline *(SAG ML)* views of the uterus demonstrate marked endometrial thickening *(calipers)*, measuring approximately 23 mm. Biopsy revealed endometrial carcinoma.

transvaginal sonogram of the uterus). In less advanced cases, there may be mild generalized endometrial thickening (5–8 mm) or focal areas of endometrial irregularity. Fluid may be present in the uterine cavity because endometrial carcinoma can obstruct the outflow of blood or secretions from the uterine cavity.

The SIS finding most suggestive of endometrial carcinoma is a poorly distensible uterine cavity lined by a diffusely irregular and thickened endometrium. Endometrial carcinoma may also present on SIS as a focal area of endometrial thickening. Sonography and SIS can suggest endometrial cancer, but definitive diagnosis can only be made by pathologic examination of endometrial tissue.

26.4. GESTATIONAL TROPHOBLASTIC DISEASE

Description and Clinical Features

Gestational trophoblastic disease includes several related pathologic entities that develop from trophoblastic tissue, including complete hydatidiform mole, partial mole, trophoblastic tumor, and choriocarcinoma.

Complete hydatidiform mole is an abnormality characterized by a large amount of trophoblastic tissue and absence of fetal tissue. Pathologically, the tissue has diffuse hydatidiform swelling of villi, trophoblastic hyperplasia, and trophoblastic atypia. The chromosomes are usually 46XX with both sets of chromosomes originating from the father. Risk factors include Asian background, advanced maternal age, and history of miscarriage. Women with hydatidiform moles typically present with bleeding during the first trimester. On physical examination, the uterus is often large for gestational age and the beta-human chorionic gonadotropin levels are elevated.

Complete hydatidiform moles are treated by evacuation of the uterus. In some cases, the molar tissue recurs, requiring a second evacuation procedure. Recurrence or persistent disease is common, occurring in approximately 20% of cases. Infrequently, choriocarcinoma develops after molar evacuation. This aggressive malignancy can metastasize to the liver and lung as well as to other organs.

Partial molar pregnancies are a form of gestational trophoblastic disease in which both fetal tissue and abnormal placental tissue are present. These gestations are typically triploid. The fetus is usually sonographically abnormal or dead by the time of diagnosis. At pathology, the placenta is characterized by focal hydatidiform swelling of trophoblastic villi, focal trophoblastic hyperplasia, and focal atypia of trophoblasts. Women with partial molar pregnancies are less likely to have elevated beta-human chorionic gonadotropin levels than women with complete moles. The diagnosis is often not made until the pathologic specimen is examined.

Partial molar pregnancies are almost always successfully treated with uterine evacuation. Recurrences are uncommon and distant metastases extremely rare.

Trophoblastic tumor is a rare form of gestational trophoblastic disease that develops in the placental bed, most often after a normal pregnancy.

Sonography

A complete hydatidiform mole is characterized sonographically by a large complex mass within the endometrial cavity. The mass usually has multiple small cystic spaces surrounded by echogenic tissue (Figure 26.4-1).

Recurrent or persistent complete hydatidiform mole appears as a poorly defined mass or masses in the uterus, with hypoechoic areas that represent vessels. Color Doppler demonstrates the highly vascular nature of these recurrent lesions (Figure 26.4-2).

With a partial molar pregnancy, a gestational sac containing a fetus is seen in the uterus. Often there is a fetal demise at the time of the sonographic examination (Figure 26.4-3). Sometimes an abnormal fetus with features of triploidy is seen. The placenta in these cases may be markedly thickened with focal cystic spaces (Figure 26.4-4). Because

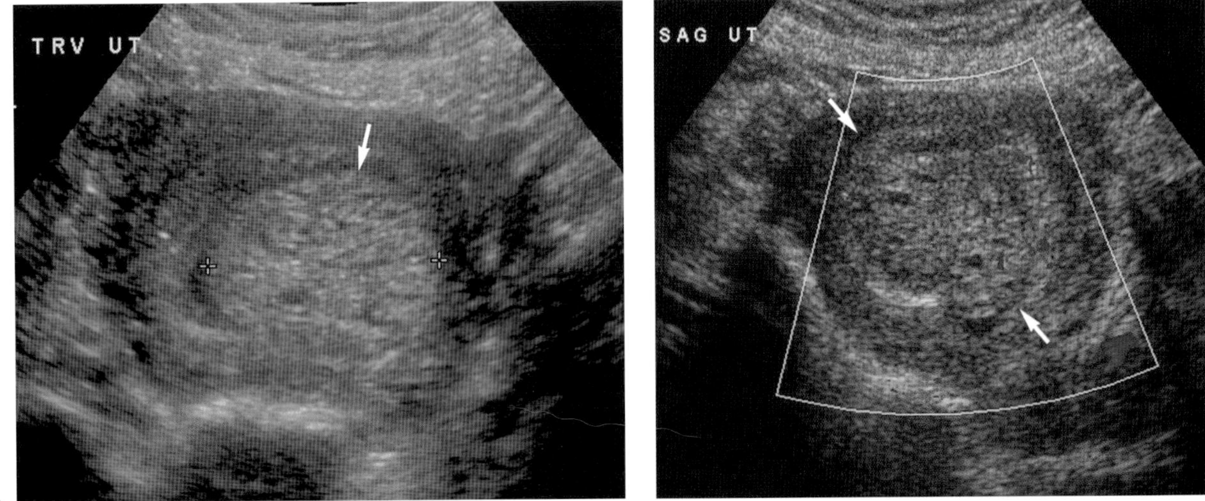

FIGURE 26.4-1. Complete hydatidiform mole. A: Transverse image of uterus *(TRV UT)* demonstrates the uterine cavity filled with an echogenic mass *(arrow, calipers)* containing small cystic spaces. **B:** Sagittal image of the uterus *(SAG UT)* with color Doppler demonstrates the mass *(arrows)* within the uterine cavity, with blood flow visible within it.

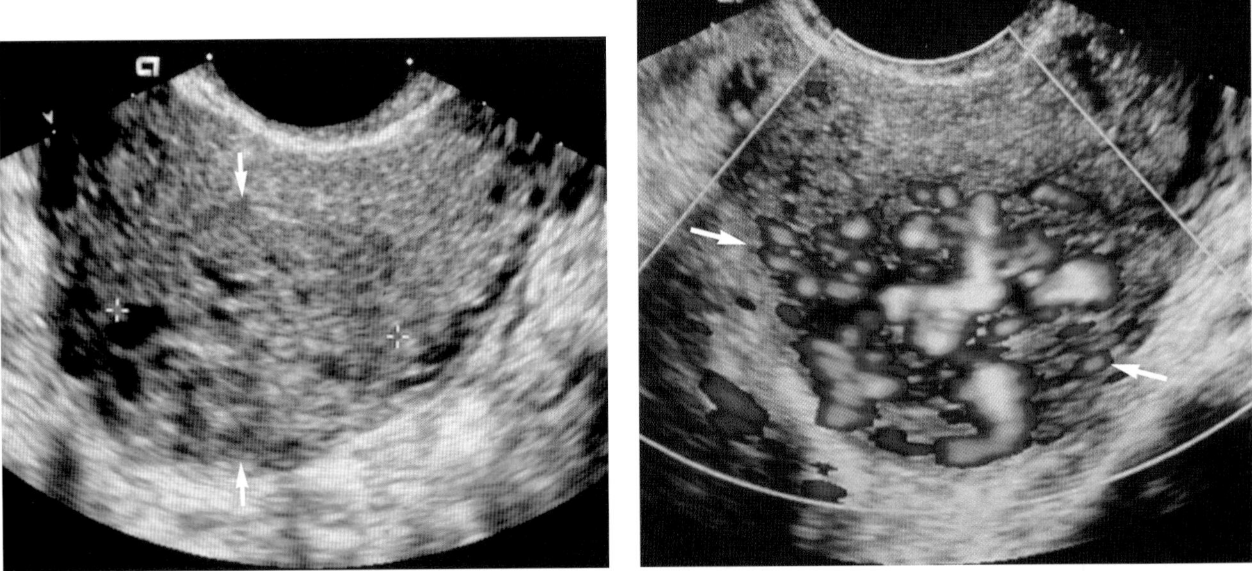

FIGURE 26.4-2. Recurrent hydatidiform mole. A: Transverse image of the uterus demonstrates a poorly defined multicystic mass *(calipers, arrows)* invading the posterior uterine wall. **B:** Power Doppler image shows hypervascularity of the mass *(arrows),* representing recurrent molar tissue.

A 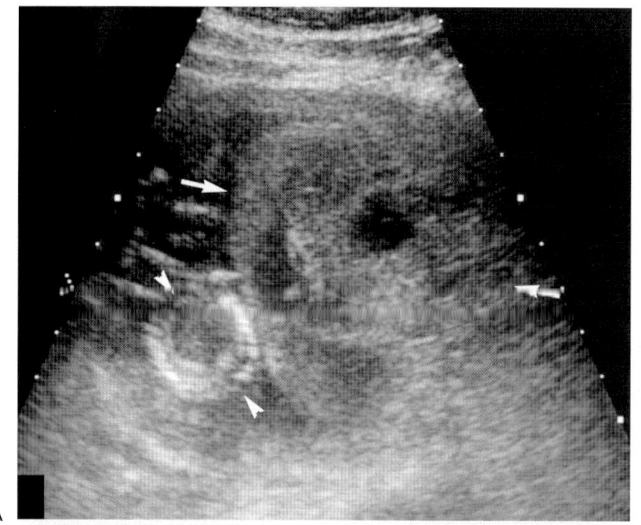

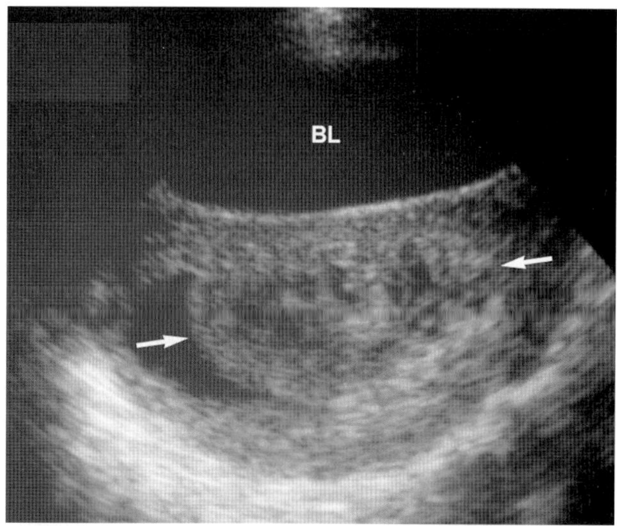 B

C 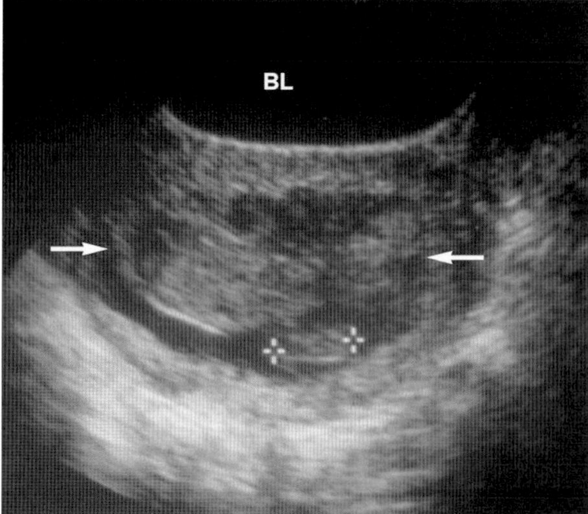

FIGURE 26.4-3. Partial mole with fetal demise. A: A markedly thickened placenta *(arrows)* with cystic spaces is seen adjacent to a dead fetus *(arrowheads)*. **B and C:** Transabdominal scans through the full maternal bladder *(BL)* in another patient demonstrate a very thick placenta *(arrows)* with cystic areas. **C:** A small dead fetus *(calipers)* is visible.

A 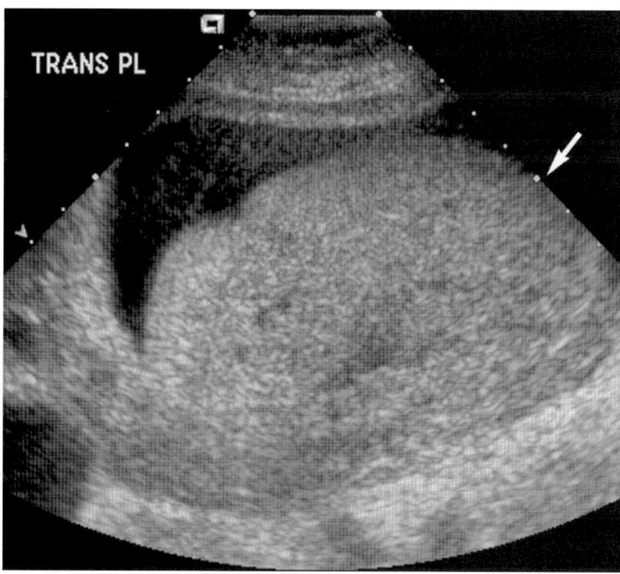

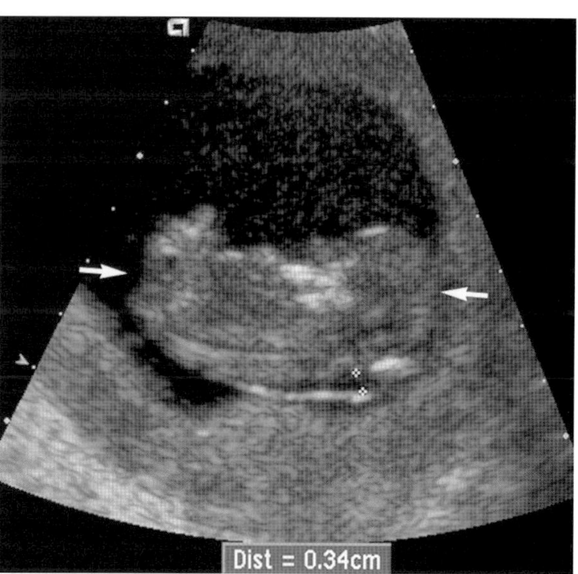 B

FIGURE 26.4-4. Partial mole with an abnormal triploid fetus. A: Image of the placenta *(arrow)*, which is very thick and contains tiny cystic spaces. **B:** The triploid fetus *(arrows)* was abnormal, with a thickened nuchal lucency *(calipers)* to 3.4 mm.

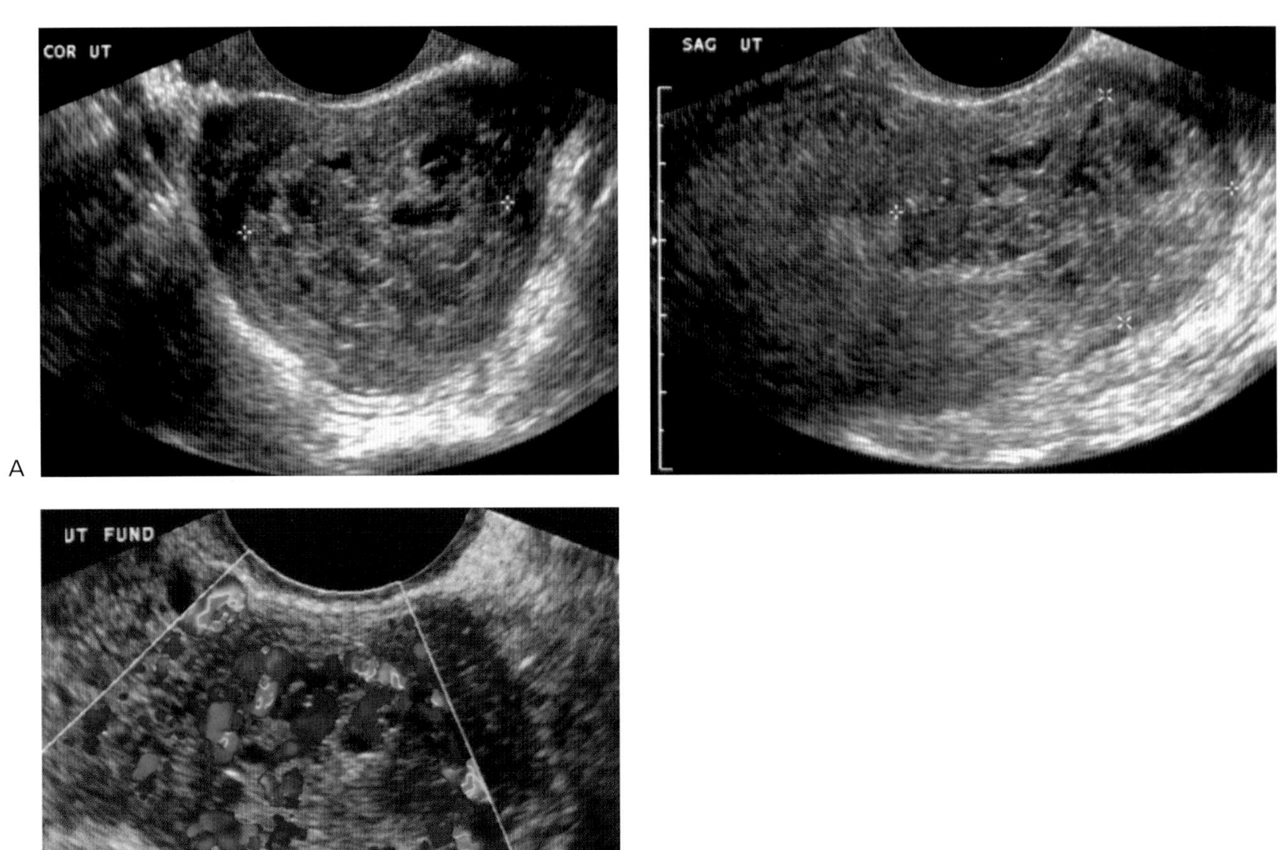

FIGURE 26.4-5. Gestational trophoblastic tumor. Coronal *(COR UT)* **(A)** and sagittal *(SAG UT)* **(B)** images of the uterus demonstrate a poorly defined mass *(calipers)* containing small cystic spaces. **C:** Color Doppler image of the uterine fundus *(UT FUND)* demonstrates hypervascularity of the mass.

the placental findings can be similar to those of a hydropic placenta with a fetal demise, it is often not possible to make the diagnosis of a partial mole by ultrasound.

Trophoblastic tumors of the placental bed appear similar to recurrent or persistent complete moles. Poorly defined hypervascular masses are seen in the uterus (Figure 26.4-5).

SUGGESTED READINGS

1. Benson CB, Genest DR, Bernstein MR, et al. Sonographic appearance of first trimester complete hydatidiform pregnancy. *Ultrasound Obstet Gynecol* 2000;16:188–191.
2. Berkowitz RS, Im SS, Bernstein MR, et al. Gestational trophoblastic disease: subsequent pregnancy outcome, including repeat molar pregnancy. *J Reprod Med* 1998;43:81–86.
3. Bourne TH, Campbell S, Whitehead MI, et al. Detection of endometrial cancer in postmenopausal women by transvaginal ultrasonography and colour flow imaging. *BMJ* 1990;301:369–370.
4. Bourne TH. Evaluating the endometrium of postmenopausal women with transvaginal ultrasonography. *Ultrasound Obstet Gynecol* 1995;6:75–80.
5. Cacciatore B, Ramsay T, Lehtovirta P, et al. Transvaginal sonography and hysteroscopy in postmenopausal bleeding. *Acta Obstet Gynecol Scand* 1994;73:413–416.
6. Caspi B, Elchalal U, Dgani R, et al. Invasive mole and placental site trophoblastic tumor: two entities of gestational trophoblastic disease with a common ultrasonographic appearance. *J Ultrasound Med* 1991;10:517–519.
7. Doubilet PM. Vaginal bleeding—postmenopausal. In: Bluth EI, Arger PH, Benson CB, et al., eds. *Ultrasound: a practical approach to clinical problems.* New York: Thieme, 2000:237–244.
8. Desai RK, Desber AL. Diagnosis of gestational trophoblastic disease: value of endovaginal color flow

Doppler sonography. *AJR Am J Roentgenol* 1991;157:787–788.
9. Doubilet PM. Commentary: Society of Radiologists in Ultrasound consensus conference statement on postmenopausal bleeding. *J Ultrasound Med* 2001;20:1037–1042.
10. Dueholm M, Forman A, Jensen ML, et al. Transvaginal sonography combined with saline contrast sonohysterography in evaluating the uterine cavity in premenopausal patients with abnormal uterine bleeding. *Ultrasound Obstet Gynecol* 2001;18:54–61.
11. Epstein E, Ramirez A, Skoog L, et al. Transvaginal sonography, saline contrast sonohysterography and hysteroscopy for the investigation of women with postmenopausal bleeding and endometrium > 5 mm. *Ultrasound Obstet Gynecol* 2001;18:157–162.
12. Fleischer AC, Jones HW. Sonography of trophoblastic diseases. In: Fleischer AC, Manning FA, Fraser-Hill MA, et al. Gestational trophoblastic neoplasia. In: Rumack CM, Wilson SR, Charboneau JW, eds. *Diagnostic ultrasound*, 2nd ed. St. Louis: Mosby, 1998:1359–1370.
13. Fleischer AC. Transvaginal sonography of endometrial disorders. In: Fleischer AC, Manning FA, Jeanty P, et al., eds. *Sonography in obstetrics & gynecology: principles and practice*, 6th ed. New York: McGraw-Hill, 2001:979–1000.
14. Goldstein RB, Bree RL, Benson CB, et al. Consensus report: evaluation of the woman with postmenopausal bleeding. *J Ultrasound Med* 2001;20:1025–1036.
15. Granberg S, Wikland M, Karlsson B, et al. Endometrial thickness as measured by endovaginal ultrasonography for identifying endometrial abnormality. *Am J Obstet Gynecol* 1991;164:47–52.
16. Hulka CA, Hall DA, McCarthy K, et al. Endometrial polyps, hyperplasia, and carcinoma in postmenopausal women: differentiation with endovaginal sonography. *Radiology* 1994;191:755–758.
17. Jauniaux E. Ultrasound diagnosis and follow-up of gestational trophoblastic disease. *Ultrasound Obstet Gynecol* 1998;11:367–377.
18. Jauniaux E. Diagnosis and follow-up of gestational trophoblastic disorders. In: Callen PW, ed. *Ultrasonography in obstetrics and gynecology*, 4th ed. Philadelphia: WB Saunders, 2000:847–856.
19. Karlsson B, Granberg S, Wikland M, et al. Transvaginal ultrasonography of the endometrium in women with postmenopausal bleeding—a Nordic multicenter study. *Am J Obstet Gynecol* 1995;172:1488–1494.
20. Levine D, Gosink BB, Johnson LA. Change in endometrial thickness in postmenopausal women undergoing hormone replacement therapy. *Radiology* 1995;197:603–608.
21. Osmers R, Volksen M, Schauer A. Vaginosonography for early detection of endometrial carcinoma? *Lancet* 1990;335:1569–1571.
22. Parsons AK. Evaluation of postmenopausal endometrium. *Ultrasound Obstet Gynecol* 1998;12:295–300.
23. Richenberg J, Cooperberg P. Ultrasound of the uterus. In: Callen PW, ed. *Ultrasonography in obstetrics and gynecology*, 4th ed. Philadelphia: WB Saunders, 2000:814–846.

27

OVARIES AND ADNEXA

27.1. SIMPLE OVARIAN CYSTS

Description and Clinical Features

The normal ovary typically contains small cysts less than 2 cm in size, usually representing developing follicles. Larger cysts, those greater than 2 cm, sometimes develop in the ovary. These cysts may represent unusually large follicles, nonfunctional ovarian cysts, or a cystic neoplasm of the ovary. Simple cysts are virtually always benign ovarian lesions. Except for a cystic neoplasm of the ovary, simple ovarian cysts tend to resolve on their own without intervention.

Sonography

A simple cyst of the ovary is an anechoic lesion with thin, smooth walls and enhanced through-transmission (Figure 27.1-1). Normal ovarian tissue is usually visible around a portion of the cyst, proving its intraovarian location.

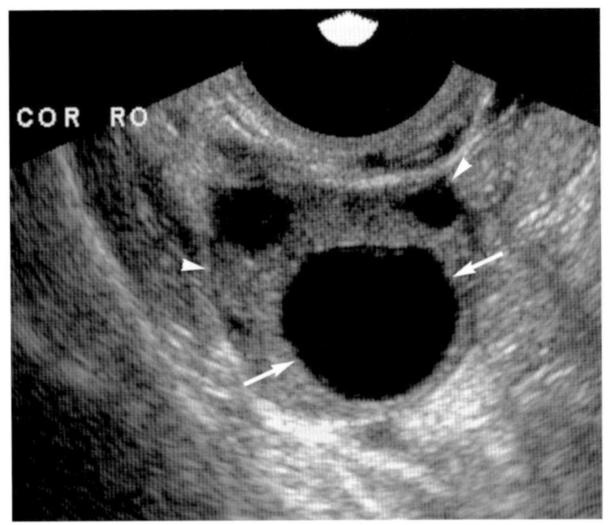

A

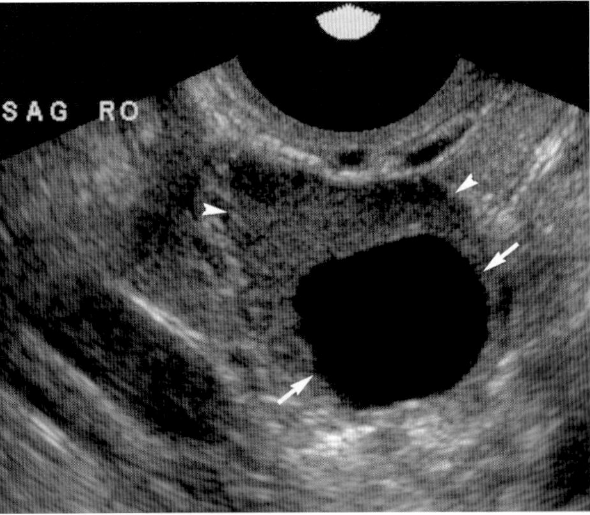

B

FIGURE 27.1-1 Simple ovarian cyst. Coronal *(COR RO)* **(A)** and sagittal *(SAG RO)* **(B)** images of the right ovary demonstrate a simple ovarian cyst *(arrows)*. Normal ovarian tissue *(arrowheads)* is seen around a portion of the cyst.

27.2. HEMORRHAGIC OVARIAN CYSTS

Description and Clinical Features

It is not uncommon for a functional ovarian cyst to contain blood. This is termed a hemorrhagic cyst. These cysts, like simple ovarian cysts, are benign lesions of the ovary that most often resolve spontaneously, without requiring surgical intervention. Occasionally, acute hemorrhage into a cyst will cause sudden onset of pelvic pain. Rarely, a hemorrhagic cyst ruptures.

Sonography

Hemorrhagic cysts appear as complex ovarian lesions. They are typically round with thin, smooth walls. The appearance of the cyst varies with the time since hemorrhage. After acute hemorrhage, the cyst may appear as a heterogeneous mass containing multiple echoes. As the cyst begins to resolve, it may develop fine septations, sometimes forming a reticular pattern throughout the cyst (Figure 27.2-1). The fluid in the cyst often has scattered echoes. With continued involution, the cyst decreases in size and becomes simpler in appearance, with fewer septations and internal echoes (Figure 27.2-2).

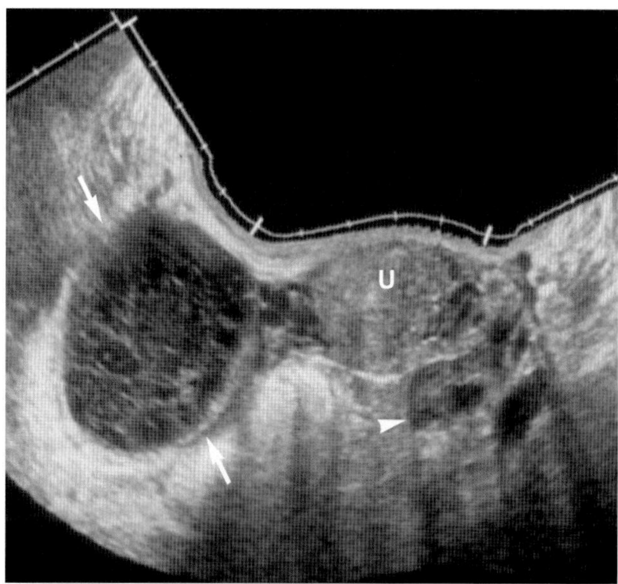

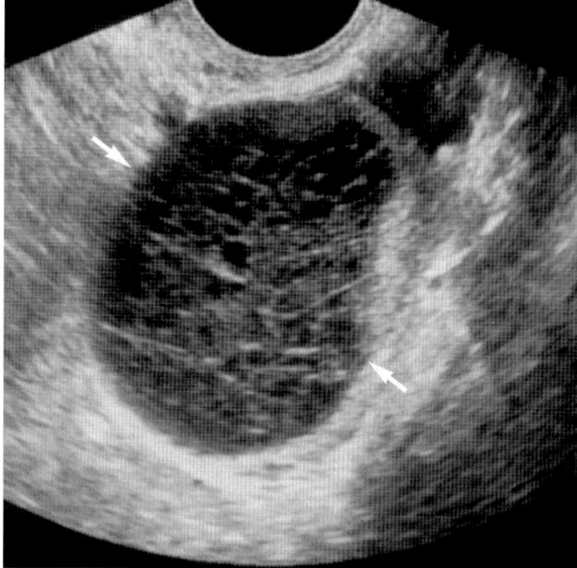

FIGURE 27.2-1. Hemorrhagic ovarian cyst. A: Transvaginal panoramic view demonstrates a complex right ovarian cyst *(arrows)* adjacent to a normal uterus *(U)* and left ovary *(arrowhead).* **B:** Magnified view of the right hemorrhagic ovarian cyst *(arrows)* shows internal septations forming a reticular pattern throughout the cyst.

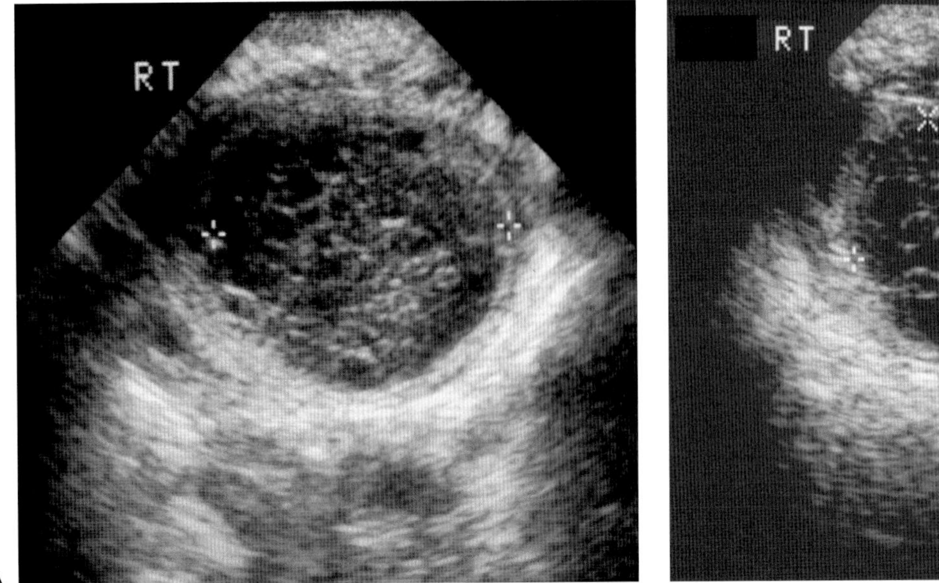

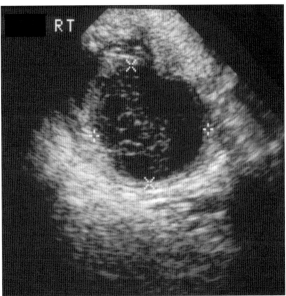

FIGURE 27.2-2. Evolving hemorrhagic cyst. A: Image of a right ovary *(RT)* demonstrates a hemorrhagic cyst *(calipers)* with a reticular pattern of fine septations throughout the cyst. **B:** On a follow-up scan, the hemorrhagic cyst *(calipers)* has more anechoic areas and fewer fine septations within it.

27.3. OVARIAN TERATOMAS

Description and Clinical Features

The most common benign neoplasm of the ovary is a dermoid cyst, also called a mature cystic teratoma. This tumor is of germ cell origin and is often found in women of reproductive age. It is bilateral in 10%–15% of cases. Most dermoid cysts are asymptomatic,

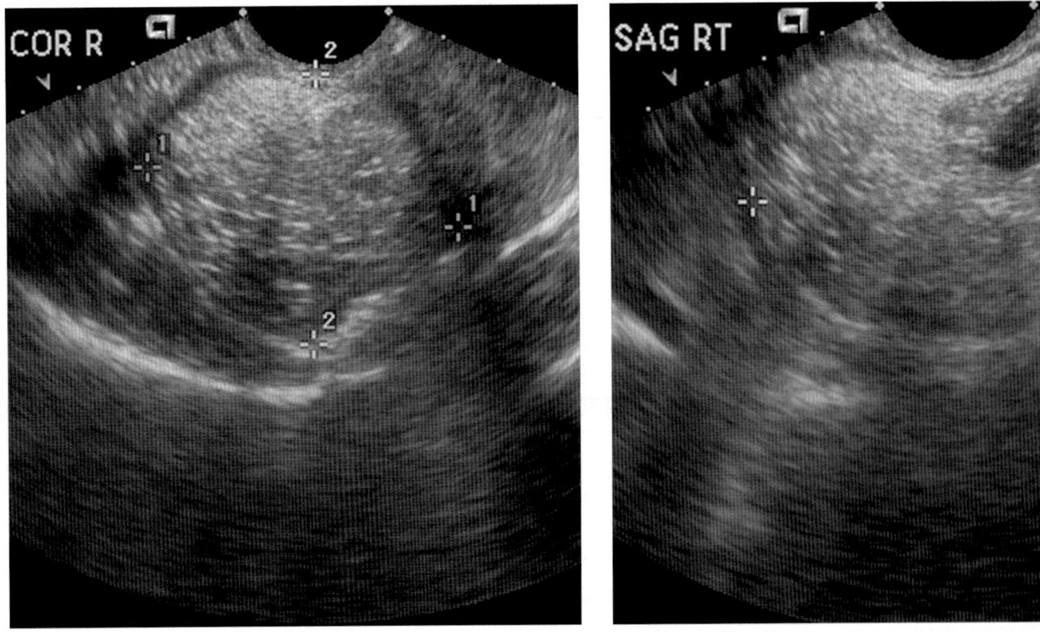

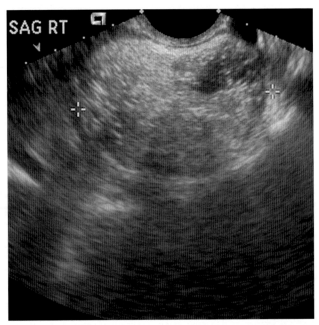

FIGURE 27.3-1. Ovarian dermoid cyst containing fat. Coronal *(COR R)* **(A)** and sagittal *(SAG RT)* **(B)** transvaginal images of a mass *(calipers)* in the right ovary filled with complex, highly echogenic material representing fat.

but occasionally they cause lower abdominal pain, swelling, and irregular menses. Ovaries containing dermoids are at risk of torsion. Surgical excision is the usual treatment of these lesions. At pathology, the tumor may be found to contain fat and sometimes bone, teeth, or hair. Rarely, an ovarian teratoma is malignant.

Sonography

Mature cystic teratomas of the ovary often have a typical sonographic appearance that allows them to be differentiated from other ovarian neoplasms. The characteristic appearance is a complex, partially cystic mass in the ovary that contains one or more highly echogenic regions that may shadow (Figure 27.3-1). Some of these echogenic regions represent fat within the tumor. In some cases, the fat floats on top of other fluid in the lesion, leading to the sonographic finding of a fluid-fluid level. Other echogenic regions that may be seen include solid nodules of tissue in the wall of the dermoid (Figure 27.3-2) and densely calcified structures representing teeth or bone.

A

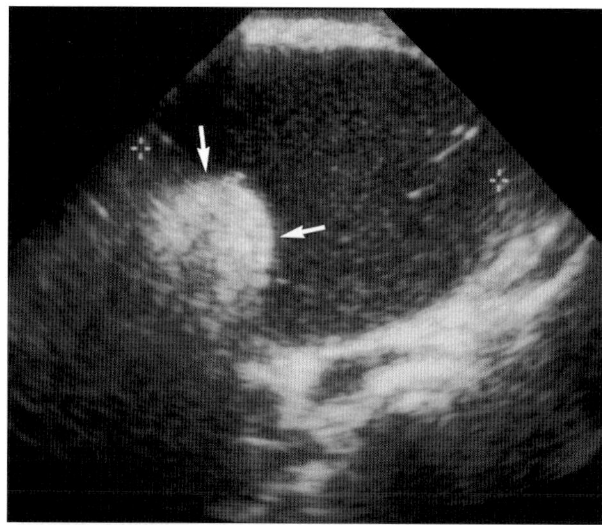

B

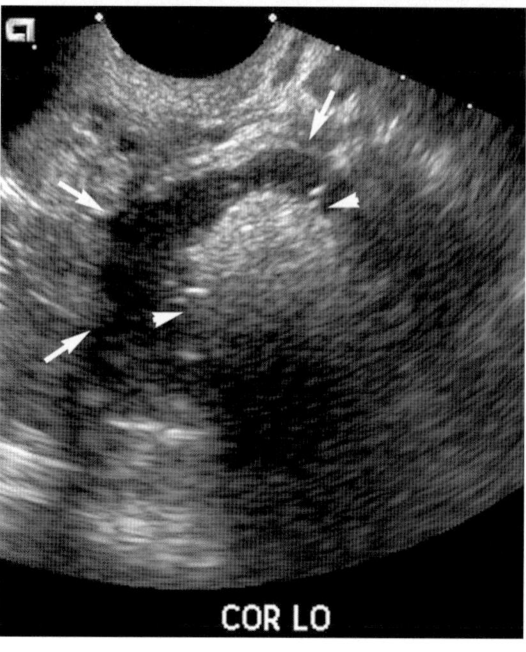

C

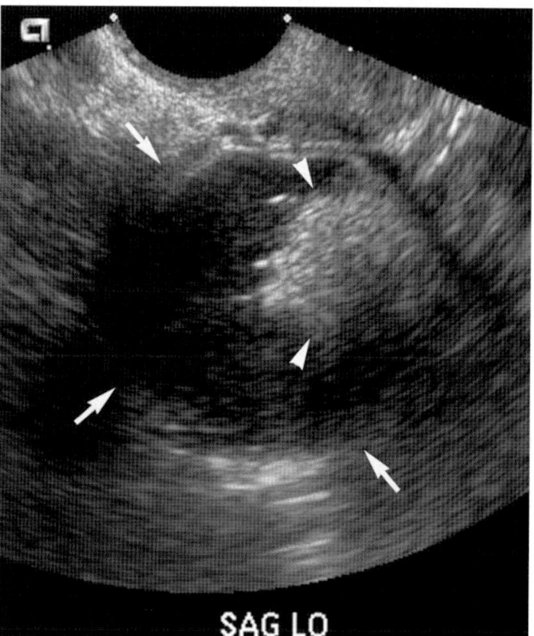

FIGURE 27.3-2. Ovarian dermoid cyst with a highly echogenic solid nodule of tissue in the wall. A: Transvaginal image of an ovary demonstrates a complex, predominantly cystic mass *(calipers)* with an echogenic solid nodule of tissue *(arrows)* protruding from the wall into the mass. Coronal *(COR LO)* **(B)** and sagittal *(SAG LO)* **(C)** images of the left ovary in another patient demonstrate a complex cystic mass *(arrows)* with an echogenic, shadowing solid nodule *(arrowheads)* protruding into the tumor.

27.4. OVARIAN BENIGN NEOPLASMS OTHER THAN TERATOMAS

Description and Clinical Features

Ovarian neoplasms that arise from epithelial cells and surrounding stromal cells can be malignant or benign. The most common benign neoplasms are mucinous or serous cystadenomas. Less common benign tumors arising from these cells include transitional cell (Brenner) tumors. Benign ovarian neoplasms can also arise from granulosa, theca, and Sertoli and Leydig cells. These neoplasms include ovarian fibromas, granulosa cell tumors, thecomas, and Sertoli-Leydig cell tumors.

The distinction between benign and malignant ovarian neoplasms cannot be made with certainty based on clinical presentation or imaging findings.

Sonography

Serous and mucinous cystadenomas of the ovary are typically complex ovarian lesions with septations separating areas of anechoic fluid (Figure 27.4-1). Blood flow can often be identified in the septations with color Doppler. Some benign tumors contain both anechoic cystic regions and solid or complex cystic areas (Figure 27.4-2). Occasionally, solid tumor nodules, containing vessels visible with color Doppler, are seen in the wall of the neoplasm, although this finding is more frequently seen with malignant than benign neoplasms.

A

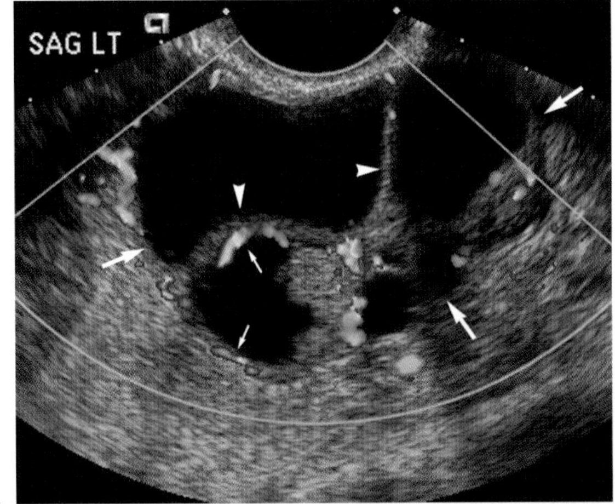

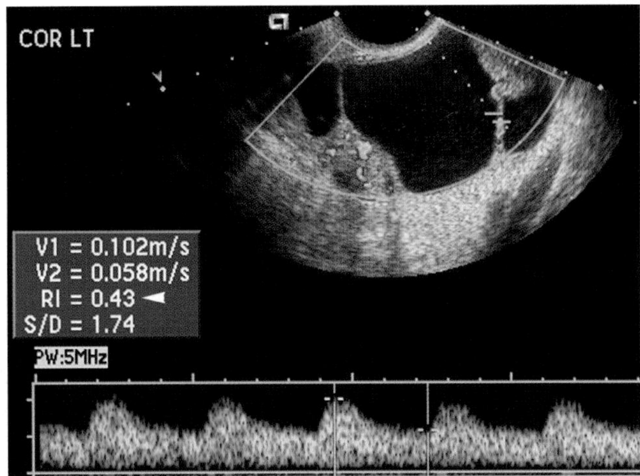

B

FIGURE 27.4-1. Ovarian serous cystadenoma. A: Transvaginal sagittal image of a left ovary *(SAG LT)* that contains a multilocular cystic lesion *(large arrows)* with thick septations *(arrowheads)*. Color Doppler shows blood flow *(small arrows)* within the wall and in the septations. **B:** Doppler gate placed on blood flow in a septation demonstrates a fairly high resistance arterial waveform *(calipers)*, with a resistive index of 0.43 *(RI arrowhead)*.

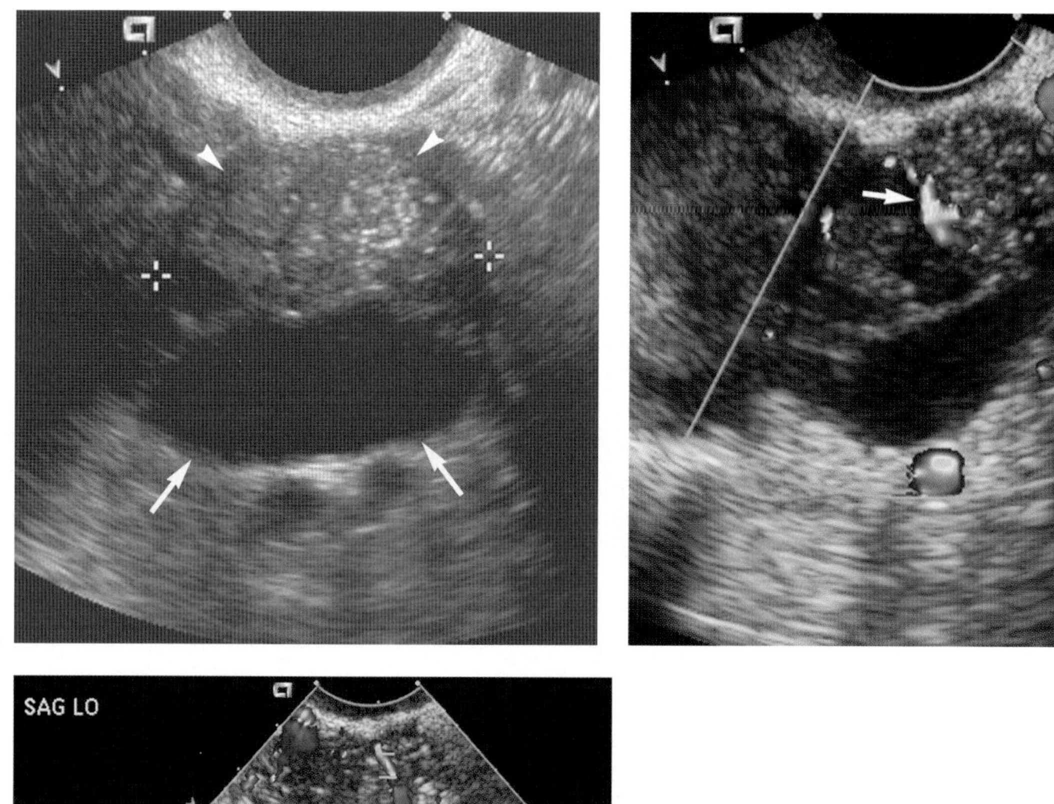

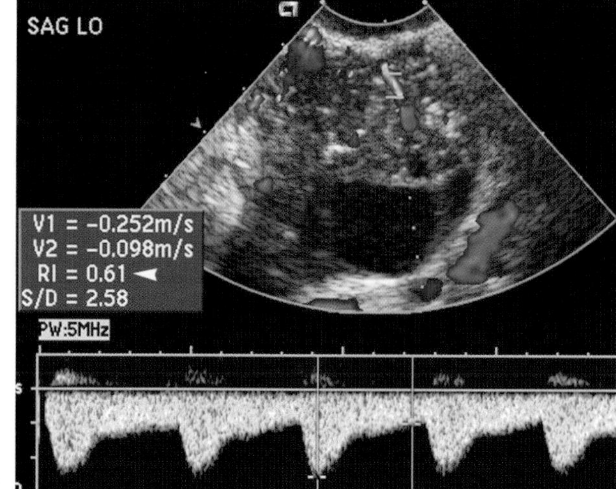

FIGURE 27.4-2. Ovarian papillary serous cystadenoma. A: Transvaginal image of an ovary containing a complex mass *(calipers)* with anechoic areas *(arrows)* and more complex, solid-appearing areas *(arrowheads)*. **B:** Color Doppler demonstrates blood flow *(arrow)* within a solid portion of the tumor. **C:** Spectral Doppler of flow within the mass demonstrates high-resistance flow *(calipers)*, with a resistive index of 0.61 *(RI arrowhead)*.

Some benign tumors, such as fibromas and granulosa cell tumors, appear as solid ovarian masses. These tumors are typically hypervascular with color Doppler (Figure 27.4-3).

Spectral Doppler arterial waveforms from the vessels of a benign tumor typically have a high-resistance pattern, with a resistive index above 0.4 (Figures 27.4-1 and 27.4-2). Although arteries in malignant tumors often have a resistive index below 0.4, Doppler cannot reliably differentiate benign from malignant lesions.

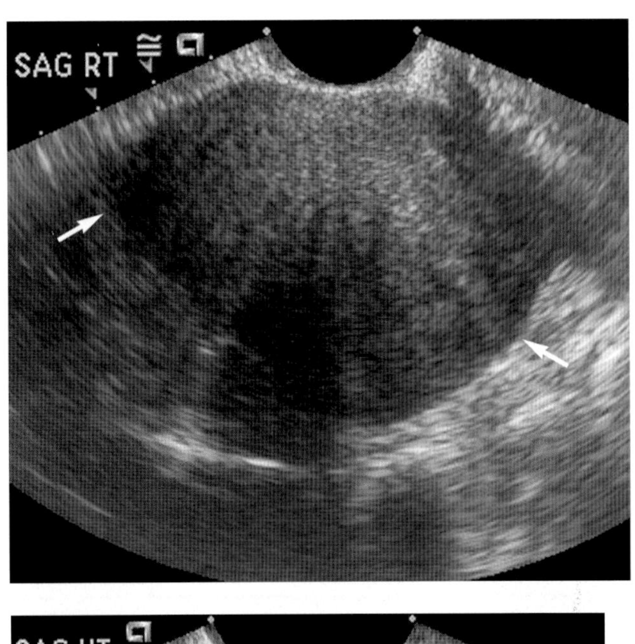

A

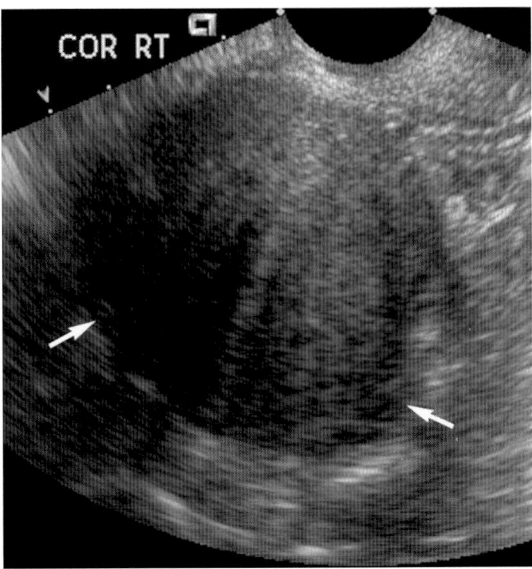

B

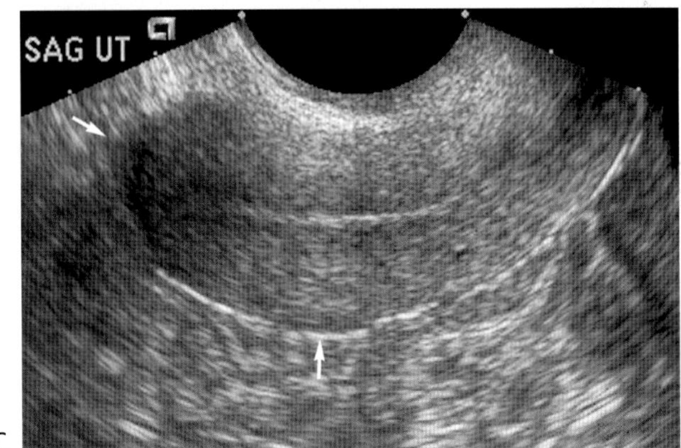

C

FIGURE 27.4-3. Ovarian fibroma. Sagittal *(SAG RT)* **(A)** and coronal *(COR RT)* **(B)** images of the right ovary demonstrate a solid mass *(arrows)* with a homogeneous echotexture. The mass has sonographic features similar to those of a uterine fibroid. **C:** Sagittal image of the uterus *(SAG UT arrows)*, which was completely separate from the ovarian mass in **(A)** and **(B)**.

27.5. OVARIAN CANCER

Description and Clinical Features

Ovarian cancer is an aggressive tumor. It is the leading cause of death among gynecologic malignancies. One of the reasons for the high death rate is that ovarian cancers are usually not detected until the disease is advanced. Seventy-five percent of cases have spread outside the ovary by the time of diagnosis. Those cases that are detected in the early stages have an excellent prognosis, with 5-year survival rates of as high as 90%.

Several centers have instituted screening programs in an attempt to diagnose ovarian cancers in their early stages. Such programs are probably beneficial for high-risk patients, such as those with a positive family history of ovarian cancer in two or more first-degree relatives and those with hereditary cancer syndromes. Their value is questionable in low-risk populations, however, because of the low incidence of ovarian cancer and the poor specificity of ultrasound.

Sonography

The gray-scale sonographic features of a complex ovarian mass that are worrisome for cancer include solid nodules in the wall of the mass, thick septations, irregularity of the wall, and poorly defined margins of the lesion (Figures 27.5-1, 27.5-2, and 27.5-3). Blood flow is usually seen with color Doppler within the septations, in the wall, and in solid nodules.

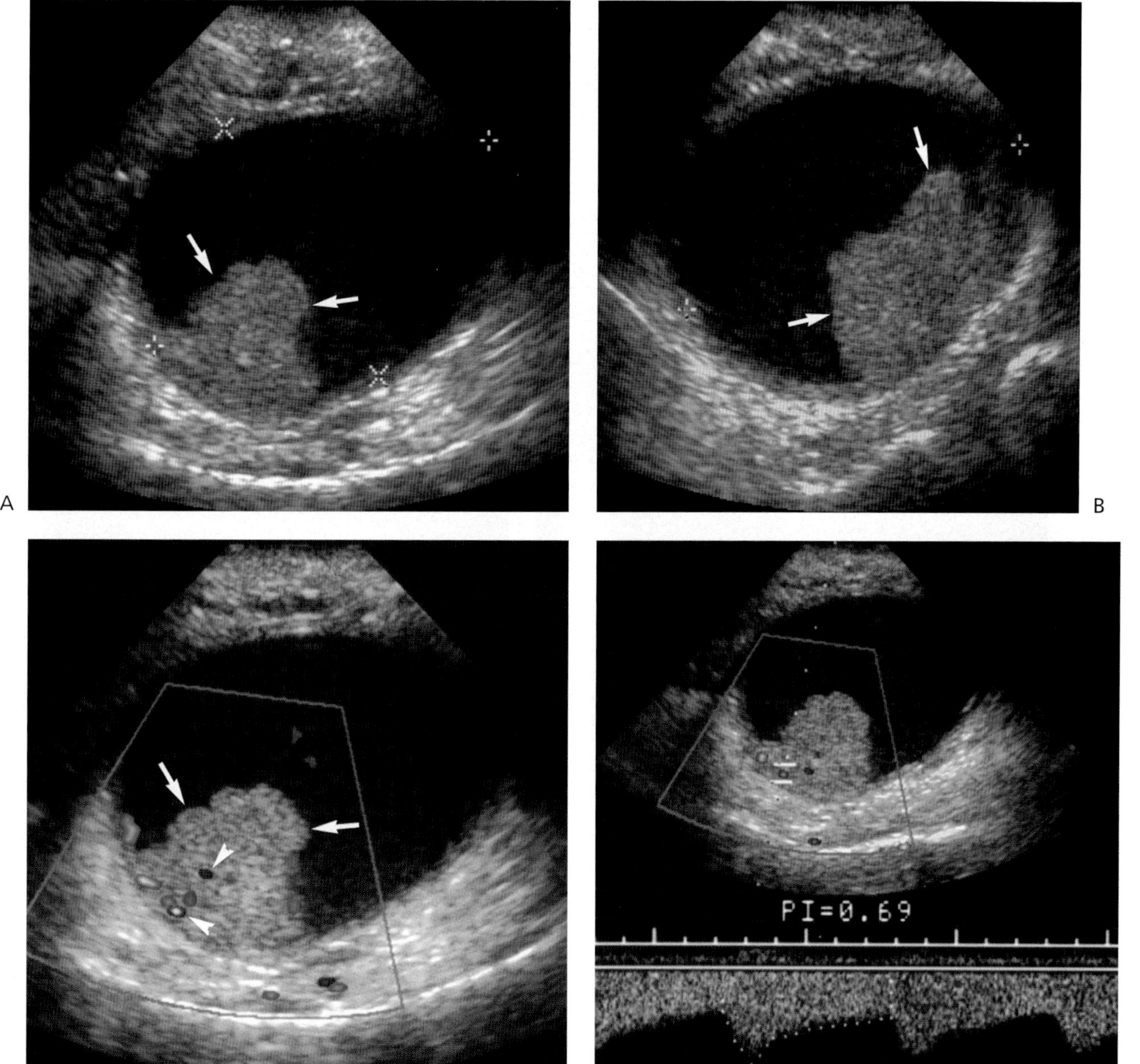

FIGURE 27.5-1. Ovarian papillary cystadenocarcinoma with solid nodule in wall. A and B: Images of an ovarian mass *(calipers)* with a solid nodule *(arrows)* projecting from the wall into the cystic portion. **C:** Color Doppler demonstrates flow *(arrowheads)* within the solid nodule *(arrows)* and wall of the tumor. **D:** Spectral Doppler of vessel within mass demonstrates low-resistance flow with a low pulsatility index *(PI)* of 0.69.

Because there is an overlap between the sonographic features of benign and malignant ovarian tumors, the sonographic diagnosis of ovarian cancer cannot be made with confidence based on ultrasound findings alone.

With Doppler sonography, malignant ovarian masses tend to demonstrate lower resistance flow than do benign tumors. In particular, malignant lesions often have resistive indices less than 0.4 and pulsatility indices less than 1.0 (Figures 27.5-1 and 27.5-2). Unfortunately, there is considerable overlap between Doppler characteristics of benign and malignant lesions, so that Doppler criteria are not reliable predictors of malignancy. In fact, Doppler findings are less accurate than gray-scale sonographic findings in the diagnosis and exclusion of ovarian cancer.

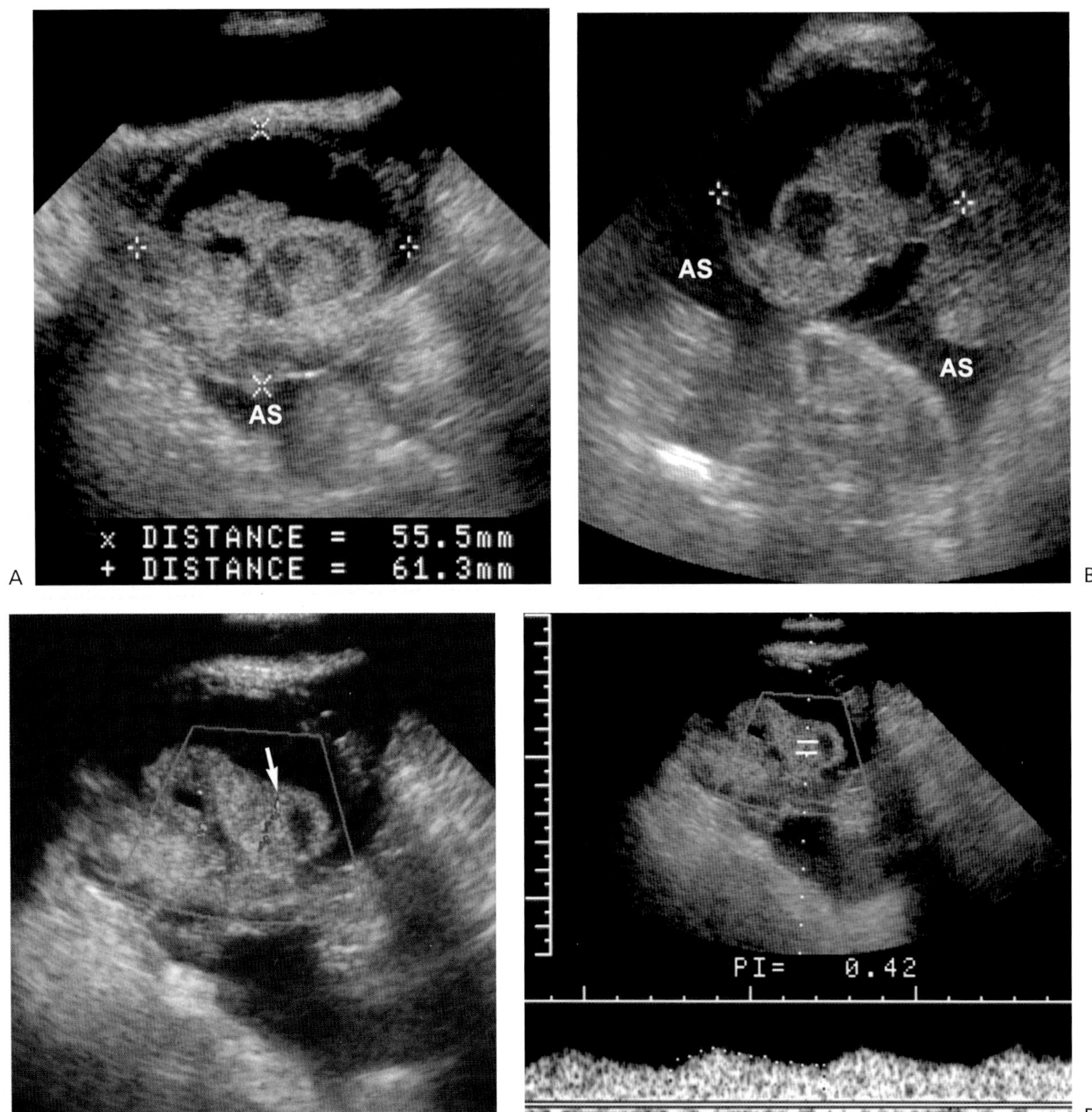

FIGURE 27.5-2. Ovarian mucinous cystadenocarcinoma with thick septations and ascites. A and B: Transvaginal images of ovary demonstrate a large, complex mass *(calipers)*. Ascites (AS) was present in the abdomen. **C:** Color Doppler demonstrates flow *(arrow)* within a solid portion of the tumor. **D:** Spectral Doppler of flow within the mass demonstrates low-resistance flow with a low pulsatility index *(PI)* of 0.42.

A 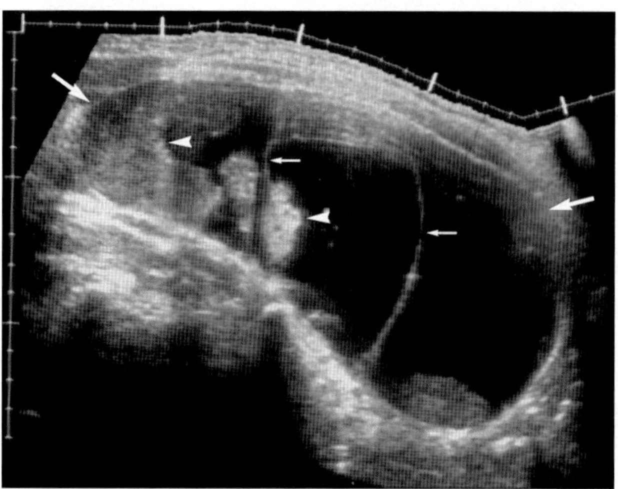 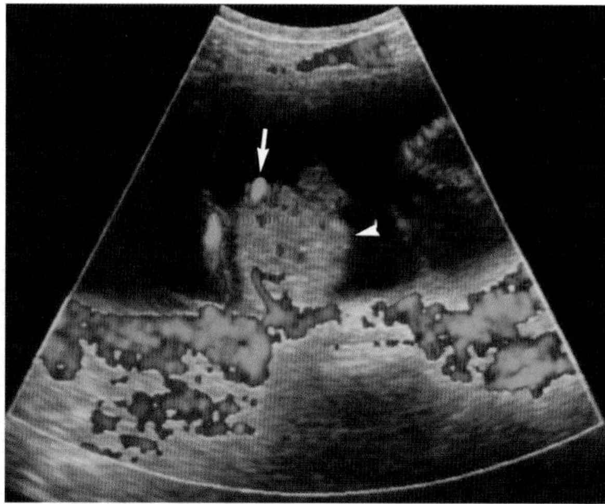 B

FIGURE 27.5-3. Ovarian malignant mixed germ cell tumor with solid and cystic components. A: Extended field of view image of an ovarian cystic mass *(large arrows)* containing solid areas *(arrowheads)* and septations *(small arrows)*. **B:** Power Doppler image demonstrates flow *(arrow)* in a solid nodule *(arrowhead)* in the tumor.

27.6. ENDOMETRIOSIS

Description and Clinical Features

Endometriosis refers to the presence of endometrial glandular tissue outside the uterus. This glandular tissue is typically located at sites inside the peritoneal cavity, such as on the ovary, attached to the fallopian tubes, or in the cul-de-sac. The ectopic endometrial tissue responds to the hormones of the menstrual cycle and may bleed periodically, causing bloody ascites and focal masses of hemorrhage called endometriomas. Patients with endometriosis may have chronic pelvic pain, back pain, dyspareunia, and infertility. Scarring and pelvic adhesions often result from endometriosis.

Sonography

Endometriosis, in the absence of endometriomas, is not visible sonographically. When an endometrioma is present, however, the lesion is easily identified if it is located in the pelvis, but its sonographic appearance is variable and may be indistinguishable from that of other pelvic lesions. The most characteristic appearance of an endometrioma is an adnexal cyst filled with homogeneous low-level echoes (Figure 27.6-1), sometimes called a "ground glass" appearance. In other cases, endometriomas appear as cysts with fine septations or a reticular pattern of septations, an appearance similar to that of hemorrhagic cysts. Endometriomas can be multilocular, with areas of anechoic fluid and other areas of complex fluid, separated by septations (Figure 27.6-2). Fluid-fluid levels may be seen (Figure 27.6-3). In many cases, more than one endometrioma is present at the time of examination.

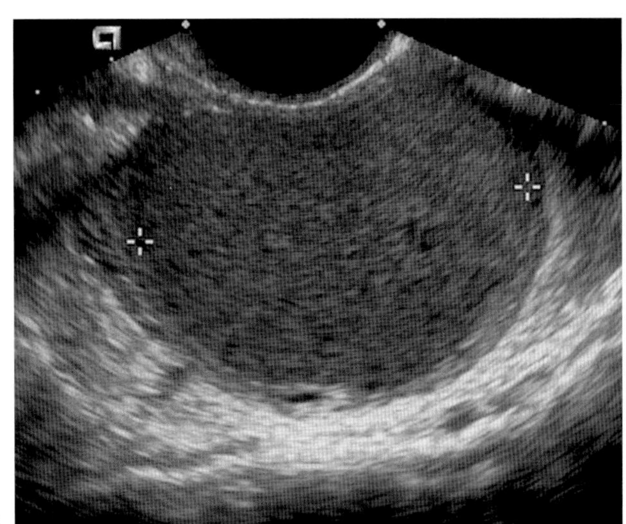

A

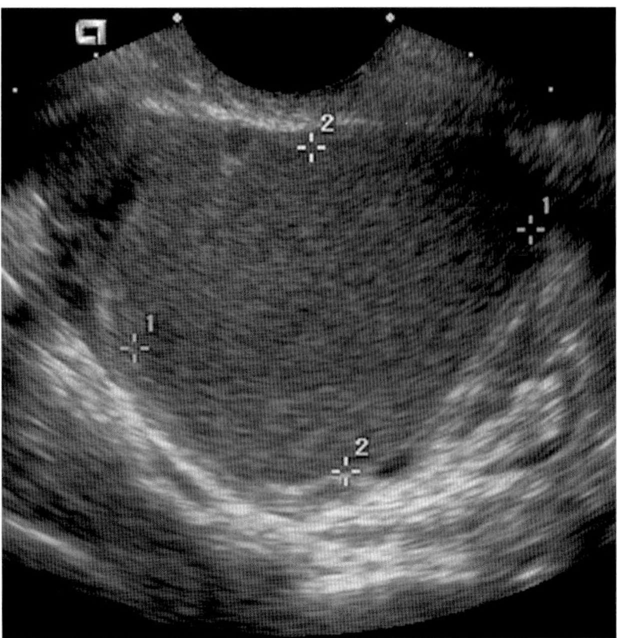

B

FIGURE 27.6-1. Endometrioma filled with homogeneous echoes. A and B: Images of cystic adnexal mass *(calipers)* filled with homogeneous echoes, characteristic of an endometrioma.

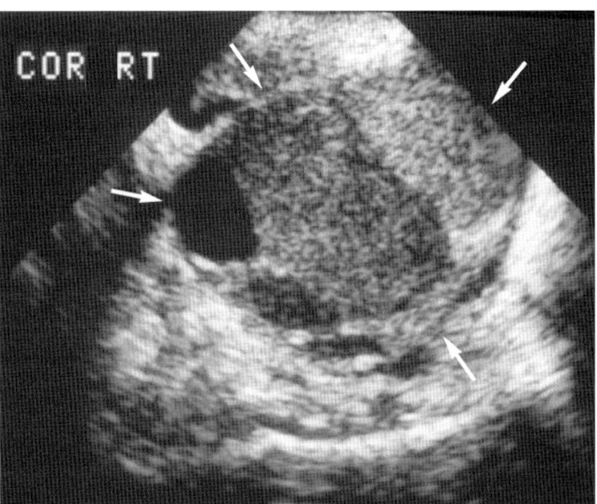

FIGURE 27.6-2. Multilocular endometrioma. Coronal image of a right *(COR RT)* adnexal cystic lesion *(arrows)* with an anechoic area and separate areas of homogeneous echoes.

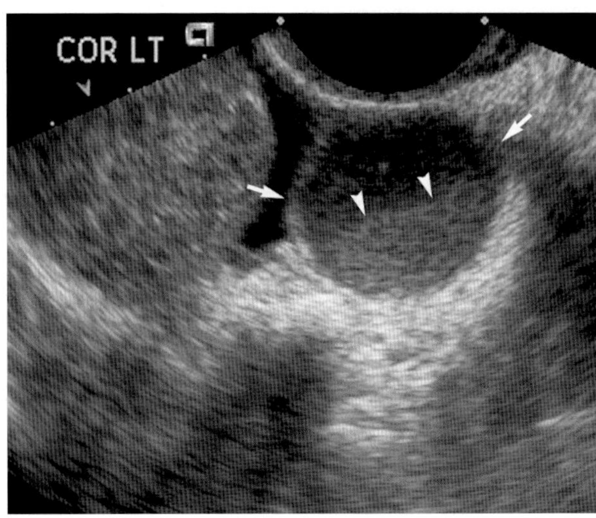

FIGURE 27.6-3. Fluid-fluid level in an endometrioma. Coronal image of a left *(COR LT)* adnexal cystic lesion *(arrows)* containing a fluid-fluid level *(arrowheads)*.

27.7. HYDROSALPINX

Description and Clinical Features

Hydrosalpinx is a fluid-filled fallopian tube that results from obstruction of the distal end of the tube. It usually occurs as a result of pelvic inflammatory disease or endometriosis, leading to adhesions at the fimbriated end of the fallopian tube that obstruct the peritoneal opening of the tube. Fluid collects in and expands the ampullary portion of the fallopian tube, sometimes extending medially along the tube. The fluid may become infected, resulting in a pyosalpinx.

Sonography

Hydrosalpinx appears as an elongated cystic structure in the adnexa, separate from the ovary. It typically has thin, smooth walls and is filled with anechoic fluid. Incomplete septations may be seen crossing the tubular structure, representing folds in the tube (Figure 27.7-1). Occasionally, the fluid within the tube contains echoes, representing either debris or pus (Figure 27.7-2).

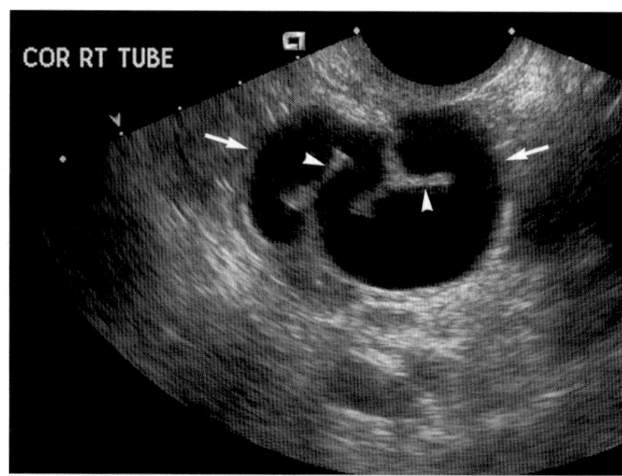

FIGURE 27.7-1. Hydrosalpinx. Coronal image of a dilated right fallopian tube *(COR RT TUBE arrows)* shows a tortuous, fluid-filled configuration with folds *(arrowheads)*.

A
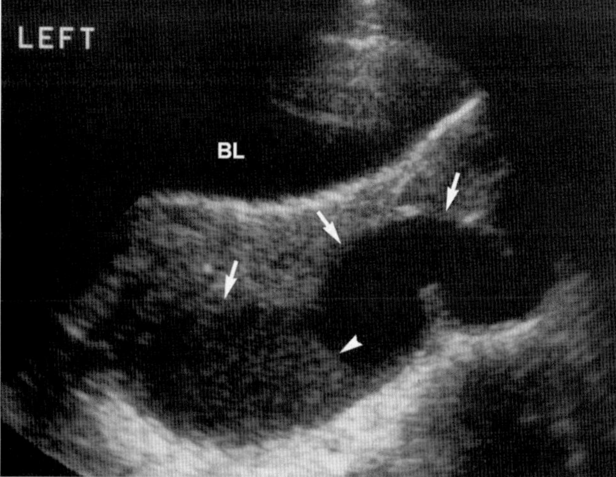

B
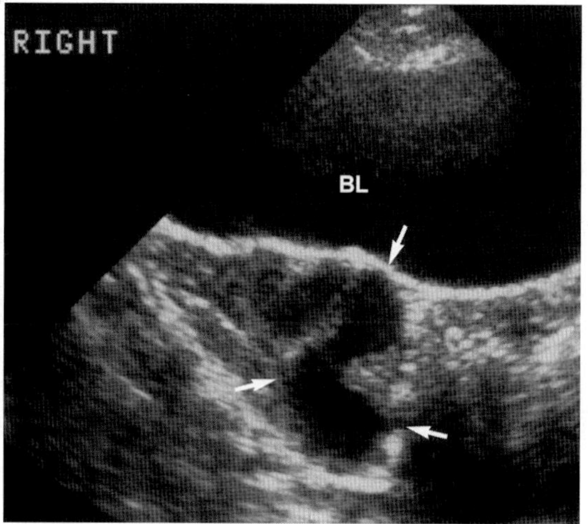

FIGURE 27.7-2. Bilateral hydrosalpinges. Transabdominal images through a full bladder *(BL)* of left **(A)** and right **(B)** hydrosalpinges *(arrows)*, both appearing as folded, fluid-filled adnexal structures. In the left hydrosalpinx **(A)** is a fluid-fluid level *(arrowhead)* due to debris or pus within the tube.

27.8. TUBO-OVARIAN ABSCESS

Description and Clinical Features

Tubo-ovarian abscess is a severe form of pelvic inflammatory disease that involves the ovary and fallopian tube on one or both sides. The abscess results from disruption of the ovaries and distal tube, with the formation of a complex inflammatory mass containing anaerobic bacteria. Patients at risk for pelvic inflammatory disease include those with multiple sexual partners, a history of sexually transmitted disease, and an intrauterine device in place. Patients typically present clinically with fever, pelvic pain, and an elevated white blood cell count.

Tubo-ovarian abscesses are usually bilateral, especially when the infection occurs as a result of bacterial spread from the lower genital tract. When unilateral, the cause is usually spread from an adjacent infection, such as diverticulitis or appendicitis, rather than from the lower genital tract. A tubo-ovarian abscess with a large cystic component can sometimes be treated successfully with transvaginal aspiration or transvaginal placement of a drainage catheter.

Sonography

A tubo-ovarian abscess appears as a complex, multiloculated adnexal mass. The margins are usually poorly defined (Figures 27.8-1 and 27.8-2). Fluid components of the complex mass are filled with echoes from debris and pus, and there may be thick septations crossing the mass. Typically, the ovary cannot be identified in the adnexa because it is encased by the inflammatory tissue of the abscess. With transvaginal scanning, patients are very tender on the affected side. When pressure is applied with the transvaginal probe, adnexal structures appear adherent to each other.

Sonography alone cannot always distinguish between a tubo-ovarian abscess and other adnexal lesions. The diagnosis is usually established based on both the clinical presentation and sonographic findings.

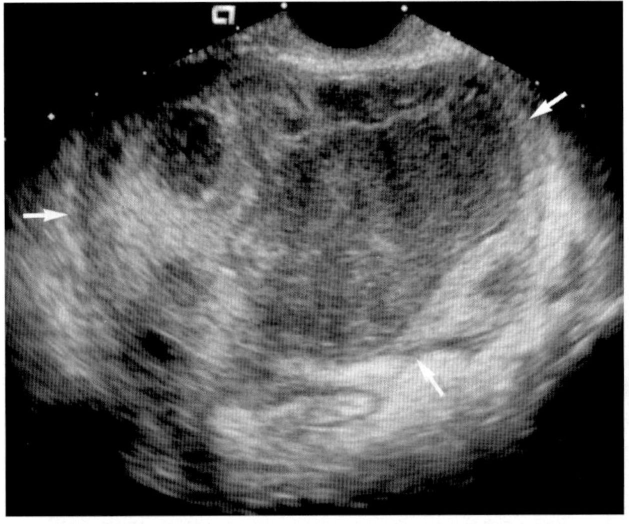

A

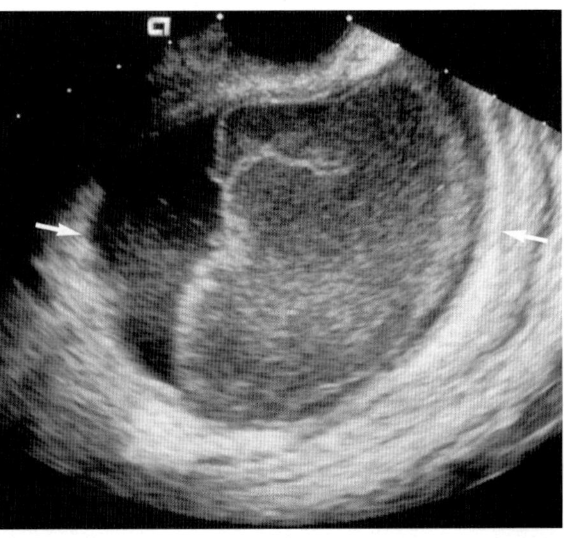

B

FIGURE 27.8-1. Tubo-ovarian abscess. A: Transvaginal image of a complex adnexal mass *(arrows)* with poorly defined margins and regions with complex fluid. **B:** Transvaginal image of the mass *(arrows)* shows predominantly cystic areas of the abscess.

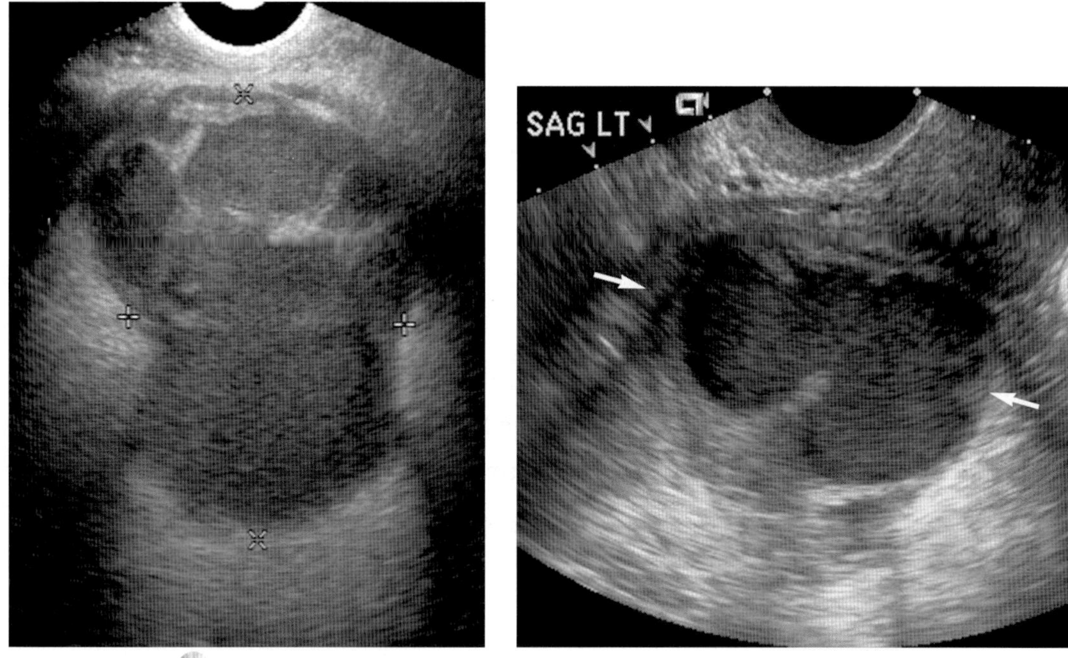

FIGURE 27.8-2. Tubo-ovarian abscess decreasing in size after antibiotic treatment. **A:** Transvaginal image of a large, complex cystic mass *(calipers)* representing a tubo-ovarian abscess. **B:** Transvaginal image of the abscess after 1 month of antibiotics shows that the complex mass *(arrows)* is smaller but still contains complex fluid.

SUGGESTED READINGS

1. Brown DL, Doubilet PM, Miller FH, et al. Benign and malignant ovarian masses: selection of the most discriminating gray-scale and Doppler sonographic features. *Radiology* 1998;208:103–110.
2. Brown DL, Frates MC, Laing FC, et al. Benign versus malignant ovarian masses. Can they be distinguished by color and pulsed Doppler ultrasound. *Radiology* 1994;190:333–336.
3. Brown DL. The abnormal ovary. In: Goldstein SR, Benson CB, eds. *Imaging of the infertile couple*. London: Dunitz M, 2001:65–69.
4. Dill-Macky MJ, Atri M. Ovarian sonography. In: Callen PW, ed. *Ultrasonography in obstetrics and gynecology*, 4th ed. Philadelphia: WB Saunders, 2000:857–896.
5. Fleischer AC, Entman SS. Sonographic evaluation of pelvic masses with transabdominal and/or transvaginal sonography. In: Fleischer AC, Manning FA, Jeanty P, et al., eds. *Sonography in obstetrics & gynecology: principles and practice*, 6th ed. New York: McGraw-Hill, 2001:883–911.
6. Fleischer AC, Jones HW. Early detection of ovarian and endometrial cancer with transvaginal and color Doppler sonography. In: Fleischer AC, Manning FA, Jeanty P, et al., eds. *Sonography in obstetrics & gynecology: principles and practice*, 6th ed. New York: McGraw-Hill, 2001:1001–1017.
7. Shwayder JM. Endometriosis. In: Goldstein SR, Benson CB, eds. *Imaging of the infertile couple*. London: Dunitz M, 2001:13–23.
8. Swayne LC, Love MB, Karasick SR. Pelvic inflammatory disease: sonographic-pathologic correlation. *Radiology* 1984;151:751–755.
9. Timor-Tritsch IE, Monteagudo A. Inflammatory diseases of the female pelvis. In: Goldstein SR, Benson CB, eds. *Imaging of the infertile couple*. London: Dunitz M, 2001:25–35.

28

ECTOPIC PREGNANCY

28.1. TUBAL ECTOPIC PREGNANCY

Description and Clinical Features

Approximately 0.5%–1% of all pregnancies are ectopic (i.e., implanted at a site other than within the uterine cavity). More than 90% of ectopic pregnancies are located in the fallopian tubes, with most in the isthmic or ampullary portion.

Women whose tubes are scarred or whose pregnancies were achieved by means of assisted reproductive techniques (e.g., *in vitro* fertilization) are at elevated risk of ectopic pregnancy. Because the incidence of pelvic inflammatory disease and the use of assisted reproductive techniques have increased over the past two to three decades, ectopic pregnancy has become more frequent.

Ectopic pregnancy typically presents clinically with pelvic pain and vaginal bleeding. Internal bleeding is not unusual and may be severe enough to cause hypovolemic shock or death, especially if the diagnosis is delayed.

Sonography

Ultrasound is the primary diagnostic modality for ectopic pregnancy. When a woman of childbearing age presents with pelvic pain or bleeding and has a positive pregnancy test (often termed a "rule-out-ectopic" patient), ultrasound should be performed emergently and its interpretation should take into account the clinical presentation. In particular, the most likely cause of a complex adnexal mass in a "rule-out-ectopic" patient is ectopic pregnancy, whereas this diagnosis is highly unlikely in a woman with the same sonographic finding but a negative pregnancy test.

The sonographic finding that is definitive for ectopic pregnancy is visualization of a fluid-filled sac that lies outside the uterine cavity and contains either an embryo with cardiac activity (Figures 28.1-1 and 28.1-2) or a yolk sac (Figure 28.1-3). A more common, although less definitive, ultrasound finding in a woman with ectopic pregnancy is a complex extraovarian adnexal mass. In some cases, the outer rim of the adnexal mass is echogenic (tubal ring) (Figure 28.1-4), whereas in other cases, the mass has a solid or mixed solid and cystic appearance (Figure 28.1-5). There is sometimes a large amount of free intraperitoneal fluid (Figure 28.1-6).

The adnexal mass representing ectopic pregnancy often has high-volume, low-impedance blood flow around it when interrogated by color or spectral Doppler (Figure 28.1-7). Doppler, however, does not usually help significantly with the diagnosis of ectopic pregnancy because sonographic demonstration of an extraovarian mass and no intrauter-

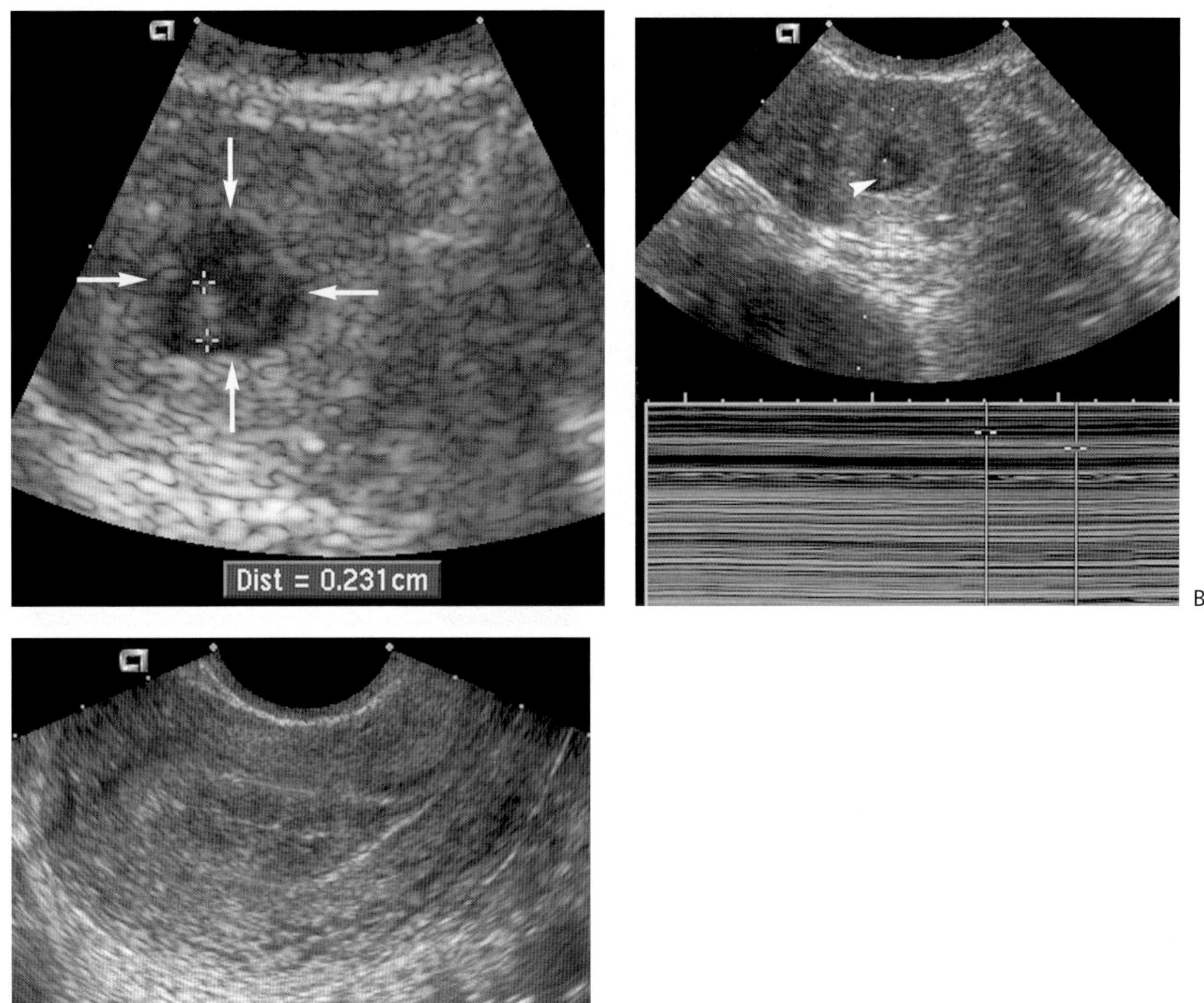

FIGURE 28.1-1. Ectopic pregnancy with an extrauterine gestational sac containing a live embryo. A: Coronal transvaginal view of the right adnexa demonstrates an extrauterine gestational sac *(arrows)* containing an embryo *(calipers)*. **B:** The embryo *(arrowhead)* has cardiac activity documented by M-mode *(dotted line on portion of the image that is the source of the M-mode, calipers measure a single heartbeat)*. **C:** Sagittal transvaginal view of the uterus reveals no evidence of an intrauterine gestational sac.

ine gestational sac in a "rule-out-ectopic" patient indicates a high likelihood (>90%) of ectopic pregnancy regardless of the Doppler findings.

There may be blood or secretions in the uterine cavity in a woman with ectopic pregnancy (Figure 28.1-2). This sonographic finding has been termed a pseudogestational sac because it can potentially be mistaken for a gestational sac. This error can be avoided by noting that such a fluid collection has none of the characteristics of a gestational sac: no yolk sac or embryo within it and no double echogenic ring surrounding it.

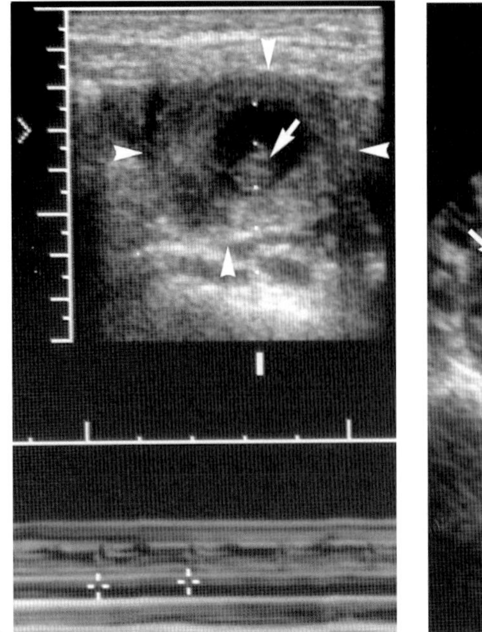
A

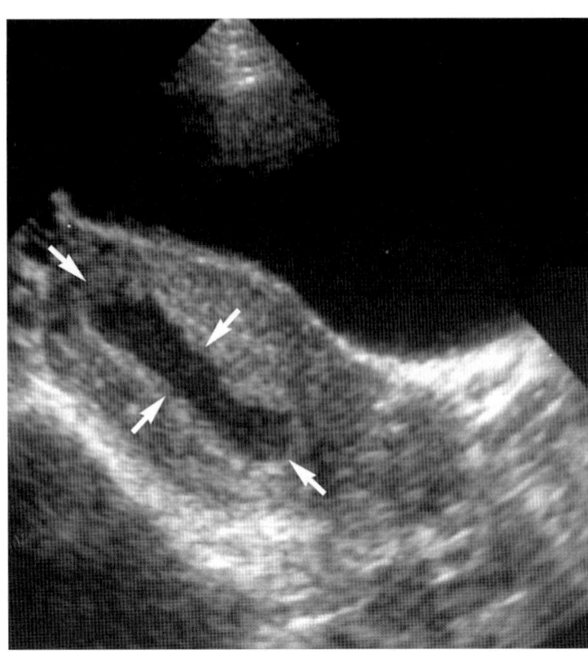
B

FIGURE 28.1-2. Ectopic pregnancy with a live embryo and an intrauterine pseudogestational sac. A: Sagittal view through the right adnexa demonstrates a complex cystic mass *(arrowheads)*. The mass contains an embryo *(arrow)* with cardiac activity documented by M-mode *(dotted line on portion of the image that is the source of the M-mode, calipers measure a single heartbeat)*, indicating that the complex mass is a gestational sac. **B:** Sagittal transabdominal view of the uterus demonstrates a fluid collection *(arrows)* in the uterus, with none of the characteristics of a gestational sac (no yolk sac or embryo within it, no double echogenic ring surrounding it). Such a fluid collection, representing blood or secretions in the uterine cavity in a patient with an ectopic pregnancy, has been termed a pseudogestational sac.

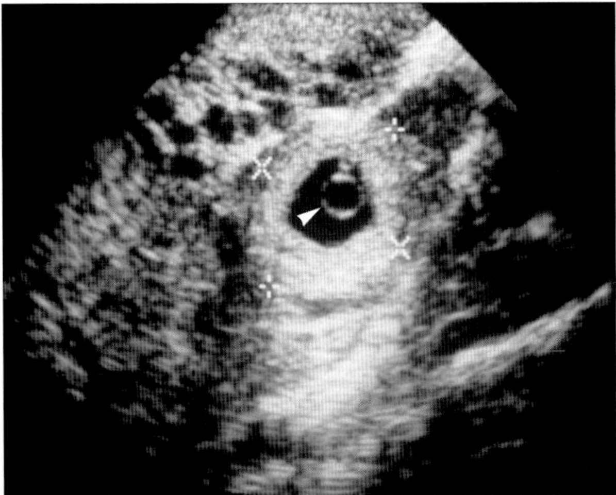

FIGURE 28.1-3. Ectopic pregnancy containing a yolk sac. Sagittal transvaginal view through the left adnexa demonstrates a thick-walled fluid collection *(calipers)* diagnosable as a gestational sac because it contains a yolk sac *(arrowhead)*.

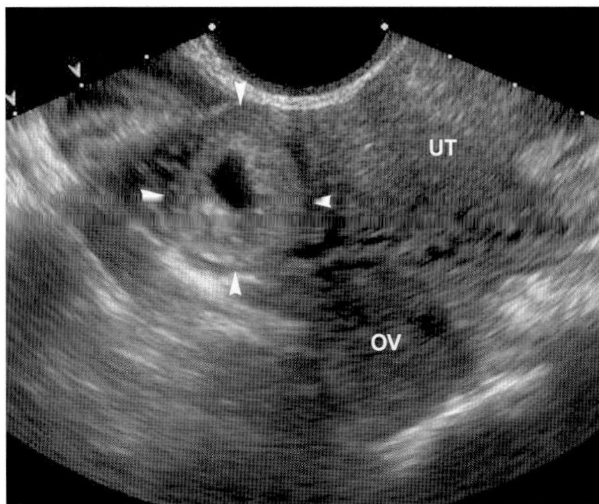

FIGURE 28.1-4. Ectopic pregnancy with an adnexal tubal ring. Coronal transvaginal view of the right adnexa demonstrates a mass *(arrowheads)* adjacent to the uterus *(UT)* and separate from the right ovary *(OV)*. The mass consists of a fluid collection surrounded by a thick echogenic rim of tissue (tubal ring).

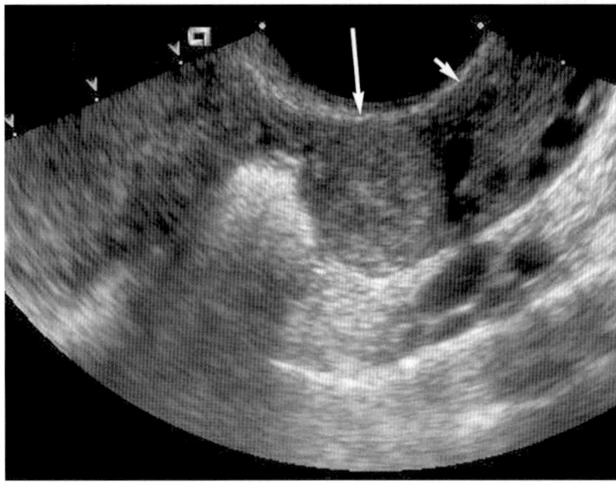

FIGURE 28.1-5. Ectopic pregnancy with an adnexal mass. Coronal transvaginal view of the left adnexa reveals a fairly homogeneous mass *(long arrow)* adjacent to the left ovary *(short arrow)*. The mass moved separately from the ovary when pressure was applied by the transvaginal transducer.

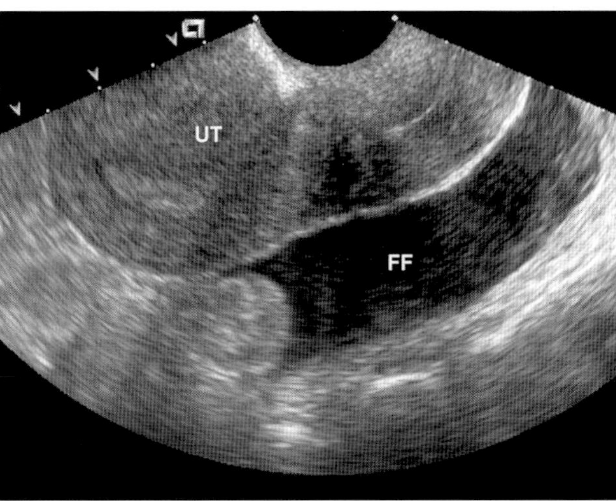

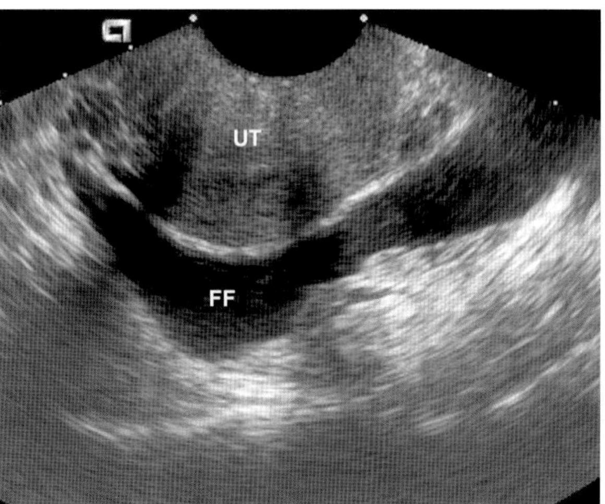

FIGURE 28.1-6. Ectopic pregnancy with free intraperitoneal fluid. Sagittal **(A)** and coronal **(B)** transvaginal views of the pelvis in a woman with a positive pregnancy test demonstrate a moderate amount of free fluid *(FF)* in the cul-de-sac and no evidence of a gestational sac within the uterus *(UT)*.

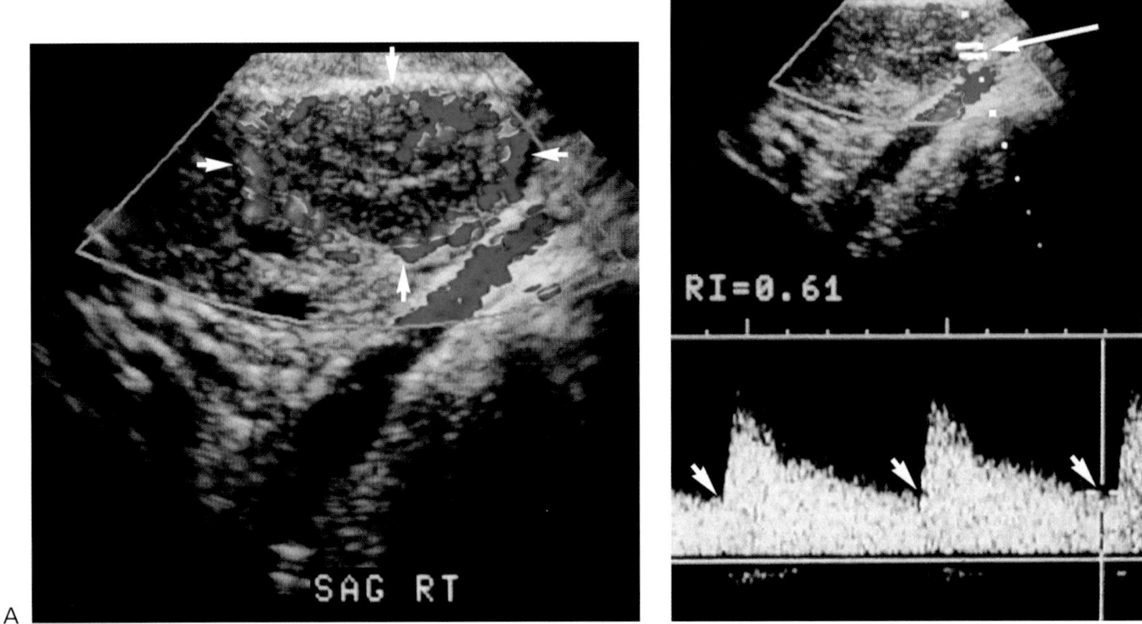

FIGURE 28.1-7. Ectopic pregnancy with adnexal mass: Doppler findings. A: Sagittal *(SAG RT)* transvaginal view through the right adnexa with color Doppler demonstrates a soft-tissue mass *(arrows)* surrounded by considerable blood flow. **B:** Spectral Doppler waveform, with the Doppler gate *(long arrow)* on a region of blood flow at the periphery of the mass, demonstrates a large amount of blood flow at end diastole *(short arrows)*, indicative of low-impedance flow around the mass.

28.2. CORNUAL (INTERSTITIAL) ECTOPIC PREGNANCY

Description and Clinical Features

Cornual ectopic pregnancy is one that implants in the intramural portion of the fallopian tube, the part of the tube that traverses the cornu of the uterus. This is an uncommon form of ectopic pregnancy but, like other ectopics, occurs more frequently in pregnancies achieved via assisted reproductive techniques than those achieved naturally.

A gestational sac in the cornu can grow for a period of time, but the cornu has a far more limited ability to expand than does the body of the uterus. Once the cornu has reached its maximal size, further sac growth will lead to cornual rupture and potentially life-threatening bleeding. Fortunately, pain usually occurs earlier than rupture, so that prompt diagnosis when the patient presents with symptoms can save the patient's life or spare her from a hysterectomy. Ultrasound-guided ablation is one of the treatment options.

Sonography

On ultrasound, cornual ectopic pregnancy appears as a gestational sac located in the superolateral portion of the uterus, separate from but contiguous with the body of the uterus. Little or no myometrium is seen around the lateral or superior aspect of the gestational sac (Figures 28.2-1 and 28.2-2). A high volume of blood flow may be seen around the sac on color Doppler (Figure 28.2-3).

Distinguishing between cornual ectopic pregnancy and an eccentrically located intrauterine gestation (e.g., a gestational sac in one horn of a bicornuate uterus) can present a diagnostic dilemma. Because the management of these two entities is markedly different—cornual ectopic pregnancy requires emergent treatment and an eccentrically

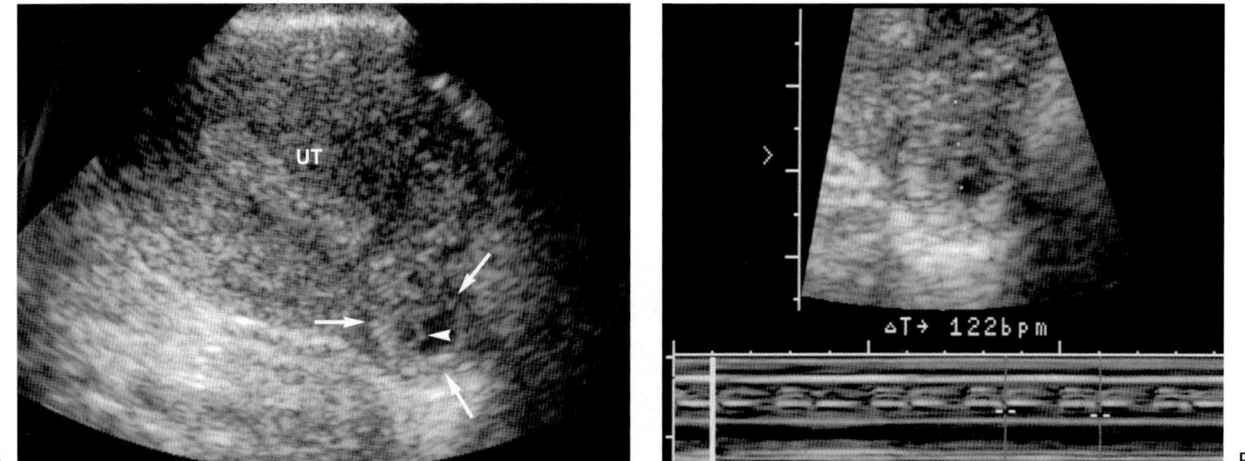

FIGURE 28.2-1. Cornual ectopic pregnancy with a live embryo at 6 weeks gestation. A: Coronal transvaginal view of the uterus *(UT)* reveals a gestational sac *(arrows)* with a yolk sac *(arrowhead)* in the left superolateral aspect of the uterus, a region corresponding to the left cornu. No gestational sac is seen within the body of the uterus. **B:** M-mode through the gestational sac (*dotted line* indicates region in which M-mode is obtained) reveals embryonic cardiac activity *(calipers)* at a rate of 122 beats per minute.

placed intrauterine gestational sac requires no treatment—it is extremely important to be accurate in distinguishing between them. The most useful sonographic feature in making this distinction is the appearance of myometrium around the sac. If an eccentrically located sac has myometrium of normal thickness (5 mm or greater) all the way around it, the pregnancy is intrauterine. If little or no myometrium is seen around a portion of the sac, the diagnosis of cornual ectopic pregnancy is established.

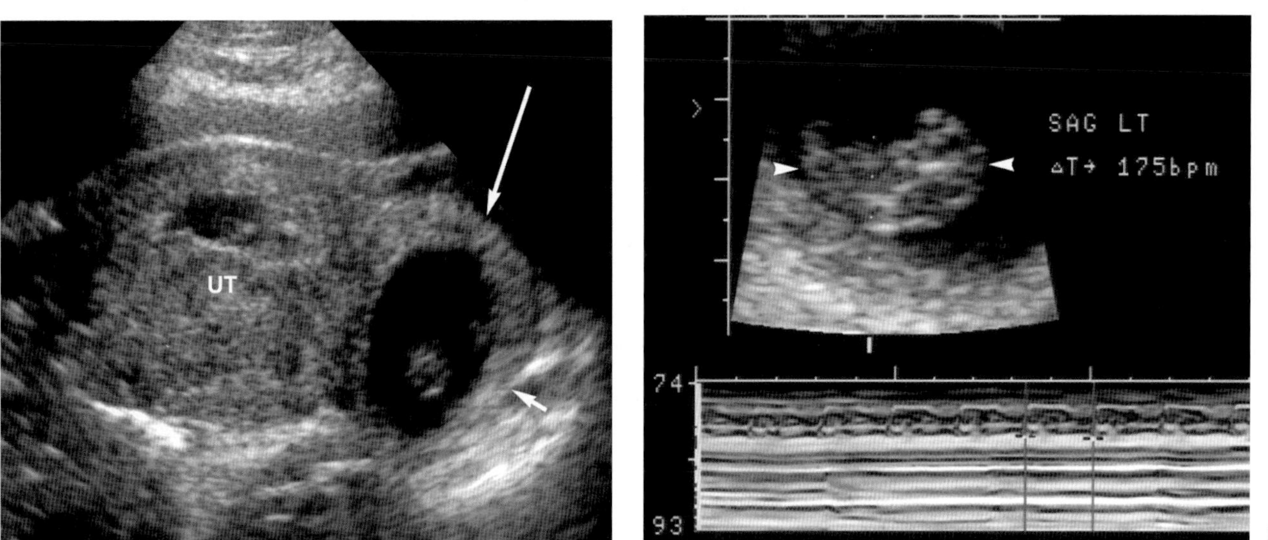

FIGURE 28.2-2. Cornual ectopic pregnancy with a live embryo at 8 weeks gestation. A: Transverse transabdominal view of the uterus *(UT)* reveals a gestational sac *(long arrow)* on the extreme left lateral aspect of the uterus. No myometrium is seen around the lateral aspect of the gestational sac *(short arrow)*. **B:** Sagittal view *(SAG LT)* through the gestational sac in the left adnexa reveals a live embryo *(arrowheads)*, with M-mode documenting its cardiac activity (*dotted line* through the embryo, *calipers* on the M-mode tracing) at a heart rate of 175 beats per minute.

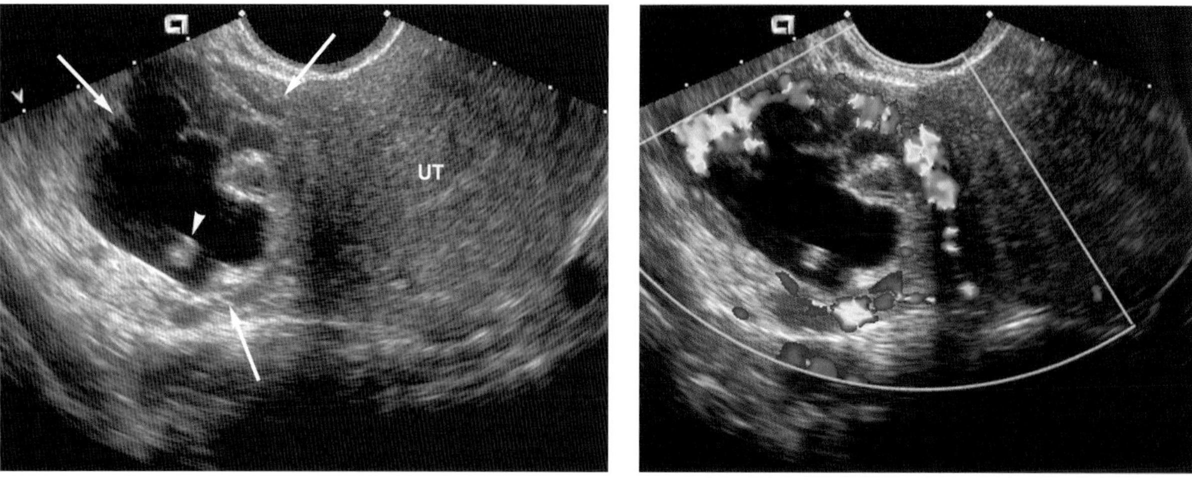

FIGURE 28.2-3. Cornual ectopic pregnancy surrounded by a high volume of blood flow. **A:** Coronal transvaginal view through the uterus *(UT)* reveals an irregular fluid collection *(arrows)* in the region of the right cornu. A small echogenic structure *(arrowhead)*, likely representing a dead embryo, is noted within the sac. **B:** Color Doppler reveals a large amount of blood flow around the right cornual gestational sac.

28.3. CERVICAL ECTOPIC PREGNANCY

Description and Clinical Features

Cervical ectopic pregnancy is one that implants in the cervix. This form of ectopic pregnancy is very rare in naturally conceived pregnancies. Although it is found more frequently in pregnancies achieved via assisted reproductive techniques, it is still an extremely uncommon occurrence. A gestational sac, with its developing embryo, implanted in the cervix can grow until about the middle of the first trimester. As the cervix stretches around the enlarging gestational sac, the patient experiences pelvic pain and vaginal bleeding. The bleeding can be heavy enough to be life-threatening to the mother if not treated promptly.

Before the availability of ultrasound, the diagnosis of cervical ectopic pregnancy was often made from the surgical specimen after a woman underwent a hysterectomy for uncontrollable vaginal bleeding. With ultrasound, the diagnosis can be made earlier and noninvasively, thus permitting treatments that leave the uterus intact.

Sonography

With cervical ectopic pregnancy, ultrasound demonstrates a gestational sac in the cervix, often containing a yolk sac or embryo (Figures 28.3-1 and 28.3-2). Two diagnostic dilemmas can arise in the sonographic diagnosis of cervical ectopic pregnancy: (1) distinguishing between cervical ectopic pregnancy and a spontaneous abortion in progress and (2) distinguishing between a sac implanted in the cervix and one implanted in the lower uterine segment. The first distinction can usually be made based on the appearance of the intracervical gestational sac. A well-formed, round or oval sac surrounded by a thick echogenic rim is highly suggestive of cervical ectopic pregnancy. This diagnosis is even more likely if an embryo with cardiac activity is seen within the sac. If, conversely, the sac is flattened, has little or no echogenic rim, and is empty or has a dead embryo within it, the likely diagnosis is a spontaneous abortion in progress. When there is uncertainty about the correct diagnosis, rescanning a day later will likely clarify the matter: an

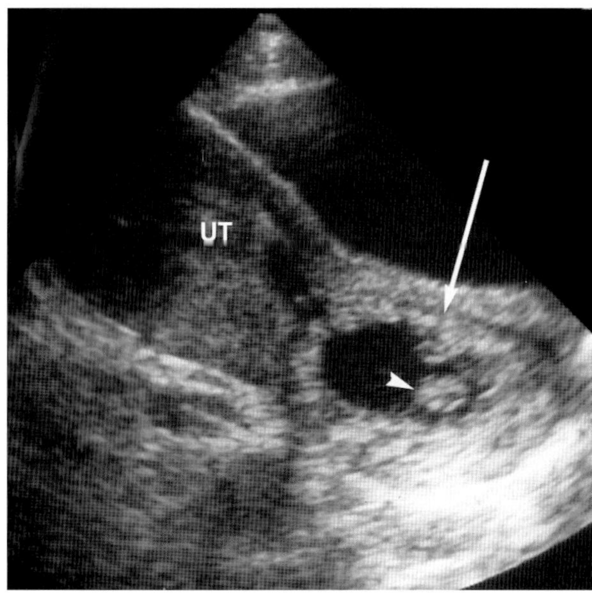

FIGURE 28.3-1. Cervical ectopic pregnancy. Sagittal transabdominal view of the uterus *(UT)* demonstrates a gestational sac in the cervix *(long arrow)*. There is an embryo *(short arrow)* within the sac, and cardiac activity was noted on real-time sonography. (From Doubilet PM, Benson CB. Obstetrical radiology: the abnormal pregnancy. In: Taveras JM, Ferucci JT, eds. *Radiology: diagnosis-imaging-intervention*. Philadelphia: Lippincott Williams & Wilkins, 2000, with permission.)

unchanged appearance is indicative of cervical ectopic pregnancy, whereas the disappearance or marked change in appearance of the sac indicates a spontaneous abortion in progress.

Distinguishing between cervical and lower segment implantation can usually be made by transvaginal ultrasound based on the distance between the gestational sac and the transducer. With cervical ectopic pregnancy, the sac is generally within 1–2 cm of the transducer.

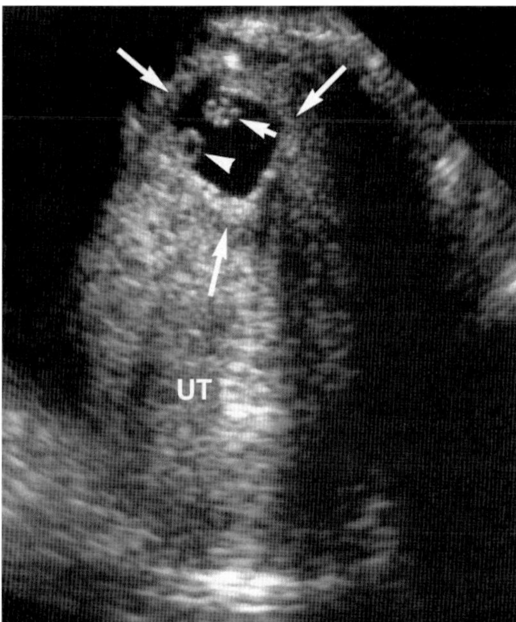

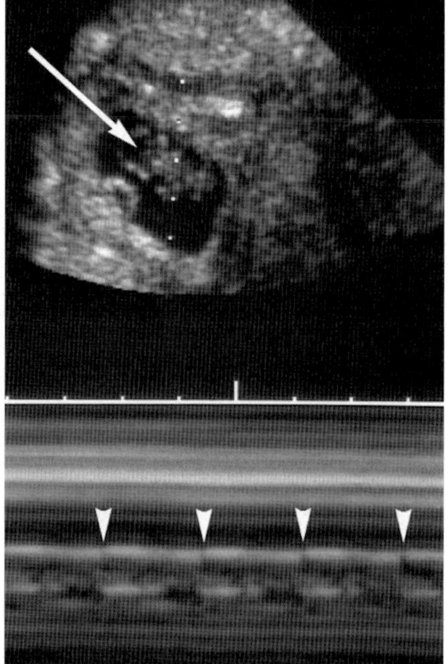

FIGURE 28.3-2. Cervical ectopic pregnancy with M-mode documentation of a live embryo. A: Sagittal transvaginal view of a retroverted uterus *(UT)* demonstrates an intracervical gestational sac *(long arrows)* containing a yolk sac *(arrowhead)* and embryo *(short arrow)*. **B:** M-mode through the intracervical fetus *(arrow)* documents cardiac activity *(arrowheads)*.

28.4. ABDOMINAL ECTOPIC PREGNANCY

Description and Clinical Features

Abdominal ectopic pregnancy is a rare form of ectopic pregnancy in which the gestational sac implants in the peritoneal cavity. This form of ectopic pregnancy can occur in two ways. In some cases, the pregnancy implants directly in the abdomen. In other cases, the pregnancy begins as a tubal ectopic and then reimplants in the abdomen after either the fallopian tube ruptures or the gestational sac is expelled through the end of the tube. The maternal mortality rate with abdominal pregnancies is several-fold higher than with other forms of ectopic pregnancy due to the high incidence of internal hemorrhage. In many abdominal pregnancies, the fetus dies early in gestation. In some cases, however, the fetus can remain alive until the second or even the third trimester. Treatment consists of surgical removal of the fetus and placenta, unless the latter cannot be safely resected from the major blood vessels or abdominal organs. If some or all of the placenta is left in place, it may take several months to resorb.

Sonography

In the early-to-mid first trimester, abdominal pregnancy may be indistinguishable from tubal ectopic pregnancy on ultrasound. In the late first trimester and beyond, demonstration of a live fetus outside the uterus is highly suggestive of abdominal pregnancy because the fallopian tube cannot contain a pregnancy that large. Because abdominal pregnancy may be contiguous with the fundus of the uterus, it is essential to delineate the margin of the uterus carefully to demonstrate that the gestational sac lies outside the uterus (Figure 28.4-1). Transvaginal scanning may be required to establish this (Figure 28.4-2).

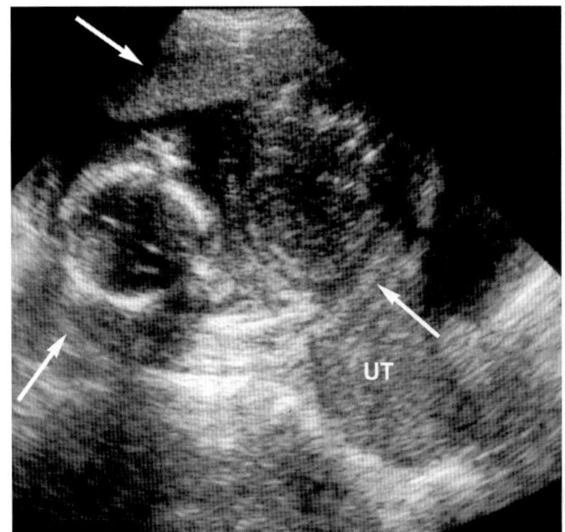

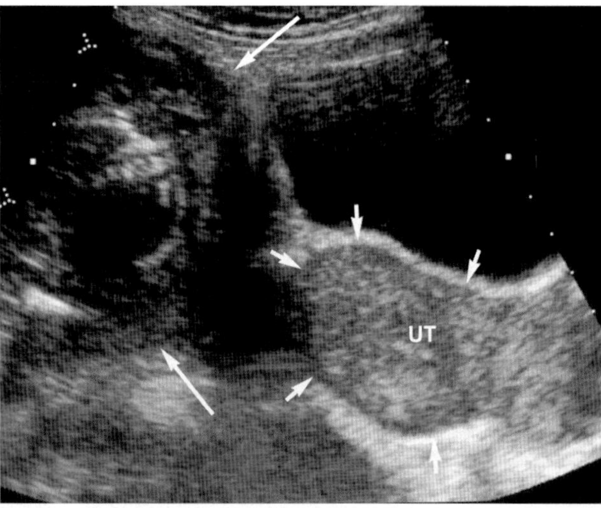

FIGURE 28.4-1. Abdominal pregnancy. A: Sagittal transabdominal view of the pelvis and lower abdomen reveals a gestational sac *(arrows)* containing a fetus, situated superior to the uterus *(UT)*. **B:** This sagittal view more clearly delineates the uterine contour *(short arrows)*, demonstrating that the gestational sac *(long arrows)* is above and separate from the uterus.

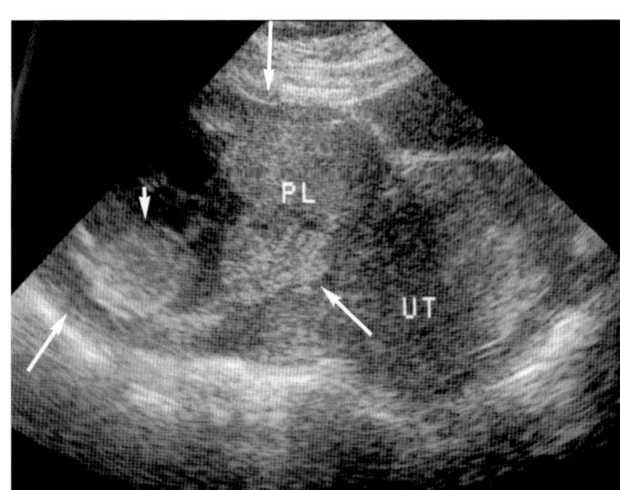

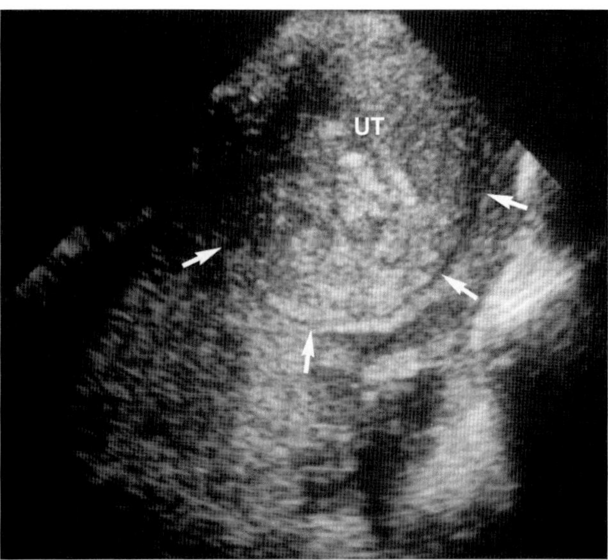

A B

FIGURE 28.4-2. Abdominal pregnancy. A: Sagittal transabdominal view of the pelvis and lower abdomen reveals a gestational sac *(long arrows)* containing a fetus *(short arrow)* and placenta *(PL),* situated superior to the uterus *(UT).* **B:** Sagittal transvaginal view of the pelvis more clearly delineates the contour *(arrows)* of the uterus *(UT)*, demonstrating that there is no gestational sac within the uterus.

If surgery is performed and the placenta cannot be removed in its entirety, ultrasound plays a useful role in monitoring the patient. In particular, ultrasound can follow the placenta until it resorbs completely, and can assess for complications of the retained placenta such as abscess or hemorrhage.

28.5. HETEROTOPIC PREGNANCY

Description and Clinical Features

Heterotopic pregnancy refers to the coexistence of intrauterine and ectopic pregnancies (i.e., there is at least one gestational sac implanted within the uterus as well as at least one ectopic gestation). Heterotopic pregnancy is very rare in natural conceptions, occurring with an incidence of at most 1:5,000. As with other forms of ectopic pregnancy, heterotopic pregnancy occurs with increased frequency in pregnancies achieved by means of assisted reproductive techniques.

Heterotopic pregnancy can lead to potentially life-threatening maternal bleeding. Accurate and early diagnosis can lead to treatment that both saves the life of the mother and preserves the intrauterine gestation.

Sonography

The sonographic finding that is definitive for heterotopic pregnancy is visualization of both an intrauterine and an ectopic gestational sac, each containing a yolk sac (Figure 28.5-1) or an embryo with cardiac activity (Figure 28.5-2).

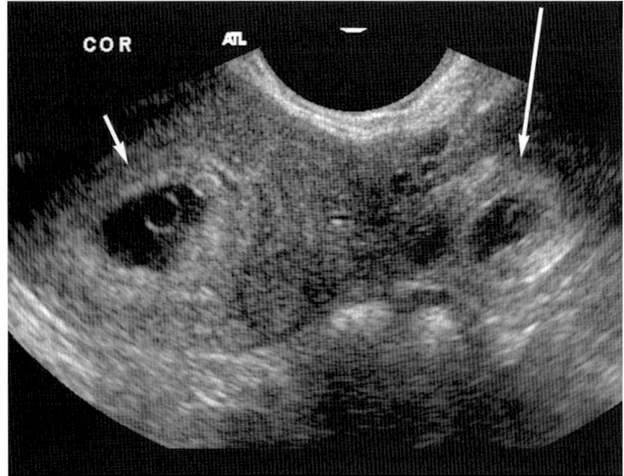

A

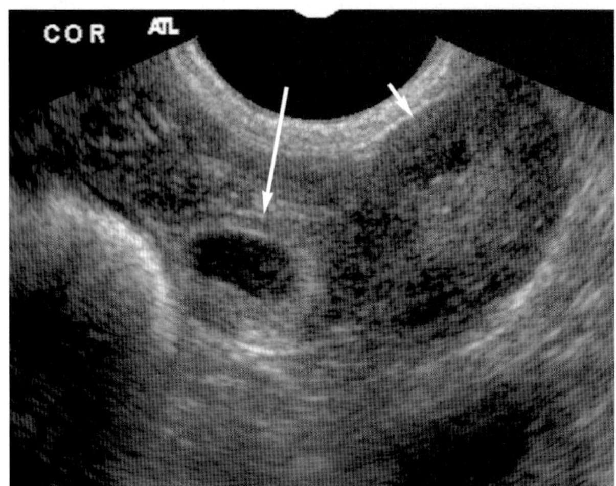

B

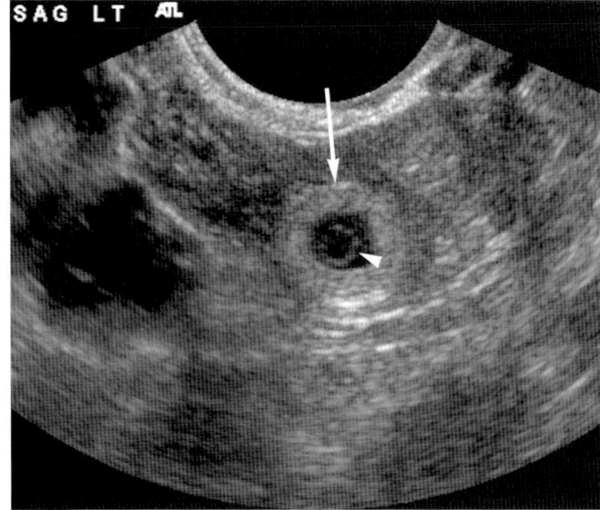

C

FIGURE 28.5-1. Heterotopic pregnancy. A: Coronal *(COR)* transvaginal view through the uterus and left adnexa demonstrates two gestational sacs, one within the uterus *(short arrow)* and one ectopically located in the left adnexa *(long arrow)*. **B:** Coronal view through the left adnexa demonstrates that the ectopic gestational sac *(long arrow)* lies adjacent to the left ovary *(short arrow)*. **C:** Sagittal *(SAG LT)* transvaginal view through the left adnexa demonstrates a yolk sac *(arrowhead)* within the ectopic gestational sac *(arrow)*.

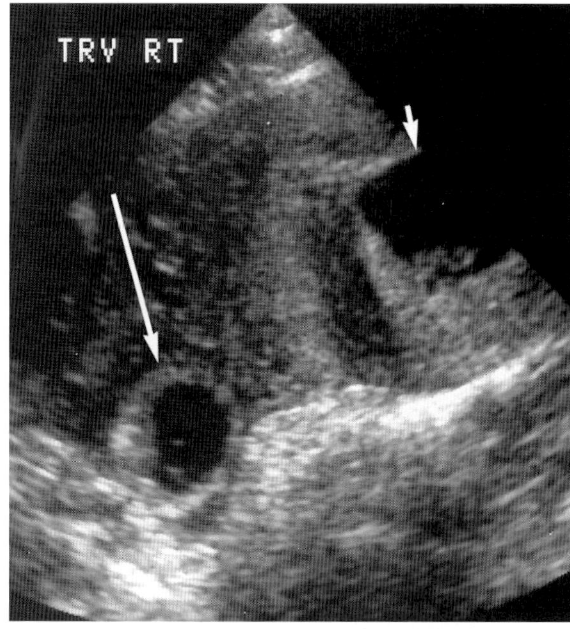

A

FIGURE 28.5-2. Heterotopic pregnancy with two live embryos. A: Transverse *(TRN RT)* view through the uterus and right adnexa demonstrates two gestational sacs, one within the uterus *(short arrow)* and one ectopically located in the right adnexa *(long arrow)*. Sagittal *(SAG ML)* view through the intrauterine gestational sac **(B)** and sagittal *(SAG RT)* view through the right adnexal gestational sac **(C)** demonstrate that each contains an embryo *(arrow)* with cardiac activity documented by M-mode *(dotted line and calipers)*.

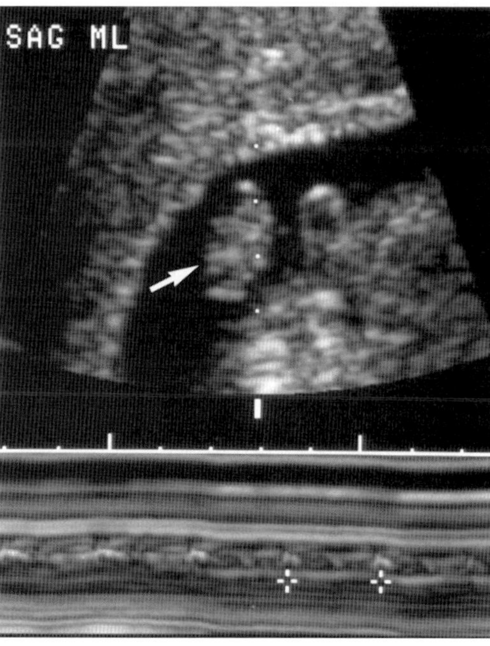

B

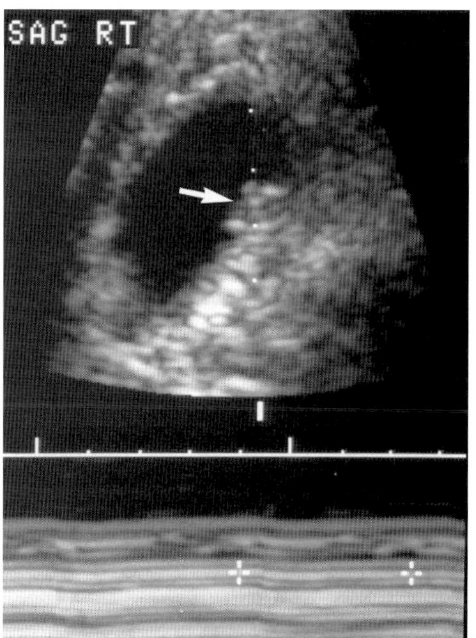

C

SUGGESTED READINGS

1. Brown DL, Doubilet PM. Transvaginal sonography for diagnosing ectopic pregnancy: positivity criteria and performance characteristics. *J Ultrasound Med* 1994;13:259–266.
2. Coleman BG. Transvaginal sonography in extrauterine and intrauterine pregnancy. *Semin Roentgenol* 1991;26:63–74.
3. Doubilet PM, Benson CB. Emergency obstetrical ultrasound. *Semin Roentgenol* 1998;33:339–450.
4. Emerson DS, Cartier MS, Altieri LA, et al. Diagnostic efficacy of endovaginal color Doppler flow imaging in an ectopic pregnancy screening program. *Radiology* 1992;183:413–420.
5. Filly RA. Ectopic pregnancy: the role of sonography. *Radiology* 1987;162:661–668.
6. Frates M. Ectopic pregnancy. In: Goldstein SR, Benson CB, eds. *Imaging of the infertile couple.* London: M Dunitz, 2001:195–203.

7. Frates MC, Visweswaran A, Laing FC. Comparison of tubal ring and corpus luteum echogenicities—a useful differentiating characteristic. *J Ultrasound Med* 2001;20:27–31.
8. Ginsburg ES, Frates MC, Rein MS, et al. Early diagnosis and treatment of cervical pregnancy in an in vitro fertilization program. *Fertil Steril* 1994;61:966–969.
9. Laing FC, Frates MC. Ultrasound evaluation during the first trimester of pregnancy. In: Callen PW, ed. *Ultrasonography in obstetrics and gynecology*, 4th ed. Philadelphia: WB Saunders, 2000:105–145.
10. Nyberg DA, Filly RA, Laing FC, et al. Ectopic pregnancy: diagnosis by sonography correlated with quantitative HCG levels. *J Ultrasound Med* 1987;6:145–150.
11. Pellerito JS, Taylor KJW, Quedens-Case C, et al. Ectopic pregnancy: evaluation with endovaginal color flow imaging. *Radiology* 1992;183:407–411.
12. Pisarka MD, Carson SA. Ectopic pregnancy. In: Scott JR, Di Saia PJ, Hammond CB, et al., eds. *Danforth's obstetrics and gynecology*. Philadelphia: Lippincott Williams & Wilkins, 1999:155–172.
13. Tanbo T, Dale PO, Lunde O, et al. Heterotopic pregnancy following in vitro fertilization. *Acta Obstet Gynecol Scand* 1991;70:335–338.

29

DIAGNOSTIC GYNECOLOGICAL PROCEDURES

29.1. SALINE INFUSION SONOHYSTEROGRAPHY

Description and Clinical Features

Saline infusion sonohysterography (SIS) is a procedure in which the uterus is scanned during and immediately after instillation of saline into the uterine cavity. By outlining the inner surface of the endometrium, this procedure enhances the ability of ultrasound to detect and characterize endometrial pathology. As such, SIS can be helpful in a number of settings, including the following:

A woman (pre- or postmenopausal) with abnormal endometrial thickening on standard sonography: SIS can determine whether the thickening is focal or diffuse, thus aiding in the diagnosis or in the selection of a biopsy technique.

A woman with a normal-appearing endometrium on standard sonography but with a high clinical suspicion of endometrial pathology: SIS is more sensitive for endometrial pathology and hence may detect pathology that was not found on standard sonography.

A woman clinically suspected of having endometrial adhesions: Adhesions are visible on SIS but not on standard sonography.

Sonography

The SIS procedure begins with the insertion of a catheter through the cervix into the uterine cavity. Some practitioners use a catheter with a balloon near its end, and inflate the balloon with saline to prevent the catheter from being dislodged as well as to decrease saline runout through the cervix. Once the catheter is in place, a transvaginal transducer is inserted and the endometrium is scanned in sagittal and coronal (transverse) planes during and after instillation of approximately 3–10 ml saline through the catheter. Care must be taken to visualize the entire endometrium, sweeping from one side to the other sagittally and from anterior to posterior coronally. Because the saline generally drains out of the uterine cavity fairly quickly (via the fallopian tubes and/or cervix), several instillations of saline are often needed during the procedure. If the catheter has an inflated balloon, it should be deflated toward the end of the procedure so that the lower segment endometrium can be adequately assessed (Figure 29.1-1).

On a normal SIS, the endometrium is homogeneous in appearance and has a smooth inner surface (Figure 29.1-1). In a woman of menstrual age, the endometrial thickness varies with the menstrual cycle; it is thinnest in the early proliferative phase and thickest in the secretory phase. In a postmenopausal woman, the endometrium is normally less than 2 mm in thickness (note that this refers to single-thickness measurement as opposed to the double-thickness measurement used to measure the endometrium on a standard sonogram without saline).

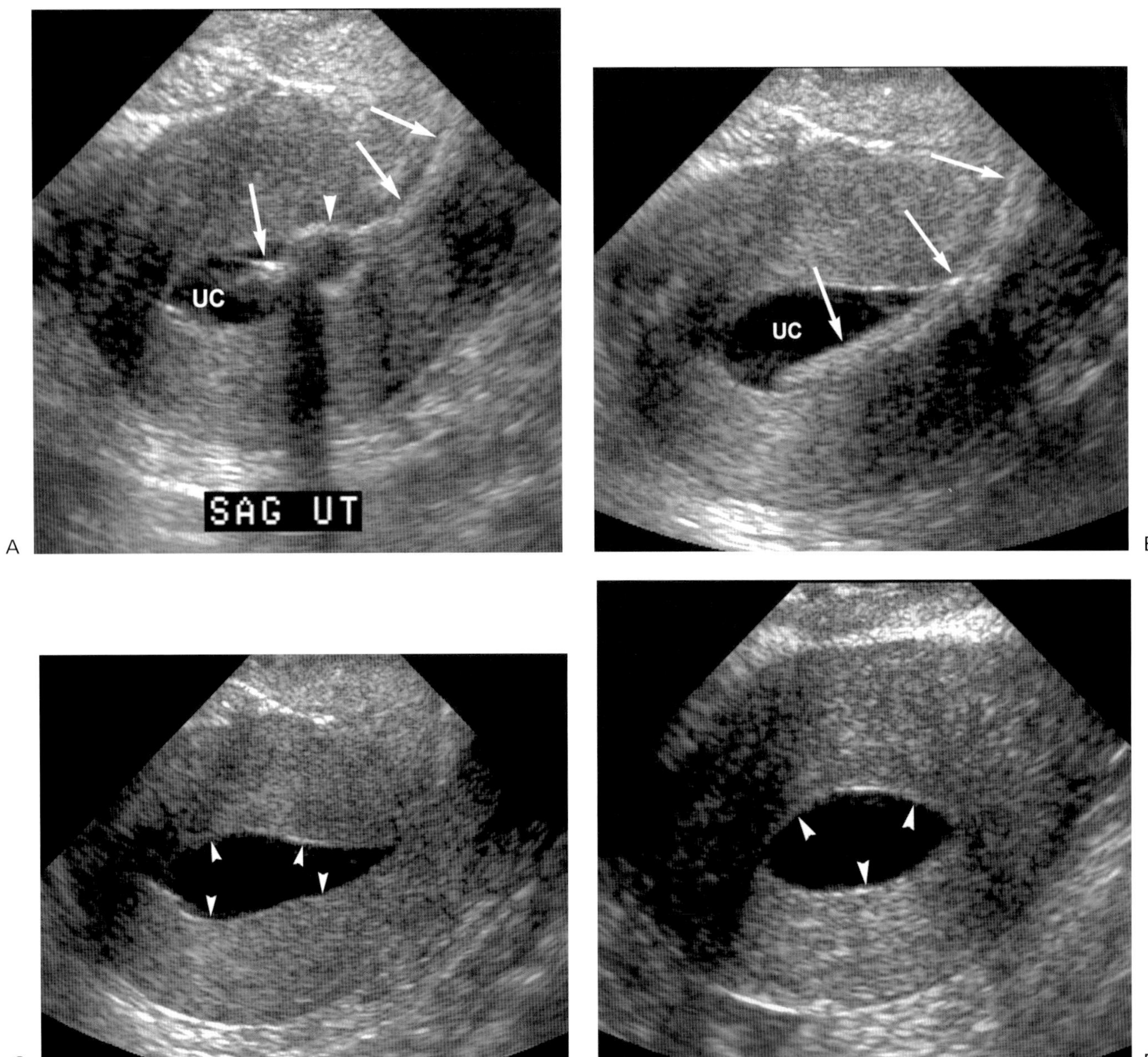

FIGURE 29.1-1. Normal saline infusion sonohysterogram. A: Sagittal *(SAG UT)* transvaginal view of the uterus demonstrates a pediatric Foley catheter *(arrows)* with a fluid-filled balloon *(arrowhead)* in the uterine cavity *(UC)*. Saline has been instilled into the uterine cavity through the catheter. **B:** The saline-filled uterine cavity *(UC)* is more completely visualized after the balloon has been deflated before removal of the catheter *(arrows)*. Sagittal **(C)** and coronal **(D)** views immediately after removal of the catheter reveal smooth, thin endometrium *(arrowheads)* outlined by saline.

Endometrial abnormalities detectable by SIS include carcinoma, which most often appears as either a focal area of irregular thickening or a diffusely thickened, irregular, and poorly distensible endometrium; polyps, which appear as focal sessile or pedunculated projections into the saline-filled uterine cavity (Figure 29.1-2); hyperplasia, which appears as a diffuse, usually homogeneous, thickening; submucosal fibroids, which appear as hypoechoic or heterogeneous masses indenting or projecting into the uterine cavity; and adhesions, which appear as linear structures crossing the uterine cavity.

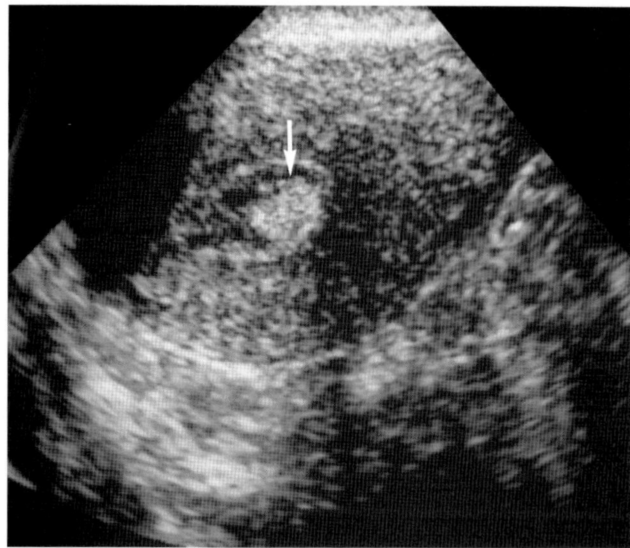

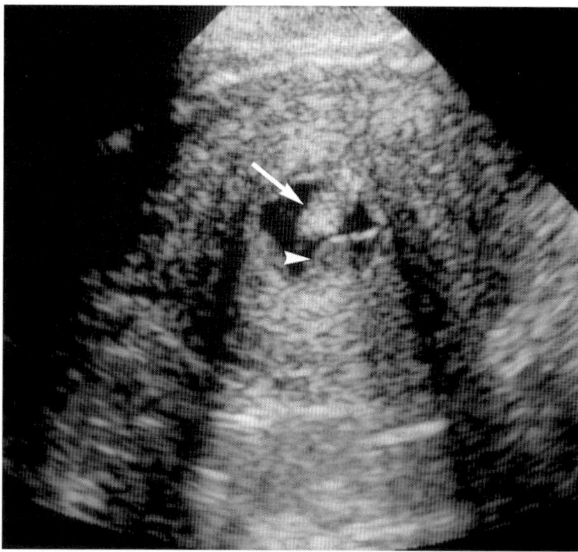

FIGURE 29.1-2. Saline infusion sonohysterogram delineating endometrial pathology. A: Sagittal transvaginal view of the uterus reveals a focal echogenic lesion *(arrow)* in the endometrium. **B:** After instillation of saline, the endometrial abnormality is more clearly defined. There is both a polyp *(arrow)* and a broad-based area of endometrial thickening *(arrowhead).*

One of the main benefits of SIS is the distinction between focal and diffuse thickening when endometrial tissue sampling is planned, because diffusely thickened endometrium can be sampled by a blind biopsy technique (office biopsy or dilation and curettage), whereas hysteroscopic guidance may be needed to perform a biopsy or resect focal lesions. This is especially important in women with abnormal postmenopausal bleeding because such women have a fairly high risk of endometrial cancer.

SUGGESTED READINGS

1. Bree RL, Bowerman RA, Bohm-Velez M, et al. Ultrasound evaluation of the uterus in patients with postmenopausal bleeding: a positive impact on diagnostic decision making. *Radiology* 2000;216: 260–264.
2. Cohen JR, Luxman D, Sagi J, et al. Sonohysterography for distinguishing endometrial thickening from endometrial polyps in postmenopausal bleeding. *Ultrasound Obstet Gynecol* 1994;4:227–230.
3. Cullinan JA, Fleischer AC, Kepple DM, et al. Sonohysterography: a technique for endometrial evaluation. Radiographics 1995;15:501–514.
4. Dubinsky TJ, Parvey R, Gormaz G, et al. Transvaginal hysterosonography in the evaluation of small endoluminal masses. *J Ultrasound Med* 1995;14:1–6.
5. Dueholm M, Forman A, Jensen ML, et al. Transvaginal sonography combined with saline contrast sonohysterography in evaluating the uterine cavity in premenopausal patients with abnormal uterine bleeding. *Ultrasound Obstet Gynecol* 2001;18:54–61.
6. Epstein E, Ramirez A, Skoog L, et al. Transvaginal sonography, saline contrast sonohysterography and hysteroscopy for the investigation of women with postmenopausal bleeding and endometrium > 5 mm. *Ultrasound Obstet Gynecol* 2001;18:157–162.
7. Goldstein SR. Use of ultrasonohysterography for triage of perimenopausal patients with unexplained uterine bleeding. *Am J Obstet Gynecol* 1994;170:565–570.
8. Parsons AK, Lense JJ. Sonohysterography for endometrial abnormalities: preliminary results. *J Clin Ultrasound* 1993;21:87–95.

30

THERAPEUTIC GYNECOLOGICAL PROCEDURES

30.1. OVARIAN CYST ASPIRATION

Description and Clinical Features

Ultrasound-guided ovarian cyst drainage can be useful in a number of clinical situations. It should not be done, however, when there is a clinical suspicion of ovarian malignancy because of the possibility of tumor seeding. Indications for ovarian cyst drainage include the following:

Follicular aspiration (oocyte retrieval) for in vitro fertilization.

Pain relief: Draining a large cyst can provide at least temporary pain relief. In some cases, the fluid will reaccumulate, and surgery would be needed for permanent relief.

In other patients, the fluid will not recur or will reaccumulate slowly enough to be managed by repeated cyst punctures, thus obviating the need for surgery.

Differentiating an infected from a noninfected cyst.

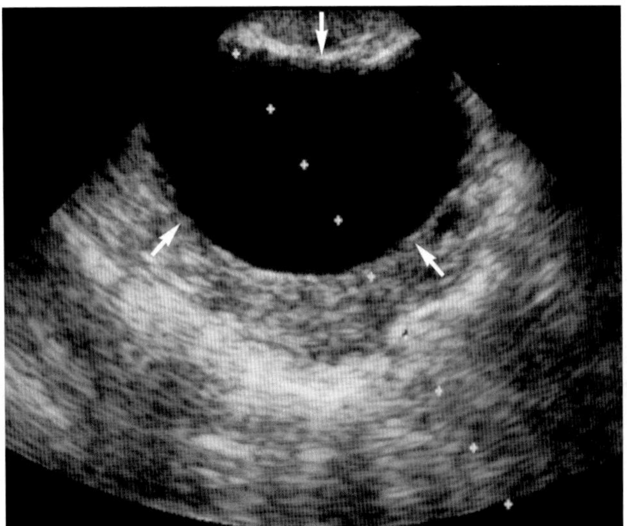

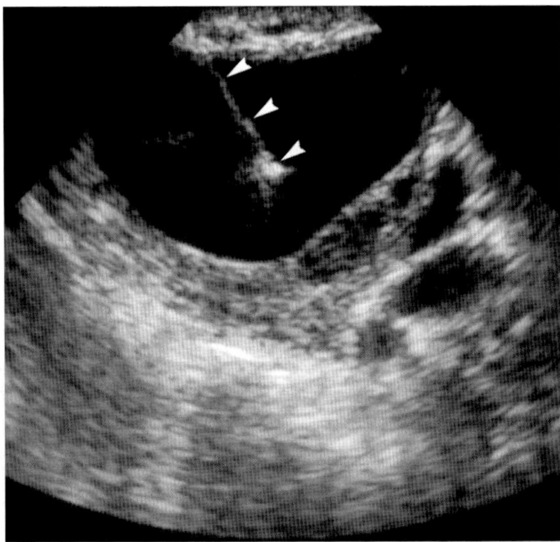

FIGURE 30.1-1. Transvaginal ultrasound-guided aspiration of a unilocular cyst. A: Transvaginal view of the right adnexa demonstrates a simple unilocular cyst *(arrows)*. There is a needle guide on the transducer, and the guide marks on the image indicate the path that will be taken by a needle inserted through the guide. **B:** A needle *(arrowheads)* has been inserted to drain the cyst.

Sonography

Ovarian cyst drainage can be done transvaginally or transabdominally, with the optimal approach depending on the location of the cyst. In most cases, the transvaginal approach is better.

Transvaginal cyst drainage is performed by cleaning the vagina with an antiseptic solution, inserting a transvaginal transducer equipped with a needle guide, and inserting a needle through the guide. Using continuous real-time guidance, the needle is advanced into the cyst (Figure 30.1-1). Once it is within the cyst, the stylet is removed, the syringe attached, and the cyst drained. If the cyst is multilocular, all (or at least the several largest) locules can be drained by redirecting the needle into different areas (Figure 30.1-2).

If the cyst extends close to the anterior abdominal wall, percutaneous puncture using transabdominal ultrasound guidance may be the optimal approach (Figure 30.1-3). Guidance can be done with or without a needle guide attachment on the transducer.

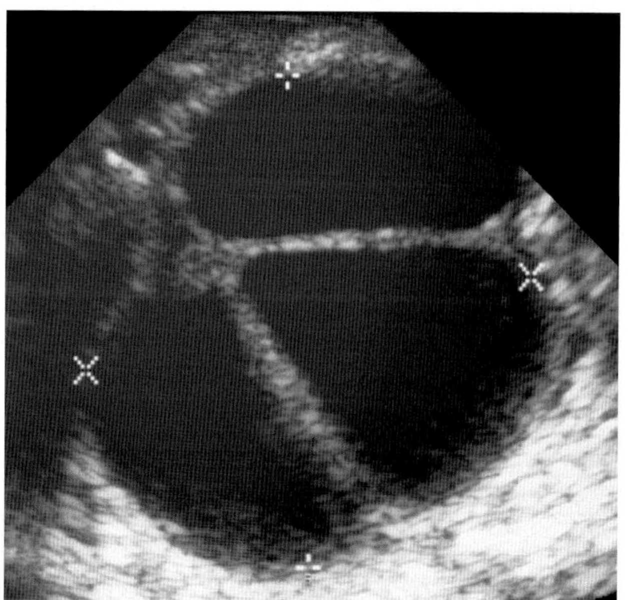

A

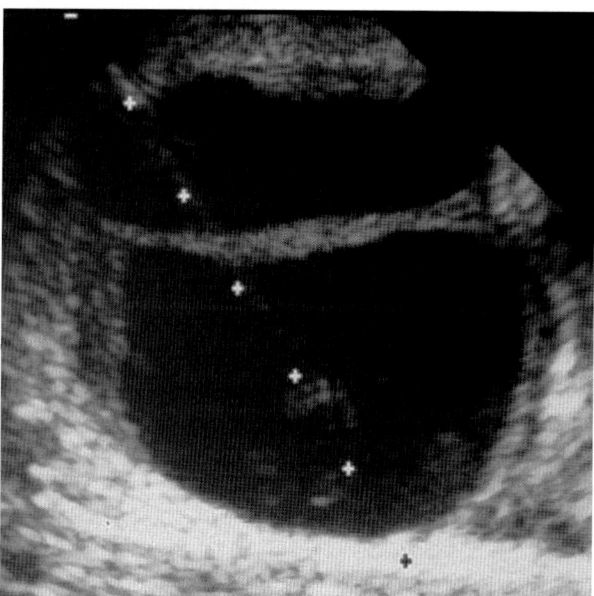

B

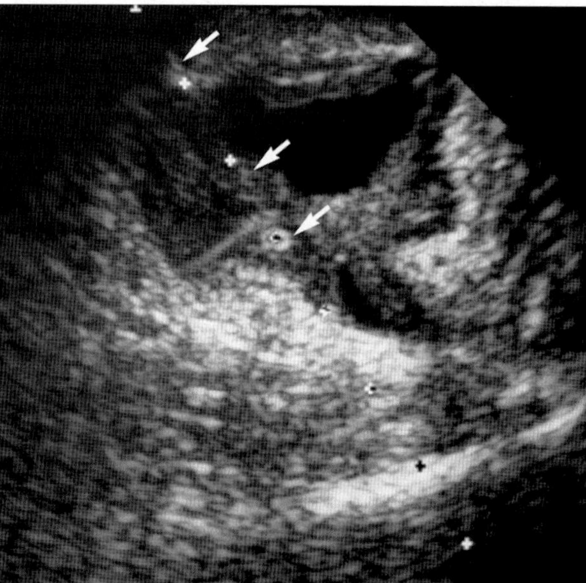

C

FIGURE 30.1-2. Transvaginal ultrasound-guided aspiration of a multilocular cyst. A: Coronal transvaginal view of the right adnexa demonstrates a cystic lesion *(calipers)* with at least three locules. **B:** A needle guide has been inserted on the transducer, and guide marks on the image indicate the path to be taken by the needle. **C:** A needle *(arrows)* ends in what was the largest locule, now drained of fluid.

(continued)

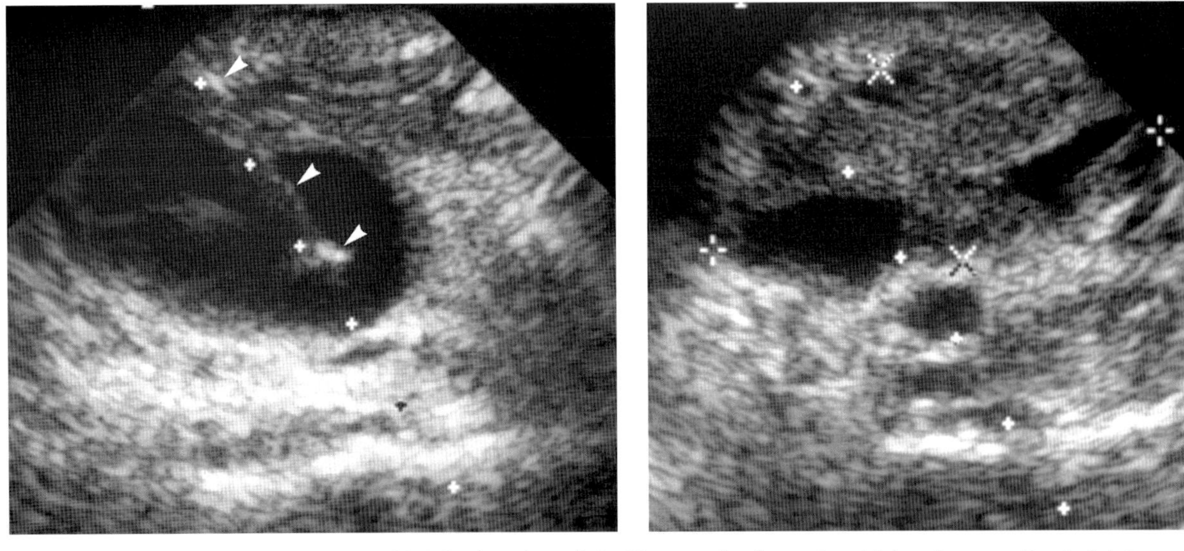

FIGURE 30.1-2. *(continued)* **D:** The needle *(arrowheads)* has been redirected into another locule. **E:** At the end of the drainage procedure, almost all fluid has been drained from the multilocular cyst *(calipers)*.

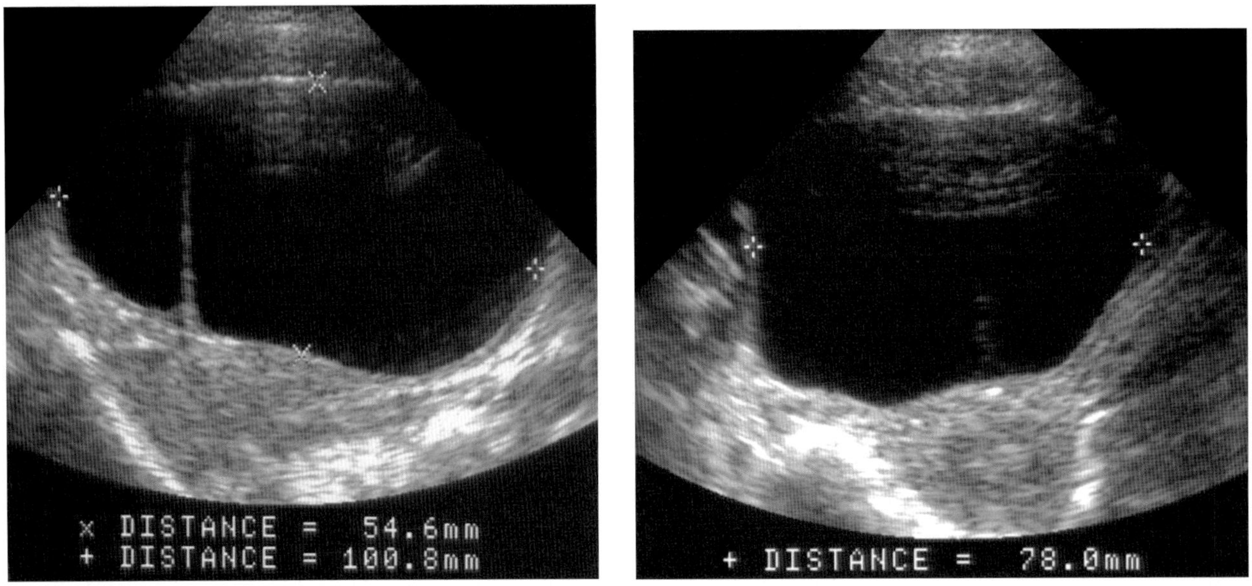

FIGURE 30.1-3. Transabdominal ultrasound-guided aspiration of a multilocular cyst. Sagittal **(A)** and transverse **(B)** transabdominal views of the right adnexa demonstrate a septated cystic lesion *(calipers)*. **C:** A needle *(arrowheads)* has been inserted in the larger locule under free-hand transabdominal ultrasound guidance without the use of a needle guide attachment.

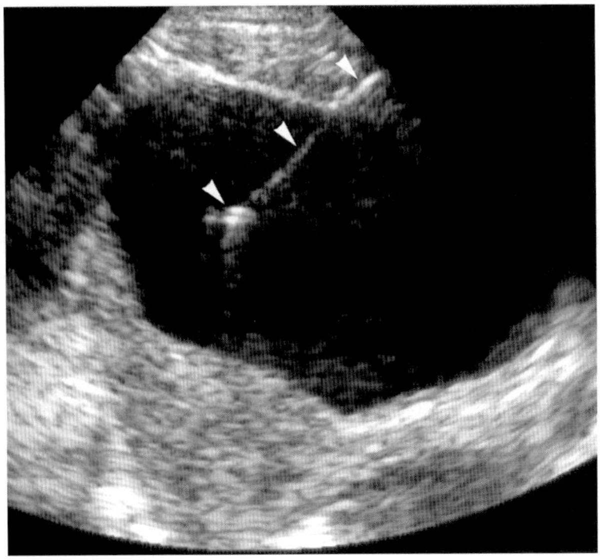

30.2. ULTRASOUND-GUIDED UTERINE INSTRUMENTATION THROUGH THE CERVIX

Description and Clinical Features

Uterine instrumentation procedures, such as dilation and curettage and office endometrial biopsy, are generally performed blindly. There are several situations in which ultrasound guidance is valuable, including the following:

- Difficulty passing an instrument through the cervical canal (e.g., cervical stenosis or sharply ante- or retroverted uterus).
- Ensuring complete evacuation of abnormal uterine cavity contents.
- Assisting in the removal of an intrauterine device (IUD).

Sonography

Guidance of uterine instrumentation is performed using transabdominal ultrasound. It is done through a completely or partially filled urinary bladder.

When a dilation and curettage or other procedure is hindered because of the inability to pass an instrument through the cervix, ultrasound can assist by determining the cervical orientation and directing the instrument along the long axis of the cervix. If necessary, the cervical orientation can be modified by filling or emptying the bladder. Once the instrument and cervix are properly aligned, forward pressure on the device will usually complete the task of getting it through the cervical canal (Figure 30.2-1).

When suctioning purulent material, retained products of conception, or other abnormal contents from the uterine cavity, ultrasound monitoring is useful to determine when the cavity is empty. This ensures that the drainage procedure is not terminated prematurely when there is still material left in the cavity, nor prolonged unnecessarily after the cavity is empty (Figure 30.2-2).

Occasionally, an IUD will fail to prevent a gestational sac from implanting in the uterus, resulting in the combined presence of a gestational sac and an IUD within the uterine cavity (Figure 30.2-3). If an attempt is made to extract the IUD, the procedure is best performed under ultrasound guidance (Figure 30.2-4) to make sure that the instrument used to grasp the IUD is properly directed so that it does not rupture or dislodge the sac.

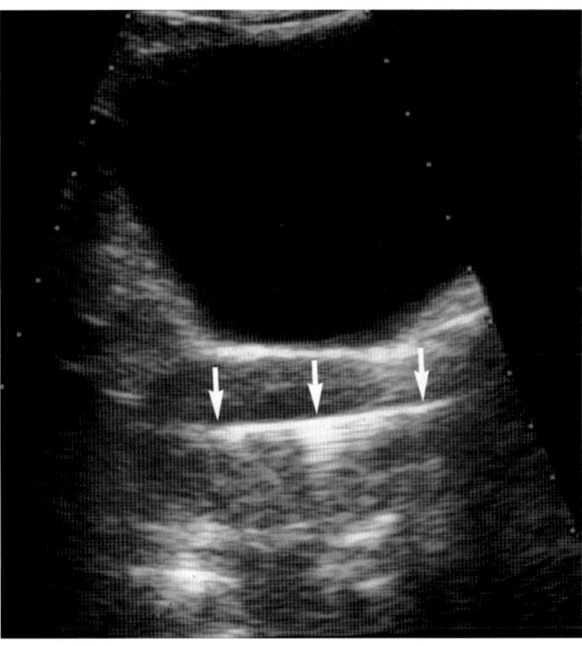

FIGURE 30.2-1. Ultrasound-guided dilation and curettage. Sagittal transabdominal view of the uterus demonstrates a curette *(arrows)* within the uterine cavity after it was passed through the cervix using sonographic guidance.

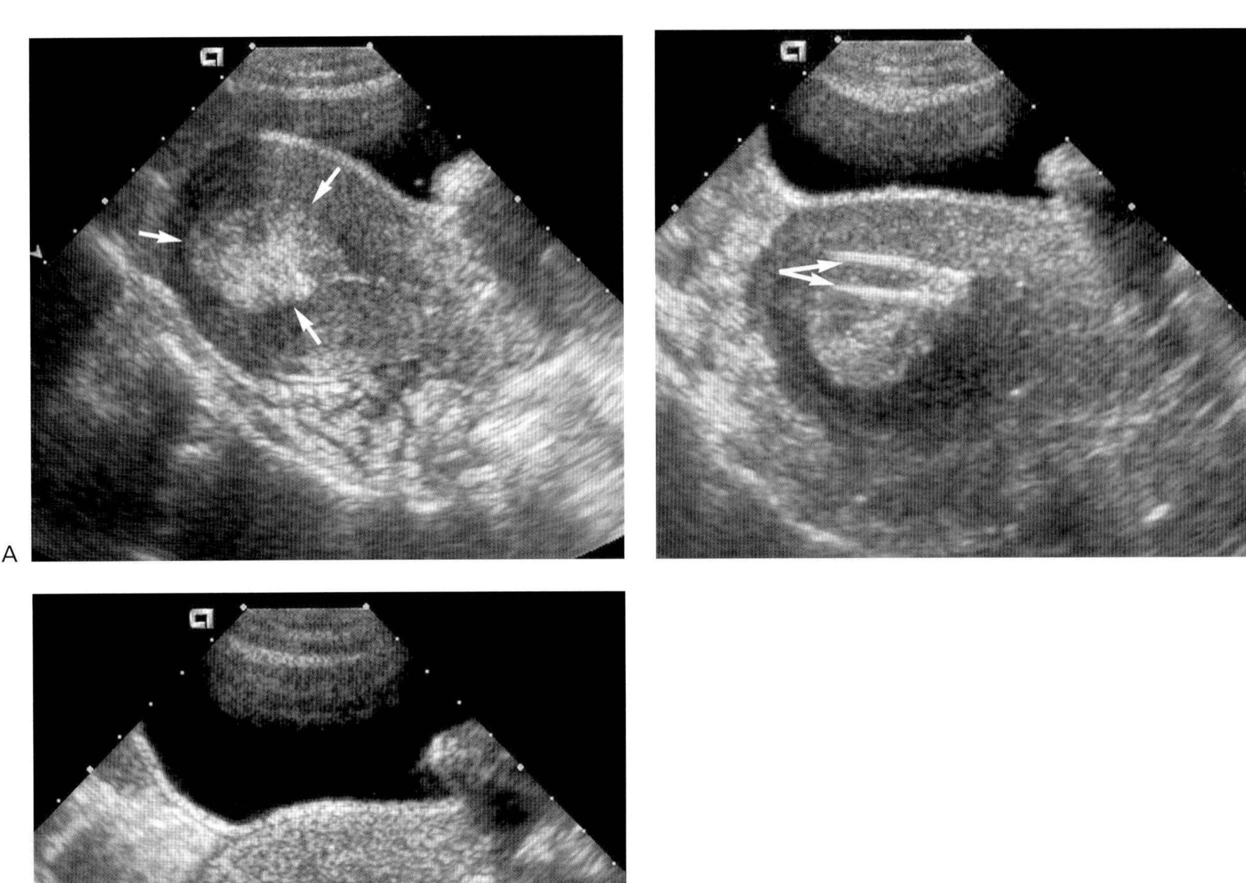

FIGURE 30.2-2. Ultrasound-guided evacuation of retained products of conception. A: Sagittal transvaginal view of the uterus demonstrates a soft-tissue mass *(arrows)* in the uterine cavity, representing retained products of conception. **B:** Under ultrasound guidance, a suction device *(arrows)* has been placed adjacent to the retained products of conception. **C:** At the end of the procedure, no abnormal tissue remains in the uterine cavity.

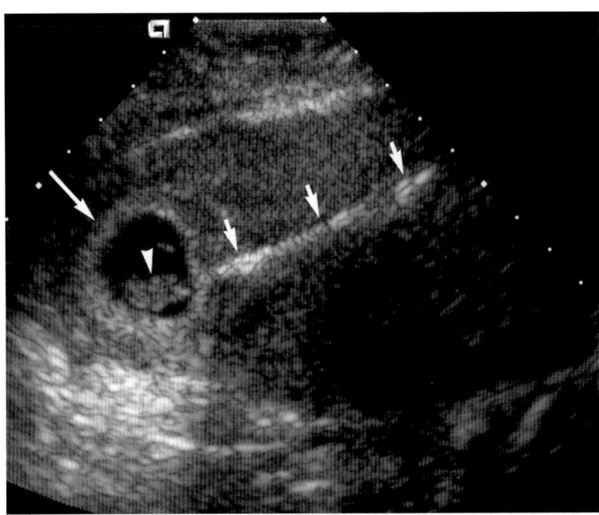

FIGURE 30.2-3. Intrauterine device adjacent to an intrauterine pregnancy. There is an intrauterine device *(short arrows)* adjacent to a gestational sac *(long arrow)* containing an embryo *(arrowhead)*.

A 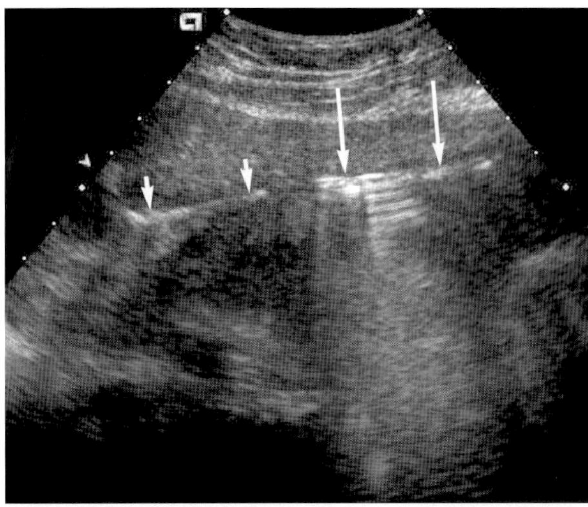
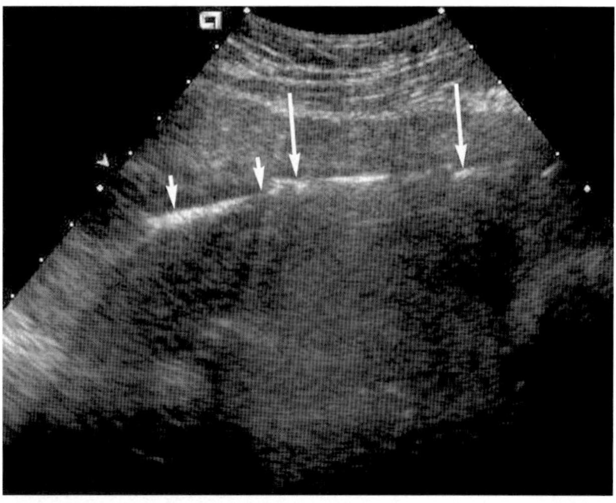 B

FIGURE 30.2-4. Ultrasound-guided removal of an intrauterine device during pregnancy. An attempt was made to remove the intrauterine device shown in Figure 30.2-3. **A:** Under ultrasound guidance, a clamp *(long arrows)* is directed toward the intrauterine device *(short arrows)*. **B:** The intrauterine device *(short arrows)* is being snared by the clamp *(long arrows)*.

30.3. ECTOPIC PREGNANCY ABLATION

Description and Clinical Features

When ectopic pregnancy is diagnosed, several treatment options are available, including intramuscular methotrexate injection and laparoscopic surgery. These work well for tubal ectopic pregnancy but may be ineffective for cervical and cornual ectopic pregnancies. An alternative approach for these types of ectopic pregnancy is ultrasound-guided ablation by injecting potassium chloride (KCl) into the embryo, if possible, or into the gestational sac. This can be performed on an outpatient basis and has been shown in a number of case series and case reports to be a safe and effective treatment. (Note: Methotrexate injected into the embryo or gestational sac can also be effective, but KCl may be preferable because a small amount of KCl injected locally is completely nontoxic to the mother.)

Sonography

Cervical ectopic pregnancy ablation is performed under transvaginal ultrasound guidance (Figures 30.3-1 and 30.3-2). The vagina is cleansed with an antiseptic solution, and a transvaginal transducer with needle guide attachment is inserted. A 20- or 22-gauge needle is introduced through the guide and advanced into the gestational sac. If the embryo is at least 5–10 mm in length, an attempt is made to place the needle tip within the embryo. Approximately 3–5 ml KCl, at a concentration of 2 mEq/ml, is then injected through the needle. If embryonic cardiac activity is present before the procedure, cessation of the heartbeat is the end point of the injection.

Cornual ectopic pregnancy ablation can be performed in a similar manner if the cornu can be safely accessed by a needle inserted transvaginally (Figure 30.3-3). An alternative approach is to insert the needle through the maternal anterior abdominal wall and use transabdominal ultrasound guidance to position the needle in the cornual gestational sac or embryo.

During the first 1–2 weeks after the ablation procedure, the gestational sac in the cervix or cornu will be replaced by ill-defined echogenic material (Figure 30.3-2). Over the next 1–2 months, this material will resorb, and the cervix or cornu will revert to normal.

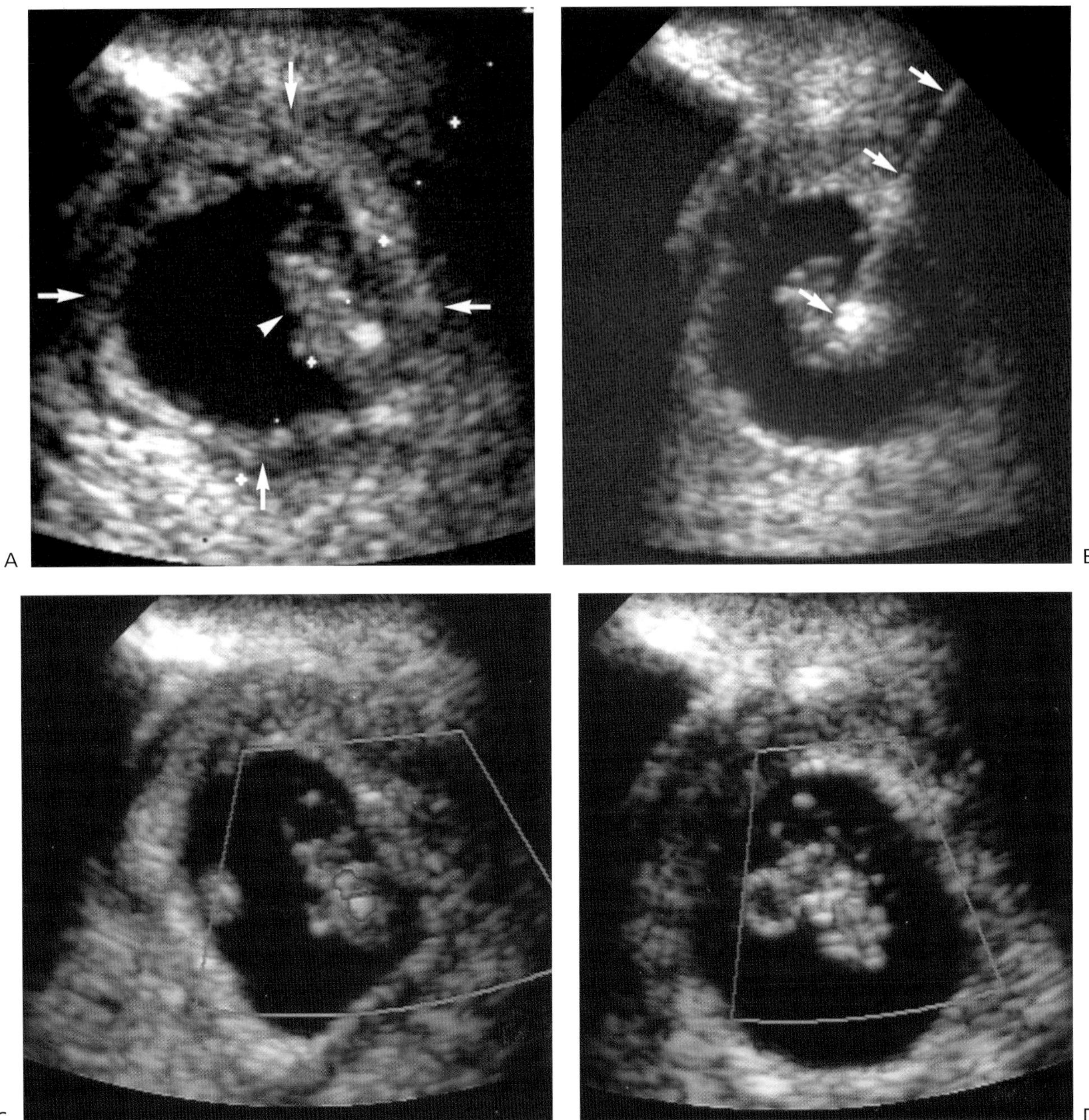

FIGURE 30.3-1. Ablation of cervical ectopic pregnancy. A: Transvaginal sonogram demonstrates a gestational sac *(arrows)* that is located in the cervix and contains an embryo *(arrowhead)*. A needle guide is on the transducer and guide marks indicate the path that will be taken by a needle inserted through the guide. **B:** A needle *(arrows)*, inserted through the guide, ends with its tip in the embryo. Potassium chloride was injected through the needle into the embryo, stopping the fetal heart. **C:** Color Doppler of the embryo before the procedure demonstrates blood flow in the beating heart. **D:** Color Doppler of the embryo after the procedure reveals no blood flow because there is no longer fetal cardiac activity.

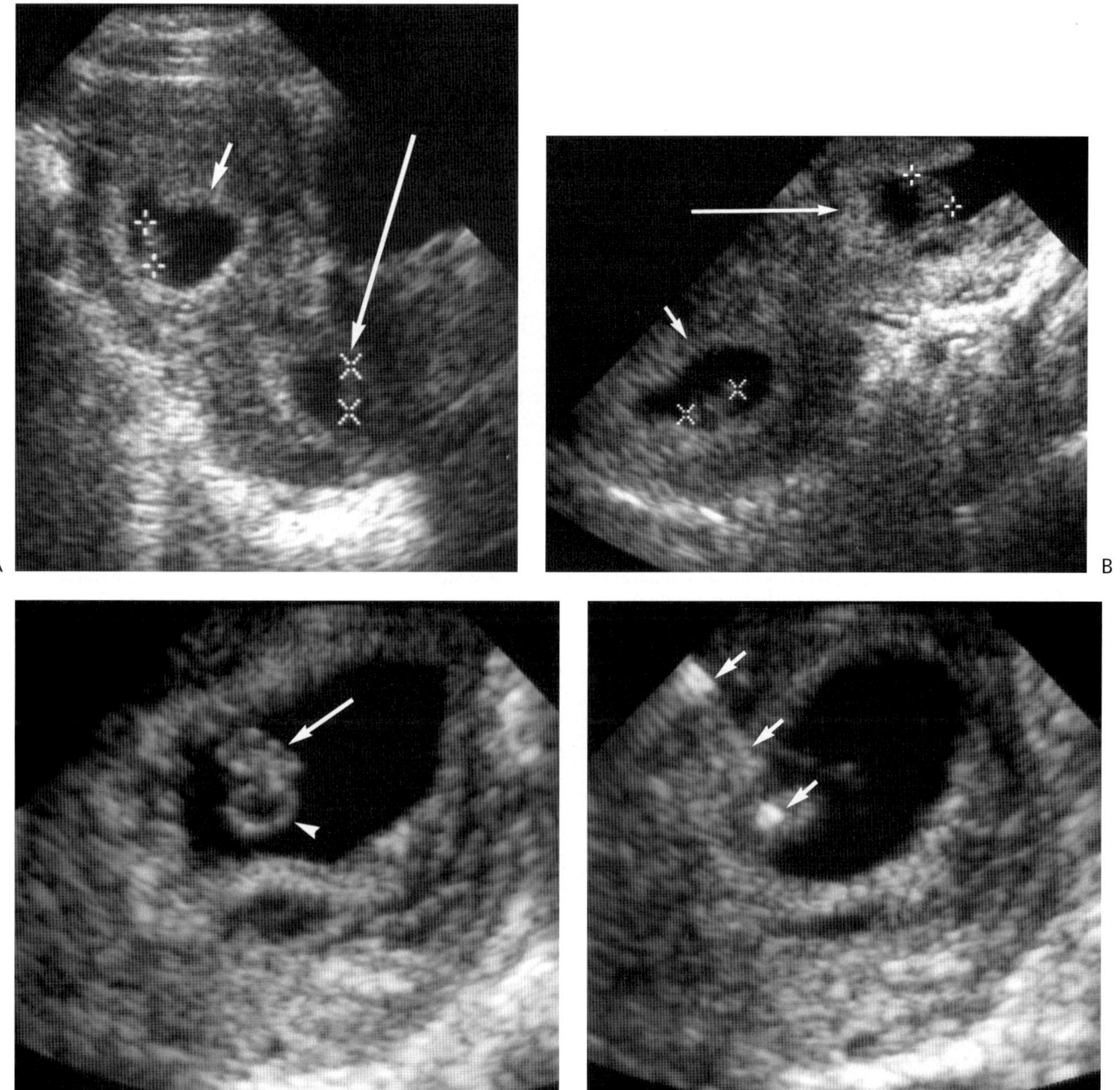

FIGURE 30.3-2. Ablation of cervical ectopic pregnancy in a patient with coexistent cervical and intrauterine gestational sacs. Sagittal transabdominal **(A)** and transvaginal **(B)** views of the uterus reveal two gestational sacs, one in the uterus *(short arrow)* and one in the cervix *(long arrow)*. Each of the two gestational sacs contains an embryo *(calipers)*. **C:** Transvaginal view of the intracervical gestational sac demonstrates an embryo *(arrow)* and yolk sac *(arrowhead)*. **D:** A needle *(arrows)* has been inserted through a guide on the transvaginal transducer to end within the embryo in the intracervical gestational sac. Potassium chloride was injected, leading to cessation of cardiac activity. *(continued)*

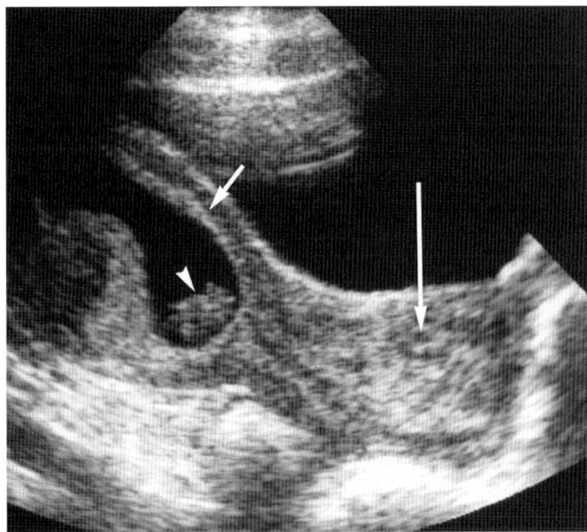

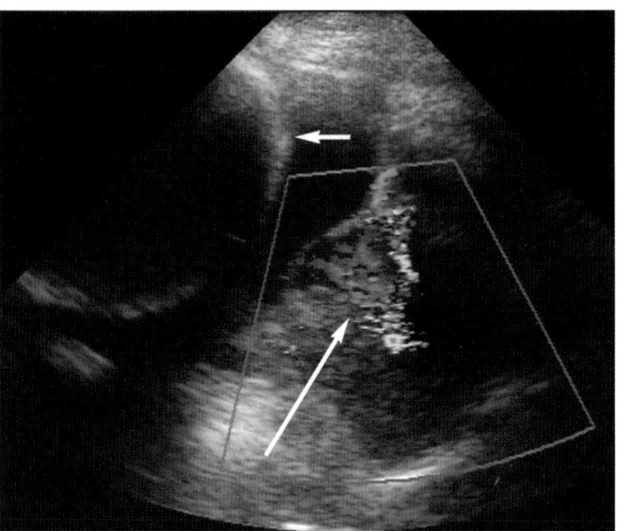

FIGURE 30.3-2. ***(continued)*** **E:** On a follow-up sonogram 1 week later, there was echogenic material *(long arrow)* but no identifiable gestational sac within the cervix. A normal gestational sac *(short arrow)* with an embryo *(arrowhead)* is seen within the body of the uterus. **F:** Follow-up sonogram in the late third trimester with color Doppler demonstrates the presenting fetal head *(short arrow)* adjacent to the cervix, which is highly vascular *(long arrow)*. Cesarean section was performed, yielding a normal baby.

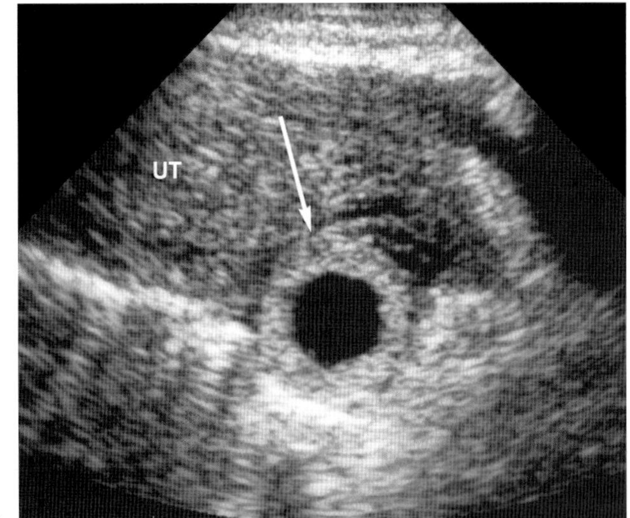

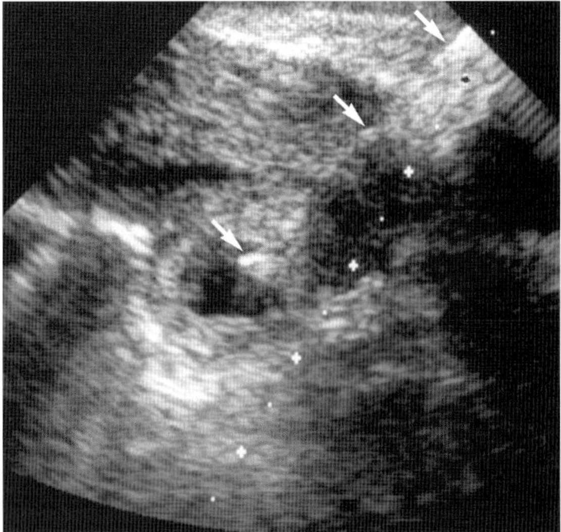

FIGURE 30.3-3. Ablation of cornual ectopic pregnancy. A: Coronal transvaginal view of the uterus reveals a gestational sac *(arrow)* in the left superolateral aspect of the uterus *(UT)*, a location corresponding to the left cornu. On other views, an embryo with cardiac activity was seen within this gestational sac. **B:** A needle *(arrows)* inserted through a guide on the transvaginal transducer ends in the cornual gestational sac. Potassium chloride was injected, leading to cessation of cardiac activity. Follow-up sonograms over the next several weeks demonstrated resorption of the cornual gestational sac, and the uterus appeared normal 2 months after the procedure.

30.4. PELVIC ABSCESS DRAINAGE

Description and Clinical Features

Several types of pelvic abscesses can occur, including tubo-ovarian, diverticular, and periappendiceal abscesses. Abscesses can also occur as a postoperative complication of pelvic surgery. Regardless of its cause, a pelvic abscess may resolve with antibiotic therapy alone.

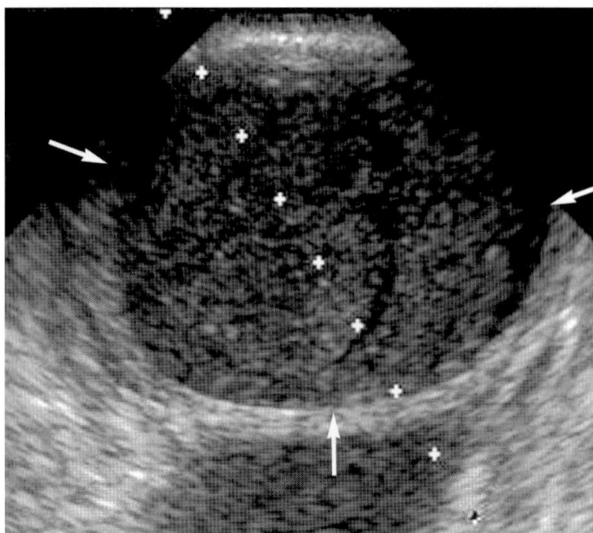

FIGURE 30.4-1. Ultrasound-guided drainage of a pelvic abscess. Transvaginal sonogram demonstrates a large, complex pelvic fluid collection *(arrows)*. Based on the sonographic appearance and clinical presentation, the collection was diagnosed as an abscess. A needle guide is attached to the transducer, and the guide marks on the image indicate the path that will be taken by a needle inserted through the guide.

If the abscess fails to resolve with antibiotic therapy, drainage is necessary. In many cases, image-guided drainage (using either ultrasound or computed tomography for guidance) can spare the patient from surgery.

Sonography

Pelvic abscess drainage under ultrasound guidance can be done transabdominally, transvaginally, or transrectally, with the optimal approach depending on the location of the abscess in relation to bowel and other adjacent structures. Deep abscesses are usually best drained transvaginally.

Whichever approach is used, options include either a simple aspiration (Figures 30.4-1 and 30.4-2) (insert the needle, drain the abscess, remove the needle, and prescribe antibiotics based on culture results) or placement of an indwelling catheter (Figure 30.4-3).

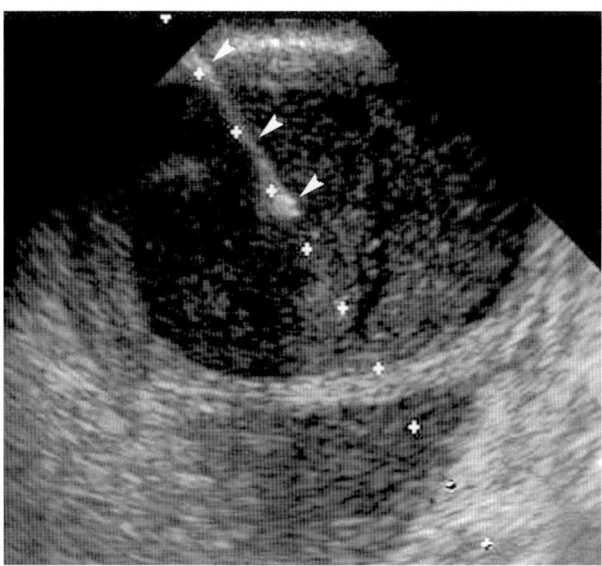

FIGURE 30.4-2. Ultrasound-guided drainage of a pelvic abscess. A needle *(arrowheads)* has been inserted to drain the abscess shown in Figure 30.4-1.

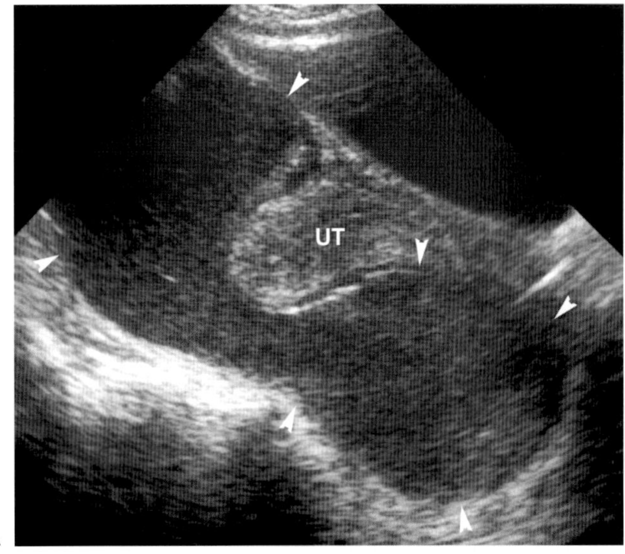

A

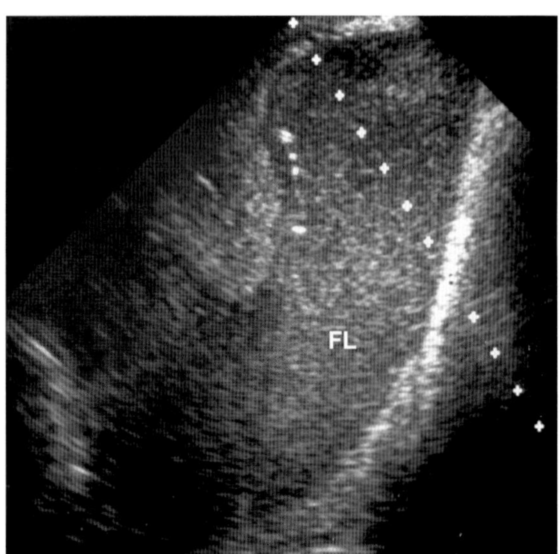

B

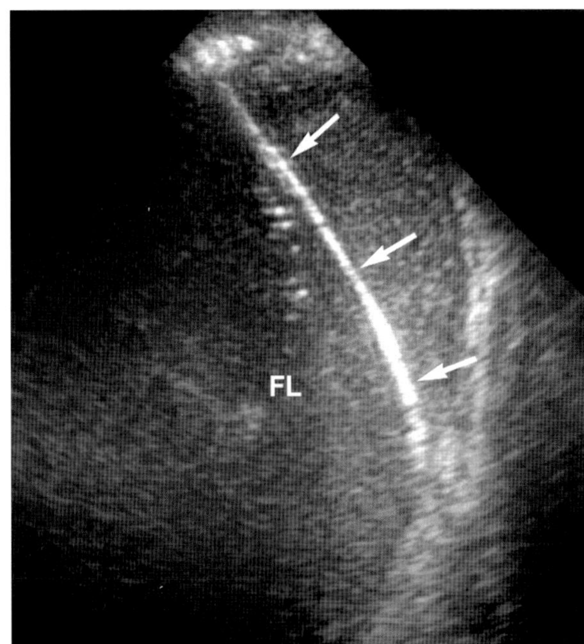

C

FIGURE 30.4-3. Ultrasound-guided placement of an indwelling drainage catheter in a pelvic abscess. A: Sagittal transabdominal view of the pelvis reveals a large, complex fluid collection *(arrowheads)* surrounding the uterus *(UT)*. **B:** Transvaginal sonogram with a needle guide attachment demonstrates pelvic fluid *(FL)*, and guide marks indicate the needle path. **C:** A needle was directed into the fluid collection *(FL)* through the transvaginal needle guide, and a guidewire *(arrows)* was inserted through the needle. **D:** A catheter *(arrows)* was inserted over the guidewire into the collection, as shown on this postprocedure radiograph. **E:** Follow-up sonogram 1 day later demonstrates the catheter *(arrows)* posterior to the uterus *(UT)*. The pelvic fluid collection has been almost completely drained.

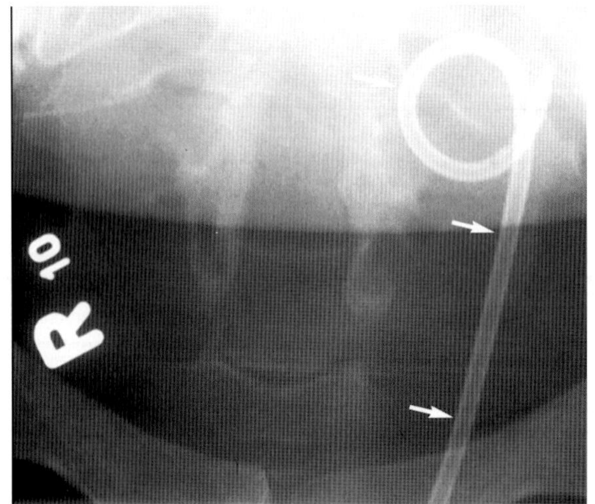

D

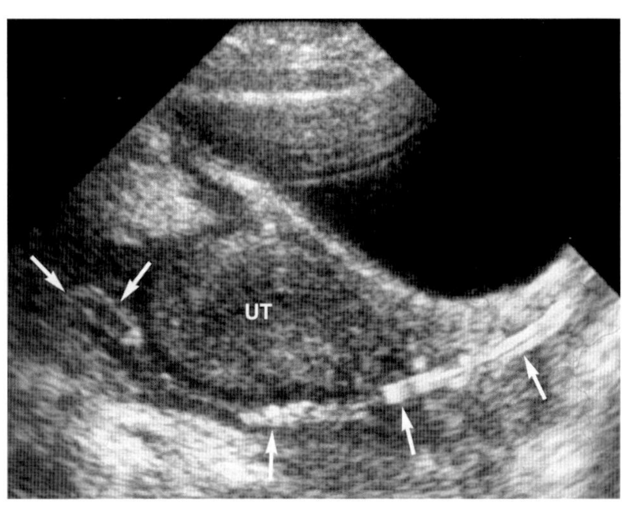

E

SUGGESTED READINGS

1. Benson CB, Doubilet PM. Strategies for conservative treatment of cervical ectopic pregnancy. *Ultrasound Obstet Gynecol* 1996;8:371–372.
2. Bret PM, Guibaud L, Atri M, et al. Transvaginal ultrasound-guided aspiration of ovarian cysts and solid pelvic masses. *Radiology* 1992;185:377–380.
3. Caspi B, Goldschmit R, Zalel Y, et al. Sonographically guided aspiration of ovarian cyst with simple appearance. *J Ultrasound Med* 1996;15:297–300.
4. Fleischer AC, Burnett LS, Jones HW, et al. Transrectal and transperineal sonography during intrauterine procedures. *J Ultrasound Med* 1995;14:135–138.
5. Frates MC, Benson CB, Doubilet PM, et al. Cervical ectopic pregnancy: results of conservative treatment. *Radiology* 1994;191:769–772.
6. Hunter RE, Reuter K, Kopin E. Use of ultrasonography in the difficult postmenopausal dilatation and curettage. *Obstet Gynecol* 1989;73:813–816.
7. Jurkovic D, Hacket E, Campbell S. Ultrasound diagnosis and conservative management of cervical pregnancy. *Ultrasound Obstet Gynecol* 1996;8:373–380.
8. Lerner JP, Monteagudo A, Timor-Tritsch IE, et al. Guided procedures using transvaginal, transperineal, and transrectal sonography. In: Fleischer AC, Manning FA, Jeanty P, et al., eds. *Sonography in obstetrics & gynecology: principles and practice*, 6th ed. New York: McGraw-Hill, 2001:1163–1184.
9. Nosher JL, Winchman HK, Needell GS. Transvaginal pelvic abscess drainage with ultrasound guidance. *Radiology* 1987;165:872–873.
10. Reuter K. Critical uses of intraoperative gynecologic sonography. *AJR Am J Roentgenol* 1997;169: 541–546.
11. Timor-Tritsch IE, Monteagudo A, Mandeville EO, et al. Successful management of viable cervical pregnancy by local injection of methotrexate guided by transvaginal ultrasonography. *Am J Obstet Gynecol* 1994;170:737–739.
12. Van Sonnenberg E, D'Agostino HB, Casola G, et al. Ultrasound-guided transvaginal drainage of pelvic abscesses and fluid collections. *Radiology* 1991;181:53–56.

SUBJECT INDEX

Note: Page numbers followed by *f* and *ff* indicate figures.

D

E